SAMUEL S. WHITE CATALOGUE

OF

DENTAL INSTRUMENTS AND EQUIPMENT

SAMUEL S. WHITE CATALOGUE
OF
DENTAL INSTRUMENTS
AND EQUIPMENT

by

SAMUEL S. WHITE

With a new introduction on
Samuel S. White and the
S. S. White Dental Company

by

Audrey B. Davis
Exhibition Curator, Dr. Samuel D. Harris National Museum
of Dentistry, Baltimore, Maryland
and
Former Curator of Medical Sciences,
Smithsonian Institution

NORMAN PUBLISHING
in assocation with
SMITHSONIAN INSTITUTION LIBRARIES
SAN FRANCISCO
1995

Library of Congress Cataloging-in-Publication Data
White, Samuel S. (Samuel Stockton), 1822-1879.
[Catalogue of dental materials, furniture, instruments, etc.]
Samuel S. White catalogue of dental instruments and equipment / by Samuel S. White ; with a new introduction on Samuel S. White and the S.S. White Dental Company by Audrey B. Davis.
p. cm.
Originally published: Catalogue of dental materials, furniture, instruments, etc. Philadelphia, 1876.
Includes bibliographical references and index.
ISBN 0-930405-63-3
1. Samuel Stockton White Dental Manufacturing Company--Catalogs. 2. Dental instruments and apparatus--United States--Catalogs.
I. Davis, Audrey B. II. Samuel Stockton White Dental Manufacturing Company. III. Title. IV. Title: Catalogue of dental instruments and equipment.
[DNLM: 1. White, Samuel S. (Samuel Stockton), 1822-1879. 2. Dental Equipment--catalogs. 3. Dental Equipment--history. W 26 W588c 1876a]
RK686.W57 1995
681'.761--dc20
DNLM/DLC
for Library of Congress 94-43672
CIP

Norman Surgery Series, No. 8

This book was printed from the original 1876 edition lent by the Smithsonian Institution Libraries. Irregularities in the printing appear exactly as they do in the original edition. It is printed on acid-free paper and its binding materials have been chosen for strength and durability.

Manufactured in the United States of America.

Copies may be ordered from:
NORMAN PUBLISHING
720 Market Street
San Francisco, CA 94102-2502
Phone: 1-800-544-9359
Outside USA and Canada: (415) 781-6402
Fax: (415) 781-5507

INTRODUCTION

SYNOPSIS

Samuel Stockton White (1822–1879) was an extraordinarily talented porcelain tooth mold carver who began to manufacture teeth on a full-time basis in 1844. Equally important was his ability to select administratively and mechanically skilled men who helped him build the first American dental supply house with an international reputation for excellence that remained the largest tooth supplier in the world for three quarters of a century. Esteem and a reputation for excellence, which was in short supply for dentists, were crucial to the company's success and essential to the technological and aesthetic advances in dental products engineered by the company. Educated as a dentist, White continually stimulated and responded to requests for changes and improvements in his products, thus building a dental supply business that both respected and advanced dental practice. Dentists offered ideas for new devices and purchased those they could afford. Founded in a period of individual craftsmanship, the company developed into a large factory enterprise typical of the age of mass production and industrialization during which it prospered. White's greatest personal achievement was to produce teeth with the idiosyncratic structure of natural teeth, making it possible for the dentist to esthetically arrange them in the mouth.

Prior to the eighteenth century, teeth carved from ivory and bone were common substitutes for lost human teeth. They resembled natural teeth whenever the skillful carver provided sufficient nuances in their design; however, ivory and bone taken from a whale, elephant, hippopotamus, or other animals is easily stained by food and beverages, so even the best of these teeth did not last, and soon became foul-smelling and discolored because they could not be adequately cleaned. The resistance to stains and durability of porcelain presented the tooth maker with an opportunity to make more lasting, better functioning, and more comfortable teeth.

In the United States, Philadelphia became a center for porcelain manufacture beginning in 1769. White's uncle, Samuel Wesley Stockton (1800–1872) was among the earliest Philadelphians to make porcelain teeth and was the first to produce them in large quantities, a skill he passed on to his nephew. For several decades Stockton and

White produced teeth independently. Stockton's teeth gradually lost their quality while White's teeth gained in sophistication. The records are silent on the relationship between Stockton and White during the twenty-eight-year period that their teeth competed on the American market. Because they were among the few to produce acceptable artificial porcelain teeth in quantity it seems unlikely that they exhausted the demand for well-made teeth.

There is evidence that White treated his employees fairly, and that they were liberally paid for their services. White hired skilled mechanics and designers and, like his uncle, trained a tooth maker who would become one of his major competitors, Henry D. Justi, whose contributions will be discussed later.

White and the company that succeeded him, the Samuel Stockton White Dental Manufacturing Company, contributed to or were major manufacturers of some of the outstanding innovations of nineteenth- and early twentieth-century dentistry. Among these are a variety of improvements in artificial teeth: gutta percha soft rubber stopping for temporarily filling teeth, especially Hill's gutta percha; the Revelation Bur; a series of dental chairs including the Wilkerson, Morrison, and the Forsyth Clinic children's unit; and finally, the greatest income-producing product: flexible cable that was applied to dental hand pieces and eventually to a variety of implements including automobile cables. These outstanding products ensured the company's financial success and permitted staff to experiment with numerous dental devices and to provide a number of customized items.

Advertising literature in the usual form was not adequate to inform nineteenth-century dentists about the changing techniques of tooth repair and replacement. Therefore, through a newsletter and a journal, White provided more extensive information concerning the scientific basis and technology required to diagnose and treat dental pathology. By providing a forum for discussion of new methods and technology White helped to raise the standards of dentistry and paved the way for selling the required implements that he manufactured. The newsletter, journal, and dental supplies and implements were all equally important parts of White's plan to develop dentistry into an effective and significant profession.

During the last decade of his life as spokesman for the dental profession, White spent time and funds on opposing, unsuccessfully, the fees charged each dentist who used vulcanite, the premier substance discovered in the nineteenth century for making denture plates. His estate paid $175,000 in court costs and damages assessed for "interfering" with the rights guaranteed to the patent holder, The Dental Vulcanite Company. White's most enthusiastic efforts during the last years of his life were devoted to "venture capitalism," specifically investment in Pennsylvania oil wells and telephone and telegraph lines. He died before any of these investments earned a profit.

SAMUEL STOCKTON WHITE AND FAMILY BECOME DENTAL MANUFACTURERS

Born on June 19, 1822, in Hulmesville, Bucks County, Pennsylvania, Samuel Stockton White was the eldest child of William R. and Mary Stockton White. His mother was descended from Richard Stockton, a signer of the Declaration of Independence.[1] White's youngest brother, James William, who would play a major role in the management and promotion of the dental company, was born in 1826. Upon the death of their father when Samuel was eight years old, the family moved to Burlington, New Jersey. At ages sixteen and fourteen respectively, Samuel and James were indentured to their maternal uncle, Samuel Wesley Stockton (1800–1872), a dentist in Philadelphia "to learn the art and mystery of the manufacture of incorruptible teeth."[2]

The life of Samuel Wesley Stockton has been largely unrecorded. Son of Samuel and Hannah Gardner Stockton of New Jersey, he married twice and became the father of twenty-one children. He began as a clock and watchmaker in 1823 and is first listed as a dentist in 1833.[3] However, a contemporary newspaper advertisement proves he made teeth as early as 1825. Stockton's office remained at 160 Vine Street between 1832–1842 until he eventually moved to 116 Chestnut Street in 1846. The name Samuel W. Stockton and Company appeared in 1847 and remained at least until 1850. Stockton's teeth are highlighted by Paul Goddard in his classic text on the anatomy of the teeth published in 1844.[4] A few of Stockton's children entered dentistry including E. C. Stockton, who began to manufacture incorruptible teeth in 1855; John M. Stockton, who was listed as a mechanical dentist; and Ezekiel G. Stockton, who was a dentist at 704 Arch Street in 1861. Another relative, Thomas H. Stockton, Jr., son of Reverend Thomas Hewlings Stockton, Chaplain to Congress, opened a dental depot at 114 North 9th Street in 1863.[5]

While under his uncle's tutelage Samuel also studied dentistry under John De Haven White (1815–1895)(no relative) in whose class he met Thomas W. Evans (1823–1897). White maintained a close professional association with John White and Thomas Evans, both of whom would contribute to the growth of White's manufacturing business. Evans strengthened White's European connections;[6] beginning in the early 1850s, White began to export teeth, becoming part of the phenomenon honored in Europe as American dentistry. White sold a considerable portion of his teeth abroad until World War I.

Evans is the most famous of a number of American dentists who set up practices in Europe. Christopher Starr Brewster, the first American to open a dental office in Paris in 1835, invited Evans to join his practice, which was so successful that Evans bought the practice in 1850 and was soon joined by his brother Theodore. The Evans brothers became dentists to the courts of France, Russia, Bavaria, Württemburg, Belgium, and Saxony. Dozens of American dentists and European dentists who trained in the United States practiced in Europe. Some of them had trained with Brewster and were in contact with Evans.[7]

White began to practice dentistry at the age of twenty–one in his uncle's office at 160 Vine Street while superintending the tooth factory. A year later he opened his own office and business at 116 North 7th Street in Philadelphia. Two assistants, one of whom was White's brother James, worked in the attic while White treated patients in the office below. The office also served as a store to sell the teeth they made. When demand for teeth increased, White moved to larger quarters at 273 Race Street above 8th Street. To obtain capital while he continued to improve the teeth he made and to support his wife, Sarah Jane Carey, whom he married on March 31, 1846, he formed a partnership with the dentists Asahel Jones (d. August 1866) of New York City and John R. McCurdy (d. January 27, 1867) of Philadelphia in 1845. Jones became the manager of the first branch of the company, which was established in New York in 1846. The first name of the firm as a partnership was Jones, White and Company (1847–1852), followed by Jones, White and McCurdy (1853–1859), and finally, Jones and White (1859–1861). For the following two decades the company retained the name of its founder Samuel Stockton White. The Jones firm continued in New York under the management of E. S. and M. J. Jones and issued a dental catalog in 1867.

Samuel's brother James graduated from the University of Pennsylvania Medical School and received an honorary D.D.S. from the Pennsylvania College of Dental Surgery. He confined his dental patients to family and friends whom he treated without charge. His publications include several books on dentistry and a chapter "Diseases of the First Dentition" in *The American System of Dentistry*. His pamphlet on the care of teeth sold one million copies. In his will Samuel placed the control of the company in the hands of three people: his brother James; Samuel's eldest son, J. Clarence; and Henry M. Lewis, hired by White in 1868 to help him manage the company. James became president in 1881, serving until his death in 1891 at age sixty-five. J. Clarence White remained as secretary until he resigned in 1901.[8]

Until 1915 company leadership remained in the hands of the White family and others associated with Samuel. William H. Gilbert (1847–1912), who was hired by Samuel in 1862, left White shortly thereafter for a few years to work in a variety of jobs: a wholesale dress business; his father's machine shop; and the wholesale druggists, French, Richards and Company. He also enlisted in the Pennsylvania Volunteer Infantry, returning in 1865 to work in the White factory. At the time of White's death Gilbert was the company's buyer. After the company was reorganized and enlarged in 1881, Gilbert was appointed general superintendent of manufacturing and branch houses. His detailed study of each product resulted in improvements in the manufacturing process and monetary savings. Upon James White's death, Gilbert became General Manager and Henry Lewis became President. Gilbert's next major task was to restructure the finance department. After Lewis's death in 1906 Gilbert became the president, a post he held until his death in 1912, at which time the company employed seventeen hundred people. W. Littell White assumed Gilbert's position as general manager in 1906, remaining in office until 1917 when the position was abolished.[9]

Samuel S. White's son, Samuel Jr. (1855–1937), was elected president in 1912 after not being in the employ of the company for thirty-two years. From an early age Samuel S. was groomed to follow in his father's footsteps by learning to distinguish and sort teeth at the age of ten. He left school in 1872 to learn the business. His first job was working in the electric mallet department. He became so skilled with this device that his father assigned him the task of taking a new mallet over to the Vienna Exposition in 1873. He then spent a few years in the retail department on Chestnut Street but resigned on July 1, 1880, after his father's death, to pursue his private interests and hobbies. He married on April 6, 1881. His son, Stockton (b. 1885) was employed by the White Company in 1907 after graduating from Harvard University. Tired of shouldering the president's responsibilities, Samuel Jr. resigned in 1915 to be succeeded by Frank Taylor, who had been associated with Yale and Towne Manufacturing Company.

During his tenure with the White Company Taylor became chairman of the United States Army's Dental Supplies Committee in World War I. His presidency lasted until 1926, when he and the heirs of Johnston Brothers favored selling the declining dental company to the investment firm of Dillon, Read and Company for five million dollars, a deal that the stockholders vetoed. T. E. Dick (Ned) Hinkson, a very popular employee from the time he joined the firm in 1888 as a clerk, was elected to succeed Taylor but died within three weeks and the presidency passed to Charles Henderson, an employee with extensive service at the company. Henderson, who was a leader in the American Dental Trade Association, retired in 1932 after forty years with the company to be succeeded by Fred E. Steen, who was born in the year of Samuel S. White's death (1879) and remained president until 1952.[10]

J. Clarence White's son, Samuel S. White III (1876–1952) had a distinguished career with the dental company. Educated at Princeton University and Cambridge, where he was a student of the physical culturist Eugene Sandow, he won a prize for his physical development in 1899. Interested in art, he and his wife Vera, an artist, traveled to Paris, where he attracted the attention of Auguste Rodin who enlisted him to pose for the famous statue, *The Athlete.* After serving in the Spanish-American War he joined the company in 1903 and for thirty years was an export manager in the tooth department, concentrating on South American countries. As well as being on the board of directors of the company, he served on the boards of the Philadelphia Museum of Art, the Union League, the Racquet Club, the Art Alliance, and the Bachelors Barge Club.[11]

There are only a few references in the White family records that discuss differences of opinion between family members and company officers. One of these sources is a letter written in 1912 by Samuel III asking for a raise from his uncle, Samuel Stockton White Jr., who was president of the company. Samuel Stockton White III complained that no one was working on his behalf to further his career in the firm. His work in Central and South America had been praised but he had not received any monetary reward. He pointed out that in the past Gilbert had promoted the interests of his brother, W. Littell White, to combat the ambitions of Henry Lewis and his son. Futhermore, he argued on behalf of family solidarity, pointing out that although White family members owned most of the company stock, there were few Whites employed by the company.[12]

SAMUEL STOCKTON WHITE AS TOOTH MANUFACTURER

Samuel Stockton White's teeth set the standard by which artificial teeth were judged worldwide in the nineteenth century. Public acclaim for White teeth was manifested within a few years in the medals obtained at numerous trade fairs and exhibitions. Porcelain teeth first attracted attention in the United States in the 1830s when a specimen was awarded the first gold medal ever bestowed on a manufactured item. The American Institute of New York presented a gold medal in 1833 to Dr. D. C. Ambler for his set of porcelain teeth. Ambler was a dentist and physician whose mentor was the celebrated New York physician, Valentine Mott.[13] Illness in his family prevented Ambler from pursuing his promising teeth-making career in New York, but the award spurred others to manufacture porcelain teeth. The first gold medals awarded for teeth made by White were presented in 1848 by the American Institute and the Maryland Institute in Baltimore. A gold medal was awarded by the Pennsylvania Society of Dental Surgeons in 1849 "for the greatest improvement in the manufacture of porcelain teeth."[14] The first international medal White obtained came from the Crystal Palace Exposition in London in 1851. The Exposition brought together a wide variety of innovations in arts and sciences, with exhibits of chemistry and physics as well as exhibits of furniture and household items. Although a bronze medal, it was the highest medal awarded to a dental manufacturer.[15] By 1876 White had collected sixty-two "first premiums" for manufactured teeth. White's teeth were admired by Europeans who used the term *American teeth* to denote their special quality.

White fostered a collegial relationship with dentists and used the resources of his manufacturing business to entice and support dental innovations in education, diagnostic methods, and treatment. White's company advanced the work of enterprising dentists by publishing their reports and inventions in the company-sponsored newsletter entitled *The Dental News Letter*, which was first published in 1847. For this endeavor, White's uncle Samuel Stockton had provided a model by publishing the first proprietary dental periodical named *Stockton's Dental Intelligencer* in 1843.

The Dental News Letter was organized for a purpose: "That the profession of theU. S. and Europe may be informed of the improvements which have been made and are being made in the manufacture of artificial teeth, the various tools and aids in the workshop and instruments for the operating room."[16] Samuel's dental tutor, John D. White, was appointed editor. The enlarged newsletter became an internationally distributed journal in 1859 named *The Dental Cosmos*. John D. White served as editor-in-chief and was assisted by James H. McQuillen, George J. Ziegler, and James White. McQuillen served as editor-in-chief between 1865 and 1871, when he resigned to be succeeded by James White. Articles, letters, meeting and conference proceedings, lists of graduates from dental colleges, obituaries, and critiques of new implements regularly appeared in the *Dental Cosmos* reflecting the major issues of concern to American dentists in this period. White products and those of other manufacturers were cited for their quality as well as faulted for their shortcomings. Competitors' advertisements regularly appeared in each issue.[17]

Articles ranged over a wide spectrum of scientific and sociopolitical issues of importance for dentistry: studies which bore on the patient's appearance, such as an individual's temperament, a modern form of the Galenic humoral theory; anthropology; phrenology; and other emerging studies growing out of the doctrine of evolution were published in the *Dental Cosmos*. Institutions that provided access to dentists were discussed. The physician H. Meredith White encouraged the establishment of dental dispensaries to serve the poor and lower-income people of the country. Because dental colleges did not operate throughout the year, people without means, who were normally treated in college dental clinics, were left without dental care. England provided the model for American dental dispensaries at mid-century.[18]

Space to manufacture and sell dental goods expanded with the growth and success of the White Company. The central administration building located on 12th and Chestnut Streets in Philadelphia since 1868 became a monument to the company's leadership in dental technology. The most expensive and largest building in the city, it was the last company building erected during White's lifetime and is illustrated in the 1876 catalog. The first floor was rented for the display of jewelry to the firm of Barley, Banks and Biddle. Dental hardware, instruments, and teeth were displayed on the second floor. These sumptuous quarters were widely admired and impressed inventors who sought White's endorsement and development of their ideas for new dental items.

In the catalog of 1867 the White trademark (consisting of two capital *S*'s superimposed on a capital *W*) was introduced and applied to steel instruments, a measure taken to ensure that customers would not be confused by similar instruments sold by other surgical and dental instrument manufacturers. Trademarks were applied to dental equipment to quickly delineate instruments whose manufacturer was not obvious by superficial observation and to call attention to White's new fine steel implements previously unavailable to dentists from any manufacturer.[19]

The 1876 catalog appeared at the time when White produced approximately two-thirds of the world's supply of artificial teeth, roughly four million teeth. By 1900 the stock of teeth maintained in Philadelphia would rise to between seven and one-half and eleven million. To make this number of teeth many molds for the same tooth were required, in fact, twice as many molds as other manufacturers used. White provided unusual teeth like smoker's black teeth and hand-stained teeth, which were abandoned early in the twentieth century.[20] Catalogs increased in size as stock multiplied and special issues devoted to specific items appeared. Twice as large as the first major catalog published by White in 1867 (the first company catalog had appeared in 1862 under the name of Samuel S. White, [successor to Jones and White]) the 1876 catalog, which was reprinted in 1877 and 1878, was the last catalog produced during White's lifetime, except for an appendix published in 1878.[21] The volume listed and in some instances depicted in line drawings White's important contributions to the manufacture of teeth and dental implements.

The catalog of 1876 is noted for advertisements of materials, instruments, and furniture sought after by skillful and well-trained dentists in a period when American dentistry was increasingly recognized as superior to dentistry in other countries. White's enterprise became a technological foundation for the evolution of American dentistry from an unorganized, erratically, if not opportunistically, adopted craft into a core group of professionals educated through apprenticeships or in dental colleges. Modern dentists used well-made, specialized instruments to execute new methods of tooth repair, and install natural-looking artificial teeth. The 1876 catalog documents White's achievements in the year of the nation's centennial, the celebration that inspired its publication. At the trade fair that occurred during the celebration White constructed "an exceedingly elaborate display in the Main Exhibition Building" and subscribed five thousand dollars toward the event.[22] The deluxe trade catalog became a permanent record of the exhibition and the final document of White's manufacturing legacy. On Pennsylvania Day, part of the Centennial festivities, White dismissed his employees for the day and gave each person fifty cents to spend at the Centennial Exhibition.[23]

THE MANUFACTURE OF PORCELAIN TEETH

The carving of artificial teeth remained largely in the hands of private dentists until two important events occurred. First was the discovery of anesthesia by dentists in the 1840s, which permitted dentists to shift their efforts toward saving partially decayed teeth by removing debris and filling the natural tooth in a comfortably sedated and therefore cooperative patient. Second was a steady supply of attractive manufactured teeth. These new resources in dentistry led to the abandonment by individual dentists of mechanical dentistry, the time-consuming and laborious practice of making porcelain or other artificial teeth. Instead, the busy operative dentist purchased manufactured teeth to install in the edentulous patient's mouth. The time dentists saved by not making teeth was considerable: carving the mold for teeth in the dentist's laboratory consumed most of a day, then the furnace had to be prepared for baking and fusing the teeth. However, in a small factory one could produce at least fifteen sets daily and the furnace of a large factory could fire at most 250 full sets, or approximately 7,000 teeth.[24]

All ceramic or porcelain items are made of essentially the same materials: feldspar, quartz, and kaolin; however, these items differ in the purity of each substance, the amount used, and the firing procedure.[25] Several properties of porcelain made it an ideal substance for artificial teeth: it is chemically impervious to mouth fluids, may be colored, and remains strong when compressed. Porcelain is easily cleaned, a property that most endeared it to the first person to wear porcelain teeth, Alexis Duchâteau. A French apothecary who wore teeth carved from hippopotamus ivory, Duchâteau was sufficiently annoyed with the difficulty of keeping his teeth clean and his mouth odor-free to seek another tooth substitute. He found a material with the requisite properties in his own laboratory in a common utensil, his porcelain mortar. Observing that a mortar was easily cleaned after it had been used to grind a variety of substances, he realized that porcelain had a number of suitable characteristics, including the property to resist stains. Although his first teeth were not practical, the chain of events that led to White's phenomenal career began with Duchâteau in Paris in 1774.[26]

Stockton began to sell porcelain teeth in 1825, within several decades after John Greenwood and Antoine A. Plantou brought the first porcelain teeth from Paris to Philadelphia. Stockton became the first commercially successful manufacturer of artificial teeth in America.[27] He was able to make the teeth more realistic in appearance, thus making them more popular with patients as well as dentists. During the period of White's apprenticeship Stockton's teeth were acknowledged as the finest factory-made teeth.[28] Stockton continued to make teeth after White opened his own office in 1844. By 1845 Stockton produced half a million teeth annually. The teeth Stockton made in his early years were lauded by dentists,[29] including Chapin A. Harris, who testified to their superiority. In the first edition of his acclaimed text, *The Dental Art: A Practical Treatise on Dental Surgery*, Harris described his experience: "During the last four years past, I have used, almost exclusively, the teeth made by Mr. Stockton of Philadelphia, and have no hesitation in recommending them, as superior to any that I have ever used."[30]

Dentists who carved teeth for their patients as needed criticized the lack of individuality of teeth made from standard molds in a factory. However, the demand for the natural-looking teeth he carved led White, after two years, to abandon his dental practice to concentrate on the manufacture of teeth. One of his achievements could only be accomplished by devoting full time to the endeavor of providing a stock of hundreds of different molds to produce teeth that would closely duplicate the differences in shape and size of natural teeth.

In the 1876 catalog White boasted that porcelain teeth were "the largest and most important department of our business."[31] By this time other dental manufacturers and suppliers emulated and competed with White in declaring that teeth were also their most important products. White touted those qualities of teeth singled out by expert judges, which included the important visual characteristics of shape, color, texture, translucency, and those physical attributes essential to their function such as strength, lightness, and the capability to resist both chemical changes and heat required to prepare the tooth.

White reprinted a chapter on porcelain teeth from the tenth edition of Chapin Harris's *Principles and Practice of Dentistry*, 1871–72, edited by P. H. Austen, in the 1876 catalog. Harris had cautioned that it would be impossible to instruct anyone in the actual methods used to make porcelain teeth without demonstrating the process in the laboratory. Harris explained in 1858 that "more time, and close, and persevering application are necessary to obtain a thorough knowledge of this then almost any other branch of practical dentistry. . . . The slightest error in the preparation or mixing of the materials, will often give a result entirely different from the one aimed at, and teeth made by different persons, from the same recipe, frequently differ very widely in appearance, depending on the manner in which they have been worked."[32]

White could not improve on the discussion of porcelain teeth manufacture that Harris published because they both realized that the art of working with porcelain to make teeth could only be acquired with practice and experimentation. Harris reported that as few as one in fifteen individuals who made porcelain teeth succeeded, and only those who, like White, devoted full time to the activity. Whereas previously dentists were reluctant to share the secrets of their tooth-making operations to protect themselves from competitors, now the process of making teeth out of porcelain was too demanding for practicing dentists who did not need to know the details of making these teeth. At first, financial motivation to manufacture porcelain teeth was lacking because there was little demand, in part because until 1833, porcelain teeth were unattractive, lacking natural color, translucency, and the animation and sparkle of natural teeth.[33]

In the nineteenth century, only a few manufacturers understood how to prepare the type of porcelain required to manufacture the best-quality teeth. Manufacturers of ceramic pottery, dishes, and other crockery did not make porcelain teeth. Nevertheless, proximity to ceramic manufacturers undoubtedly ensured the success of Stockton and White, who worked in a city that had been an American center of porcelain manufacture since the eighteenth century, boasting such important makers as the Abraham Miller family and William Ellis Tucker (1800–1837).[34] Susan Myers, historian of early Philadelphia ceramic makers, has suggested that White and Stockton might have exchanged ideas with ceramicists at the Franklin Institute, which was the setting for lectures, and a sponsor of awards to talented ceramic manufacturers.[35] White was indeed a member of the Franklin Institute.[36]

High-quality feldspar provided 80 percent of the minerals used to produce teeth; therefore, White and others looked for mines that produced better feldspar to buy for making teeth. White's artificial teeth were made from a well-known variety of highly purified feldspar from Chester County, Pennsylvania. White had discovered the feldspar quarry by chance while on a walk during a visit to his wife's family, who lived in the region. This particular feldspar is believed to have provided the special appearance that made White's teeth become famous so quickly.[37]

Although Harris, White, and other dentists did not publish a full account of making teeth in a factory, a ceramicist named Arthur S. Watts explained in 1915 how the Dentists Supply Company of York, Pennsylvania, manufactured artificial teeth.[38] For constructing the body of the tooth several earthy materials colored with metallic oxides were used: feldspar, silex, and kaolin; to apply the enamel surface, feldspar with traces of silex and metallic oxides was added. There were several grades of porcelain used to make artificial teeth; these differed in the flux elements and the temperature at which they matured. A basic mineral formula for porcelain teeth consisted of 68% Si02, 17% A1203, 10% K20, 2.5% Na20, and traces of other mineral oxides. The ingredients consisted of 81% feldspar, 4% clay, and 15% flint. Materials that could be fused at low temperatures made it possible for the dentist to fuse teeth in his small laboratory furnace, which, however, could not withstand the temperature required to make the best artificial teeth. Feldspar was brought from the quarry and crushed to quarter-inch sized particles and then hand sorted to remove discolored and unwanted pieces. The selected portion was placed in a drag mill of thirty inches in diameter, where a metal piece was dragged over the feldspar, grinding it to a desired degree of fineness. The size of the feldspar particles was essential in determining the tooth's transparency. If ground too fine the transparency of the teeth was reduced, while more coarse particles raised the temperature needed to fuse the substance, thus increasing the wear on the furnace, obviously an important factor for a commercial maker. Feldspar was mixed with kaolin and quartz to achieve the desired shrinkage and to provide mechanical strength in the teeth. Because use of too much clay made it difficult to remove the mold without cracking the teeth, a small amount of starch and gum arabic or tragacanth was added instead, which helped to fill the mold and make it easier to release the tooth after it had cooled in the mold. Varied colored porcelain mixtures were required to match the ever-varying tints of natural human teeth. To obtain different shades, oxides of iron, titanium, cobalt, copper, chromium, manganese, and gold were blended in during the molding process.

An original model of the tooth was first produced in plaster of Paris of a larger size than required to allow for shrinkage of the porcelain in the burning process. Finding the correct proportion between the size of the cast and final product was difficult, a difficulty Duchâteau never solved. Models were made in two parts to facilitate the tooth's removal from the mold. The final mold into which the porcelain materials were inserted was made of bronze and produced in a manner similar to bronze castings. We know little about the details of White's craftsmanship except that he was a master metal mold maker. He ground crude metals in a hand mortar and compounded these into the finished metal block.[39] He then carved molds from solid blocks of metal using natural teeth, rather than plaster molds, as the patterns.

By himself White could not make the seven to eight hundred molds used to make the ten thousand shapes of teeth he manufactured by 1865.[40] Therefore he hired assistants and among them were a few who eventually became his competitors. White introduced the man who would become his closest competitor to the business of metal mold carving. Henry Justi immigrated to Philadelphia from Germany and was employed by Jones, White and McCurdy in 1852. Although Justi was an experienced metallurgist in Germany, he had no training in dentistry or teeth making. At the time Justi joined the dental company, White had assembled a collection of artificial teeth made by all other makers in the world. A collection that may be White's exists in the holdings of the

Science Museum of the University of Utrecht; however the source of the collection is not known. Experience gained with White led the ambitious Justi to seek the aid of a Philadelphia dentist who was an expert in taking impressions of the mouth, including alignment of the upper and lower teeth that resulted in better articulation when chewing. Justi then carved molds based on the patterns provided by the dentist. He enlarged the dentist's arsenal of manufactured artificial teeth by introducing sectional teeth,which were teeth mounted in segments of two or more that were used to replace a few missing teeth. Previously it had been more common to pull all teeth, including sound teeth, to provide the space for a full denture.[41]

To form the tooth, a small amount of light-colored raw porcelain was laid into the mold at the point forming the biting edge of the tooth. The darker-colored portion that constitutes the body of the tooth was then added. To provide an uninterrupted flow of porcelain, each color was introduced by a separate operator working as a member of a team. The material was put into the molds with the fingers and when the two half-molds were filled they were placed together immediately, and clamped to insure the union of the body of the tooth. By subjecting the mold to heat and pressure, the tooth was baked into a tough mass, only slightly shrunken. At this stage the tooth resembled a very soft biscuit or low-temperature porcelain. The teeth were then rapped out of the mold and the bur edges filed off and polished.

Burning was the last and most delicate step in the manufacturing process. The biscuited teeth were carefully placed in an inverted position in fused silica trays. The tray was placed in a gas muffle furnace and heated to the required temperature. It was essential to subject the teeth to heat for the shortest possible time to ensure that the tooth surface would fuse and become smooth without the heat penetrating into and deforming the teeth. The teeth were taken from the furnace when the operator observed the appropriate brilliance produced by the fusion. Upon annealing the teeth were cooled and graded to eliminate imperfect specimens.

Due to the high heat required to fuse porcelain teeth, the pins that were imbedded in the teeth and used to attach the teeth to the plate had to be made from a substance resistant to high temperatures. Platinum, one of the most expensive metals, was the most desirable material. Tooth makers speculated that if a lower-fusing porcelain could be used to make teeth, a metal less expensive than platinum might be used, thus reducing the cost of artificial teeth.

Correspondence beginning in 1856 between White and the tooth designers W. G. Oliver and Thomas Harrison confirms White's continual search for perfection and his ability to improve upon the teeth he manufactured. In several letters details are presented of some of the steps White was asked to take to produce individual teeth shaped to match those of a "well formed mouth of 25 or 30 years of age." The gum line was to be carefully traced and the block of teeth put into a furnace with a soft heat during the biscuit process, after which the teeth would be separated. White made changes in the teeth following Oliver's suggestions over several years, until in a letter of February 24, 1857, Oliver exclaimed: "I am very much pleased with this lot of gum teeth, in fact, they are perfectly beautiful. I never saw such handsome teeth either of yours, or any other makers. The plain teeth look remarkably well and I think will do in every respect."[42]

White's ability to make teeth to satisfy various patients and designers may have contributed to an increasing neglect of some dentists to skillfully place artificial teeth in their patients' mouths. At the time of White's death, prosthetic dentistry, also called mechanical dentistry, was disparaged within the dental profession. In turning over the tooth-making part of dentistry to manufacturers, practitioners seem to have abdicated their role as patient advocate in the final appearance of the artificial tooth-bearing face. Apparently, many dentists no longer wished to be compared to jewelers and seemingly lost their esthetic sense. Saving teeth soon became the primary mission of a "good" dentist. Manufacturers were blamed for the poor appearance of those who wore artificial teeth. W. Warrington Evans of Washington, DC, studied the problem and discovered that manufacturers made a greater variety of beautiful teeth than most dentists purchased. Generally, only a few styles of teeth were in demand among dentists, who frequently turned over their mechanical work to an assistant or student. Evans claimed that dentists were not taught the anatomy of the tooth well enough to appreciate its intricacies and its esthetic dimensions.[43] James White as editor of the *Dental Cosmos* welcomed discussion of the dentist's role in mechanical dentistry. "It is entirely possible, by the study of physiognomy, of the muscles of expression, of esthetic anatomy, to avoid the glaring incongruities so constantly met with in artificial dentures and to add to usefulness the charm of naturalness."[44]

Few dentists who were exceptionally skilled porcelain teeth makers were willing to work for many hours in a laboratory. One of these experts whose teeth remain in the National Museum of American History collections was Dr. Jacob Burkholder Bauman (1827–1907) of Columbus, Ohio. Excelling in continuous gum work he also perfected an all-porcelain plate to avoid using vulcanite and paying the royalties for its use. He used a high-fusing porcelain similar to the type used in continuous gum sections for which he purchased the unmixed porcelain materials from White. He also mixed his own gum colors. In some instances, biscuited White continuous gum teeth were placed in the porcelain he had mixed and fused together in the oven. Frequently Bauman carved the teeth out of the same porcelain as the plate. C. A. Hawley, Bauman's student who later practiced in Washington, DC, watched Bauman fuse his teeth in an old-fashioned coke oven, often working until three or four in the morning. Bauman's dentures that had been worn for years released no odor when placed over a slow fire.[45]

DENTAL MANUFACTURERS AND TRADE FAIR EXHIBITS

Trade fairs provided the venue to display the latest dental innovations, and by giving prizes, encouraged craftsmen to share their methods and find a market for their products. Prizes provided the winners with a unique advertising message, and teeth were among the most attractive and macabre items exhibited at trade fairs. J. R. McCurdy reported in *The Dental News Letter* his observations of the Crystal Palace Exposition in 1851. McCurdy was dissatisfied with European-made teeth, but above all with the disdain the judges expressed regarding manufactured dental items. His comments provide an informal view of the fair and the insights of a manufacturer. McCurdy summed up his impression that "dentistry in Europe . . . is after the same style, although with different degrees of finish, and in describing one collection all are described."[46]

Among those exhibitors singled out by McCurdy were the Swiss, French, Prussian, and English. Carved Swiss teeth were chiefly made of the tooth carvers' favorite form of ivory, hippopotamus canine teeth; Swiss porcelain teeth were fitted into a bone base, a combination of materials first developed in France. The clasps used to fasten the teeth were, according to McCurdy, placed in such a position that they could injure or destroy the gums and natural teeth to which they were fastened. Only one well-made specimen of human teeth was mounted on gold plate. According to McCurdy spiral springs were more commonly applied to European teeth than to those manufactured in America Three-quarters of a century after John Greenwood made a set of artificial teeth with spiral springs for George Washington, American manufacturers had abandoned this awkward contrivance for retaining artificial teeth in the mouth.

The French exhibit was startling. It contained fifty specimens, of which nine sets were in active operation, "chewing away lustily." To demonstrate the effect of replacing missing teeth in the mouth, a model jaw was arranged to open while two or three teeth in the upper jaw slowly moved out of sight, "leaving an ugly space, particularly remarkable when the jaws come together, then when the jaws open again, these two or three teeth come back to their place, and show the beauty of a perfect set of teeth. Another case revolves slowly, by pivots on the sides, thus showing the shape and workmanship all around. . . ."[47] Parisian dentists also displayed their personally crafted artificial teeth in cases mounted at the doors of their offices.[48]

The Prussian exhibition was similar to the French except that the teeth were not as well formed. The English collection consisted mostly of teeth made from hippopotamus canines, beautifully carved and very accurately fitted. However, as stated before, ivory teeth were subject to decay, discoloration, and assimilated bad odors, thus forcing the owner to have them replaced annually, a condition, McCurdy reasoned, that would not suit most Americans "as we could not spare the time, and would not like to spend the means, to have a new operation yearly."[49]

VULCANIZED RUBBER DENTURES

Improvement in artificial teeth increased the demand for more natural-looking and less expensive substances than gold and silver for making the denture plates to which the teeth were attached. The first recorded search for a better denture substance began in Europe in the laboratory of an American dentist. Thomas W. Evans was forced to discontinue his dental practice in Paris and stay in London in 1848 because of the revolution, and he used the time to test the properties of metals and minerals as possible denture materials. He discovered a form of hard rubber, which due to the impurities in his source was black. On one of his early samples he wrote, "I searched for ivory and found ebony."[50]

Several years after his experimentation Evans was introduced by the dentist Charles Morey to Charles Goodyear, who discovered the vulcanization, or stabilization, of rubber and had received his first patent in 1844.[51] Goodyear's brother Nelson was able to "convert the soft flexible material into the hard ebonite substance"[52] and received a patent in the United States for his method of creating hardened rubber, which he called vulcanite, in 1851. Goodyear came to Paris after attending the Crystal Palace Exposition in London. He offered Evans exclusive rights to use his patent to make denture bases in Europe, which Evans declined. Evans was among those dentists who acted on the belief that dentists should share their discoveries freely, therefore he did not seek a patent for the substance. Then, Morey obtained a French patent for vulcanite. Morey was apparently convinced of Evans's priority in the discovery of hard rubber to be used in dentures, a fact his widow testified to in 1867.[53] In the United States, an obscure Boston dentist, Dr. John Cummings, received a patent for both vulcanite to be used in dentures and also the denture itself in 1864, after three previous unsuccessful attempts, beginning in 1852, with the filing of a caveat on "an invention not fully perfected. . . ."[54] During the period of Cummings's efforts, Goodyear's son visited Evans on a number of occasions to study his methods of making vulcanite.

Evans became aware of the financial and professionally awkward consequences for American dentists of the Goodyear-Cummings patents early in the controversy. Evans's decision not to seek a patent was to lead to a state of affairs in which the American patent was to be controlled by a singularly profit-centered individual who was not a dentist, and whose assiduous methods of collecting fees to use vulcanite in dentures became a major burden to Samuel Stockton White and thousands of dentists. The patent for denture vulcanite was acquired by the Goodyear Dental Vulcanite Company from Cummings in 1864 and assigned in 1866 to Josiah Bacon of Boston. Malvin Ring discusses the scenarios played out by Bacon, who ruthlessly and persistently hounded dentists to pay license and per-item use fees to make vulcanite dentures.[55] Bacon, who devised the plan to charge a fee for each vulcanite denture installed, insisted that dentists keep a list of their patients to be inspected whenever a representative of the Dental Vulcanite Company deemed it necessary. The patient's privacy as well as the dentist's ethical position in acceding to this demand were further issues that increased the profession's opposition to the Dental Vulcanite Company.

John Dehaven White, editor of the *Dental Cosmos*, contacted Evans when the latter returned to the United States in 1864 on a diplomatic mission for the Emperor of France to determine the possible outcome of the Civil War.[56] Evans became aware of the unsatisfactory financial arrangement for using vulcanite imposed on American dentists and testified to his priority in the discovery of vulcanite for dentures in an effort to assist dentists who were contesting the validity of the American patent, and therefore, the fee system imposed on them. The Massachusetts Dental Association had discovered Evans's claim to priority through J. Pashud-Shaw, a British dentist, who learned of Evans's work through the Ash Dental Company, which was a pioneer in the manufacture of a portable vulcanizer designed by C. S. Putnam of London.[57] Shaw had brought vulcanized rubber to England in 1857 and consulted Ash about the patent. Shaw was then directed to Evans.[58]

In his statement, sent upon request to the Massachusetts Dental Association, which made Evans an honorary member, Evans explained his role in the development of hard rubber for dentures and his refusal to accept the exclusive European right to a patent from Charles Goodyear.[59] Evans explained that he had not announced his discovery immediately because past experience in announcing a discovery prematurely had made him cautious. Evans's explanation might have appeared in White's *Dental News Letter*, for which he was a foreign correspondent. Among Evans's early discoveries was an amalgam paste made of tin, cadmium, and mercury, which he had touted as a better filling material. It was rejected by dentists. Subsequently Evans retracted his promotion of the filling amalgam and decided against recommending other substances, including hard rubber, until they were thoroughly tested. Had Evans published his discovery of vulcanite in *The Dental News Letter*, the history of hard rubber in American dentistry might have included a chapter on an earlier development and wider use of the substance without penalty of a fee for each use and without a protracted threat of criminal prosecution and a suit for damages.

Vulcanite provided dentists with a good substance for constructing partial dentures, which were becoming more in fashion as dentists learned to preserve partially decayed teeth. Henry Justi realized the potential of vulcanite for creating a more life-like gum line. He introduced artificial teeth made in blocks or sections in which the gums were more realistically curved around the teeth and differentiated in color.[60] Justi's new teeth provided dentists with another option for fitting patients with partial dentures and it became an immediate success.

Whatever the complications in using vulcanite, White realized that vulcanite was the best material for making less-expensive dentures. In fact vulcanite remained a major source of denture material until the mid-twentieth century. White prepared a superior form of vulcanite, and as early as 1862 advertised his rubber as being equal to or better than any other rubber available for vulcanizing into dentures.[61] White also sold the implements to work with vulcanite, including the steaming chambers, also called vulcanizers; spatulas; and gauges, as listed in the 1876 catalog. White stamped his dental rubber with a trademark in the shape of an Indian bow and arrow, which was registered on June 23, 1874. In the catalog White noted that "those of us who are still willing to use Rubber as a base for Artificial Dentures are naturally desirous of producing the best results of which the material is capable; but satisfaction in the working and meaning of it depends not alone on the skill and care of the manipulator, but, to a very great extent, on the quality of the material."[62]

In the meantime, White encouraged dentists to protest and even refuse to pay the fees imposed on them for making vulcanite dentures because he reasoned that those dentists who bought vulcanite enabled the Vulcanite Company to use the income to bring suits against other dentists for not complying with the company's demands.[63] The *Dental Cosmos* became White's bully pulpit for articles, notes, and correspondence on the subject.[64] White was not successful in having the fee eliminated nor against a judgment arising from a slander suit for $175,000 brought by Josiah Bacon against White for "false and defamatory publications which dissuaded dentists from purchasing licenses."[65] According to White, Bacon charged him with "malice against them and inducing 3000 dentists to refuse to take the license and furnishing them [the dentists] with advice to suits which I knew the company were [*sic*] going to bring against the dentists."[66]

Publicly and privately dentists attempted to circumvent the vulcanite denture patent as Ring has demonstrated.[67] However, the resources and resolve of Josiah Bacon were insurmountable. In a letter to White of October 24, 1879, Dr. C. De Montreville of St. Paul, Minnesota, described how in the summer of 1873 Josiah Bacon had called upon him and boasted of the way he could continue to use the patent law to win judgments against infringing dentists. Among the issues discussed was the Simpson rubber patent that "Hale of Bridgeport, Connecticut, agreed to warrant and defend the user against any suits of the Rubber Company."[68] Edwin L. Simpson owned a patent for removing the bad taste of vulcanized rubber dentures by adding oil to the substance, an improvement essential to denture wearers. Bacon commented on Hale's bold offer to De Montreville: "Ah Doctor we had all of your letters to Hale, Simpson and Co. in our Iron Safe and we knew to a Doctor what you were worth, and we knew a judgment against you was worth every cent it called for."[69] When taken to court by Henry B. Goodyear, Nelson Goodyear's administrator, the Simpson patent was ruled unenforceable and subject to the prior Goodyear patent.[70]

Josiah Bacon, treasurer of the company, whose tactics to enforce his patent dentists considered to be abusive, was murdered by a dentist he had pursued across the country. Dr. Samuel Chalfant, who had recently relocated his office to San Francisco in April of 1879, shot Bacon after an argument in his hotel room. Samuel S. White's death has been attributed, in part, to the stress and weariness resulting from his protracted litigation with Bacon. White died eight months after Bacon's death.

White was not only involved with the legal mechanism of using the vulcanite patent, but with disseminating information on how to solve a serious problem generated in the preparation of vulcanite dentures: explosion of the device in which the dentures were hardened. To prepare the denture the rubber had to be subjected to high temperature and pressure in a special cooker equipped for the purpose called a vulcanizer. Dr. George E. Hayes and Dr. Benjah T. Whitney of Buffalo designed the two most popular vulcanizers: the Hayes, patented in 1861 and again in 1866, and the Whitney in 1867. The two dentists founded the Buffalo Dental Manufacturing Company to manufacture both vulcanizers. (The Buffalo Dental Manufacturing Company is the third oldest dental company in the United States; the second oldest dental manufacturer founded in the United States was Lee S. Smith of Pittsburgh, which was organized a year earlier in 1866.) Reports of explosions were sent to White, who published them in the *Dental Cosmos.*

Alarmed by the increasing number of catastrophes and wanting to ward off more disasters, the Odontographic Society of Philadelphia assigned William H. Trueman of Philadelphia the task of investigating the causes of these explosions. Trueman contacted the Buffalo Dental Manufacturing Company and received replies from Hayes and Whitney, all of which were published in the November 1869 issue of the *Dental Cosmos.* Hayes' earliest vulcanizers were made with an iron chamber, the strongest material for the purpose. Whitney's vulcanizer was made from copper, which made the boiler lighter and therefore easier to handle. Whitney, whose vulcanizer was involved in most of the explosions by virtue of its popularity among dentists, responded that all units were tested by the manufacturer before they were shipped to customers. The walls of the Whitney were made of sufficiently thick copper to withstand a higher temperature than it was likely to receive while in use. Whitney attributed all the exploded vulcanizers he had inspected to mishandling by the dentist—that is, overuse, overheating, and improper cleaning. Trueman concurred, concluding that more safety features were not needed; rather, dentists had to change their methods and heed the precautions required in working with steam boilers.[71]

RUBBER DENTAL INSTRUMENTS

Rubber was a versatile substance, which in its soft and pliable state provided the material that solved a major problem in repairing teeth with gold. In 1857 Robert Arthur of Baltimore invented the most practical and widely used technique for the installation of gold fillings. Gold in thin slices was packed or cold welded into the tooth cavity layer by layer. However, the cavity had to remain dry throughout the tedious process, which could take hours to complete. Sanford C. Barnum, in 1864, was inspired to punch a hole in a piece of rubber and slip it over a lower molar, thus sealing it from the saliva. He had invented the rubber dam, which remains an essential part of the gold filling process.[72]

Hard rubber or vulcanite was quickly applied to instrument handles by several dentists. A short announcement published in the *Dental Cosmos* of 1862 pointed out that a Dr. Buckingham in Philadelphia, a Dr. Richardson in Cincinnati, and a Dr. Wheat in Connecticut had attached vulcanite handles to dental instruments. Buckingham found the vulcanite handles superior to those made of leather, while Richardson had been using pluggers with vulcanite handles, and Wheat, perhaps even earlier, had handles made of hard rubber for his dental instruments. However, in the early 1860s, dental instrument manufacturers had a stock of metal handles and a staff accustomed to working with metal, and lacked sufficient funds to invest in new products; therefore, manufacturers had not yet begun to make hard-rubber handles.[73] White soon produced vulcanite handles for instruments, which were considerably less attractive than the pearl, ivory, and shell instruments already associated with the White label. However, this loss of aesthetic value was offset by the fact that the new vulcanite instruments were more easily manipulated by dentists.

THE DEVELOPMENT OF A DENTAL INSTRUMENT DEPARTMENT

Before the mid-century, the better dental instrument handles were made from pearl, ivory, conch shell, and bone, which White supplied in beautiful patterns. Among the best sources of ivory for handles was the dentine layer of the hippopotamus canine tooth, also prized by the dentist for carving teeth, because the material resisted stains better than other types of ivory. However, the elegant appearance of the handle did not ensure a good-quality instrument. Through the editor's column of the *Dental Cosmos* in 1861, White chastised dentists for being more concerned with the handles of their instruments than with the steel from which the instrument itself was made.[74] Therefore White set about improving the functional part of dental instruments, beginning with the search for better-quality steel.

White's goal was to make better steel and improve the designs of implements offered to the dentist, which would thus improve the latter's techniques for repairing teeth. White enlisted a mechanic named George Kaeber who worked in his building but found that although Kaeber possessed fine mechanical skills, he lacked the initiative to pursue investigations that would lead to improved dental instruments. However, White soon found a suitable manager for the shop: Henry Coy, who made dental lathes in his own small machine shop. Coy was engaged to manage the shop that was financed by

White at a time when the latter was short of money, having just contributed to the support of a Union Army regiment and owing his former partners for their share of the business that he had recently bought from them. Working on a commission basis, Coy, in 1867, introduced steel instruments and forceps with an unprecedented adaptability, temper, and finish. The Samuel Stockton White logo was first applied on these steel instruments. Coy's superior craftsmanship was acknowledged by stamping his initials beside the White logo on all the pieces manufactured under his supervision.[75] Surgeons as well as dentists admired the new White-Coy instruments and today they are rare collectors' items. Coy also helped shepherd into existence an award-winning foot-pedal dental engine in 1874. The American Institute and Franklin Institute judges praised the first flexible wire shaft and sheath engine: "This ingenious machine . . . specially designed for the Dental Practitioners . . . is the most complete instrument or machine ever made for this purpose. It . . . is a long step forward in the application of machinery to Dental operations, and is deserving of a special award as the best of its kind."[76] Coy remained with White until 1880, when he was succeeded by Levi Teal, who had previously arranged the contracts between the White Company and dealers throughout the country.[77]

Eli T. Starr (1834–1905) who had manufactured, devised, and tested dental appliances for the White Company since 1862, managed the company's patents starting in the 1870s.[78] He worked in concert with patent lawyers William and Joseph Peyton and was succeeded by lawyer Edward Simpson (d. 1928), who became a specialist in dental patents while working with the White Company. Simpson organized the patent department around 1900 and established a company museum for old dental objects. Panels of objects from this museum now reside in the collection of the National Museum of American History, Smithsonian Institution, and in the Dr. John Harris Dental Museum in Bainbridge, Ohio.

SAMUEL STOCKTON WHITE AND OTHER INVESTMENTS

In the last few years of his life White's large income from the sale of artificial teeth and dental instruments enabled him to invest in other business endeavors. Company records show that various charities and philanthropic organizations benefitted from White's generosity. White was among the first businessmen to financially support the Union Army. The company supported many private and state welfare agencies guided by his brother James, who was noted for his participation in civil and human rights organizations, including the Freedman's Aid Society, the Sanitary Fair, and the Maternity Hospital. James was appointed the first president of the Board of Charities and Correction of Philadelphia.

White's interests were centered on innovative technologies. One of the most intriguing was his investment in Elisha Gray's Harmonic Telegraph, a venture actively pursued during the last year of his life. Correspondence with Charles Rudd, an engineer who strung wire between stations for a telegraph system, shows that White kept informed about the details and progress of the telegraph project, and in return for the information supplied by Rudd, sent him hundreds of dollars on a number of occasions to keep him on the job. In March of 1879, White's accountant H. M. Lewis submitted a report stating that the company did not make any money from its telegraph investments. Lewis testified that "the business has been depleted, drained to exhaustion by the Gray venture, nearly $33,000 solid money having been withdrawn for that purpose during 1878, until my diagnosis is not 'How much longer can this depletion process be continued?' but 'Has the patent enough vitality left to rally from the present exhaustion?'" The loss from the money invested in the Elisha Gray patents amounted to $110,000.[79] White also was a large stockholder in the American Speaking Telephone Company—an outgrowth of the Harmonic Telegraph. He adjudicated disputes between rival claims for the telephone and prevented costly litigation.[80]

White's son, Samuel F. White, Jr., who had not spent much time on company business except for three years when he served as president between 1912 and 1915, recalled in 1933 that his father planned to form a company with Dr. Norman Green, president of Western Union Telegraph Company, for five or ten million dollars. However, Samuel S. White died before he could form the company. The company was to use Elish Grig's [*sic*, Elisha Gray's] patents for the Duplex and Harmonic Telegraph. White was to purchase half interest in the telegraph business.[81]

At his death in 1879, White's estate was worth 1.5 million dollars, which was shared by his wife who lived until August 5, 1904, and four surviving children. In his will the management of the company was placed in the hands of three survivors: his brother James; his oldest son, J. Clarence; and his business manager Henry M. Lewis. Because Lewis was S. S. White's close business associate, he probably knew White's plans for the business better than anyone else. Lewis delineated the duties of the three partners in a letter of May 11, 1880. James would be in charge of manufacturing and editorial matters, J. Clarence would manage the clerks and purchase of supplies, while Henry would supervise commercial dealings because he had twelve years of experience with the accounts and knew when to give credit.

The partnership worked well. Soon they agreed to accept the offer of Johnston Brothers to purchase the their firm, which was located in Staten Island, New York. S. S. White and Johnston Brothers were combined into a joint stock company in 1880, with a paid-in capital of one million dollars. The Staten Island plant doubled the manufacturing capacity of S. S. White and provided facilities that enabled the Samuel Stockton White Dental Manufacturing Company (SSWDMC, the new name of the joint company) to produce a greater variety of instruments, office furniture, and appliances. Johnston's factory produced items that would make a great deal of money for the White Company over the next fifty years.

Johnston Brothers, founded in 1865, issued its first catalog in 1881, having delayed publication in order to prepare a more extensive edition. The company claimed priority in manufacturing one thousand fine gold foil, power instruments to replace hand tools, liquid nitrous oxide, an adjustable table bracket, an adjustable fountain spittoon, cone socket instruments, and the easily adjustable Morrison and Wilkerson chairs.[82] The Morrison chair was the first internationally popular dental chair, and its patent was sold abroad as well. In 1871, shortly after its invention, Ash and Sons (established 1822) purchased from Mr. Morrison, at considerable cost, the right to manufacture and supply these chairs in Europe.[83]

White had worked for ten years on perfecting a dental chair with only modest results in creating one that was maneuverable. He introduced the first metal frame chair, called the Harris chair, in 1871. Although heavy, it replaced an equally heavy wooden chair already in production. In 1876 the handsome White chair was placed on the market; however, it was soon surpassed by an easier to manipulate hydraulically controlled chair. In 1878 the White pedal-level, or "pump" chair, was first manufactured.

In an industry where skillful mechanics sold their implements to innovative and dexterous dentists, patents were particularly important in stabilizing the manufacturing process, at least for a few years. Because manufacturers and dentists were continually modifying their instruments, one vital test of the extent of the change and the claim of the manufacturer to exclusive rights to produce an item was the interpretation of the patent in the courts. Carolyn C. Cooper has demonstrated that "lawsuits were a normal feature of the [nineteenth-century] patent system, not a symptom of its malfunctioning nor of cranky personal temperaments." Cooper concluded that the process of determining a new invention's originality "became a matter of social construction through patent management."[84]

One special concern of dental patent holders in defending their claims was locating a patent examiner and judge who could understand the intricacy of the terminology and technology. Previous unfavorable experience with an examiner or court could persuade a litigant to seek justice in another setting. Lawyers continually worked with designers, mechanics, and dentists to advise, improve, and defend patents for the White Company. By the turn of the century, experience and, especially, losses led White to insist that patent holders who sold their rights to the dental company defend their claims if challenged.

By 1879, the White Company owned 150 patents or reissues of which ten were awarded to Samuel White. The range of patented items included teeth, molds, pluggers, engines, chairs, disk carriers, brackets, fans, files, chip blowers, drills, stools, gold, syringes, flasks, head rests, articulators, and foot rests. The most prolific patent holder was Eli T. Starr, who had obtained twenty-six of his eventual one hundred patents by this time.[85] The company continually defended its patents and kept a record of those who appeared to infringe upon its patent rights. When William Gilbert reorganized the factory in 1880 he discovered that Henry Justi was the worst offender in using White patents illegally. He made pluggers and handpieces that copied features peculiar to White patents.[86]

An item that caused a lot of controversy was the patenting of flexible shafting. Flexible shafting was an essential piece in transferring power from the foot pedal to an engine while permitting the dentist freedom to move about the patient. There were many arguments and patent challenges over the invention of flexible shafting, which had a number of applications in a host of industries and became a lucrative item to manufacture. The history of the development of flexible shafting as it affects dentistry is revealed in memoranda for the defense in litigation by Samuel S. White against Johnston Brothers for making flexible shafts, which occurred before the merger of the two companies in 1881. Patents obtained from the late 1850s through the 1870s reveal the major claims of each party. Among the key inventors were Thomas Welham for universal shafting (January 1865), Albert Kennedy for sheepshears (January 1866) "containing the first organized power with a loose-wire coil," and Mason Stow for a rotary wire coil shaft with a non-rotating flexible shaft (June 1874). Stow testified that in 1857 he made "a flexible shaft or cable composed of pieces of whale-bone twisted together and made a sheath for it composed of a spiral of steel wire, without any covering." He used the device to brush horses and clothes. In 1865 Stow made a flexible shaft of coiled wire and enclosed it in a flexible sheath of black leather. He attached the shaft to a foot-power device and used it as a horse brush.[87]

One elementary dental instrument in the process of being re-evaluated and redesigned by Johnston Brothers at the time of the merger was the machine-cut engine bur, the most successful dental instrument produced by the restructured White Company in the nineteenth century. Johnston was stimulated by the need for a more durable bur to use with the more powerful foot-treadle drill that Johnston had introduced in 1871 upon acquiring James B. Morrison's patent. Criticism of Johnston burs followed the introduction of the foottreadle dental engine in 1871. Edwin Sercombe, a dentist in London with whom Morrison had practiced, wrote to Morrison after the latter had returned to the United States. In March of 1871, a month after Morrison received a patent for the engine, Sercombe told Morrison that he would wait for his engine rather than buy an English "machine" even though his "busy season [was] fast approaching." In February of 1873 Sercombe was so delighted with Morrison's engine that he temporarily relinquished his own engine in order to enter Morrison's engine in the International Exhibition scheduled to open in the summer of that year in London. Sercombe demonstrated the engine at the Odontological Society meetings, published his comments in the Society's journal, and promoted its features to the London instrument maker and dealer, Claudius Ash. Sercombe, who obtained his Morrison engines from Johnston, complained about the size of some burs that did not stay in place in the handpiece and the poor resistance to wear and cutting quality of others.[88]

In the meantime, Samuel White's achievements in bur making were modest; he first produced steel burs in 1872 and introduced modifications including the hand-cut stoned burs in 1878. A less expensive honed bur was produced by the SSWDMC in 1882. Experiments to improve the bur were done in the factory on Staten Island, which culminated in a major design change and a very effective multi-purpose bur-drill. White had also improved the foot-power dental engine in 1874 by incorporating a flexible shaft, a feature that would make it a favorite among dentists for decades.[89]

Almost two decades after the Morrison engine was developed, SSWDMC introduced a vastly improved bur. Dentists who used the bur were excited enough to select a name for it from the title of its promotional literature, *A Revelation in Burs*. Dentists asked for the bur by the name "Revelation," a term that was soon applied to the piece by its manufacturers. Revelation Burs, although changed in composition to include diamond tips and, in some instances, disposable diamonds, currently are made in Lakewood, New Jersey. There were numerous attempts to copy the original Revelation Bur's design by other manufacturers.[90]

Voluminous correspondence, patent actions, and personal testimony regarding the conception, development, protection, and sale of Revelation Burs enlighten us on the importance of this item to the SSWDMC and the evolving impetus among dentists to concentrate on saving teeth by repairing those with pockets of decay, rather than removing them. Announced on January 1, 1891, the new bur was reputed to increase the comfort for both dentist and patient during the preparation of cavities. Arthur W. Browne, inventor of the No. 7 handpiece, who was in charge of development and improving the manufacturing process, obtained the patent for the bur. Browne's claim was for a bur that was configured to function like both a bur and a drill. The novel design feature was a cutting edge on the blade carried across the very center of the bur when it was brought parallel to the surface to be removed. Up to this time, dental burs were constructed so that a hollow or non-cutting circle of space was formed at the tip where the cutting leaves of the bur ended without meeting. Previously, because of this "dead" space, another implement called a drill was used to open up the channel of a decayed tooth to the depth required; the old-fashioned bur was then applied to ream out and smooth the edges of the space into which the filling was to be inserted. The dual function of the Revelation Bur was coupled with the elimination of chatter or slippage by arranging the cutting blades so that they did not follow in the exact path. Particularly significant for the patient was a razor sharp edge that lapped or "stoned" off the dentin, the most sensitive portion of a tooth lying beneath the enamel, thus reducing the pain created during this dreaded dental operation.

Not only were the new burs considerably improved, but they were cheaper for the dentist to use because they lasted longer and were sold at a lower price. Efficiency in manufacturing the machine-made bur and its immediate popularity enabled the SSWDMC to reduce the sale price of each bur and still make a profit.

The SSWDMC proudly claimed that it required a dozen years of experimentation and an expenditure of over fifty thousand dollars to produce the new bur. To the dismay and astonishment of the factory, the original stock of the new burs was sold out in two months. By assigning men to work in two shifts of ten hours each, the factory attempted, however in vain, to supply all orders. Consequently the burs were not advertised for a year and a half to allow time for the plant to produce a sufficient quantity to meet the increased orders. Behind schedule by over one hundred thousand burs in the 1890s, the company's success with the bur continued, with sales of many hundreds of thousands per month in the mid-1920s.

Other dental manufacturers reacted quickly to the new bur. The most extreme and potentially damaging action was taken by Ash and Sons in London, who were incensed by SSWDMC's advertising literature, which claimed that all previous burs were obsolete, even though this claim may have been justified. Ash immediately began to produce its own form of the Revelation Bur. SSWDMC asserted its rights as patent owner and demanded that Ash desist from further production or agree to operate under a license from SSWDMC. Ash ignored the request and continued to make the burs, claiming that the White patent was invalid because burs had been made for years in this form for other uses, one of which was to bore out gun barrel channels. Browne's patent was not defended after White employees visited a Dr. Rutherford in 1895. Rutherford claimed that a Mr. Ward had made similar burs twenty years earlier and produced one hundred examples.[91]

In correspondence during the early 1890s, both companies clarified their positions in considerable detail, thus providing a record of how dentists interpreted the process of excavating tooth decay and contrasting it to other drilling actions, as well as its implications for tooth repair and patient response. In May of 1895, several years after a fruitless trip to London to discuss the matter, Henry Lewis, President of SSWDMC, agreed to dismiss the suit brought against Ash and pay litigation costs in exchange for an agreement from Ash not to contest the validity of the patent. Ash was not compelled to purchase a license to manufacture the bur. Ash did not publicize the arrangement with

SSWDMC nor claim credit for preventing the patent from being enforced. Perhaps in a gesture of conciliation Ash bought more burs from SSWDMC. Henry Lewis accepted defeat and summed up the arrangement with Ash who "seemed to think there was no necessity for any formal papers to be drawn up, as our withdrawal simply puts the matter back where it was before we commenced action. . . . By this we prevent for the present the invalidating of the patent which is all we can hope for."

ADVERTISING AND DISTRIBUTION

To distribute his artificial teeth as widely as possible White opened branch houses in New York (1846), Boston (1850), Brooklyn (1852), and Chicago (1858).[92] Soon demand prompted White to sell teeth to dealers at a discount so that dentists not located near a branch could more conveniently order White teeth. White's dealership system ensured that a large stock of artificial teeth was available throughout the country for dentists to choose from and purchase at short notice.[93]

The *Dental Cosmos* remained the most important vehicle for advertising until the twentieth century. Frank L. Hise, a savvy copy writer and author of the company's eighty-second anniversary volume, understood the commercial value of appealing to all types of dentists. He began his career with the company in the 1870s as secretary to Samuel White, but by 1880 he began to prepare most of the advertising statements. By the end of the nineteenth century, of forty-eight scrapbooks of advertisements accumulated by SSWDMC, Hise laid claim to having written the copy for 90 percent of them. During these three decades the company income increased from one million to six million dollars.

Hise claimed responsibility for the increasing success of several items, including the promotion of Hill's stopping, a type of gutta percha used for temporary and less-expensive tooth filling. Introduced by Samuel White in the 1860s, its sales increased five-fold under Hise's aggressive advertising. For many years eight to nine thousand boxes were sold annually; around the turn of the century, Hise began a special campaign to sell the material. He boasted that in 1911 forty to fifty thousand boxes were sold.[94]

For decades Hise had argued in favor of introducing new methods of encouraging dentists to try new products and convincing new dentists to try traditional White products. He advocated that the company send free samples to dentists, including samples of successful products like the Revelation Bur and guarantee every product by offering to take back any item that did not satisfy the buyer. These free-wheeling advertising suggestions did not appeal to the more conservative leaders of SSWDMC at the time. Henry Lewis and William Gilbert, presidents during this period, shared Samuel White's opinion that modesty was valuable in business. However, neither president encouraged Hise to change his advertising techniques. Hise tried to entice Gilbert by responding to one of the president's main concerns: a rising stock of goods in the company storerooms. Hise compared the amount of money that had been spent on increasing production over the last decade and the amount used for advertising expenses: the investment in machinery and buildings doubled, whereas advertising increased by a mere 10 percent. Hise envisioned an agency "whose efficacy in creating a market for the products of the Company's factories [that] has never been properly tested. Other businesses are built up and thrive by their advertising. Our house has never yet had the nerve to go at advertising in earnest. We keep on in the same old track we followed twenty years ago. The conditions have changed, and we ought to change with them. We want to make our advertising department a fitting mate for our manufacturing department."[95] Committed to continually creating new markets, Hise explained, "We can produce almost enough goods to supply the entire dental world. We reach directly, once a month, through the *Dental Cosmos*, perhaps one-sixth of that world; through the other dental journals perhaps twice as many more; say one-half of the entire number reached at varying intervals from one week to three months through the journals. There still remain a full half whom we reach only casually, if at all, most of them not more than once a year."[96]

Traditional low-key advertising methods were effective for some products, such as the White label dentrifices. Approached by dentists to produce a safe and useful tooth cleanser, White, upon consultation with dentists, physicians, and pharmacists, introduced his tooth powder in 1862. White soon added a toothpaste and soap in 1869 and sold tons of dentrifices without much advertising, but instead by relying on the recommendations of these items by dentists to their patients.[97]

At the time of White's death the company he founded and guided for thirty-five years was poised to expand its operations to manufacture much more of the hardware and furniture. White's executors, led by Henry Lewis, who brought a business training to the company, seized the opportunity to expand by purchasing a well-equipped dental plant on Staten Island, New York. With the Johnston Brothers Company came the rights to important patents in dental chairs, the staff to perfect the dental bur and dental instruments, thus making the White Company a well-rounded dental manufacturer. Having brought the White name to the pinnacle of dental goods, Samuel Stockton White left a legacy that could hardly be superceded. After World War I intense competition in teeth production and uninspiring leadership led to the decline in the White Company's dental manufacturing. However, the life of the company was prolonged by the production of one dental item: the flexible cable, which was adapted for another use required in far greater quantities when installed in automobile radios. Under the control of the White Company and until the patent was broken at the end of the 1930s, automobile manufacturers purchased cables from the White Company, thus providing the primary source of profit during this period when dental goods were being manufactured by more firms and thus reducing the White Company's role as the premier manufacturer in the dental materials market.

NOTES

The primary sources of White dental catalogs are the library of the Hagley Museum and Library, Wilmington, Delaware, and the major dental museums listed in the *Directory of Dental Collections,* prepared by Hannelore T. Loevy and Aletha A. Kowitz and published in July of 1992 as a supplement to the *Bulletin of the History of Dentistry* (*BHD*). The Samuel S. White Dental Manufacturing Company deposited the company papers and catalogs in the Hagley Museum and Library in the 1970s. The papers are catalogued and arranged in approximately three hundred boxes and maintained in the Archives Center. The catalogs reside in the main library. The papers catalogued as Manuscript 1320 consist of correspondence, patent papers, memoranda, blueprints, photographs, scattered articles about company staff and products, diaries containing advertisements, patent histories, accounts books, and family history. My citations from these papers refer to this manuscript collection. I am grateful to the Hagley Museum and Library for supporting my study of the White material during the summers of 1989 and 1990 and for the cordial and helpful manner in which the staff responded to my many requests for assistance.

The bibliography of medical and dental trade literature by Audrey B. Davis and Mark S. Dreyfuss, *The Finest Instruments Ever Made* (Arlington, Massachusetts: Medical History Publishing Associates I, 1986), includes name, date, and location of the medical instrument catalogs in American and European libraries; these were discovered by the early eighties. Undoubtedly other sources exist as institutions and private owners rearrange, discard, sell, and buy these ephemeral items. The White Company instrument museum or "morgue," created around the turn of the century, is partially preserved in the dental collections of the Division of Medical Sciences of the National Museum of American History, Washington, DC, and the Dr. John Harris Dental Museum in Bainbridge, Ohio. A list of items in the White Company museum is preserved in the Hagley Museum and Library.

1. Frank L. Hise, *82 Years of Loyal Service to Dentistry: History of the House of White,* published on occasion of the Seventh International Dental Congress at Philadelphia during the Sesquicentennial

Exposition (Philadelphia: SSWDMC, 1926), 11.

2. *Incorruptible* was the eighteenth-century term for porcelain teeth. Although these porcelain teeth were not sculpturally perfect and only poorly represented natural human teeth, they could be cleansed and kept odorless. The age at which Samuel began his apprenticeship, sometimes given as two years earlier when he was fourteen, is taken from his apprenticeship certificate reproduced in Frank L. Hise's *82 Years of Loyal Service*, 10, which indicates that he was sixteen years old.

3. Most early dentists in Europe and America came from within the ranks of jewelers, ivory turners, hairdressers, perfumers, druggists, and watchmakers. See Freda Christine Hillam, "The Development of Dental Practice in the Provinces from the Late 18th century to 1855," (Ph.D. thesis, Department of Modern History, University of Liverpool, July 1986).

4. Paul Goddard, *The Anatomy, Physiology and Pathology of the Human Teeth* (Philadelphia: Carey and Hart, 1844), vi. Stockton's teeth were widely advertised. See for example, "1700 incorruptible teeth from Dr. Stockton of Philadelphia which are pronounced by the profession to be superior to any other in use." Advertised in 1844 by W. H. Jarvis in the *Daily Evening Gazette.* Cited in *The History of Dentistry in Missouri* (Fulton, Missouri: History Committee of Missouri State Dental Association, 1938),23.

5. T. C. Stockton prepared a history of White's mother's family: *Stockton Family of New Jersey and Other Stocktons*, 1911.

6. For information on nineteenth-century dental apprenticeships in the United States see Robert J. Bruckner, J. Henry Clarke, and Janice S. Bruckner, "Dental Preceptorships of the 19th Century: What were they like? " *BHD* 36 (April, 1988): 12–21. On Thomas W. Evans, see Anthony Branch, "Dr. Thomas W. Evans: American Dentist in Paris, 1847–1897" (Ph.D. thesis, University of California at Santa Barbara, 1971), 4, 51–53. Also Malcolm Wallace Carr, D.D.S., "Thomas W. Evans: His Life and Influence on the Development of Dentistry as a Learned Profession, The First Thomas W. Evans Lecture," *American College of Dentistry Journal* 46 (1979) 87–100; W. S. Davenport, Jr., "The Pioneer American Dentists in France and Their Successors," *Revue d'histoire de l'art dentaire* 3 (1965): 99–116. Evans founded the American Dental Club of Paris in his home on October 13, 1890. There were sixteen active members. In a letter addressed to American dental instrument manufacturers dated December 1, 1865, Evans stated that because he had acquainted the French public with the organization and results of the American Sanitary commisison during the Civil War (incidentally Evans sold medical supplies to the Northen army and made a profit), he was now planning to introduce American ingenious inventions to the French, especially those that contributed to the success of the Sanitary Commission. Evans's plan was to mount an American Sanitary Museum in conjunction with the 1867 Exhibition in Paris (this international exhibition was another major event like the Crystal Palace Exposition in London). Evans requested donations of articles but offered to pay for them if necessary. Samuel S. White received a copy of this request and undoubtedly sent items. This information provides further evidence that Evans helped introduce White dental items to European dentists.

7. *The Dental Reporter,* "American Dentists in Europe," by the Paris corresponding reporter of the *New York Times* (11 January 1859). February 1859, 177–80. This article mentions twenty-two dentists. The article was also reprinted by Malvin Ring, "American Industry Abroad," *BHD* 29 (1981): 88–90.

Evans's diplomatic role seems to have had an adverse effect on his dental skill according to the prominent British dentist Edwin Sercombe (d. 1875). Sercombe wrote in a letter to James B. Morrison: "I have seen some of his [Evans's] patients having had to replace some of his stoppings. I certainly have seen much better work. I suppose he did work better at some period." March 21, 1871, Division of Medical Sciences, National Museum of American History, Smithsonian Institution, Washington, DC.

See also Davenport, "The Pioneer American Dentists," 100. In addition, on page 115, Davenport provides a chart of American dentists and their successors who practiced in Paris.

For American dentists in Germany see David E. Huff, "A Comparison of American and German Dentistry, 1850–1900," *BHD* 33 (1985): 47–53. Among the most famous American dentists in Germany were Willoughby Dayton Miller, who championed the bacterial origin of tooth decay and whose important papers were published in the *Dental Cosmos*, and William G. A. Bonwill, inventor of a popular dental drill and other items produced by the White Company.

8. Hise, *82 Years of Loyal Service*, 11. Carving teeth as part of an apprenticeship was a common practice. See Bruckner, Clarke, and Bruckner, "Dental Preceptorships," 14. The biographical details of Samuel and James White's lives and business activities are recorded most fully in Hise, *82 Years of Loyal Service*. Hise provides a chronological list that summarizes, by year, the major achievements of the company. Hise worked for over thirty years as an advertising specialist preparing copy for the announcements placed in the *Dental Cosmos* and other publications and was in a position to have access to company records. However his role as company spokesman did not place him in a position in which he could feel free to be critical of his sources and company practices in print. In 1894 on the fiftieth anniversary of the company, President Henry M. Lewis prepared a twenty-eight-page history of the achievements of the company. Superlatives dot the pages of this account—biggest, best, most, greatest—in a variety of endeavors. Lewis's account must be read with caution. Henry M. Lewis, *A Retrospect of a Half Century: A History of the Business of Manufacturing Dental Supplies in the U. S.* (Philadelphia: SSWDMC, 1894).

Shorter biographical accounts of Samuel White appear in the *Dictionary of American Biography* (New York: Charles Scribner's Sons, 1936). The article on Samuel S. White is by Louise P. Blodgett of the Library of Congress. Blodgett's sources include obituaries and B. L. Thorpe's biographical article in C. R. E. Koch, ed., *History of Dental Surgery* (1910), 3: 304–9; A. Porter Sweet, D.D.S., FAAOR, *Dental Biographical Sketches* (Pittsford, New York: The Naportan Company, 197?); S. R. Bingham was manager of the Chicago Branch House and an employee for over forty years at the time he wrote his eulogy of Samuel and James White shortly after James's death in 1891. The eulogy is appended to Henry Lewis's *Retrospect*; H. M. Lewis, "On the Duties of Trustees, Estate of Samuel Stockton White," May 11, 1880. Box 282, folder 1880–90, Hagley Museum and Library.

9. Hise, *82 Years of Loyal Service*, 132; idem, "William Henry Gilbert," 8 pages, 1912. Hagley Museum and Library.

10. Hise, *82 Years of Loyal Service*, 17.

11. Obituary, "Samuel Stockton White III (1876–1952)," *Proofs* (December 1952): 19. Samuel III was elected to the Board of Directors in 1926 and served for thirty years as an export manager. See the article about his art collection entitled "The Business Man and Picasso," *Fortune* 86 (1950).

12. Samuel Stockton White III to Samuel Stockton White, Jr., undated but contents reveal it was written nine years after Samuel III began to work for the company in 1903, therefore the year of this letter is 1912. Samuel III's father, J. Clarence, approved of his son's request. Box 3, Hagley Museum and Library.

13. Valentine Mott (1785–1865) of Long Island was a pioneer in vascular surgery. He prepared a treatise on pain and anesthesia for use by physicians attending the soldiers during the Civil War and published a catalog of his anatomical museum and a number of other medical papers and books. See Fielding H. Garrison, *An Introduction to the History of Medicine*, 3d ed. (Philadelphia: W. B. Saunders Co., 1922), 535–37.

14. Hise, *82 Years of Loyal Service*, 17.

15. The Awards Committee at the Crystal Palace Exposition decided that Jones, White, and McCurdy teeth should receive a silver medal for best manufactured teeth but was overruled by the judges, led by Professor Renwick, who concluded that a bronze medal was the highest that should be given for dentistry. J. R. McCurdy, "Report on Crystal Palace Exhibition," *Dental News Letter* 3 (1851): 139–44; idem, "The World's Fair—The Result so far as Dentistry is Concerned," *Dental News Letter* 4 (1852): 266–68; "Remarks on Above," *Dental News Letter* 4 (1852): 152–54; John Trevor, E. Parmly, and T. L. Buckingham, "Committee's Report," *Dental News Letter* 4 (1852): 150–54. Samuel Wesley Stockton's displays according to McCurdy were poorly arranged and excessively rough. "They were not what I expected to see from him, nor at all equal to specimens of his, manufactured ten or more years ago." J. R. McCurdy, "American and French Dentistry at the World's Fair," *Dental News Letter* 4 (1852): 359.

16. Stanley Gelbier, "Dentists, the Dental Trade and Development of Dental Periodicals," (M.A. thesis in Social and Industrial History, Department of Humanities, Middlesex Polytechnic London and King's College School of Medicine and Dentistry, October 1985 [published in 1986]), 81–82. Stockton's journal was known as *The Dental Intelligencer and Record* when publication ceased in 1848. When the *Dental Cosmos* published "The Human Mouth as a Focus of Infection," by Willoughby Dayton Miller, the editor was criticized for diverting so much space to "ultra-scientific, high-brow and impractical" material. "The Action of Micro-Organisms in the Decay of the Human Teeth," *Dental Cosmos* 24 (1882): 640.

17. The *Dental News Letter* is a rarely preserved journal. Copies are located in the collection of the Dr. Samuel D. Harris National Museum of Dentistry in Baltimore, Maryland, and in the collection of the National Library of Medicine (a few issues are missing). Copies of the *Dental Cosmos* are more common, although complete sets are unusual.

The importance of a forum to discuss the scientific and practical methods of tooth repair and replacement is underscored by the fact that a good proportion of dentists throughout the nineteenth century did not study in a dental college. By 1901 a survey taken by William Gies revealed that of 28,142 dentists who began to practice after 1840, 11,311 practitioners had not graduated from a dental school.

18. H. Meredith White, "Dental Dispensaries," *Dental Cosmos* 3 (1862): 364–66. The first dental clinic was opened in Philadelphia in 1910. Brochure, *Dental Dispensaries*. Department of Public Health and Charities, City of Philadelphia. Uninventoried, Hagley Museum and Library.

19. Hise, *82 Years of Loyal Service*, 26. In the 1862 White catalog White's name was stamped on dental forceps made by the surgical instrument maker J. Kern of Philadelphia. The stamp appeared as "S. S. White" in the catalog on pages 22–32.

20. *A Catalog of the World's Premium SSW Porcelain Teeth* (Philadelphia: SSW DMC, 1909 [reprinted from 1900, 1902, 1903, 1905, 1907]), 82.

21. In the 1862 catalog White offered to provide items ordered from any dental catalog to which the dentist might have access. The 1876 catalog was also reprinted in 1878 with a seventy-page appendix. For shorter and specific S. S. White catalogs see Davis and Dreyfuss, *The Finest Instruments Ever Made.* Most S. S. White catalogs are in the collection of the Hagley Museum and Library, Wilmington, Delaware.

22. "Samuel Stockton White," *Dental Cosmos* 22 (1880):62; Extracts from the General Report of the Judges of Group XIV, 1876 Dentistry (Philadelphia, 1888), 3: 6–13.

23. Samuel S. White, Jr., Diary dictated to Charles A. Thomas, May 22, 1933, page 9. Box 3, Hagley Museum and Library.

24. *A Catalog of the World's Premium SSW Porcelain Teeth* (1909): Introduction. On the emergence of the professional dental laboratory see Robert J. Rothstein, *History of Dental Laboratories and Their Contributions to Dentistry* (Philadelphia: J. B. Lippincott, 1958).

25. Robert C. Sproull, "A History of Porcelain in Dentistry," *BHD* 26 (1978): 3.

26. James H. Prothero, *Prosthetic Dentistry* (Chicago: Medico-Dental Publishing Company, 1916), 1125–26.

27. For the earliest porcelain teeth makers in America see Jerry Hershfield, "Charles H. Land and the Science of Porcelain in Dentistry," *BHD* 34 (1986): 48–54. On N. C. Keep see Malvin Ring, "The Early Life of Nathan Cooley Keep, Monumental Figure in Dentistry," *BHD* 38 (1990): 15–18. Keep began as a jeweler's apprentice and was invited to study with A. A. Plantou in 1827. Maurice D. K. Bremner relates the story that Samuel Stockton became a porcelain tooth maker because he hired someone to assist him as a jeweler who had learned to make porcelain teeth. *The Story of Dentistry* (Brooklyn, New York: Dental Items of Interest Publishing Company, 1958), 110.

See also Vincenzo Guineri, "Invention of Mineral Teeth," in *A History of Dentistry* (Philadelphia: Lea and Febiger, 1909), 344–45; R. T. Moffatt, "The Art of Carving and Baking Porcelain Teeth and Crowns," *Transactions of the New York Institute of Stomatology* (1904): 106–25. Boston dentists were the most outspoken in preferring hand-carved teeth to mass-produced artificial teeth.

28. J. F. F. [Flagg] to the Editor, "American Dentistry," *Boston Medical and Surgical Journal* 19 (1839): 3–7.

29. *Dentistry in Missouri,* 23.

30. Chapin Harris, *The Dental Art: A Practical Treatise on Dental Surgery* (Baltimore: Armstrong and Berry, 1839), 315.

31. *Catalog of Materials, Furniture, Instruments, etc. for sale by Samuel Stockton White,* 1876, 9. Claudius Ash, founder of the earliest dental manufacturing company and British rival of S. S. White, was drawn into full-time dental manufacturing earlier than White by the demand for his high-quality teeth. "By 1820 [Claudius Ash] found so many dentists were seeking his services that he could afford to specialize in dental work." "Looking back on 150 years of Looking Ahead," typescript, British Dental Association.

32. Harris, *The Principles and Practice of Dental Surgery,* 7th ed. (Philadelphia: Lindsay and

Blakiston, 1858), 779.

33. Harris, *Principles and Practice of Dentistry*, 315; idem, *Principles and Practice of Dental Surgery*, 666.

Oakley Coles commented in the American edition of his textbook that "scarcely any dental surgeon in the present day would think of making his own mineral teeth and blocks . . . however, I warn the reader that it is not to be taken as an accurate description of the actual work carried on by [those who do] . . . as in this country [England] at any rate they guard the secrets of their tooth factories with a most religious jealousy." *A Manual of Dental Mechanics* (Philadelphia: Lindsay and Blakiston, 1873), 102.

34. Phillip Curtis, "Tucker Porcelain 1826–1838: A Re-Appraisal," (M.A. thesis in early American culture, University of Delaware, June 1972), 9.

35. Susan Myers, *Handcraft to Industry: Philadelphia Ceramics in the First Half of the Nineteenth Century*, in *Smithsonian Studies in History and Technology* (Washington, DC: Government Printing Office, 1980), 43. Benjamin Tucker, William Ellis Tucker's father, was a charter member of the Franklin Institute, which enabled his son to attend lectures at the Institute. Abraham Miller was a member of the first board of managers of the Franklin Institute when it was organized in 1824. Curtis, "Tucker Porcelain," 9.

36. "Samuel Stockton White," *Dental Cosmos* 22 (1880): 62–63.

37. Hise, *82 Years of Loyal Service*, 15–16.

38. Arthur S. Watts, "Dental Porcelains," *Transactions of the American Ceramic Society* 17 (1915): 190–99. I am grateful to Reggie Blaszect for this reference.

39. Royalty Accounts Book, typescript, Hagley Museum and Library.

40. "From Philadelphia," *Chicago Tribune*, 28 October 1865. Hagley Museum and Library.

41. The dental collection currently housed in the Science Museum of the University of Utrecht contains six mounted sheets of porcelain teeth showing the evolution from those teeth made by Charles W. Peale to the early twentieth-century varieties. This is the only labeled collection of porcelain teeth that I have seen. For more on Justi's history see Rothstein, *History of Dental Laboratories*, 75.

42. The patent granted to Oliver and Harrison is dated May 20, 1856. The objective was to use these teeth in the Blandy process by which teeth are molded or poured into a tin base instead of being fastened by pins. Letter in box 30, Hagley Museum and Library.

43. W. Warrington Evans, "Esthetic Dental Prosthesis," *Dental Cosmos* 22 (1880): 343–44.

44. Editorial, *Dental Cosmos* 22 (1880): 372–73.

45. C. A. Hawley to Dr. Henry Gillett, January 26, 1928, Division of Medical Sciences, National Museum of American History Archives.

46. McCurdy, "Crystal Palace Exhibition," *Dental News Letter*, 3 (1851), 139.

47. Ibid.

48. Ibid., 140.

49. Ibid., 141.

50. Thomas W. Evans, *De la découverte de caoutchouc vulcanisé et de la priorité de son application* à *la chirurgie civile et militaire et aux opérations dentaires* (Paris: S. Racon, 1867), 14.

51. Malvin Ring, "The Rubber Denture Murder Case: The True Story of the Vulcanite Litigation," *BHD* 32 (1984): 4. Ring obtained his data from the account of the vulcanite story in the *Dental Cosmos*. The Hagley Museum and Library contains the original documents for this story in boxes 245 and 246.

52. Cornelius C. T. Yap, "Developments in Prosthetic Dentistry in the Nineteenth Century," *BHD* 35 (1987): 45.

53. Evans, *De la découverte de caoutchouc vulcanisé*, 16.

54. Ring, "The Rubber Denture Murder Case," 6.

55. Ibid., 7.

56. Carr, "Thomas W. Evans," 92–93. As an interesting sidenote, Evans met with President Lincoln and General Grant and inspected the battlefields, concluding that the Northern army would soon be victorious. He discouraged Napolean III from following England's leadership in supporting the Confederacy.

Samuel White had been delegated by the American Dental Association to meet with President Lincoln to discuss how arrangements could be made to provide dental care to the soldiers. White was repeatedly advised as he was passed down the chain of command to speak to the Medical Department which he was told "was fully competent to make the requisite decisions." White and other leading dentists were not able to get a dental corps established at this time. The spade work for a United States Dental Corps was laid during the Spanish-American War. Malvin Ring, "S. S. White, Abraham Lincoln, and the Need for Dentists in the Union Armies," *BHD* 41 (1993): 79–80. Evidence for Ring's account appeared in the *Dental Cosmos* 6 (1864).

57. Yap, "Developments in Prosthetic Dentistry," 45.

58. Evans, *De la découverte de caoutchouc vulcanisé*, 22.

59. Ibid., 17.

60. H. D. Justi, *Illustrated Price List of Dental Materials, Etc.* (Philadelphia,1888), 12.

61. Advertisement, *Dental Cosmos* 8 (1866): 49.

62. White, *Catalog of Dental Materials* (Philadelphia,1876), 33.

63. The licenses sent to White at his request by numerous dentists are preserved in the Hagley Museum and Library, box 244, folder 1872–79 and box 249.

64. Many of the court arguments are reprinted in the *Dental Cosmos* of 1873, volume 15.

65. Ring, "The Rubber Denture Murder Case," 14.

66. S. S. White to Dr. T. H. Rehwinkel, February 26, 1874, Chillicothe, Ohio. Uninventoried, Hagley Museum and Library. White said he had neglected his business for the previous nine months, spent $11,000 in lawyer's fees, and received $3500 compensation.

67. Ring, "The Rubber Denture Murder Case."

68. Ibid.

69. C. De Montreville to S. S. White, October 24, 1879, page 4. Box 247, folder 1866–79, Hagley Museum and Library.

70. Henry Coy, "Correspondence, Hard Rubber Patents," *Dental Cosmos* 11 (1869): 425.

71. William H. Trueman, "Vulcanizers—The Dangers Attending Their Use," *Dental Cosmos* 11 (1869): 561–74.

72. Arden G. Christen, "Sanford C. Barnum, Discoverer of the Rubber Dam," *BHD* 25 (1977): 2–8; Richard A. Glenner, "The Rubber Dam," *BHD* 42 (1994): 33–34.

73. J. H. McQuillan, "Hard Rubber Handles for Dental Instruments," *Dental Cosmos* 3 (1861): 499.

74. Editorial, *Dental Cosmos* 2 (1861): 501.

75. Hise, *82 Years of Loyal Service*, 26; S. R. Bingham, "Eulogy: Samuel Stockton White and James White," 30.

76. White, *Catalog of Dental Materials* (1876), 73.

77. Hise, *82 Years of Loyal Service*, 40, 51.

78. *SSWDMC v. Bonwill*, December term 1890, Philadelphia, Pennsylvania. Box 253 Complaint's Affidavit Common Pleas, No. 4. Hagley Museum and Library.

79. "Report of H. Lewis." Box 284, folder 1878–87, Hagley Museum and Library. In these files there is a memo from Dr. White describing "a new company to be formed under a new name into which all the interests of the rival telephone companies are to be consolidated. The name will be 'Consolidated Telephone Companies of North America.' Capital of the new company is $5,000,000, one million to the Bell Telephone Co. and one million to the American Speaking Telephone

Company."

80. "Samuel Stockton White," *Dental Cosmos* 22 (1880): 62.

81. Samuel S. White, Jr., dictated notes to Charles A. Thomas. May 22, 1933. Administrative Records, box 3, Hagley Museum and Library.

82. Introduction, *Preliminary Catalog of Dental Materials for Sale by Johnston Brothers* (1870). 1260 Broadway, New York.

83. *A Catalog of Artificial Teeth, Dental Materials, Instruments, Tools, Furniture, etc. manufactured, imported, and sold by Claudius Ash and Sons* (London, 1871), 29.

84. Carolyn Cooper, "Social Construction of Invention thru Patent Management, Thomas Blanchard's Woodworking Machinery," *Technology and Culture* 32 (1991): 968.

85. List of dental patents owned by S. S. White. March 21, 1879. Box 287, Hagley Museum and Library.

86. Joseph Peyton to William Gilbert, March 16, 1880, Hagley Museum and Library.

87. W. D. Bailey, "*Johnston v. White.* Memoranda for Defense." February 2, 1874. Box 251, folder 2, Hagley Museum and Library. See also Mark Wilde, "Development and Patent Policy at the SSWDMC" (*History* 886, typescript, 24 pages, spring 1981), Hagley Museum and Library.

88. Edwin Sercombe to [James] Morrison, 1871–1873. Division of Medical Sciences, National Museum of American History, Smithsonian Institution. See also Richard Glenner, *The Dental Office: A Pictorial History* (Missoula, Montana: Pictorial Histories Publishing Company, 1984), 70–71, 75–76.

89. Hise, *82 Years of Loyal Service*, 31.

90. Audrey B. Davis, "Samuel Stockton White and Claudius Ash: Porcelain Teeth Manufacturers and the Origin of Mass-Produced Teeth," *Proceedings of the 6th Congress of the European Medical Museums Association* (The Netherlands: Leiden: September 3, 1994), 28–34.

91. Legal Diary insert, page 147. Item 219, Hagley Museum and Library.

92. By 1900 branch houses also were located in Atlanta, Georgia; Rochester, New York; Berlin, Germany; Buenos Aires, Argentina; St. Petersburg, Russia; and Toronto, Canada.

93. Hise, *82 Years of Loyal Service*, 21.

94. Frank L. Hise to Mr. William Gilbert, December 29, 1911. Box 3, Hagley Museum and Library.

95. Frank L. Hise to William Gilbert, March 20, 1897, page 2, folder in uninventoried box, Hagley Museum and Library.

96. Ibid.

97. Hise, *82 Years of Loyal Service*, 34.

Low-key response to acclaim and criticism characterized the attitude of Samuel White and carried over into his business methods, which originated as a response to customer demand for his artificial teeth. Dr. Atkinson reported on an episode he observed which reveals this side of Samuel's personality. Atkinson asked Samuel why he had not defended himself from a harsh critic, and Samuel responded, "I knew I was not the man he took me for, and I felt that I could afford to wait till he would find it out." S. S. White to Dr. Atkinson, *Dental Cosmos* 22 (1880): 184. Atkinson prepared the testimonial in memoriam to White's death for the New York Odontological Society.

SPECIAL NOTICE.

☞ *The* MERCHANDISE MAIL *permits the sending of packages which do not weigh* over four pounds.

Goods that can be forwarded by this mail, when ordered at retail prices, accompanied with draft, or postal money-order, will be sent

FREE OF POSTAGE

to any part *of the* United States *from the Philadelphia House or either of our Branch Houses. With this opportunity, those at a distance from our depots, who have been unable to procure our manufactures from local dealers, can order directly, have their orders filled and packed with care, and receive the goods by return mail.*

SAMUEL S. WHITE.

CATALOGUE

OF

DENTAL MATERIALS

FURNITURE, INSTRUMENTS, ETC.,

FOR SALE BY

SAMUEL S. WHITE,

MANUFACTURER, IMPORTER, AND WHOLESALE DEALER IN ALL ARTICLES APPERTAINING TO DENTISTRY.

TRADE
SSW
MARK.

1876.

Manufactory and Principal Depot:
CHESTNUT ST., CORNER OF TWELFTH, PHILADELPHIA.

BRANCHES:

767 & 769 Broadway, New York. 13 & 16 Tremont Row, Boston.
14 & 16 E. Madison Street, Chicago.

To the Dental Profession.

TRADE

MARK.

THIS Catalogue has been copyrighted; but no copyright, it would seem, is sufficient to prevent parties' making use of that which is original, peculiar, and proprietary, as will be manifest to any who are familiar with most of the catalogues which have appeared from those in the trade, in which our cuts, numbers, classifications, and descriptions have been copied without alteration (the exact language meeting their views so well that no change was deemed necessary); embracing lists of articles of our own manufacture, arbitrarily numbered for our own convenience, and having no significance outside of that fact, and which could not therefore be supplied by other parties except through us; a course which appears more complimentary to us than honorable in the parties so acting. We have therefore secured, by law, a *Trade Mark*, which, so far as practicable, will henceforth be stamped or otherwise placed upon every article manufactured by us.

This Catalogue, which has been carefully prepared, is respectfully submitted to the Profession, in the belief that its use will prove a great convenience to buyer and seller.

Our stock is larger, more varied and complete than ever before; and our aim has been so to arrange and classify it as to enable our customers to see in detail the varieties in quality and price of any article they may desire.

A full supply of all goods named herein will be kept constantly on hand, and all new and useful improvements will be added thereto; thus enabling the dentist to find at our establishments every requisite of each department of his art.

In the department of precious metals, special care will be given to make the goods conform in fineness to the standard claimed, and in this matter we invite investigation and comparison, as all of our Gold Plate is made by the direct combination of pure metals, alloyed according to official standard; and not from the remelting of scraps and filings. Scraps and filings will be purchased at their full value, as nearly as can be determined. We will pay all that we can get for them at the Mint.

Special attention is solicited to our stock of imported goods.

It is our determination to fully meet the wants of the Profession in every department of the business.

SAMUEL S. WHITE.

Philadelphia, May 10, 1876.

Hints for Ordering Goods.

The purchaser's attention to the following hints will enable us to fill all orders, large or small, as satisfactorily to the purchaser as though he were present to make selections.

1. In ordering goods by Catalogue, specify distinctly the article desired, with price affixed; and as we have published several Catalogues, as well as a number of price-lists, during the last fifteen years, customers will please be careful to state that it is the Illustrated Catalogue of 1876 from which they make their selection.

2. Bring the various items of an order together at the beginning or close of a letter, and thus avoid the oversight which may occur when they are scattered through the body of the correspondence.

3. Do not depend on our remembrance of some previous order.

4. State how you wish your goods forwarded—by mail, express, or otherwise.

5. Write the name of your town, county, and State, and your own name, *distinctly.*

6. All orders will have prompt and careful attention. Any article needed in the practice of dentistry will be procured and furnished at advertised rates.

7. If an article not enumerated in the Catalogue is desired, be particular to give a full description, and, if possible, the price, when there is choice of qualities or styles.

8. The Catalogue of any manufacturer or dealer in dental goods may be used in ordering from us, care being taken to designate, by date or otherwise, the edition of the Catalogue, or by sending it, to be returned with the goods.

9. Should there be any misapprehension or error on our part in putting up an order, it will afford us pleasure to correct it on receiving prompt notice of the same, as it is our desire to give entire satisfaction in every transaction.

10. Every article sent by us not answering our description, or not according to order, will be taken back without loss to the purchaser.*

11. Our terms are NET CASH. Parties ordering goods who have not an open account should send the cash with their order. The most convenient method of remitting is by a *Bank Draft* or *Post-Office Order.*

* NOTE.—We are often at a loss to understand the meaning of dentists who write for one or more teeth to be selected by a sample sent, when the terms "to match" and "to correspond with" are used; as these expressions are intended sometimes to designate the *mate* and sometimes the *duplicate* of the pattern. The annoyance caused by delay, etc., can be avoided if the purchaser will be particular to name specifically the tooth desired, whether Right or Left, Superior or Inferior, Central, Lateral, Canine, Bicuspid (1st or 2d), Molar, Single or Block, Gum or Plain, for Plate or Rubber Work.

12. Remittances may be made by postal money orders, checks, or drafts drawn to our order, *without risk.* Registering letters is simply informing dishonest P. O. clerks that money is inclosed.

13. Goods sent by mail, except such articles as are advertised free, will be charged with the postage, which must accompany the remittance.

14. Goods ordered to be sent by express, bill payable on delivery, will be charged with expenses of collection. This charge insures the safe delivery of the goods to the purchaser, as well as the safe return of the money to us.

15. Strangers ordering goods C. O. D. should inclose a reasonable proportion of the bill, on account, to cover any risk of the goods not being claimed on arrival, and which may have to be returned at the expense of the shipper.

16. *None but* EXPRESS COMPANIES *collect bills on delivery of the goods.*

17. All goods are carefully packed, and can be transported safely, with careful handling, to any part of the world. They are shipped at the risk of the purchaser; therefore for all delays or damages he must look to the transporters of the goods, who alone are legally responsible to the owner for their prompt and safe delivery. We do not guarantee delivery or safe carriage of goods. We ship and take receipts for them "in good order," and they are at your risk after such receipt is signed by the transportation company. When you receive goods, if there is any loss or damage, it should be ascertained if possible before you sign a receipt, and, in any case, you should make your claims on the transportation company without delay.

18. Goods are not insured except by request, and then always at the expense of the purchaser.

19. In making use of the "merchandise mail" to send us instruments for alteration or repair, please observe that the law requires such matter to be so wrapped that it can be examined without destroying the wrapper, and forbids any *writing* inside or outside of the package, *except the address;* but a business card or the name and address of the sender may be printed, impressed, or pasted (if printed) on the wrapper.

20. We decline sending C. O. D. bulky goods, such as chairs, lathes, etc., and those of small value in proportion to their bulk, such as plaster, furnaces, gasometers, retorts, etc.

NOTICE.

At each of our Depots there is kept A BULLETIN BOARD, on which brief notices may be registered, FREE OF CHARGE, of *Dentists desiring Assistants, Parties seeking Positions in the Office or Laboratory, Partnerships, or Practices for sale or desired.*

Porcelain Teeth.

To this, the largest and most important department of our business, we desire to call special attention and critical examination—by comparison with natural teeth,—in reference to shape, color, texture, translucency, and vital appearance; and by contrast with teeth of other manufacturers in reference to strength, lightness, capability of resisting changes of temperature in soldering, and adaptability.

What is included in these terms is briefly as follows:

Shape. The preservation of the distinctive characteristics of the different teeth of the upper and lower jaws, and of the right and left sides of the mouth; their relations to each other, to those with which they antagonize, and, when properly adjusted, to the dental arch.

Color. The imitation in this respect of the colors of the natural teeth, as shown by placing them alongside of teeth in the mouth,—the nice blending of the brown or yellow base or body of the tooth with the clearer enamel of the cutting edge.

Texture. The absence of the appearance of vitrifaction; the soft, waxy, enamel-like, and natural surface which they present.

Translucency. The word indicates the close imitation of the semi-transparency of natural teeth, which contrasts so strongly with the opacity frequently found in artificial teeth.

Vital Appearance. Made up by the combination of color, texture, translucency, absence of the appearance of vitrifaction, and the blending of the colors of the body and enamel in proper relations,—especially manifest when exposed *in the mouth to an artificial light.*

Strength. As tested by riveting, and other processes of the workman, and by their legitimate use by the wearer.

Lightness. In any test of strength, the weight and thickness must be taken into account, the object being to secure the greatest strength with the least weight and bulk.

Resistance to Variations of Temperature. As ascertained by the process of soldering, in the manufacture of new dentures, or the repair of old ones.

Adaptability. In the ease with which they can be adapted to various conformations of the maxillary, with slight labor on the part of the artist in grinding and fitting.

In the *combination* of these essential characteristics we claim a marked superiority for our teeth.

Our facilities for supplying variety of shape, size, and shade in PORCELAIN TEETH are unequaled by any other establishment in the world, whether reference is had to the number of hands employed, the number of teeth made, or the number of moulds in use.

Sixty-two first premiums for our manufactures have been received from various organizations in this country and abroad.

PORCELAIN TEETH.

Our stock of Teeth is larger, more varied, and more complete than at any previous time, embracing a large assortment of sizes, shades, and forms of the following varieties:

DOUBLE-HEADED PIN.
(Patent Issued January 21st, 1862; Re-issued April 29th, 1862.)

FOOT-SHAPED PIN.
Patented September 9th, 1872.

TEETH ADAPTED FOR A VULCANIZABLE BASE.

BLOCKS IN SECTIONS OF TWO OR THREE.

SINGLE GUM TEETH, } IN SETS OF 28, 14, 6, 4, AND 2.
SINGLE PLAIN TEETH, } MOLARS AND BICUSPIDS IN SETS OF 8.

TEETH FOR MOUNTING UPON GOLD AND SILVER PLATE.

SINGLE GUM TEETH, } IN SETS OF 28, 14, 6, 4, AND 2.
SINGLE PLAIN TEETH, } MOLARS AND BICUSPIDS IN SETS OF 8.

TEETH MADE EXPRESSLY FOR CONTINUOUS-GUM WORK IN SETS AS DESIRED.

PLAIN TEETH MADE EXPRESSLY FOR THE CELLULOID BASE.

PIVOT TEETH.

WHAT WE CLAIM.

For the Teeth which we are now offering to the Profession we claim superiority over all others in the market. In all the essential characteristics which Artificial Teeth should possess we believe them to be unequaled, possessing as they do not only those qualities which render them easy of adaptation and articulation, but, with these, naturalness of form, color, and arrangement. We claim also that, by reason of their composition, and the size, number, shape, and insertion of the platinum pins, they are stronger than those of any other manufacture.

A vast variety in shape, size, color, etc., gives opportunity for selection adapted to almost any possible case, including even the extreme cases which are sometimes met with; also, a beautiful series of those various deviations from a uniform regularity which are so common in natural dentures.

We are receiving abundant testimony from the Profession as to the superiority of our Teeth, and Medals, Certificates, and Diplomas from Institutes and Fairs, the committees of which, after thorough examination, have recommended that the highest premium be awarded us for excellence and superiority over all competitors.

We claim, in brief, that our stock, in quality, quantity, and variety, cannot be approached in any other establishment in the world.

VIENNA EXPOSITION,

1873.

Grand Diploma of Honor.

Artificial Teeth, Dental Instruments, Dental Chairs (The Harris), Quarter Century Gold Foil, Globe Gold Foil, and Corundum Wheels.

ANOTHER TRIUMPH!

THE HIGHEST AWARD OVER ALL COMPETITORS.

ALL THE PRINCIPAL MANUFACTURERS IN THE WORLD REPRESENTED.

To the FIRST PREMIUMS awarded us at each of the previous GREAT WORLD'S FAIRS of

LONDON, NEW YORK, AND PARIS,

IS TO BE ADDED THE

GRAND DIPLOMA OF HONOR

FROM THE

VIENNA EXPOSITION,

Showing the estimate in which our Manufactures are still held over those of all Competitors.

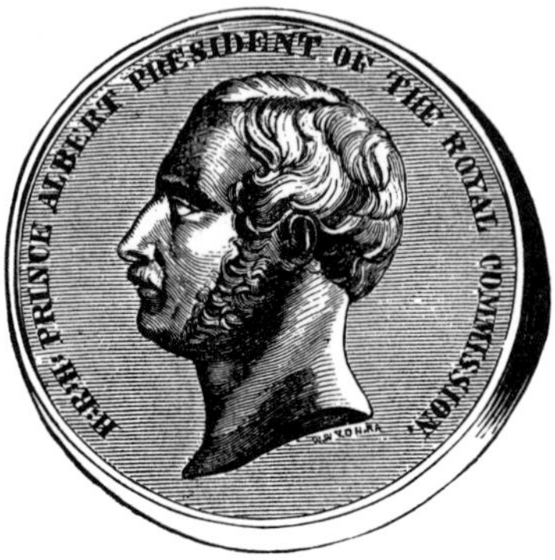
H.R.H. PRINCE ALBERT PRESIDENT OF THE ROYAL COMMISSION.

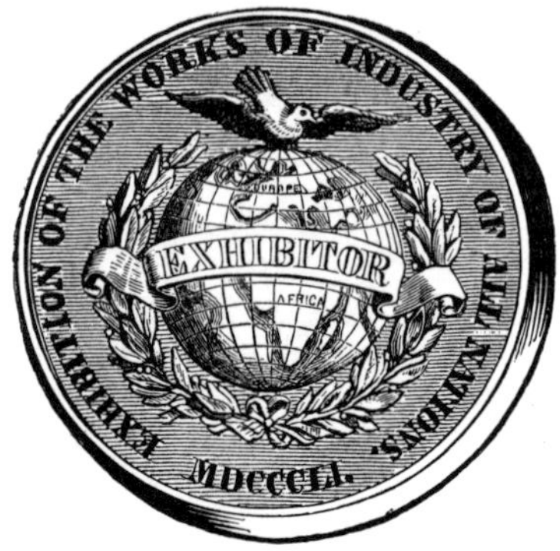
EXHIBITION OF THE WORKS OF INDUSTRY OF ALL NATIONS.
EXHIBITOR
MDCCCLI.

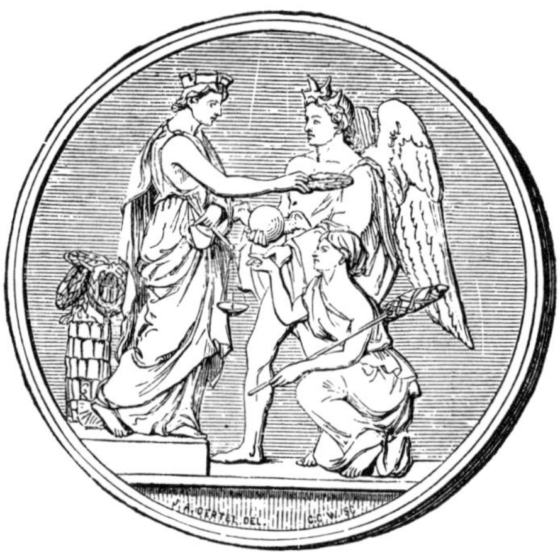

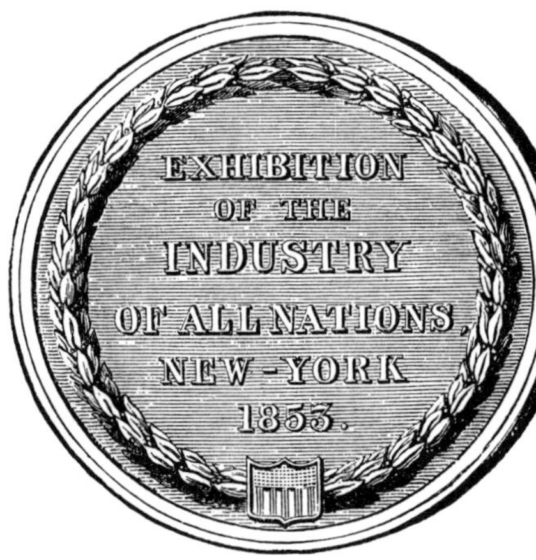
EXHIBITION
OF THE
INDUSTRY
OF ALL NATIONS,
NEW-YORK
1853.

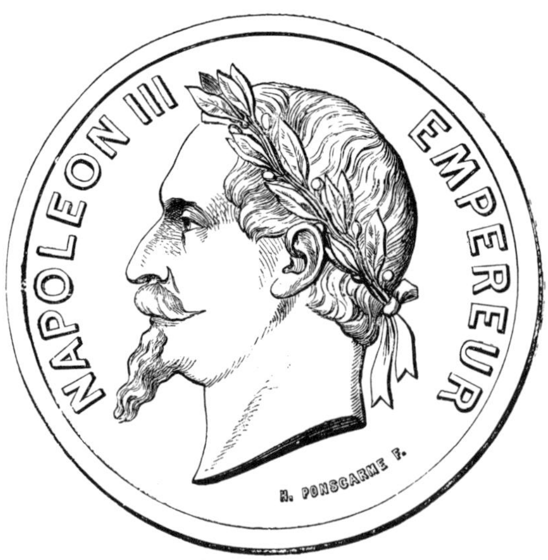
NAPOLEON III EMPEREUR
H. PONSCARME F.

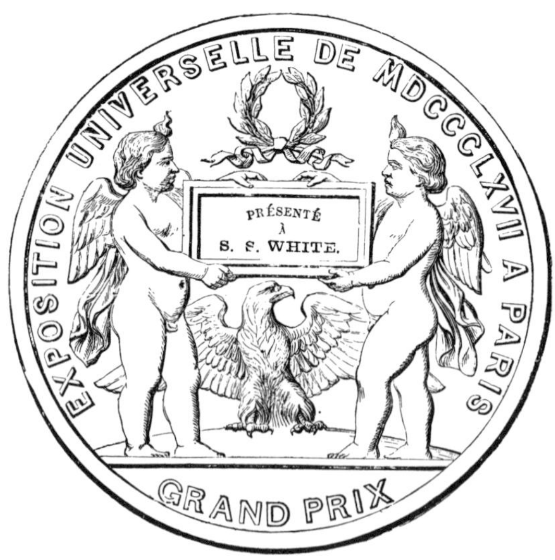
EXPOSITION UNIVERSELLE DE MDCCCLXVII A PARIS
PRÉSENTÉ
À
S. S. WHITE.
GRAND PRIX

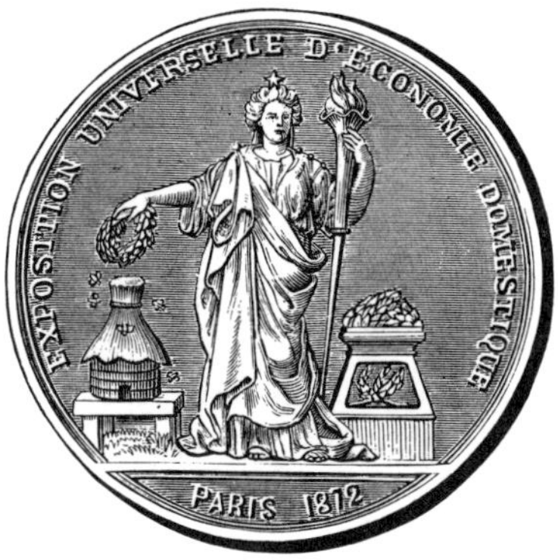

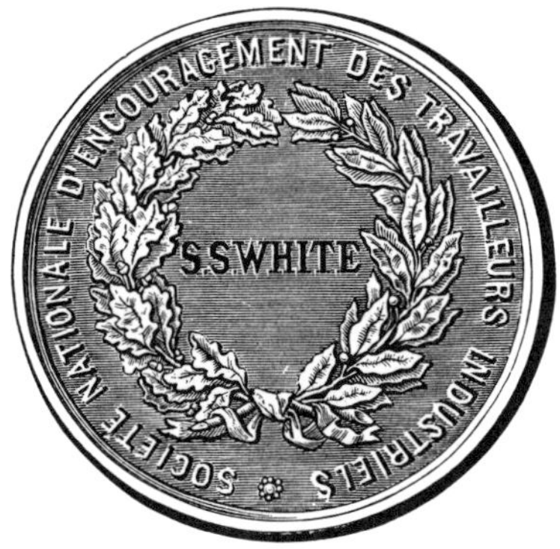

INCLUDING THE FOREGOING

INTERNATIONAL EXHIBITION MEDALS

AND THE

Grand Diploma of Honor,

AT THE VIENNA EXPOSITION, 1873,

WE HAVE RECEIVED IN ALL

SIXTY-TWO FIRST PREMIUMS.

These awards, coinciding in their recognition of the superiority of our manufactures with the judgment of the most cultured and appreciative members of the Dental Profession, justify us in claiming to

LEAD THE WORLD IN DENTAL MANUFACTURES.

Porcelain Teeth.

[THE following chapter on Teeth is taken by permission from the tenth edition of "Harris's Principles and Practice of Dentistry," edited by Professor P. H. Austen.

Some additional illustrations have been introduced, accompanied by the necessary description. These additions have been submitted to the author, and met his approval. The foot-note on page 18 is ours.

The illustrations will enable dentists practicing in cities and towns remote from dental depots to order, with some degree of certainty, styles, sizes, and shapes of teeth adapted to particular cases in hand. The numbers attached to the cuts are moulded on the reverse of the blocks.]

AS Pharmacy was once a part of Medical practice and instrument-making a part of Surgery, so the manufacture of Porcelain teeth was, at one time, confined to the dental laboratory. Until within the past twenty years, a practical knowledge of the Dento-ceramic art was considered an essential part of dental education. Galen compounded his celebrated *Theriaca* for two Roman Emperors; Paré and Wiseman made many of their surgical instruments; and necessity has compelled physicians and surgeons in all ages to imitate these examples. But the medical and surgical world have, for many years, committed the manufacture of drugs and instruments to those who, by making it a special art, can produce far better results.

The time has fully come when Dentistry should do the same with porcelain-work, for two sufficient reasons:—1. Manufacturers now offer to the Profession porcelain teeth in such variety of beautiful forms that not one dentist in a thousand could equal them. 2. Moderate proficiency in block-carving requires such an amount of preparatory training and of continuous experience, that the dentist's education and practice must suffer in the line of important duties which cannot thus be delegated to others. Hence nearly, if not quite, all of the most skillful block-carvers engaged in the general practice of Dentistry have, since the year 1850, one after another given up this art which it cost them so much to acquire. For these reasons, and also because the management of a porcelain furnace cannot be taught in books, we shall not attempt in this chapter to give a full and didactic exposition of the manner of making porcelain block or single teeth. Those who desire such knowledge, with a view to making it a specialty, require that which it no longer comes within the scope of a work on the "Principles and Practice of Dentistry" to teach.

There is, however, on the part of all students, and probably of most practitioners, a desire to know the composition of dental-porcelain, and to have some idea of the manner in which a few earthy materials and metallic oxides are made to assume such beautiful forms. Some knowledge of the component parts of porcelain is essential to a correct understanding of the necessity for their admixture, as well as of the effects thus produced.

PORCELAIN MATERIALS.

The infusible earths Silica and Alumina, and the fusible alkalies Potassa and Soda, form the bulk of all porcelain. Certain Metallic oxides, in small quantity, give color, and some varieties of pottery are modified by small proportions of Lime and Magnesia. Dental-porcelain is made from the purest compounds of silica, alumina, and potassa, colored by metallic Gold and Platina, and by the oxides of Gold, Titanium, Manganese, Cobalt, and Uranium.

SILICA.

Silica (quartz, silex, silicic acid) is, next to oxygen, the most universally diffused substance in nature, constituting fifty per cent. of all rocks. Granite, gigantic rocks, sandstones, and sand contain not less than three-fourths silica; mica-schist, clay-slate, and clay, not less than two-thirds; trap-rocks and lava, one-half. Silica is to the mineral kingdom what carbon is to the vegetable—the element of stability. In its purest forms (rock-crystal, Brazilian pebbles, or crystals of quartz), it is free from discoloration by iron or other oxides; it is absolutely infusible, and is insoluble in water; this is the kind selected for dental-porcelain, but for other varieties of porcelain flint is commonly used. It forms silicates with alumina, magnesia, lime, potassa, and soda; the most important of which, in this connection, are the silicates of alumina and potassa. Silica, as found in feldspar and kaolin, is partly pure silica, partly the silicate of alumina. Now the "behavior" in the furnace of silica and the silicate of alumina is different; hence chemical analysis can estimate only the relative purity of these substances; experiment alone can determine the proportions of each necessary for the development of any required property in porcelain.

FELDSPAR.

Next to silica, alumina (oxide of aluminum) is the most universally diffused of all minerals; but, unlike silica, it is rarely found uncombined. The gem Sapphire is pure crystallized alumina, and is the next hardest mineral to the diamond; a less pure form is well known in Dentistry, as emery or corundum; some specimens of which seem, under the lens, to be a collection of minute crystals of dark-colored sapphire. For porcelain manufacture alumina is never used in its pure state, but in its natural combinations with silica, lime, potassa, and soda. For dental-porcelain only two of these are used—Feldspar (known to the Chinese as Pe-tun-tse) and Kaolin. Feldspar is a silicate of alumina and potassa, containing a little lime and a trace of iron. A less common variety of spar contains soda in place of potassa; it makes a soft porcelain, fusible at lower heat than the potash spar. Lime feldspar is used in some kinds of pottery, but for dental purposes potash feldspar is the only variety. It is an abundant mineral, and is often found in large masses; the purest varieties alone are used for dental-porcelain; Delaware and Pennsylvania spars are most esteemed by American manufacturers. Its most extensive dissemination, however, is as one of the components of granite and granitic rocks, by disintegration of the feldspathic constituents of which large beds of porcelain clay are formed, as found in China and Japan, England, Germany, and France, and also in the United States.

KAOLIN.—Ka-o-lin (the Chinese word for clay) is the purest of these mixtures of silica and silicate of alumina, prepared in Nature's laboratory, for the manufacture of porcelain. Pipe-clay, potter's-clay, blue-clay, fire-clay, and Cornish-stone are similar in composition, but only the purest kaolin is used for dental-porcelain. It contains nine parts of silica and eight parts alumina; whereas spar has nine parts silica and only two parts alumina; also spar is made fusible by its silicate of potassa,—kaolin has none. Kaolin is therefore feldspar deprived of its soluble silicate of potassa (or soda), which has been washed out during the disintegration of the feldspathic rocks. It is soft and unctuous, and is highly plastic; pulverized spar, on the contrary, is granular or powdery, and is moulded with difficulty. Kaolin, like silex, is infusible; under intense and continued heat it shrinks greatly, and becomes extremely hard, but it is always porous and absorbent. Silex lessens the contraction of kaolin, spar gives it fusibility; both diminish its absorbent quality, so objectionable in any material that is to be worn in the mouth.

Stone-ware, China-ware, Wedgwood-ware, Parian-porcelain, and Dental-porcelain vary in their properties because of the different proportions in which kaolin and feldspar are combined; also in the kind of flux used. For instance, the Parian statuettes have kaolin and spar in equal proportions, with about half as much of a flux, made of spar, quartz, and potash. Dental-porcelain, demanding less heat, less shrinkage, and a more translucent appearance, has a very much greater proportion of spar. It has required a very extended series of experiments to combine silica, alumina, and potassa in correct proportions, and to know just which of Nature's compounds it is best to use, in order to harmonize the requisites of strength and beauty, so essential to the character of a porcelain tooth.

COLORING MATERIALS.

The foregoing materials give a pure white porcelain of greater or less translucency. It is now required to find substances which will, in the strong heat of the furnace, yield indestructible colors; by skillful combination of which the porcelain may imitate the almost endless varieties of tint in the natural teeth and gum. Of these there are three principal colors and three subordinate ones.

TITANIUM.—The purest varieties of the oxide of titanium are selected; it is found as a mineral in various localities throughout the United States. The crystals are reddish-brown, and have a bright metallic luster; they give, when ground, a beautiful yellow, or yellowish-brown color. It is used in the coloring of all *body*, and is the basis of color for the class of yellowish *enamels.*

PLATINUM.—This metal, precipitated from its solution in aqua-regia, then washed and dried, is known as platina sponge. It gives a gray-blue color, and is the basis of color for the class of grayish-blue enamels.

GOLD.—Gold precipitate is used to give life and animation to the tooth, producing often a very remarkable effect. The oxide of gold, known as *Purple of Cassius*, and generally considered to be a mixed oxide of gold and tin, is used to impart the well-known red color of the artificial gum; no less costly substitute has ever been found for this purpose.

Oxide of Manganese gives a purplish color, and is used occasionally for some shades of tooth, but not of gum. *Oxide of Cobalt* gives a bright blue color. If wrapped in best blue paper, and burned in a covered crucible, it is called the Ashes of Cobalt, and is thought to give a more desirable tint to the enamel than the simple oxide. *Oxide of Uranium* is used in its mineral form, and gives a greenish-yellow color; whilst a lemon-yellow color may be given by the oxide of silver: but this is a fugitive color at high temperatures.

These colors singly, and in combination with each other, produce a great variety of colors or shades. Thus, say forty shades of *body-color* are made by using these materials in different quantities and in different combinations; also a like number of *enamel-colors.* Then, starting with the lightest shade of body, forty different grades may be produced by using a different point-enamel; so of each of the forty shades of body, making, if required, sixteen hundred variations of shade.

The following formulas will suffice to give a correct idea of the proportions in which the preceding materials are combined to give the Body and Enamel of porcelain teeth, single or in sections:

BODY.		ENAMEL.	
Feldspar	12 oz	Feldspar	3 oz.
Quartz	2 oz.	Sponge Platina	1 to 4 grs.
Kaolin	15 dwts.	Flux	3 dwts.
Titanium	24 to 48 grs.		

The Flux here mentioned is made by fusing four ounces of finely ground quartz with Glass of Borax and Sal Tartar, each one ounce: it forms a transparent glass. The following formulas show the preparation of Gum Enamel:

GUM FRIT.		GUM ENAMEL.	
Oxide of Gold	10 grs.	Gum Frit	1 oz.
Feldspar	1 oz.	Feldspar	3 oz.
Flux	8 dwts.		

The titanium, platina, and oxide of gold must, in these recipes, of course, be modified by mixture with other colors to produce the requisite varieties of shade. We shall now briefly describe the processes by which the porcelain teeth and sections, sold to the Profession, are manufactured.

PROCESS OF MANUFACTURE.

The silex and feldspar, in their crude state, are first submitted to a red heat, then suddenly thrown into cold water. This is called "Calcining," and the effect is to render them more easily broken and pulverized. All impurities having been carefully removed, they are crushed between flint stones; when fine enough, they are put into a mill, formed of burr-millstone, with chasers of the same material. They are ground in water, then floated off, and allowed to settle. The water is then drawn off or evaporated; the silex and spar, dried and sifted, are then ready for use. The kaolin, having been already pulverized in Nature's laboratory, is prepared by washing until perfectly free from impurities, and when dry is ready for use. The Flux and Frit are coarsely ground, but the Coloring materials are reduced to an impalpable powder. All these porcelain materials are combined in proper proportions to form the body and the enamel, then mixed with water and worked into masses resembling putty. When, however, the method of *biscuiting* is adopted, the enamels are mixed in a much thinner state than the body.

The unbaked porcelain masses are now ready for the Moulding-room. The moulds in which single teeth or sections are formed are made of brass, and are in two pieces,—one-half of the tooth being represented on either side. The precise shapes desired are carved out with great care; holes are drilled to receive the platina pins in each tooth:

when the two halves are fitted accurately together, with guiding pins for exact closure, the mould is ready for use. The brass matrix must be made about one-fifth larger than the size desired, to allow for shrinkage of the porcelain paste. After greasing the moulds, the first operation is, by means of small tweezers, to place the platina pins in the holes made for them (there are many sizes of these pins, differing in length and thickness, to suit the different sizes of the teeth). As no piece of mechanism can be stronger than its weakest part, there should always be such a relation between the tooth-substance and the pins, as to shape, size, and angle of insertion, that one will be as strong as the other, and both sufficient for all legitimate uses. This strength of pin, without loss of strength in the tooth, characterizes a recent and valuable improvement made by Dr. S. S. White, and known as the "foot-shaped pin," illustrated in Fig. 1.* The thickest part of this pin is at the angle, or heel; the point, or toe, runs upward into the

FIG. 1.

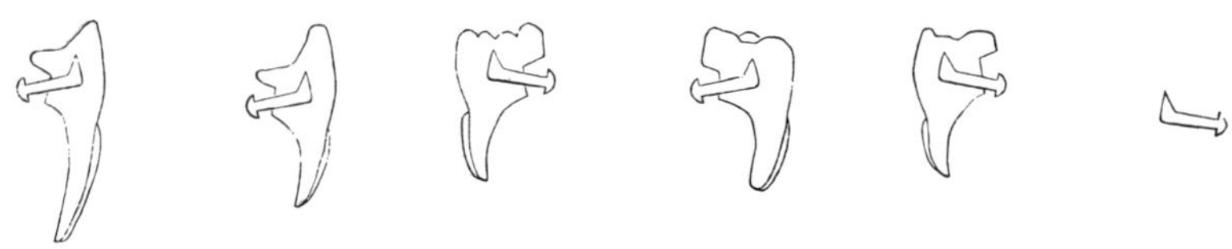

thick part of the tooth, giving additional security against its being drawn out. The insertion of the pin at an upward angle beds it in the strongest portion of the tooth-material; thus any weakening of the thin portion of the tooth is avoided, as when the headed pin is inserted in a straight line; also, the greatest amount of material is found where the greatest strain is brought to bear upon it. The force of mastication is exerted outward and toward the necks of the teeth; thus the shape and direction of this pin are best calculated directly to oppose it. It will also be noticed that its direction and unusual length of insertion permit a close grinding of the tooth, which would cause the usual short and horizontal pin very soon to break away from the porcelain. The double-headed pin, a previously patented invention of Dr. White, was a very great improvement in the shape of tooth-pins; but we think it is destined to be superseded by this new "foot-shaped pin."

The pins being properly adjusted, the enamels for the tooth and the gum are carefully placed in the moulds, by means of a small steel spatula, in the exact position and

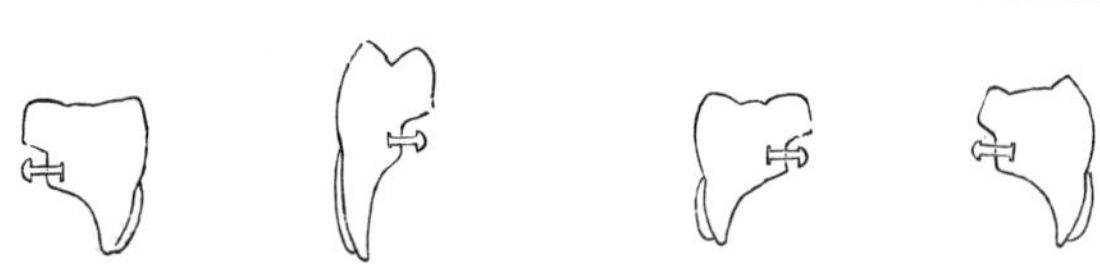

* THESE CUTS REPRESENT SECTIONS OF TEETH IN OUR POSSESSION BOUGHT FAIRLY OF OTHER MAKERS, AND GROUND DOWN TO THE MIDDLE OF THE PIN. COMPARISON OF THESE WITH THE CUTS OF OURS RENDERS COMMENT UNNECESSARY, EITHER AS TO THE SHAPE AND USEFULNESS OF THE PIN, OR THE QUANTITY OF PLATINUM USED.

WE CLAIM THAT, BY REASON OF THEIR COMPOSITION, AND THE SIZE, NUMBER, SHAPE, AND INSERTION OF THE PLATINUM PINS, OUR TEETH ARE STRONGER THAN THOSE OF ANY OTHER MANUFACTURER IN THIS OR ANY OTHER COUNTRY.

SAMUEL S. WHITE.

quantity required; the body is placed in them in lumps corresponding to the size of the teeth; the top of the mould is then put on, and the matrix laid under a press, which compacts each separate mass. They are then dried by a slow heat. When perfectly dry, the top is removed, and the teeth will now drop out. In this state they are extremely tender, owing to the large percentage of feldspar, and require very careful handling.

They are now sent to the trimmers' room, where each tooth is carefully inspected, and all imperfections removed or filled up; the spare edges left by the union of the two sides of the mould are smoothly filed, and the arch of the gum over each tooth made rounding and true with a small pointed instrument. They are then placed on beds of coarse quartz sand, on trays or slides made of fire-clay, and are ready for the furnace. Formerly, there was another process, called crucing or biscuiting, which was universally practiced, and is still used in some factories; it is also used in the making of blocks carved to order. It consists in submitting the teeth, after moulding, to a heat sufficient to harden them so that they can be cut or filed like chalk, and what is called an *outside enamel* is then applied with a camel's-hair brush; but it has been found that the composition of the tooth is injuriously affected by this partial burning, subsequent cooling, enameling, and reburning. This process is unavoidable when the blocks are carved by hand for special cases; but whenever they can be made in a matrix, the tooth is better and stronger when it is enameled in the mould, and finished in a single firing.

The furnace is built substantially on the principle of the dentist's furnace, differing chiefly in size. The trays holding the teeth are placed in the muffle, and are thus protected against injury from the gases of the fuel. There is no rule which can be given to determine the exact amount of time the teeth must remain in the furnace; the practiced eye of the burner must determine, from the appearance of the teeth, when the firing is completed. If taken out before they are done, the enamel will craze, or crack, in cooling; if a little too much done, the surface will be too glassy, and the body will not be strong. When cool, the teeth are removed from the slides, placed upon wax cards, and are then ready for the dentist.

The vast variety in shape, size, color, etc., of the teeth thus made, gives opportunity for the selection of forms suitable to nearly every case which presents itself to the practitioner. The assortment must of necessity be very large and varied, to meet the wants of the operator; in fact, the manufacturer has shown a better appreciation of the æsthetic requirements of the dental art than the practitioner. Whilst the work of the latter too often exhibits an unmeaning monotony, the former has made provision for even the extreme cases which are sometimes met with; he has also given a beautiful series of those various deviations from a uniform regularity which are so common in natural dentures. In some mouths these seem to be imperatively demanded, to restore the familiar expression; whilst in any mouth, the use of some one or other of them would go far to disarm that suspicion of artificiality, detection of which is mortifying to most patients.

Porcelain is a material in which the beauty of the result well repays the highest exercise of Art. It has been for centuries a favorite material for expressing the Poetry of Form. The famous Etruscan vases of antiquity, the exquisite gems of the *Majolica* of the sixteenth century, the marvelous works of Bernard Palissy, the prince of potters, the beautiful productions of the Sèvres and Dresden manufactories, the well-known charming designs of the Wedgwood-ware, and the still more recent Parian statuettes, may be named in proof of the fitness of Porcelain to embody the conceptions of Genius.

Dental-porcelain is worthy of such associations: not only like them does it delight the eye, and give evidence of high æsthetic cultivation, but it adds to beauty the charm of usefulness. It is customary to attribute the rapid growth of Dental Art, since 1840, to its Associations, Colleges, Journals, and its didactic Literature,—and with much truth. But to Porcelain it owes its very existence, as an æsthetic art, and the larger part of its extent and utility as a prosthetic art. It was altogether impossible for perishable human teeth, or their wretched imitations in ivory, to offer such tempting fac-similes of nature as we meet in porcelain. By thus creating that enormously increased demand for dental service, which has been the chief cause of the rapid development of its resources, it has made the Dental Profession its debtor to a greater extent than any other single influence. The depot not only renders service by the superior excellence of the surgical instruments and prosthetic materials which it supplies, but it directly benefits the science and art of dentistry, by releasing the practitioner from manufacturing toil, and giving time for the acquirement of increased knowledge and skill. Thus, if the time heretofore given to block-making were devoted to the study of dental æsthetics, patients would have the benefit of an artistic selection from a far larger variety of porcelain dentures than could otherwise be possibly made.

The illustrations of this chapter can but imperfectly convey an idea of the beauty and expression of the originals: they will, however, assist the student in his study of those principles which guide in the selection and arrangement of teeth; they may serve also to awaken practitioners to the extent of the present resources of Ceramic dentistry, and to the importance of æsthetic culture in order properly to make full use of the same.

The improvements in the Dento-Ceramic Art have sprung from a careful inquiry into the essential characteristics which artistically formed porcelain teeth should possess. Among these are (1) *Naturalness:* under which term are included shape, color, and a vital appearance; the last depending upon the precise amount of translucency, the texture of the surface, and the nice blending of the colors of the body and enamel,—an appearance which should be maintained as well under artificial as under solar light. Many teeth which will bear inspection reasonably well in daylight have a very unnatural and artificial appearance when exposed in the mouth to a light under which the wearer may be most anxious to excite admiration. (2) *Shape:* which includes a preservation of the distinctive characteristics of each tooth, securing the instant recognition of its position in the dental arch. There must be some defect or inaccuracy of form if, out of the twenty-eight teeth of a set, in unassorted confusion, an experienced eye cannot tell the place of each; for every tooth has its distinctive contour. Not only should each tooth possess the individuality which belongs to it, but it should also indicate the character of its relation to its companions on either side, and to its antagonist. The eye trained to observe nature should not be offended by the recognition of any inharmony; should not find a second bicuspid or molar in place of a first, or incisors undistinguishable from each other, or an upper tooth in place of its corresponding lower one; nor should it detect in the midst of one style of denture some incisor or canine characteristic of another. Figs. 2 and 3 exhibit very strikingly the marked peculiarities of each one of the twenty-eight teeth of an artistically designed artificial set; whilst these and subsequent illustrations demonstrate how possible it is for modern dentistry to adapt its work to the great varieties of facial expression. Probably every reader has more than once turned at the sound of a familiar voice, to see a face strangely resembling the looked-for friend. This correspondence between voice and face, often so startling, is only another one of those links between external and internal conformation, which makes the study of æsthetic anatomy essential to the success of the dental mechanism.

The great law of correspondence, which enabled Cuvier to build up the entire

FIG. 2.

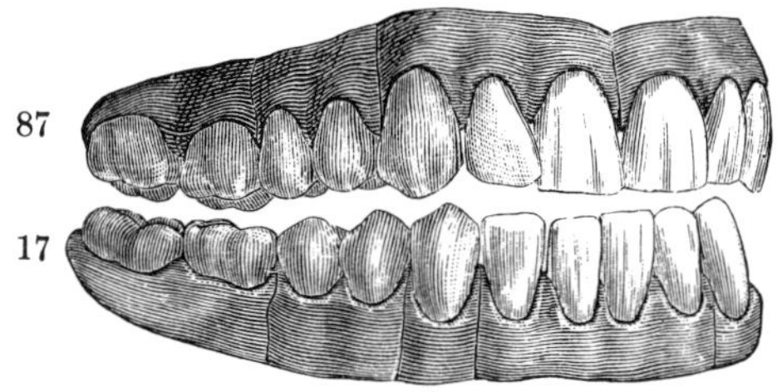

skeleton from a single bone, makes us associate the idea of intellect with certain forms of forehead, and of character with certain forms of mouth, nose, and chin; it is the same law which permits us to infer from what remains the expression of what is lost. Age, sex, temperament, and complexion; also many physical, mental, and even moral

FIG. 3.

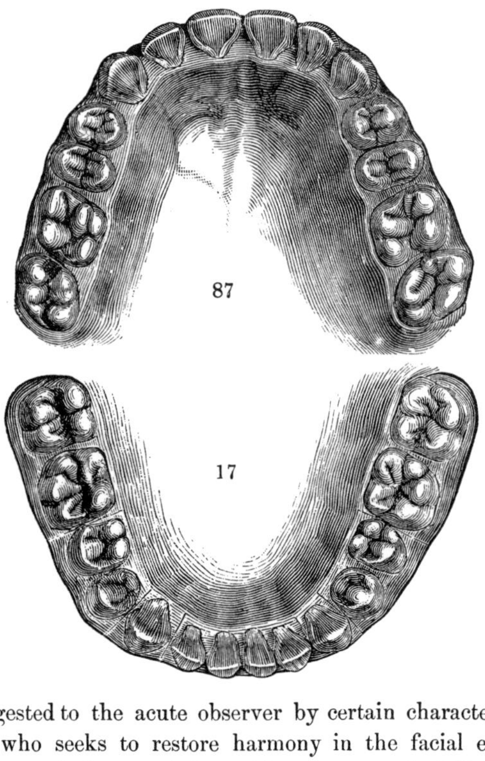

peculiarities are suggested to the acute observer by certain characteristics of the dental organs. The artist who seeks to restore harmony in the facial expression should be skilled in the observance of these varied manifestations; such skill is demanded alike in the manufacture and in the application of artificial dentures.

In addition to these æsthetic qualities, porcelain teeth should possess (3) *Strength* adequate to the legitimate use for which they are intended; this strength should come from the quality of their composition, the skillful distribution of bulk to parts most requiring it, and from the due form, position, and proportion of the pins, rather than from any increase in bulk and weight beyond that of the natural organs. They should

FIG. 4.

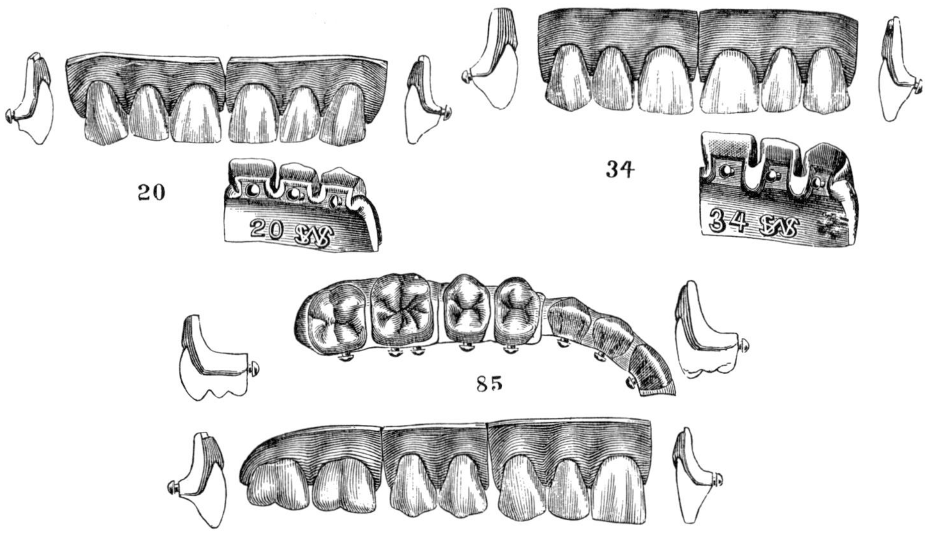

possess also, by reason of their conformation (4), *Adaptability* to the various irregularities caused by unequal absorption of the alveolar ridge, so that when judiciously selected they shall require little labor to adapt and antagonize them. Special provision should be made for the results of extreme or very irregular absorption, or for the loss, by disease or otherwise, of parts of the maxillary ridge; so that in such cases the teeth can readily be made to articulate and afford comfort to the wearer, assisting in speech and mastication, and yet not presenting any incongruous appearance.

FIG. 5.

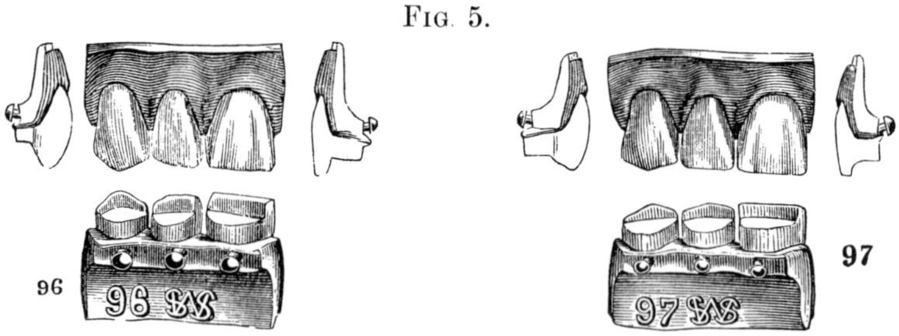

There are, moreover, special modifications demanded by many other conditions; as, for instance, in cases having a very short articulation, requiring the pins to be set in a recess near the crowns of the teeth, thus bringing the greatest resistance where there is the greatest strain in mastication, as is well shown in Fig. 4. In both these blocks the full external size of tooth is given, and its characteristic form and the expression of interdental gum preserved; this could not be done with the usual form of blocks ground down to suit such cases. The third set has a plain back without shoulder: the pins are set so as to give a longer bite in the front teeth, and in the back teeth so as to allow of grinding off the inner cusps if desirable, thus avoiding the breaking through of the thin shell which is made when an ordinary block is ground down. In Fig. 5 we have front

FIG. 6.

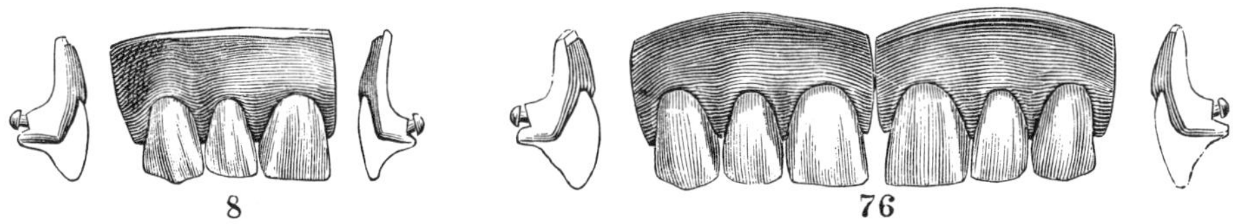

blocks for mouths, where a shoulder is required to antagonize with the lower front teeth when there are no back teeth remaining.

Where early contraction and protrusion of the upper maxillary arch has caused it to have a sharply curved projection, bringing the closure of the lower teeth much behind the upper ridge at the central incisors, or where absorption above has left a ridge

FIG. 7.

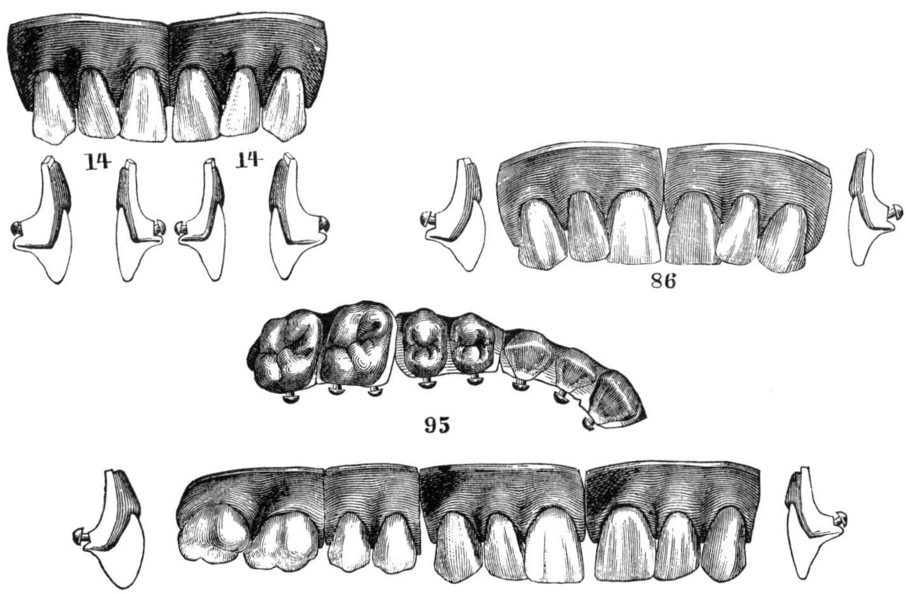

prominent at its lower edge, or margin of the gum, it becomes necessary to give a peculiar twisted form to the front blocks. Fig. 6 shows two blocks for such arches. Fig. 7 represents blocks adapted to pointed arches and crowded dentures. It is impossible to adapt blocks of ordinary form to such cases without destroying their true expression at one or other of the joints; in fact, much of both gum and tooth is often sacrificed to get correct articulation. In Fig. 8, the blocks are for cases in which absorption has taken place, especially over the canines, bringing the bite of the lower jaw outside of the upper maxillary ridge.

FIG. 8.

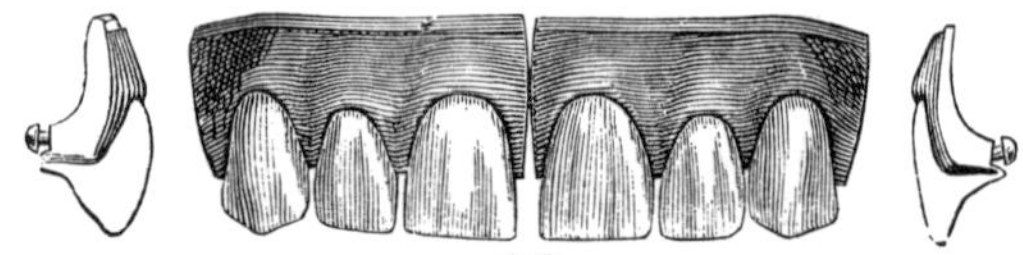

92

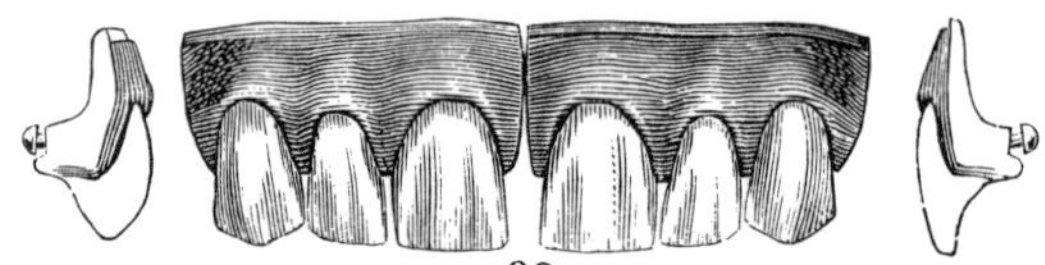

90

Where a prominence of the gum exists, from want of exterior absorption, teeth such as are shown in Fig. 9 are adapted. The same condition of the lower jaw

FIG. 9.

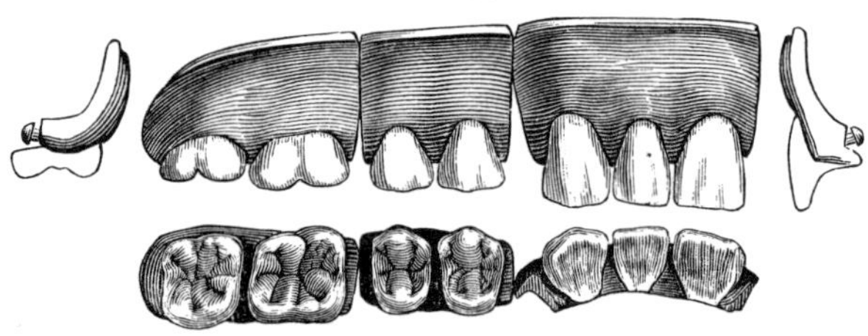

70 1/4

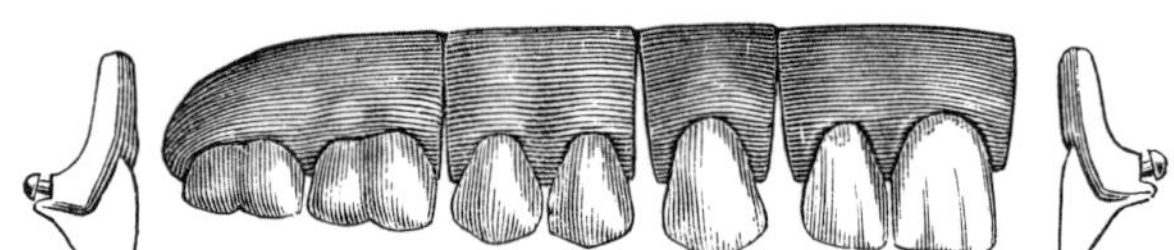

99

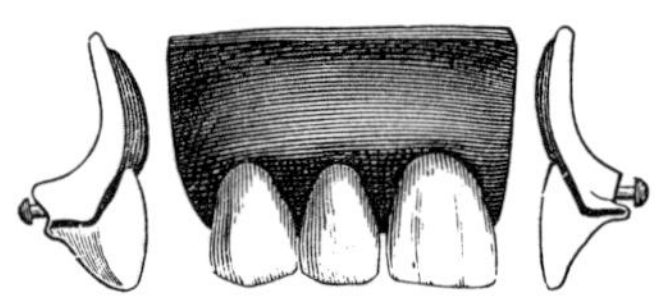

70

is designed to be met by blocks represented in Fig. 10. Where the previous wearing of a plate requires the teeth to be set directly upon the ridge, with no artificial gum

FIG. 10.

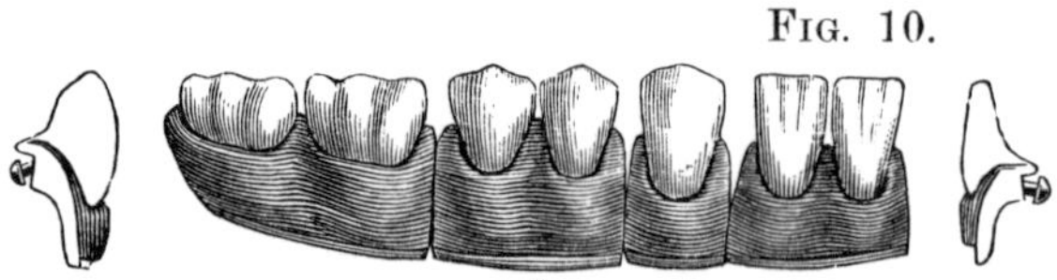

4

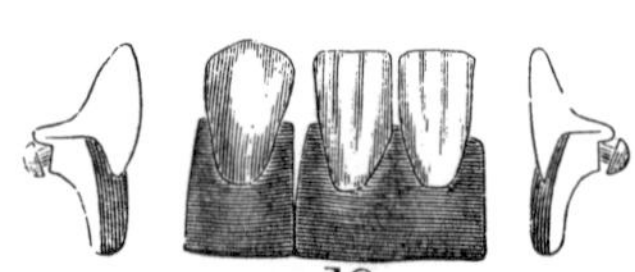

18

between it and the lip, blocks, illustrated in Fig. 11, are required. In the latter case, if the color of gum is judiciously chosen and the blocks well adapted, the triangles of artificial gum will be scarcely if at all distinguishable from the natural: we regard this as an extremely useful form of block. Sectional view of the molar, in first cut, Fig. 9, shows the curve necessary to bring its grinding surface directly under the ridge. The views of grinding and cutting surfaces, together with front views, show how each tooth has a distinctive character; as, for instance, in the bicuspids, so often chosen without regard to the difference in form between the first and second. Again, the curves of the front blocks in Figs. 9 and 11 show two of several variations required in the curvature

FIG. 11.

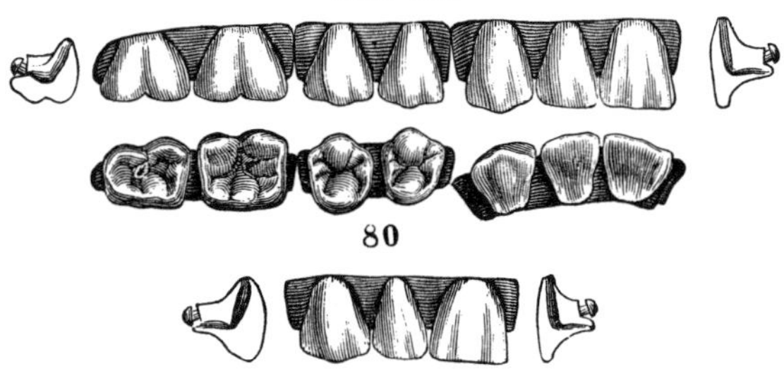

of the arch: in the upper cut in Fig. 9, the sharp turn at the canines gives a squareness across the incisors; in Fig. 11 this turn is at the central, and is adapted to a pointed arch.

When the molar block of lower sets extends to where the ramus of the jaw begins to rise, a peculiar ploughshare curve of the base is required: such that, whilst the gum of the second bicuspid lies on the outside of the ridge, the gum of the second molar

FIG. 12.

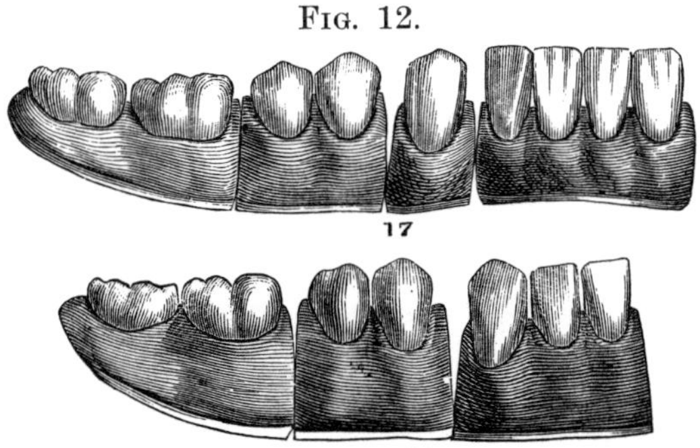

may lie partly upon the ridge, so as to give more perfect antagonism with the upper molars, as shown in Fig. 12. The molar and bicuspid teeth, from which these were drawn, are also marked by a characteristic curve of the buccal surfaces, giving not only a very natural appearance, but acting as a guard to the cheek, and preventing its being caught between the teeth.

Variations in curvature of the arch are shown also in Fig. 3 and the fourth cut in Fig. 22. Notice also the marked difference in the character of the bicuspids and molars in upper and lower cuts, and the totally different expression of the front teeth in Fig. 2.

Fig. 13 shows how the same intermaxillary space may be filled with teeth of widely different size as well as character. In the first, a very long tooth and short gum; in the second, a very long gum and short tooth. But length of teeth is by no means the only difference here; relative size of central and lateral, direction of the axis of lateral and canine, and outline of cutting edge of the block, are three features which equally mark the

FIG. 13.

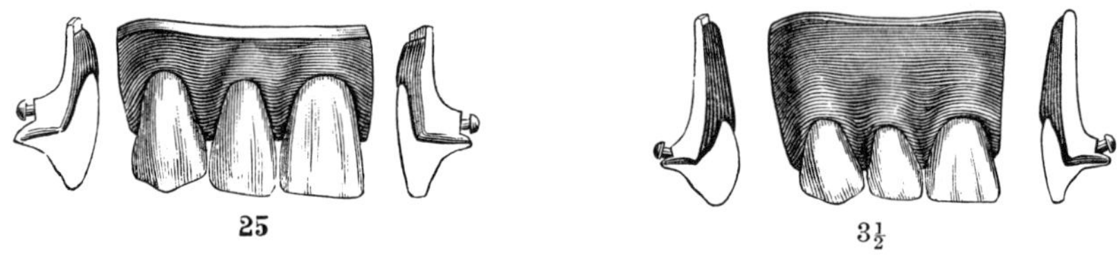

distinctness of these two styles: these also are points which demand that both long and short teeth shall differ among themselves as widely as these samples differ from each other. The lateral view of these teeth shows another marked difference in form.

FIG. 14.

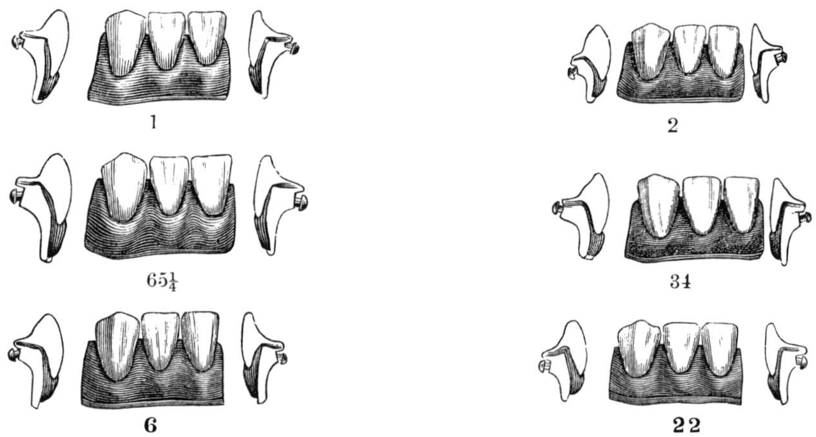

Fig. 14 gives the characteristic equality of lower incisors, or slightly greater size of the lateral; it also gives some of the diversities in length, width, shape of cutting edge, and form at arch of the gum. Although there is much less difference in the shape of the six lower front teeth than of the six upper, it is a great mistake to suppose that a given lower block will answer for any lower case, if only long enough. Side views show also a difference in the slant of the teeth, inward or outward, which has an important effect in modifying the expression of the lower arch. There are also differences in curvature of the lower arch, as well as of the upper. Fig. 3 shows the usual upper and lower curves, and Figs. 9, 11, and 22 show variations of upper curvature requiring some modifications of the lower, dependent on the character of the articulation. In Fig. 15 are five other forms of lower front blocks, the value of which will be at once recognized. The three right-hand sets differ from those of Fig. 14 mainly in the length and width of teeth. The left lower set is well suited to patients whose natural teeth, for many years before their loss, were marked by exposure of the neck: this appearance may also be increased

FIG. 15.

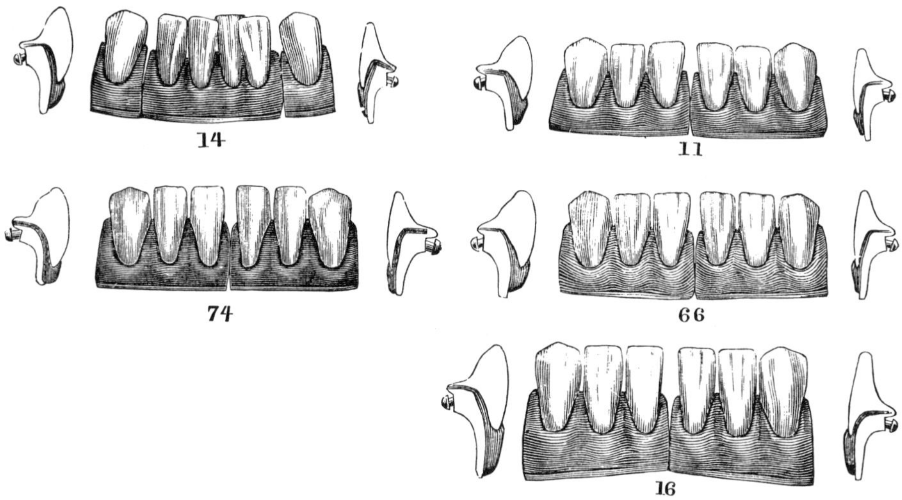

(sometimes it may be made) by judicious use of the corundum-wheel, but the block here given is invaluable for such cases. The left upper block is an admirable imitation of a very usual arrangement of incisors, resulting from crowded dentition: the drawing gives a very imperfect idea of the great beauty of the original porcelain block. When the

FIG. 16.

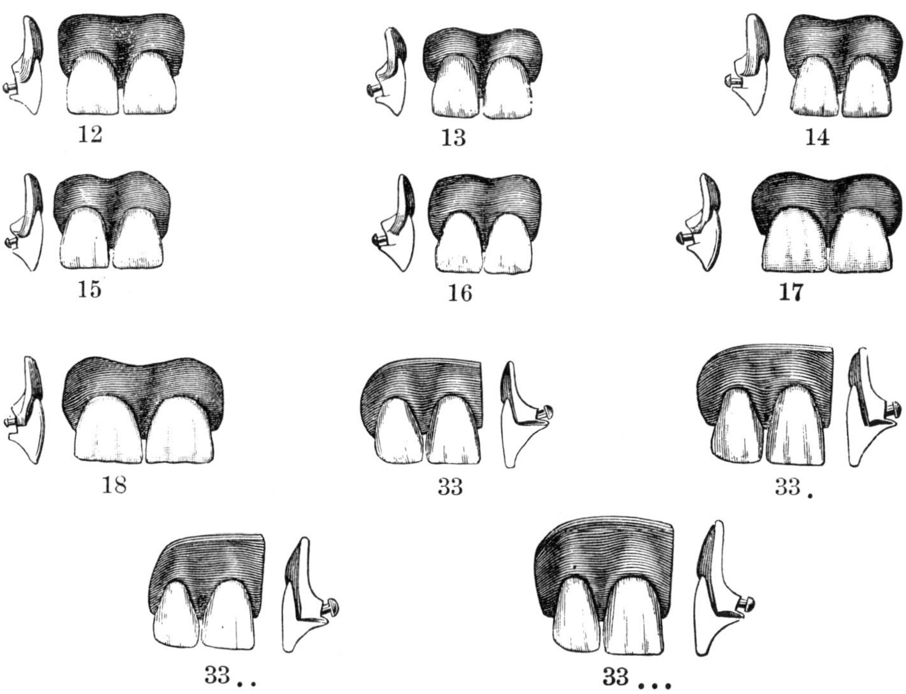

facial expression indicates its use, it will have great effect in disarming suspicion of artificiality,—a very desirable quality in artificial dentures.

In Fig. 16 we have very convenient modifications to suit front spaces of two or four teeth; the set of four being in two blocks. The peculiarity of these blocks is the lateral

FIG. 17.

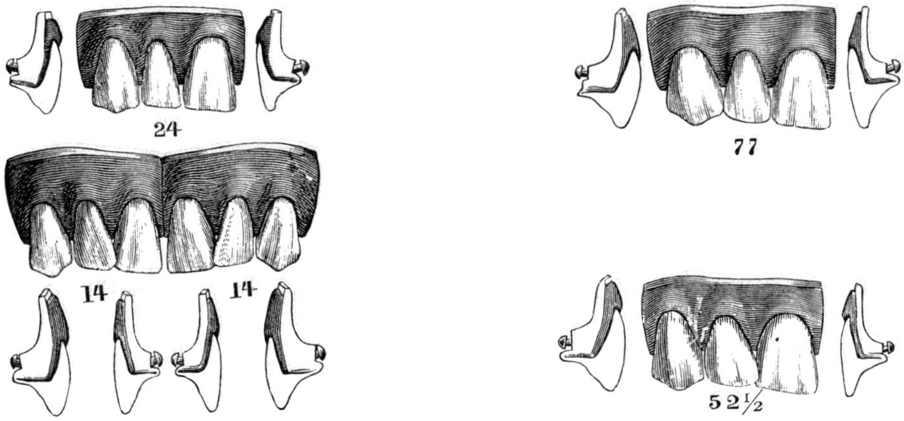

finish of the gum; instead of a square joint, for fitting to an adjoining block, they have a rounded edge of gum color that can be adapted to the curves of the absorbed natural gum. There should also be blocks of two, a lateral and central, with gum shaped like the double central, as such cases are of frequent occurrence. Besides the forms of teeth

FIG. 18.

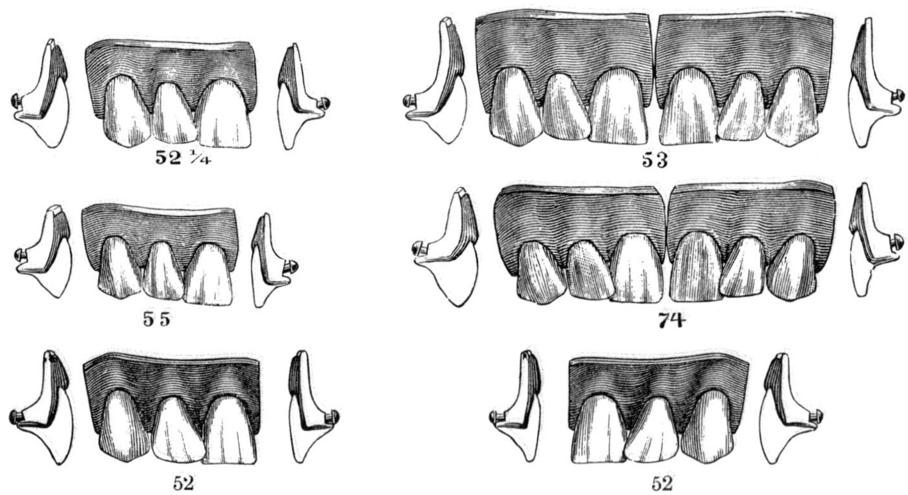

here given, there are many other varieties, in size and shape of this very useful kind of block.

Figs. 17, 18, and 19 represent a few of the great variety of forms of upper incisors and canines, designed to meet the demands of an æsthetic discrimination. In Fig. 17

we have, first, a long, delicate lateral, with sloping but not rounded edge, showing a decided space between it and the cuspid and central: then we find it wider, with corners and edge rounded and filling the space. Lastly, for want of space, the laterals, although long and narrow, overlap the centrals: this style is generally associated with a pointed arch. The fourth block, although with an overlapping incisor, has an entirely different character: it is often found in a rather flattened arch, and does not indicate a crowded denture. In these blocks the inclination and shape of the canine, as well as the shape of the incisor, help to give to each block a distinctness of character which will not permit the use of one in a case demanding either of the others.

The *celare artem* effect of overlapping or twisted laterals, like that of irregular lower incisors, is such as to tempt one to use them whenever admissible.

In Fig. 18 we have some additional varieties of this kind of block. In all these

FIG. 19.

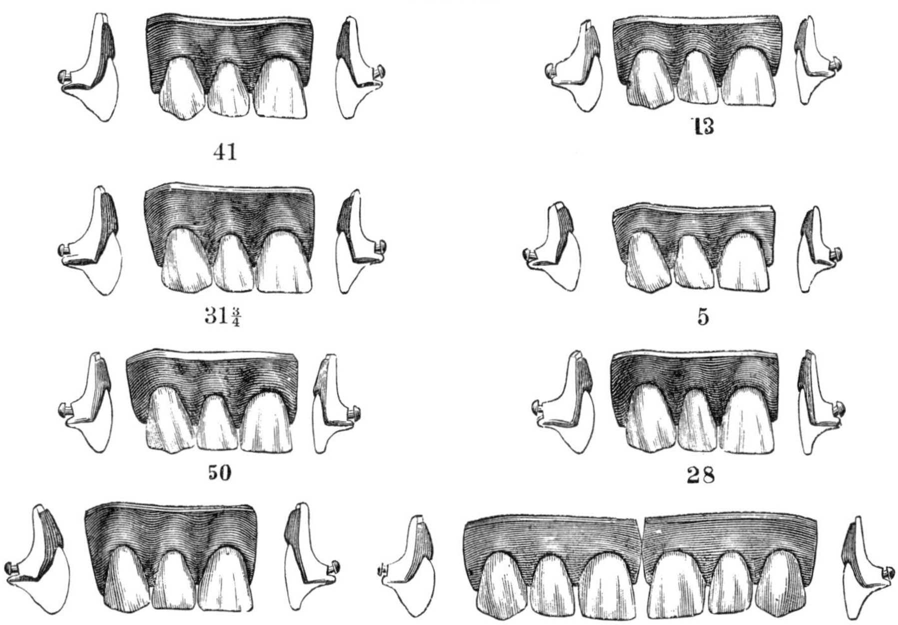

cases we find differences in the size and character of the lateral, in the extent of its lapping, and in the degree of twist given to it. A careful study of natural teeth will teach the dentist what character of face is best suited to each of these different forms, and thus he will much increase the extent to which he may properly use this kind of irregularity.

In Fig. 19 the blocks vary little in size, yet they each have a distinctive character. In the first, we have, lateral rounded on both corners, and its axis vertical; canine, with pointed cusp and edges quite rounded. In the second, we have lateral inclined, with median corner pointed, lateral corner quite round; canine with blunt cusp, also axis inclined. In the third, surface of the canine is decidedly furrowed, which, with the indented edge, gives it a marked character: the lateral and central, unlike the previous blocks, have square-cut edges, with corners but slightly rounded. In the fourth, the lateral is more nearly equal to the central, and none of the teeth have any marked

FIG. 20.

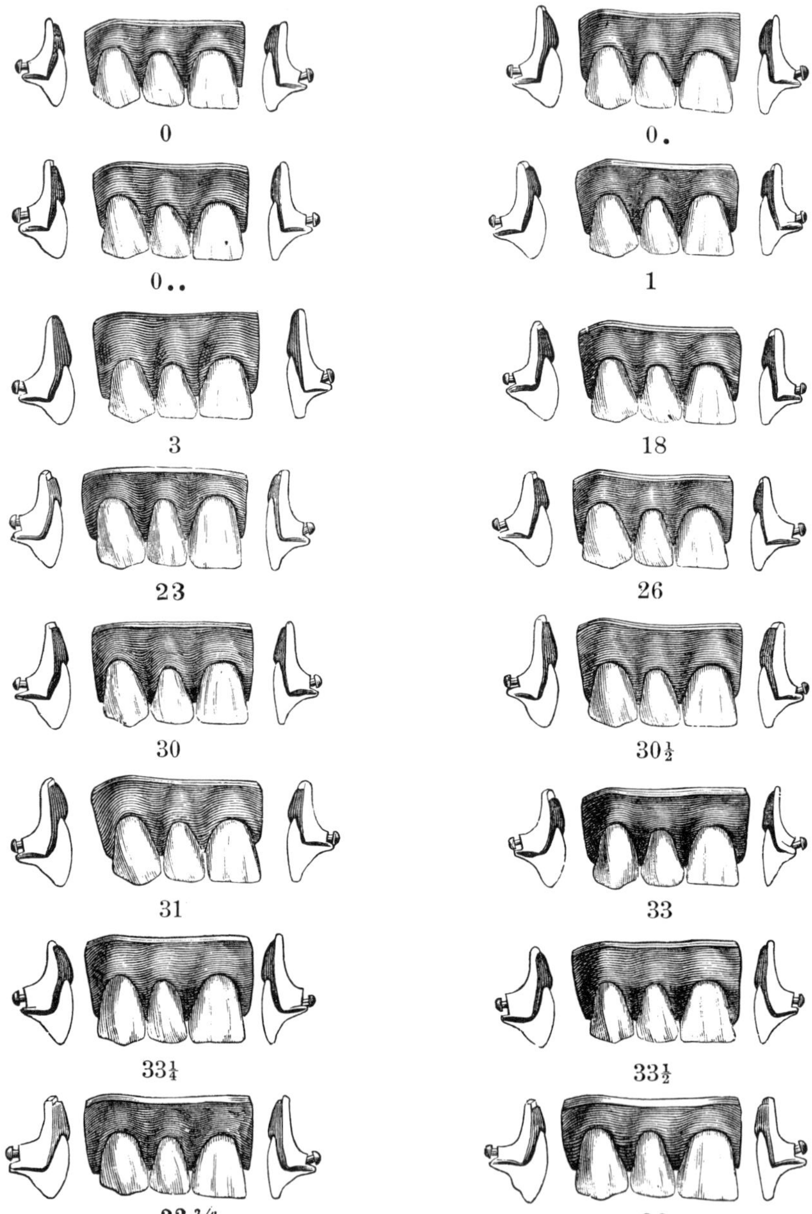

peculiarities: this style of block, in its different sizes, suits well in many cases, and is perhaps one of the best for general use by those practitioners who pay no regard, in their selection of teeth, to the indications given by the physical characteristics of the face and head. The eighth block is one of that class often met with in old age, where, by the action of the lower teeth or other causes, the arch has spread, widening the interdental

Fig. 21.

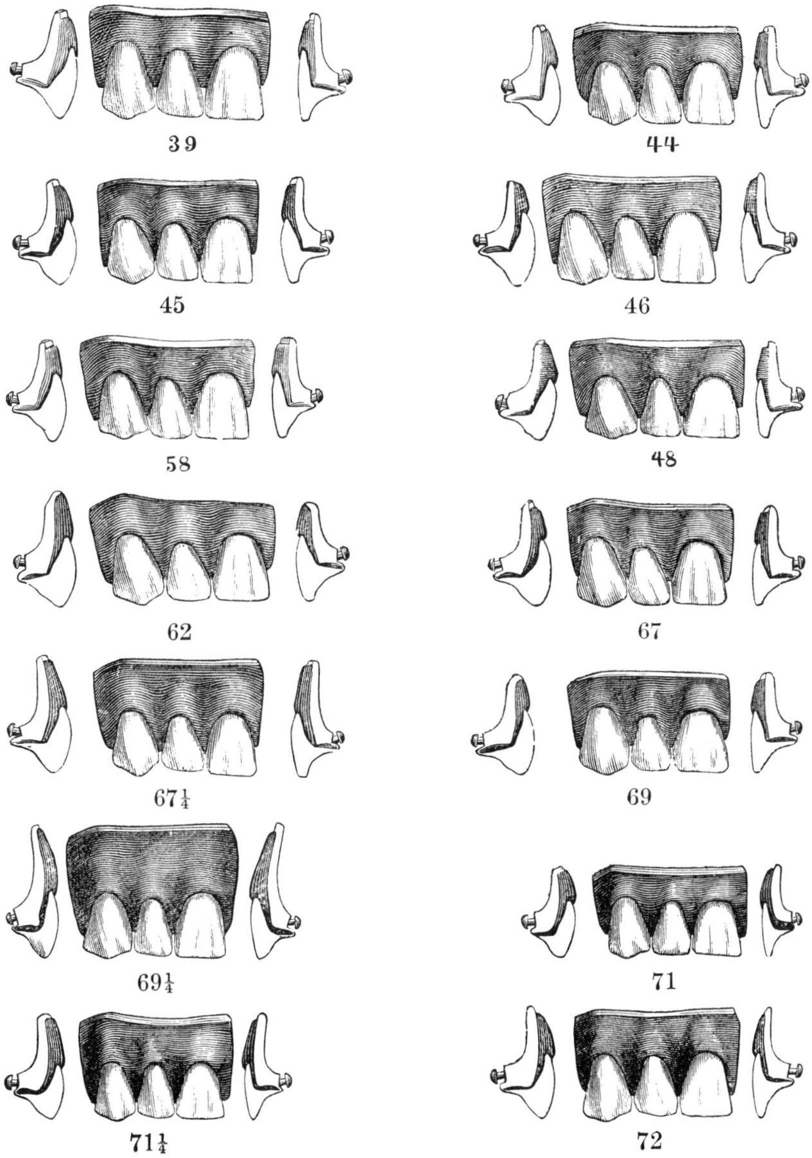

spaces. The interdental gum is also much shorter than in youth, as is finely shown in the original from which this cut is taken.

Figs. 20 and 21 illustrate additional forms of upper incisors and canines, giving a wide range of selection where teeth of this character are indicated.

In the selection of porcelain blocks, not only must the color, size, and form of the teeth be carefully considered, but reference must also be had to the curvature of the arch. For although moderate variations in curvature can be fitted by the same set of blocks, the true expression of a porcelain denture is often lost by the attempt to adapt it to a curve for which it was not designed. In Figs. 3, 9, 11, and 22 we have various curves of the alveolar arch, with corresponding variations in shape of the blocks. Sometimes the canines are made separate with a view to increase the range of application of a given set: but a joint on either side is very apt to injure the effect of this important tooth. In the lower jaw it is of less consequence because the gum is less often exposed, and it is frequently desirable to make the four incisors in one block. But in the upper jaw, it is much better to have a median joint, and another behind the canines.

In Fig. 22 the reader will notice that the centrals of the first set overlap the laterals, an arrangement of frequent occurrence in prominent and sharply-curved arches.

Fig. 22.

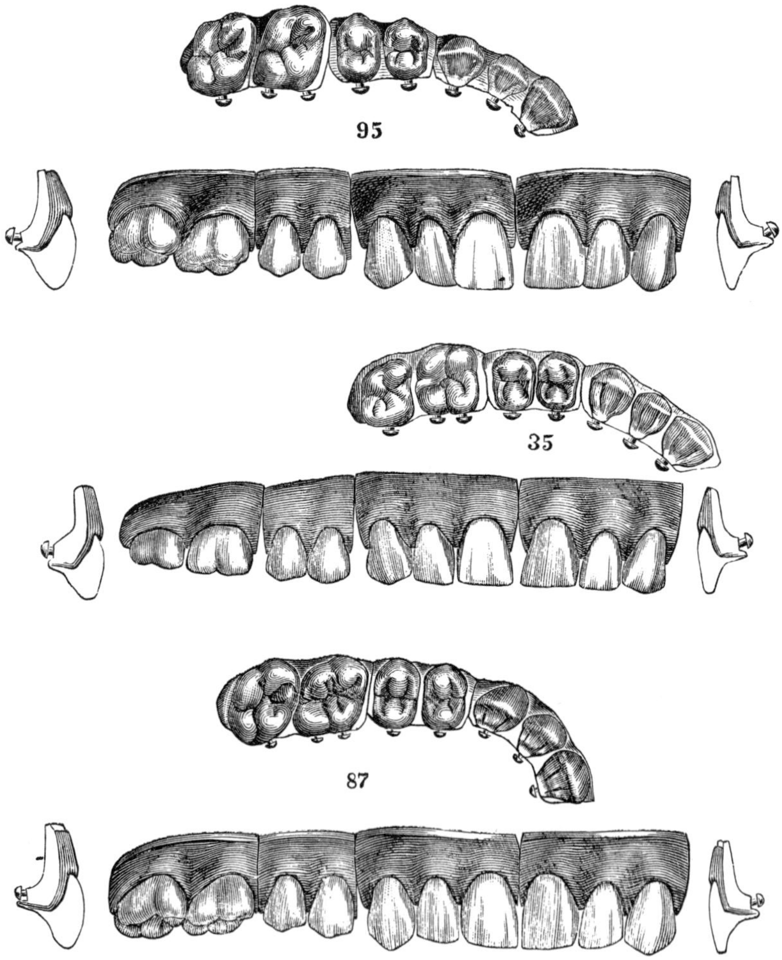

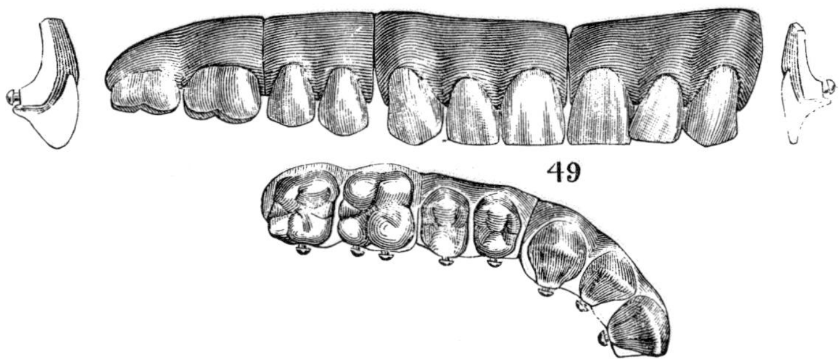

49

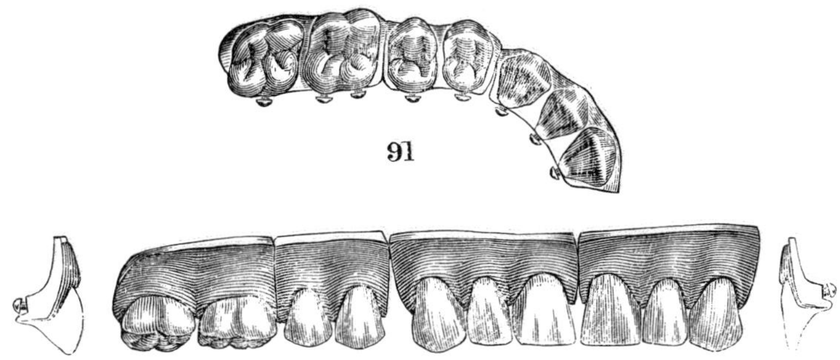

91

In the second set the blocks are so shaped that the left central overlaps its fellow. Thus we have three varieties of overlapping upper teeth; laterals over centrals, centrals over laterals, central over central; each of which may be used with great effect if applied with discrimination. In the fourth set of Fig. 22, and in a few of the preceding cuts, the gum over the cuspids is very strongly marked. This is a very characteristic feature of some mouths, and when correctly used gives a fine effect; but it would sadly belie the expression in a timid and gentle lady's face. Yet such incongruity is only one of hundreds constantly occurring where every sense of æsthetic beauty and harmony is violated,—teeth of a Russian in the mouth of a Frenchman, those of a New Englander given to a South Carolinian, or those of a Canadian to a Cuban,—the lips of age disclosing the teeth of youth, and no distinction made between a male and a female denture. These æsthetic blunders are not confined to the inexperienced tyro, but are perpetrated by many who presume to call themselves skillful mechanicians. When we consider the extensive assortment of porcelain teeth which ceramic art has placed at the disposal of the practitioner, such malpractice is without excuse.

These are only a few out of the great number of varieties, in size, form, and arrangement, of porcelain teeth; they give to the dentist a much wider range of selection than some have the ability or inclination to avail themselves of. When to variety of shape we add shades of color, the number of sets that admit of being made, distinguishable at a glance from each other, seems almost infinite. A visit to a first-class porcelain-tooth manufacturer's rooms will convince any one that incongruity or want of expression in a set of teeth is the fault of him who selects and applies rather than of him who designs and makes dental-porcelain.

It will be perceived that the foregoing illustrations of the æsthetic principles of the dento-ceramic art are taken from one class of teeth, those for vulcanite or metallo-plastic work. We have done so because the art has here had its fullest recent development, in consequence of the great demand for this form of block. But dental æsthetics is quite independent of the material of the plate so long as that which is visible in the mouth is porcelain; and dentures which show any substitute for the gum other than this, however useful they may be, cannot rank as specimens of highest art until some material for the plate shall be discovered possessing higher claims to beauty than any yet known.

Fig. 23.

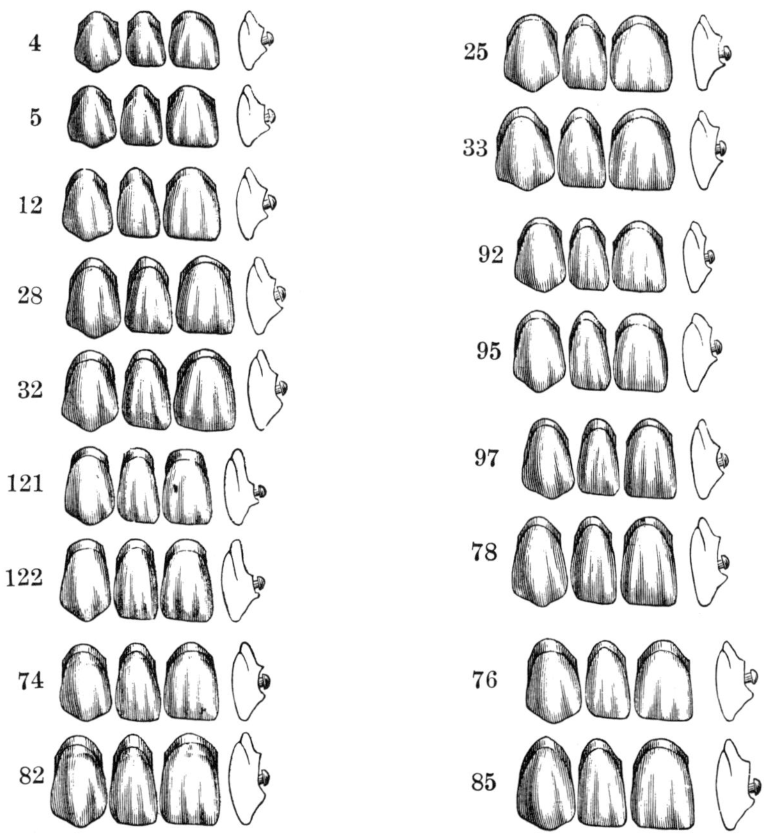

The foregoing rules will apply to the form and size of plain teeth when these are set directly upon the natural gum; but, except in case of true pivot or plate-pivot teeth, it is impossible to reproduce the precise natural arching of the gum above the tooth without some gum-colored porcelain. We must often be content, in such cases, with the nearest possible approach to nature. But when the plate is seen on the outside of the arch the artist's reputation is dependent upon the concealment of the greater part of his work; even here, however, the cutting edge and two-thirds of the tooth permit the display of great varieties of expression. Of plain teeth without gum there are four kinds.

1. Pivot teeth, shaped somewhat like the crowns of the upper incisors and canines, with a hole in the base for insertion of a wooden pivot. 2. Plate teeth, the oldest known form of porcelain teeth, having pins for attachment of a back by which to secure it to the plate. 3. Continuous-gum teeth, resembling natural teeth in having a root which is more or less serrated for better retention in the investing porcelain base; they are sometimes made without platina pins; but they are better with pins, so that they may be securely fastened to the platina plate. 4. Plain vulcanite (Fig. 23), having a small neck, by which they are held in the vulcanite or other material in which they are set. These teeth may be set directly on the gum by grinding off the neck; they may also be used adjacent to natural teeth with exposed neck, by slight alteration of this neck, so as to give to the artificial tooth the same appearance as the natural one.

There are also other forms of gum teeth besides those above represented. Formerly, single gum teeth were extensively used on gold plate, and may still be occasionally required when the supremacy of that old-fashioned material becomes once more recognized in the laboratory. The great facility of adapting blocks or sections in vulcanite work, or in vulcanite attachment to swaged plates, has led to the almost entire exclusion of this form of tooth, except for repairing. A serious objection to single gum teeth is the number of joints: these greatly mar the artistic effect which it is the design of the artificial gum to produce, especially when not kept perfectly clean, or when the material of plastic plates is allowed to enter the joints. Fig. 24 is designed to show the importance

FIG. 24.

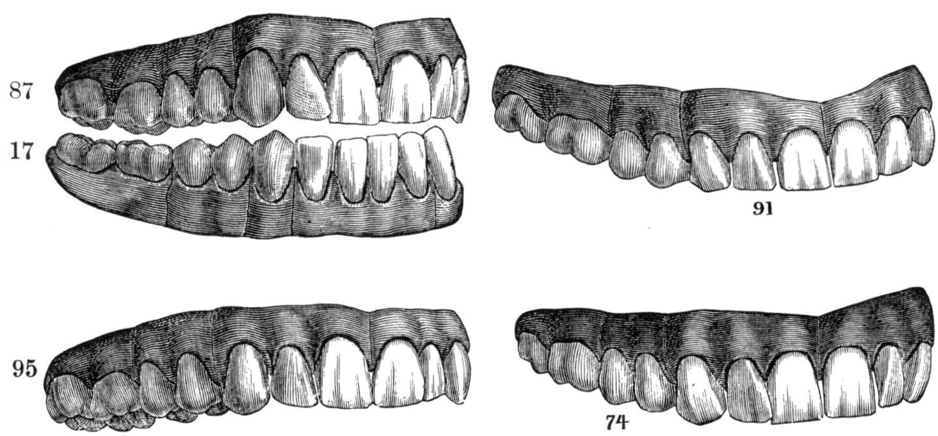

of correct and accurate grinding in order to display the true character of a set of teeth. When properly done, the joint does not interrupt the continuous surface of the gum more than the lines in the two lower sets of Fig. 24; nor should it in any case be more visible than the heavier lines of the first set. Neither should the set be so inaptly chosen as to require such grinding of joints and base as to injure its original expression. Fig. 24 should also be carefully studied by the student, on account of the varieties of form and relation of teeth presented: each of the four upper sets here displayed having a very distinctly marked character.

We cannot more appropriately close this chapter on dental-porcelain than by quoting some remarks of the great English ceramic manufacturer, Josiah Wedgwood, applicable to the art which he did so much to elevate. They have a significance beyond ceramic art; and convey, in this lesson of the past, a warning to those who may, perhaps unconsciously, be dishonoring the profession of their choice.

"All works of taste must bear a price in proportion to the skill, taste, time, expense, and risk attending their invention and manufacture. Those things called dear are, when justly estimated, the cheapest: they are attended with much less profit to the artist than those which everybody calls cheap. Beautiful forms and compositions are not made by chance, nor can they ever, in any material, be made at small expense. A competition for cheapness, and not for excellence of workmanship, is the most frequent and certain cause of the rapid decay and entire destruction of arts and manufactures."

CATALOGUE.

OPERATIVE DENTISTRY.

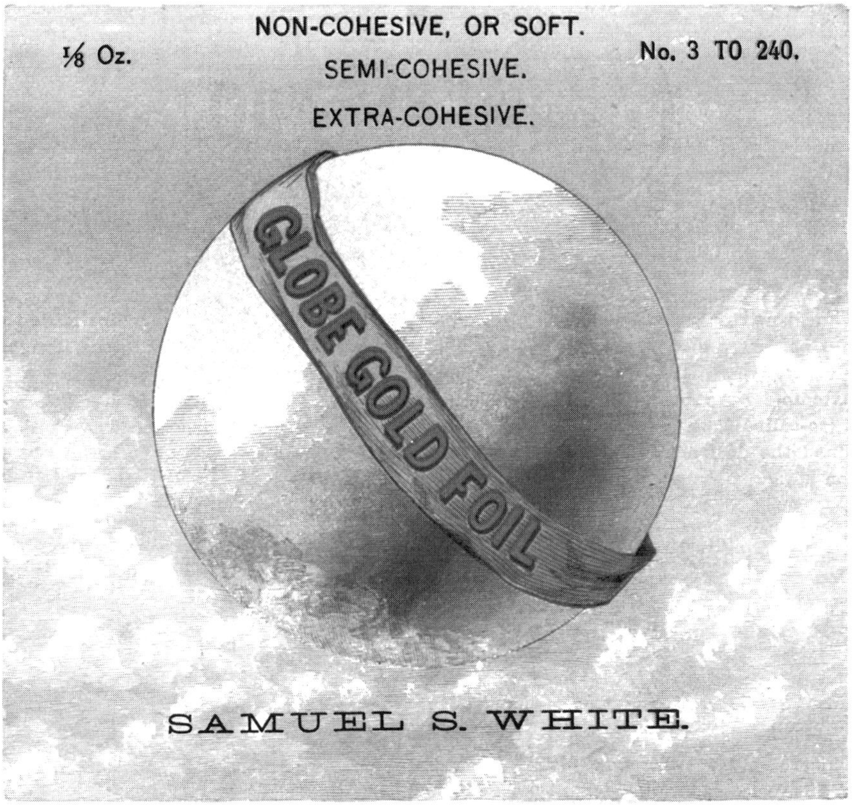

Under this distinctive title (*name and design patented March 25th, 1873*), attention is solicited to a GOLD FOIL in three distinct grades, *uniform* in their qualities, presentin , it is believed, all the variety desired in foil.

An unparalleled sale and an unprecedented unanimity in the recognition and hearty indorsement of this Foil show the appreciation by the Profession of its quality, and of the essential differences in the various grades and their varying adaptability to different operations. The terms employed to designate the several varieties are intended to express marked distinctions in their physical properties, and consequently in their relative fitness for different purposes. The term COHESIVE implies that different pieces of it will cohere or stick together by mere pressure, as if one mass. The term *adhesive*, hitherto used, rather indicates that it will adhere or stick to other things, not to itself.

THE NON-COHESIVE OR SOFT FOIL

is an exceedingly soft gold, which, when made up into masses, as blocks, cylinders, or pellets, yields readily under the instrument, without "balling," as it is termed.

THE EXTRA-COHESIVE FOIL

is a grade which, in the *stale* condition, may be worked cohesively in the form of pellets or ribbons; but when heated in the flame of an alcohol lamp, it becomes exceedingly cohesive, and can then be used successfully only by those who fully understand how to take advantage of this property. Attention is called to the unusual softness exhibited by this grade of gold under the *burnisher*, after having been packed cohesively.

THE SEMI-COHESIVE FOIL

is a grade between the soft or non-cohesive and the extra-cohesive. It will satisfy the wants of many who do not desire the greatest cohesiveness, and yet feel the need of more of this quality than can be developed by heating the soft foil.

We claim a uniformity of quality of each grade of this foil not hitherto attained.—a result of new and skillful processes, used only in the manufacture of

THE GLOBE GOLD FOIL.

☞ When ordering, state the *kind* of Foil desired. For sale in all numbers, from 3 to 240.

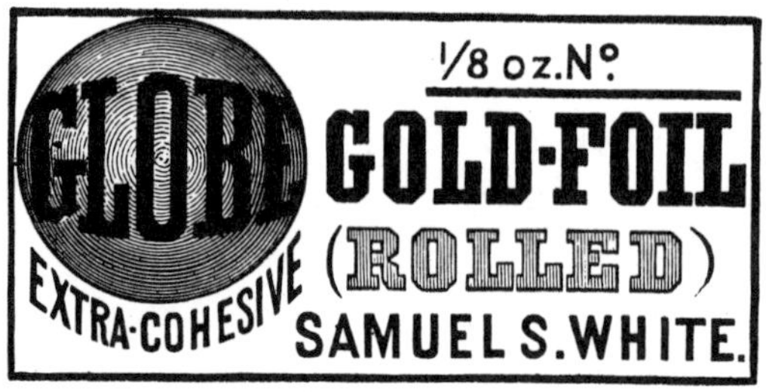

The growing use of heavy gold for finishing fillings has made it very desirable that it should possess all the cohesiveness possible, combined with all the softness, toughness, and tenacity of which gold is capable.

Attempts have been made heretofore to attain these results, but much of the rolled gold (so-called) has been reduced in part by the ordinary process of beating. We have obtained the desired qualities in the highest degree, and now have the pleasure of offering an

Extra-Cohesive Globe Gold Foil,

PREPARED WITH GREAT CARE

ENTIRELY BY ROLLING.

This rolled Foil has now been in use for several months, giving, in each case heard from, entire satisfaction.

The commendations which it has received enable us to claim that it is softer than beaten gold, and therefore greater in its adaptability to margins, and in its solidity and strength after packing; and that to produce these results it requires less labor than any heavy beaten gold previously used.

Put up in small envelopes bearing the cut which heads this page.

Nos. 30, 40, 60, and 120 kept in stock.

SAMUEL S. WHITE'S

One-Quarter of a Century

DENTISTS' SUPERIOR GOLD FOIL.

This FOIL has been known to the profession for about a quarter of a century. Under the names successively of Jones & White; Jones, White & McCurdy; Jones & White, and Samuel S. White, it has had a large and steadily increasing sale. Many who adopted it when first introduced are still using it with satisfaction. As a result of an improved method of manufacture, the Foil supplied since January 1st, 1872, has been very uniform, and superior in quality to that furnished at any previous period.

This is a SOFT FOIL when used without heating. It is made quite cohesive by heating, and must then be manipulated as cohesive foil is. Supplied in all numbers, from 3 to 10.

GOLD FOIL.

Samuel S. White's Globe Gold Foil

" " " " " " Rolled

" " " One-Quarter of a Century Gold Foil

Abbey & Sons' Gold Foil

A. J. Watts's Crystal Gold Foil

" " " or Sponge Gold

James Leslie's Crystalline Gold

Morgan's Plastic Gold

All other Foils at manufacturers' prices.

Put up in one-eighth ounce books or packages.

Prices quoted each month in the DENTAL COSMOS.

TIN FOIL.

Samuel S. White's Chemically Pure Tin Foil	per book	$0.50
" " " " " Extra Tough Tin Foil, Nos. 4, 6, 8, 10, 14 18, and 20	per book	.75

COMPOSITION FILLINGS.

Hill's Stopping, in sealed envelopes of 1 dwt., 2 dwts., and ¼ oz., 25 cts., 50 cts., and	$1.25
Houghton's Os-Artificiel, per box	1.00
" " " Gum Color, per box	1.00
Oxychloride of Zinc, Smith's, 1 oz. package, assorted Colors	4.00
" " " " 1 oz. " plain form	1.00
" " " " ¼ oz. " glass-stoppered bottle	1.00
Guillois's Cement, Nos. 0, 1, 2, 3, and 4—1 oz. package	3.00
" " Nos. 1, 2, 3, and 4—½ oz. "	1.75
" " Assorted in 1 oz. packages, Nos. 1, 2, 3 only	3.50
" " No. 5, Gum Color, 1 oz. package	3.00
" " No. 5, " " ½ oz. "	1.75
Lawrence's Amalgam, per oz.	3.00
Townsend's " "	2.00
" " Improved, per oz.	3.00
Arrington's New Amalgam, per oz.	4.00
Cement Plombe, Nos. 1, 2, 3, and 4—1 oz. package	3.00
Oehlecker's White Enamel Stopping, Nos. 1, 2, 3, 4, and 5—1 oz. package	2.00
" " " " Nos. 1, 2, 3, 4, and 5—½ oz. "	1.25

OZ.

TRADE MARK.

HILL'S STOPPING.

A. Hill D.D.S.

Registered May 11, 1875.

SAMUEL S. WHITE,
SOLE AGENT,
Philad'a, New York, Boston, Chicago.

BEWARE OF COUNTERFEITS!
The genuine is sold (in any quantity) in Sealed Packages only, bearing the above TRADE MARK.

"In consequence of a *spurious* article thrown upon the market, under the title of '**Hill's Stopping,**' and the shameless course of certain individuals who prefer fraud to honesty and fair dealing, and in order that those who desire it may be saved from deception, I hereby announce to all whom it may concern, that

SAMUEL S. WHITE

will hereafter have the EXCLUSIVE AGENCY OF THIS MATERIAL.

"*All dealers will hereafter be able to purchase of him at the same rates as heretofore of myself;* and all so purchasing will have the assurance of getting the *genuine* article.

"A. HILL.

"NORWALK, CONN., Feb. 8th, 1872."

Since the death of Dr. Hill, we have received information, believed to be reliable, that an imitation, externally, of Hill's Stopping, but of very poor quality, has been offered for sale by travelers in some portions of New England. We therefore republish the above caution, written by Dr. Hill because of similar practices, reminding the Dental Trade and Profession that this House is still the SOLE AGENCY for the sale of the genuine Hill's Stopping.

Hill's Stopping is now *sold only in sealed envelopes*, bearing the label which heads this page, containing 1 dwt., 2 dwts., and ¼ oz.

Prices, 25 cts., 50 cts., $1.25; per oz., $5.00.

GUILLOIS'S CEMENT.

"Dealers and dentists are cautioned against imitations and counterfeits of this Cement. In order that all who desire may have a guarantee of the genuineness of my Cement, I have appointed Mr. SAMUEL S. WHITE EXCLUSIVE AGENT for the United States and Canada, who will fill all orders from the trade.

"A. GUILLOIS."

CEMENT PLOMBE.

THE CELEBRATED GERMAN CEMENT FILLING.

"Dealers and Dentists are cautioned against imitations and counterfeits of our Cement. In order that all who desire may have a guarantee of the genuineness of our preparation, we have appointed Mr. SAMUEL S. WHITE EXCLUSIVE AGENT for the United States and Canada, who will fill all orders from the trade.

"GRASS & WORFF."

WHITE ENAMEL STOPPING.

"Dealers and Dentists are cautioned against imitations and counterfeits of this Stopping. That all who desire to use it may have a guarantee of its genuineness, I have appointed Mr. SAMUEL S. WHITE EXCLUSIVE AGENT for the United States and Canada, who will fill all orders from the trade.

"F. OEHLECKER."

Dental Instruments.

At the Fair of the American Institute, New York (Exhibition October, 1869), the First Premium was awarded to us for SUPERIOR DENTAL INSTRUMENTS.

At the Fair of the Maryland Institute, Baltimore (Exhibition November, 1869), a Gold Medal was awarded to us for EXCELLENCE OF DENTAL INSTRUMENTS.

At the Cincinnati Industrial Exposition (Exhibition of October, 1870), the Premium was awarded for Superiority in Dental Instruments, the Judges reporting as follows:

"In the competition for Dental Instruments, we unhesitatingly recommend S. S. White *as first in merit.*"

EXTRACT FROM REPORT OF THE COMMITTEE ON INSTRUMENTS OF THE AMERICAN INSTITUTE:

"We have carefully examined the Dental Instruments exhibited by S. S. White, and find them of superior finish and excellent temper. We would particularly mention the perfection with which the burs and the serrations on the points of the filling instruments are cut: the shapes of the various kinds of filling instruments are admirable. In accordance with the wish expressed by the Board of Managers, we were very particular in testing the temper of these instruments, to ascertain if this important point had been attended to with the same care and skill as were evident in the other parts of their construction, and we found that in this particular their manufacture had been as carefully conducted as in the other parts, and that the instruments had the varieties of temper best suited to the purposes for which they were constructed. And we pronounce them to be the best we have ever seen produced by any manufacturer of Dental Instruments."

REPORT TO ILLINOIS STATE DENTAL SOCIETY, BY COMMITTEE ON INSTRUMENTS AND APPLIANCES:

"Some of the finest specimens of Instruments the Committee have ever seen are exhibited by S. S. White."

EXTRACT FROM A REPORT OF THE STATE DENTAL SOCIETY OF PENNSYLVANIA, JUNE, 1870:

"The fine points were examined by the members present with the aid of a magnifying-glass, and universal commendation expressed of the superiority in their manufacture."

REPORT OF THE COMMITTEE APPOINTED BY THE SOUTH CAROLINA DENTAL ASSOCIATION TO EXAMINE THE INSTRUMENTS AND SPECIMENS PRESENTED BY S. S. WHITE:

"They have examined the instruments with care and severe scrutiny. They have magnified the serrations of the mallet pluggers, and find them *regular*, *smooth*, *even*, *sharp*, *well-defined*, and *well-tempered*.

"The excavators were subjected to severe pressure,—many times greater than they would be put to in any operation in the mouth. One delicate hatchet excavator cut with ease a piece out of the untempered handle of another without exhibiting any dullness, mar, or hack. The finish of all these instruments is beyond our criticism."

All of the Dental Instruments and Machinery exhibited at these Fairs and Associations were selected out of regular stock on hand and for sale.

CLEVELAND, Dec. 29th, 1870.

SAMUEL S. WHITE.

DEAR SIR:—Please accept sincere thanks for the new set of finely-wrought Pluggers. They are *now* up to my present conception of the highest degree of excellence of a Mallet Plugger. I am highly pleased with the entire features of the instrument, especially the serrating. No other copies of my points or instruments that are in the market have ever received my approbation, they being inferior in manufacture, having been made without my patterns. As ever, C. R. BUTLER.

NEW YORK, February 9th, 1870.

SAMUEL S. WHITE.

DEAR DR.:—Please accept my heartiest thanks for those *exquisitely-wrought* Pluggers. They come so near my present ideal in their manufacture, that I have nothing to wish in that direction. No other copies of my points that have come under my observation will successfully stand anything but careless or hasty examination. Heretofore I have felt *obliged* to make my own plugger points, but that necessity no longer exists, as your recent productions "fill the bill"; and as the price you have put on the set is so reasonable to the mind that appreciates their *delicate accuracy* of serration, no amateur can afford to spend his time and eyesight in making his own. I am truly, etc., R. W. VARNEY.

Forceps.

OCTAGON JOINTS, EXTRA QUALITY.

These Forceps, for quality and adaptation, are not equaled by those of any other manufacturer. In ordering, state the number of the cut.

Price, per pair (excepting Nos. 29, 30, 62, 66, 67)	. . . . . .	$3.00
" " Nos. 29, 30, and 62	. . . .	2.75
" " Nos. 66 and 67	. . . .	3.50

Nickel-Plated, 50 cents each additional. Silver-Plated, $1.00 each additional

ROOT FORCEPS.

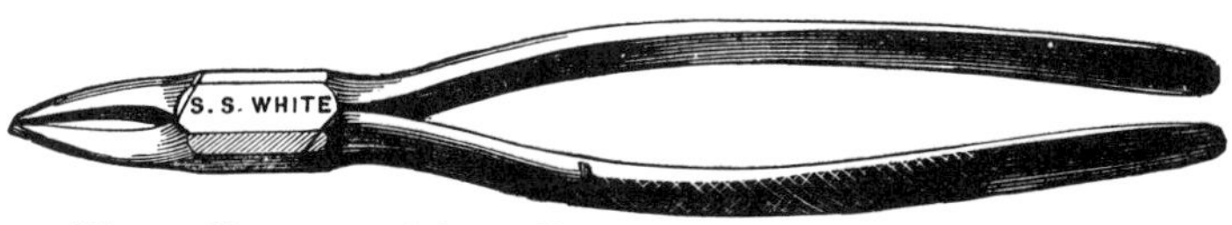

No. 1—Root, Upper Front, straight. Four sizes: Long slender, large, medium, and small.

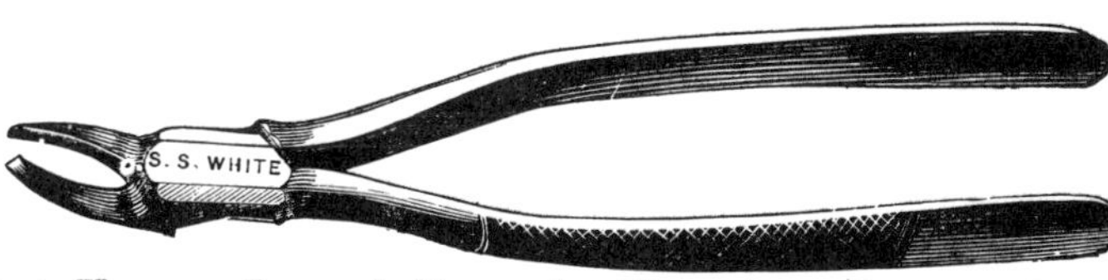

No. 2—Root, Upper or Lower, half curved. Three sizes: Large, medium, and small.

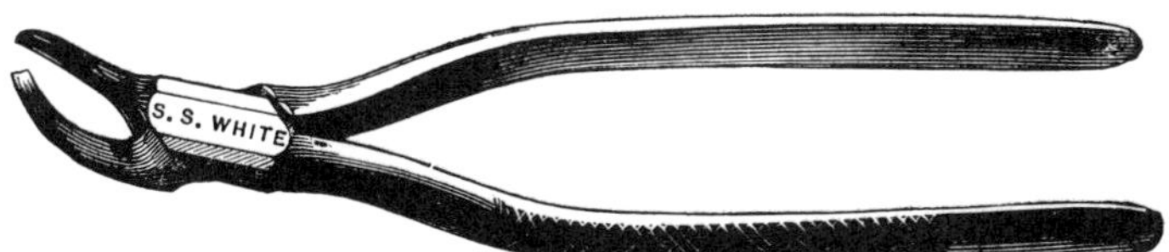

No. 3—Root, Lower, full curved. Three sizes: Large, medium, and small.

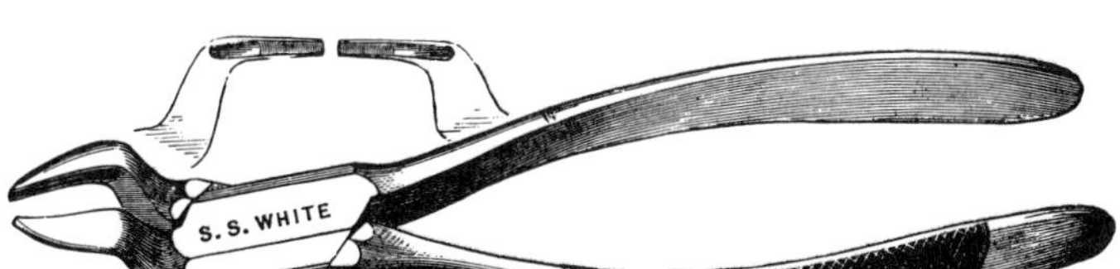

No. 35—Root, bayonet-shape.

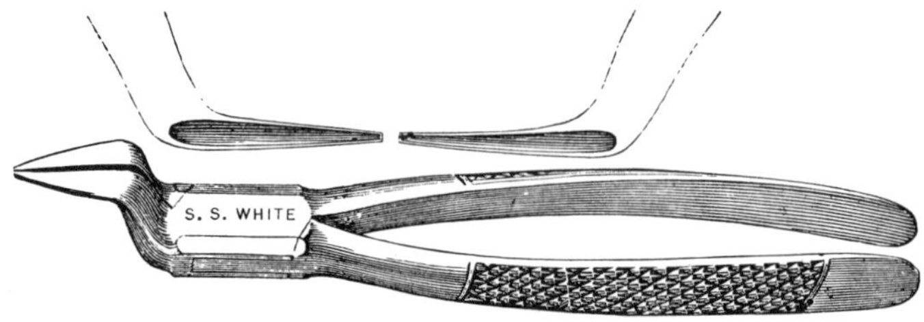

No. 65—Root, bayonet-shape, slender beak, for difficult roots in the Upper Jaw, and roots of Front Teeth in the Lower Jaw (Arrington's).

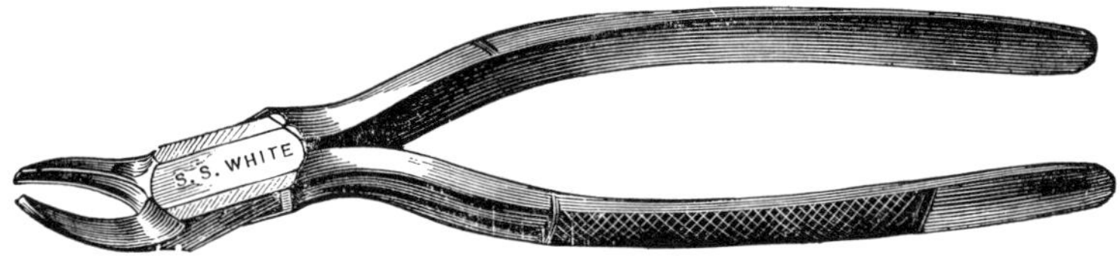

No. 7—Root, Upper Back, universal.

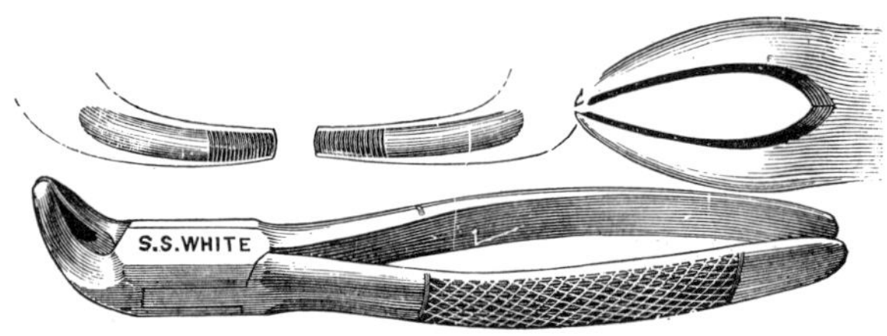

No. 49—Root, Lower Molar, with crowns, for either side.

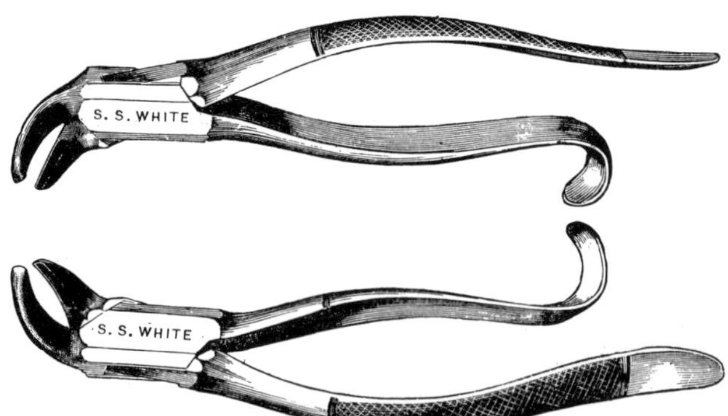

No. 50—Root, Lower, right and left,—two pairs.

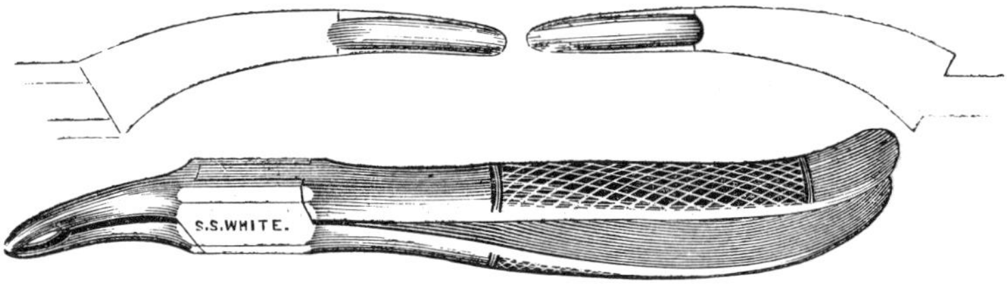

No. 63—Spicula, universal.

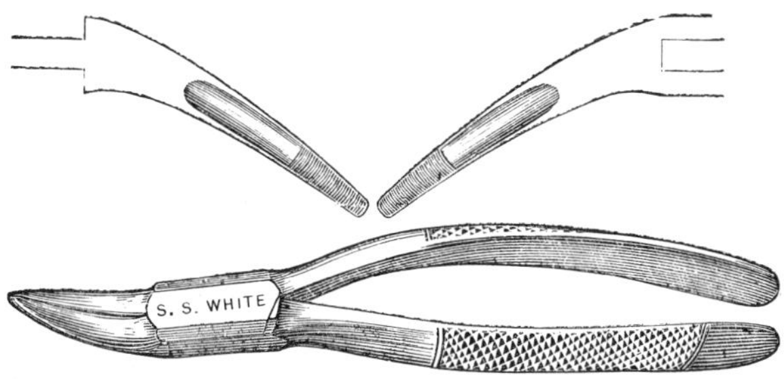

No. 69—Fragment or Small Root, universal (Tomes's).

ALVEOLAR FORCEPS.

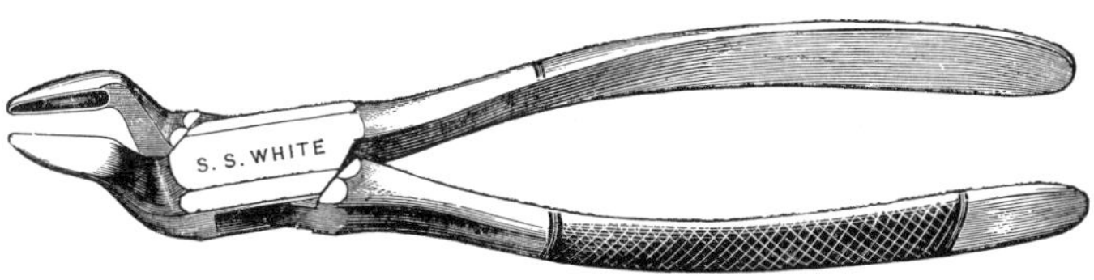

No. 32—Alveolar, bayonet-shape (Parmly's).

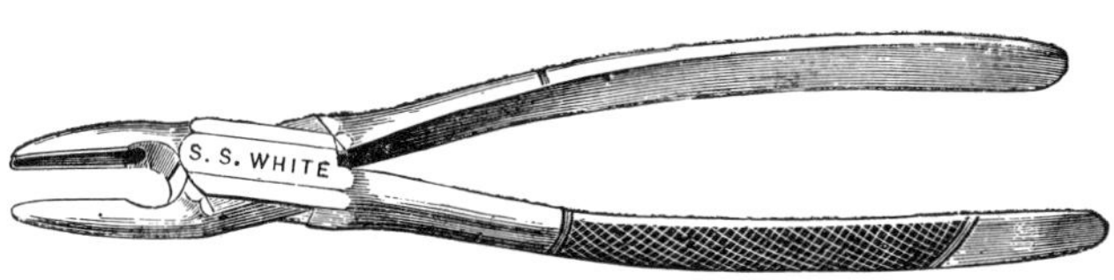

No. 33—Alveolar, straight beak (Parmly's).

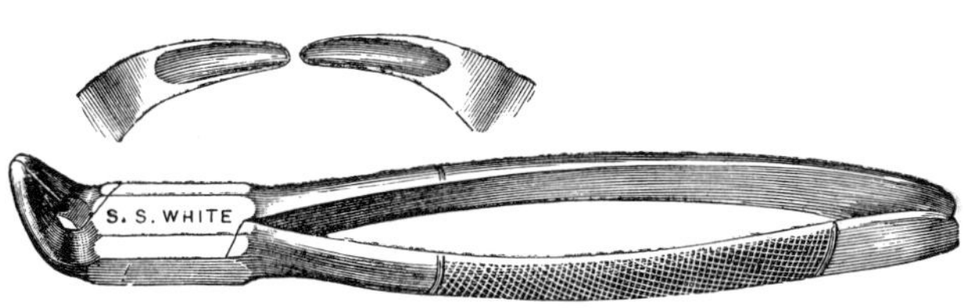

No. 34—Alveolar, curved beak (Parmly's).

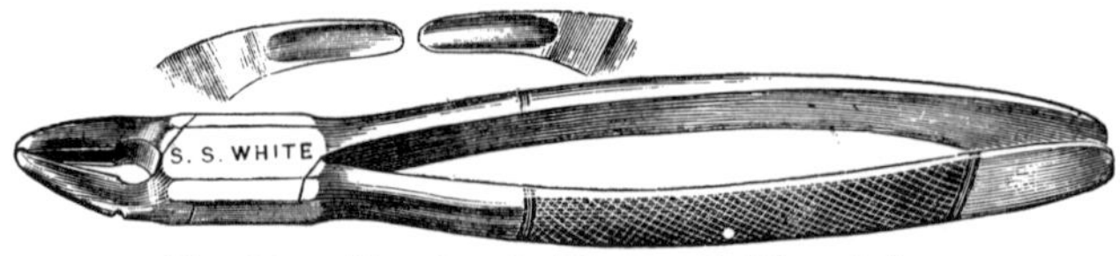

No. 39—Alveolar, half curved (Parmly's).

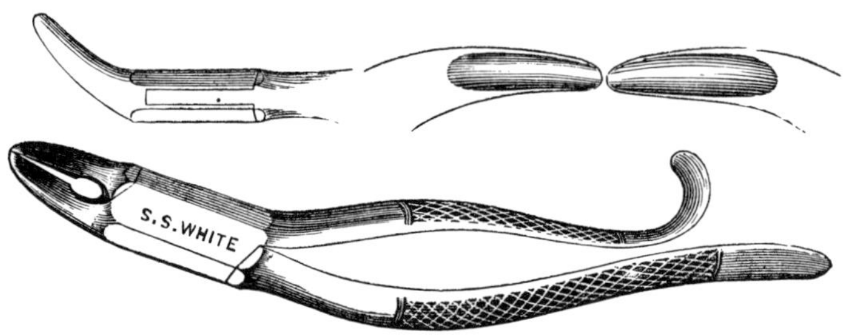

No. 52—Alveolar, Lower, for either side (Parmly's).

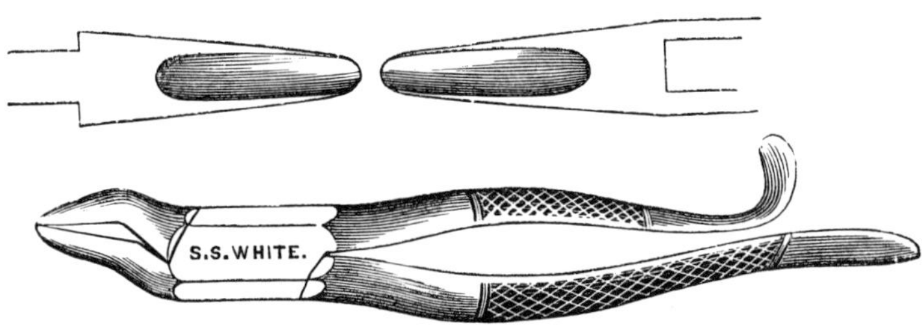

No. 58—Alveolar, Upper Incisor and Cuspid.

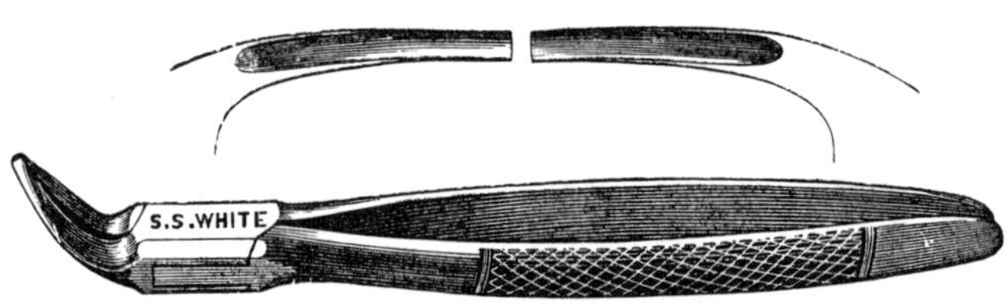

No. 41—Alveolar, long beak, half curved.

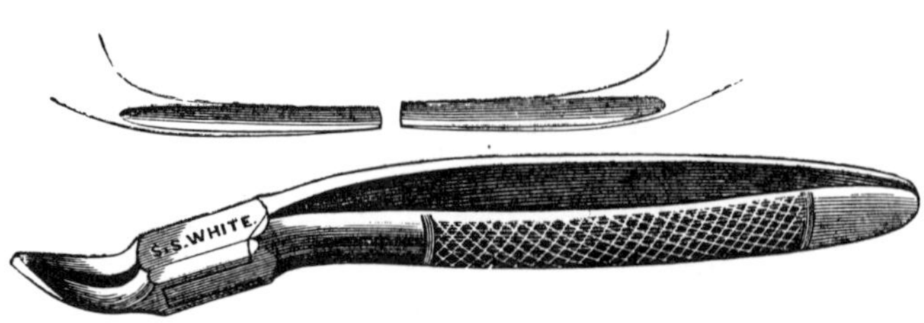

No. 42—Alveolar, Upper Back, long beak.

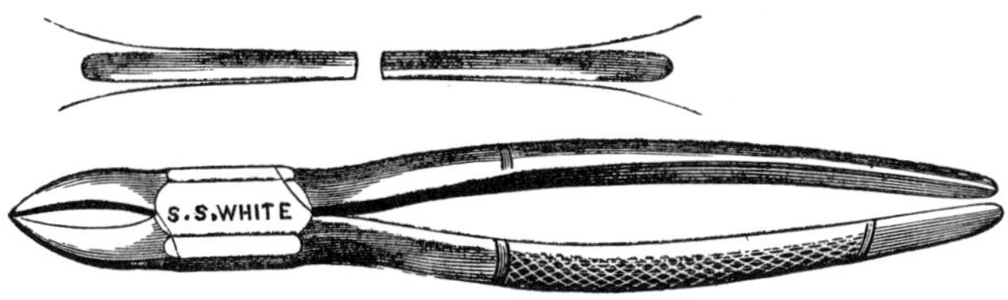

No. 43—Alveolar, long beak, straight.

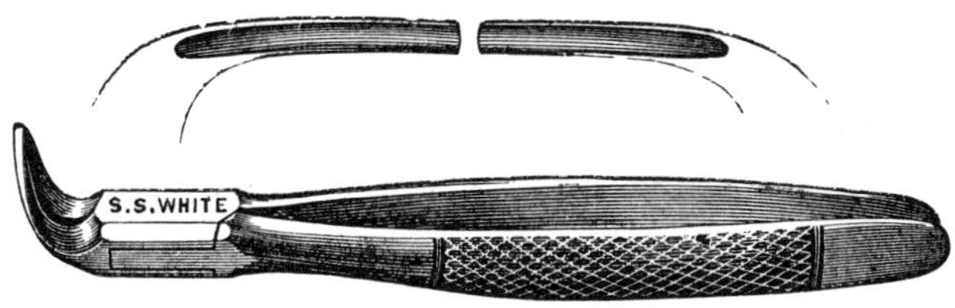

No. 44—Alveolar, long beak, full curved.

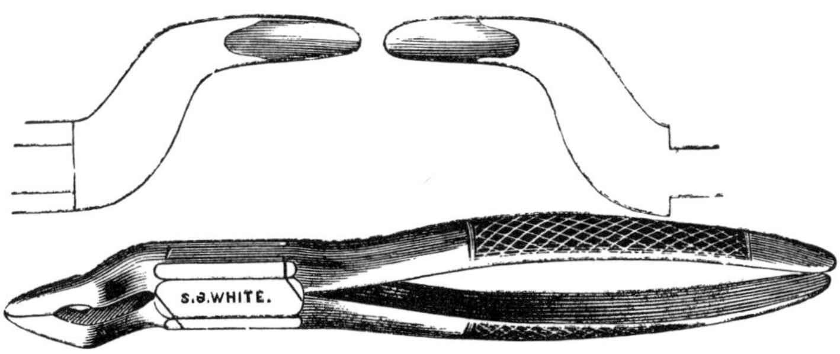

No. 61—Alveolar Nipping, Back, for cutting away processes after extraction.

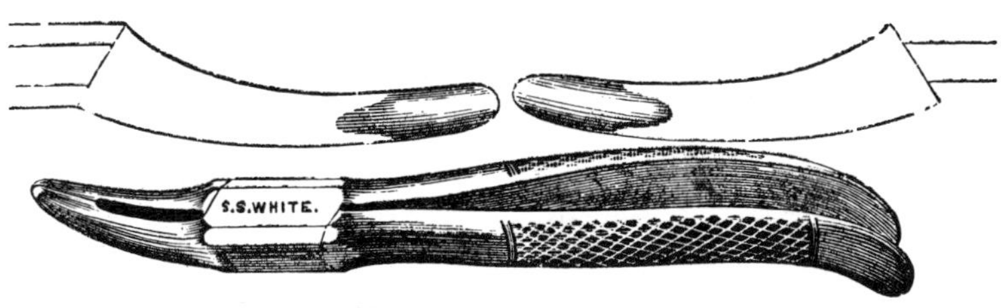

No. 64—Alveolar Nipping, Front, for cutting away processes after extraction.

FORCEPS FOR CROWDED TEETH.

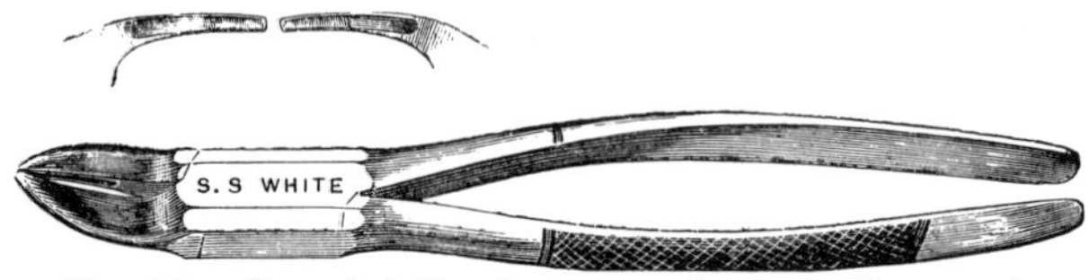

No. 36—Crowded Teeth, narrow beak, half curved.

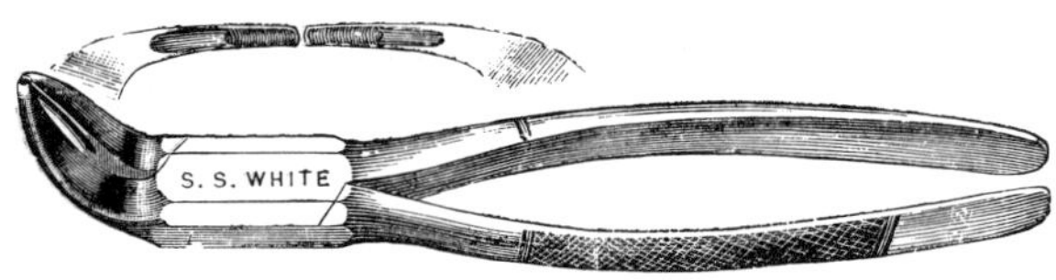

No. 37—Crowded Teeth, narrow beak, full curved.

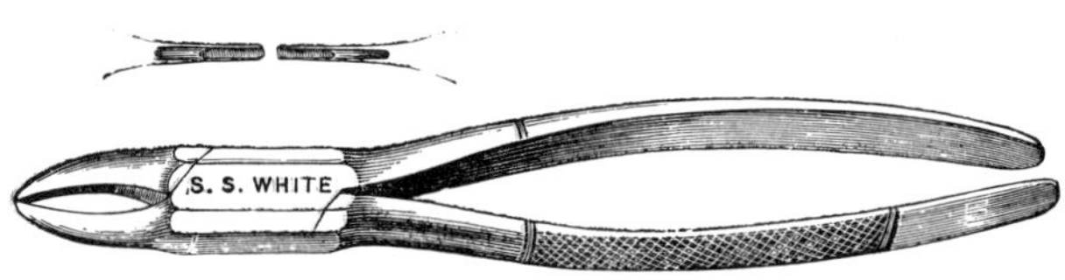

No. 38—Crowded Teeth, narrow beak, straight.

INCISOR FORCEPS.

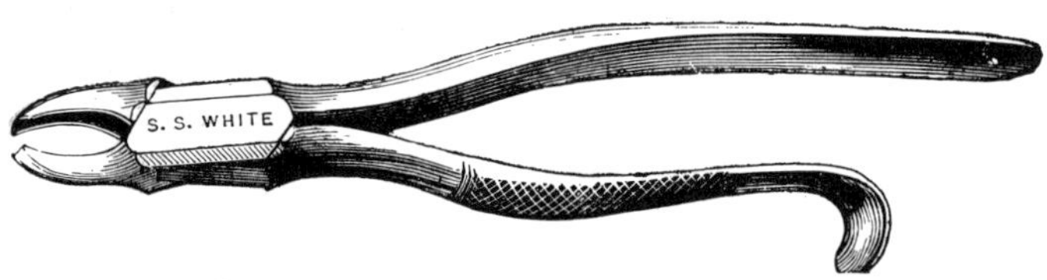

No. 13—Incisor, Upper, with or without hook on handle.

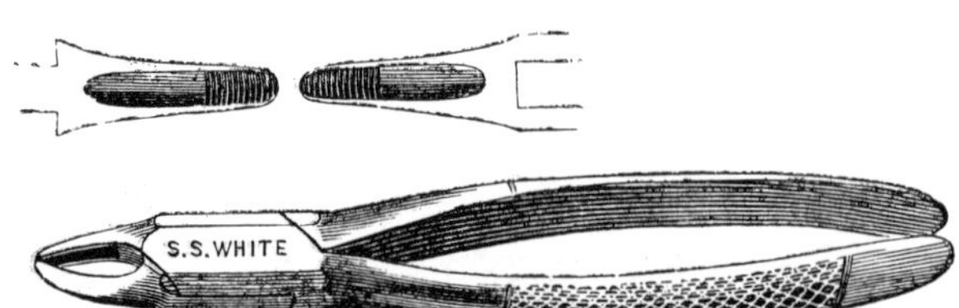

No. 48—Incisor, Upper Lateral.

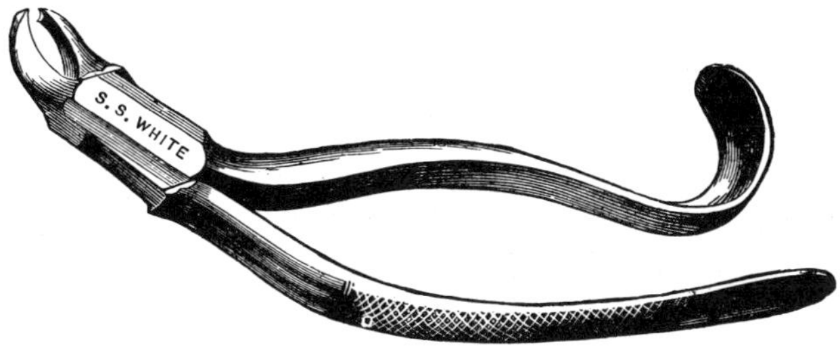

No. 9—Incisor, Lower, hawk bill.

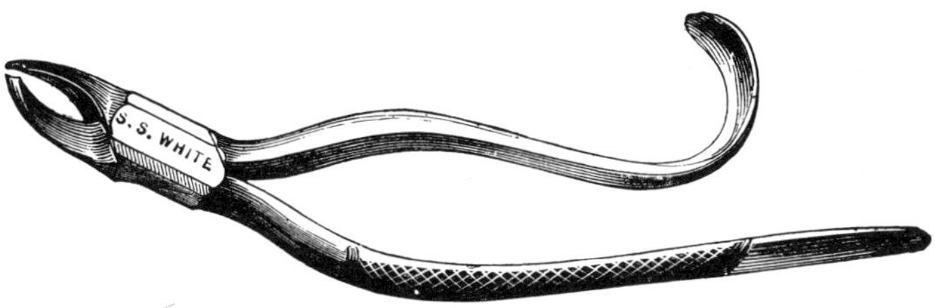

No. 14—Incisor or Bicuspid, Lower, for either side.

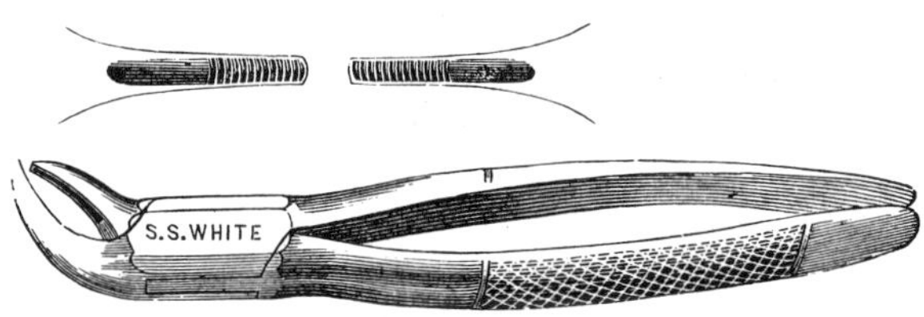

No. 46—Incisor, Lower, and Crowded Teeth, hawk bill.

BICUSPID FORCEPS

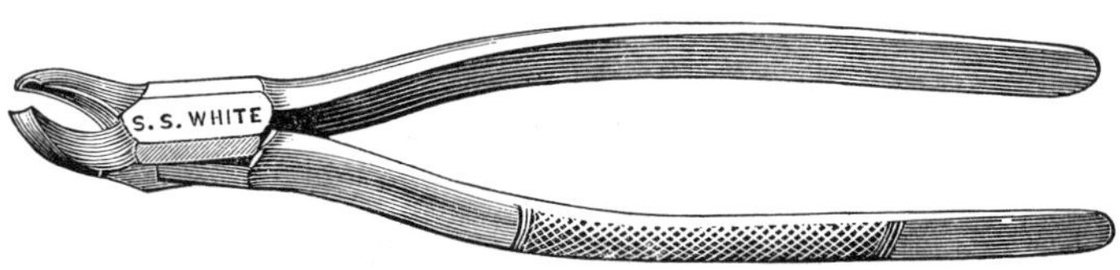

No. 4—Bicuspid, Upper or Lower, half curved.

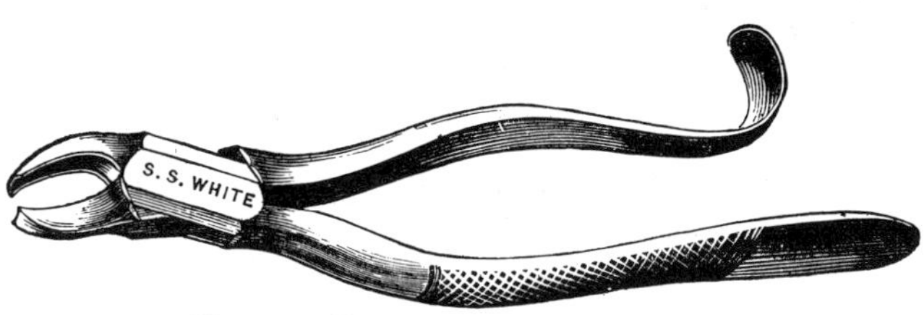

No. 11—Bicuspid or Canine, Upper.

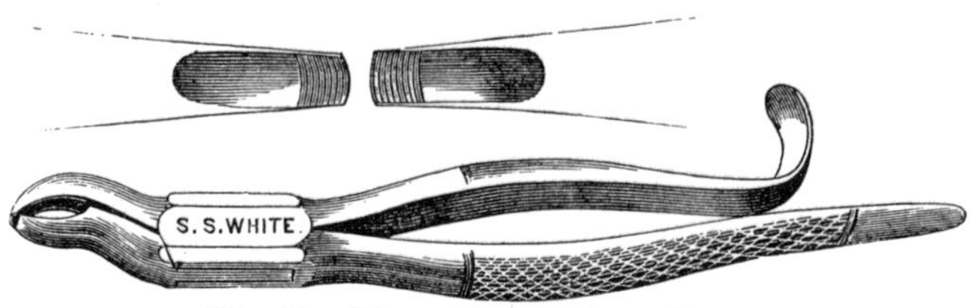

No. 40—Bicuspid or Incisor, Upper.

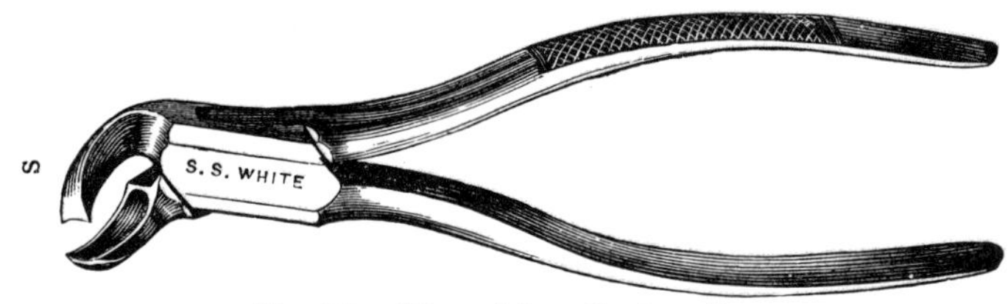

No. 21—Bicuspid or Canine, Lower.

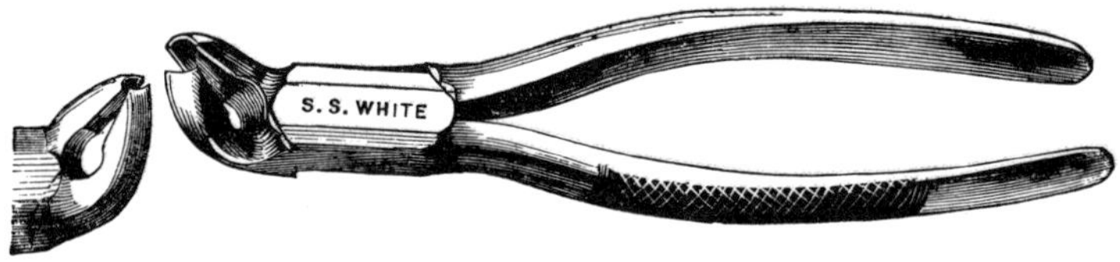

No. 25—Bicuspid, Lower, safety.

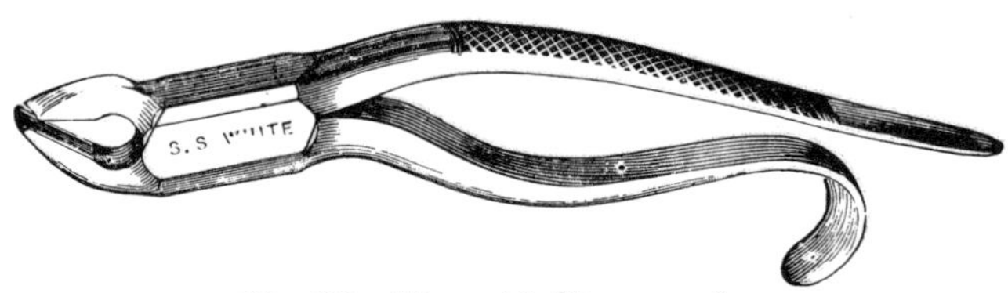

No. 26—Bicuspid, Upper, safety.

MOLAR FORCEPS.

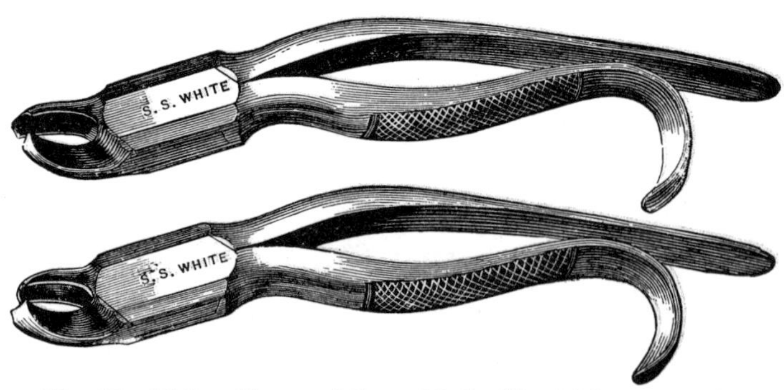

No. 18—Molar, Upper, right and left (Harris's),—two pairs.

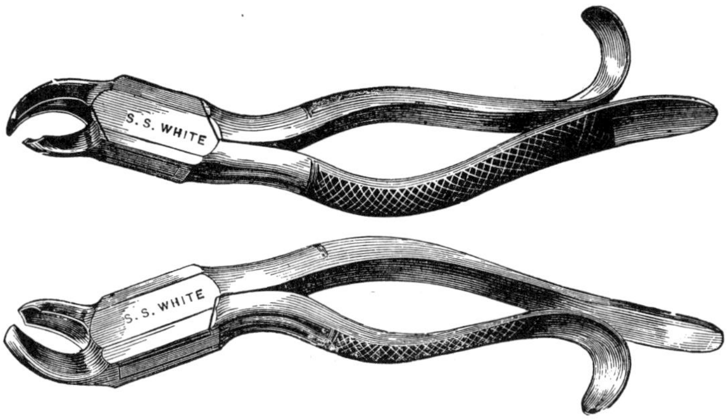

No. 19—Molar, Upper, right and left,—two pairs.

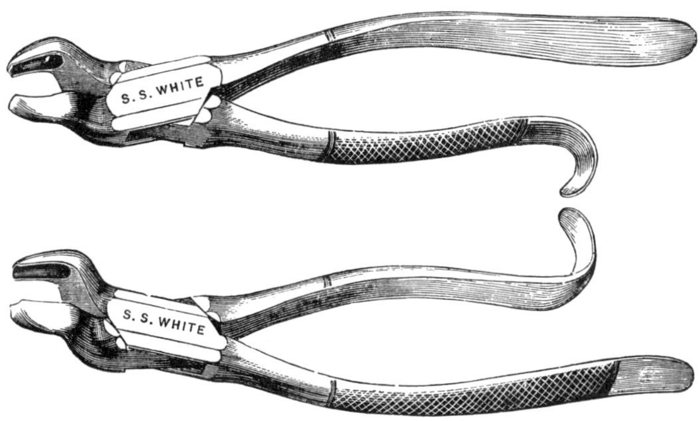

No. 53—Molar, Upper, right and left, with or without hook on handle,—two pairs.

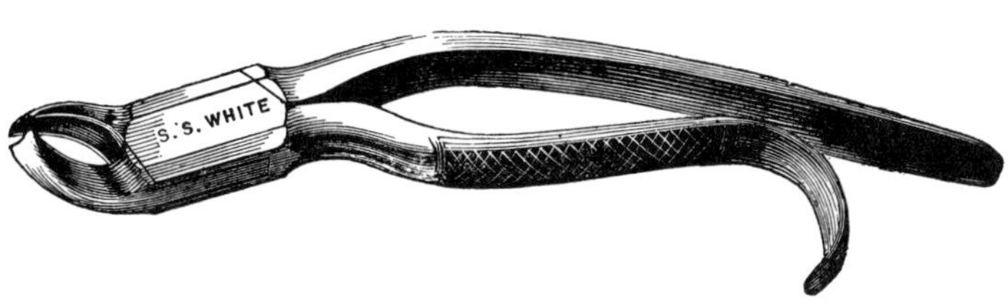

No. 24—Molar, Upper, for either side.

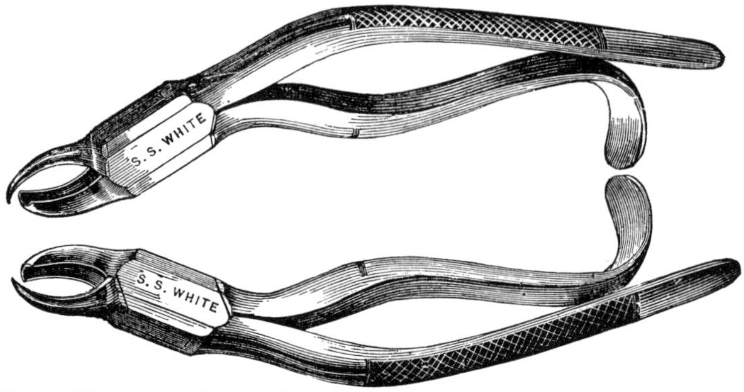

No. 20—Molar, Upper, cow horn, right and left,—two pairs, which, with No. 16, make an invaluable set for the extraction of Molar Roots when the crowns are decayed below the process.

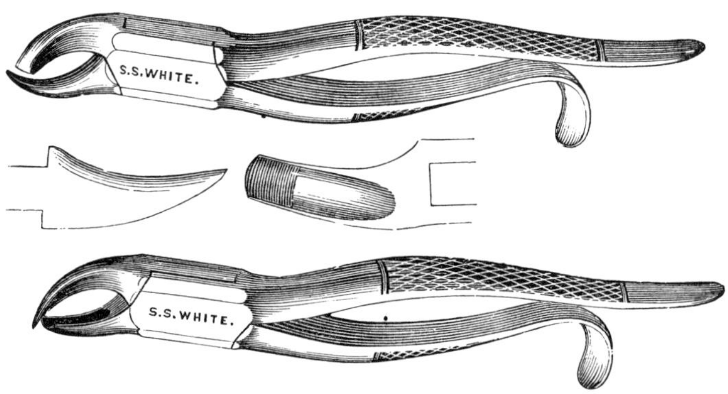

No. 59—Molar, Upper, cow horn, right and left,—two pairs.

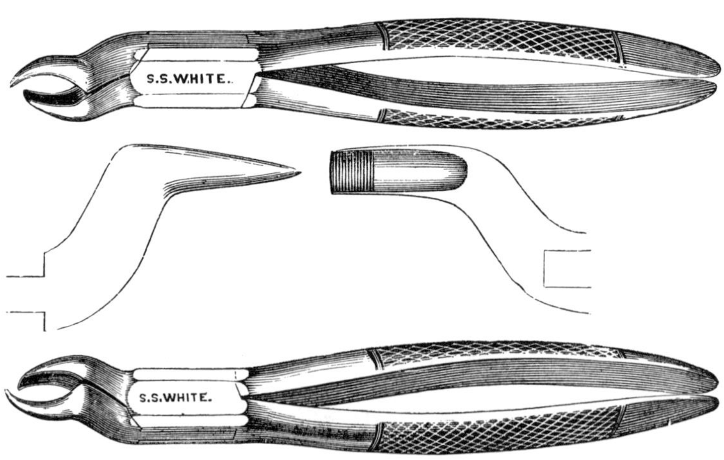

No. 57—Molar, Upper, cow horn, right and left, with or without hook on handle,—two pairs.

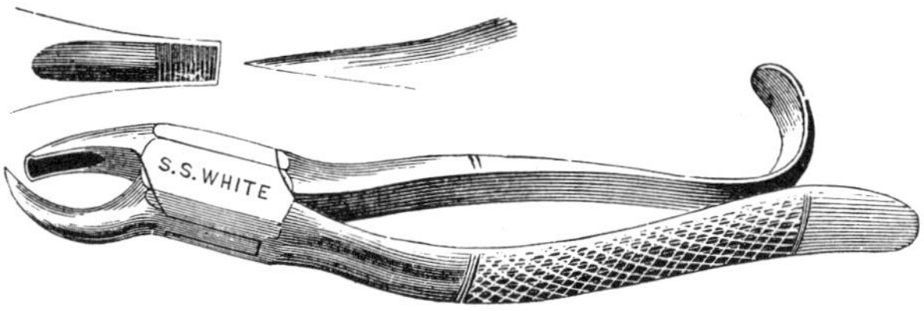

No. 45—Molar, Upper, cow horn, for either side.

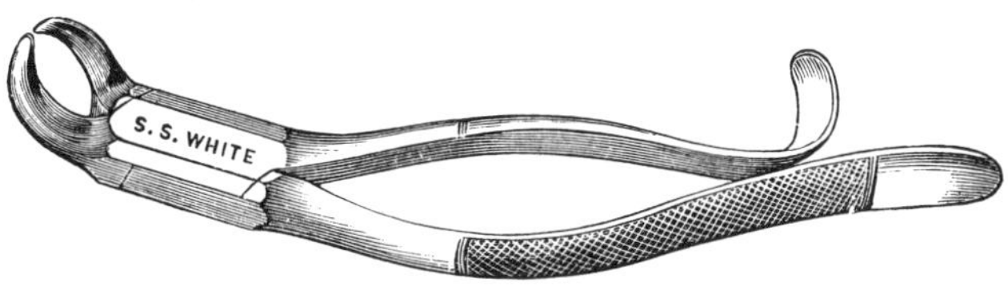

No. 55—Molar, Lower, cow horn, right side.

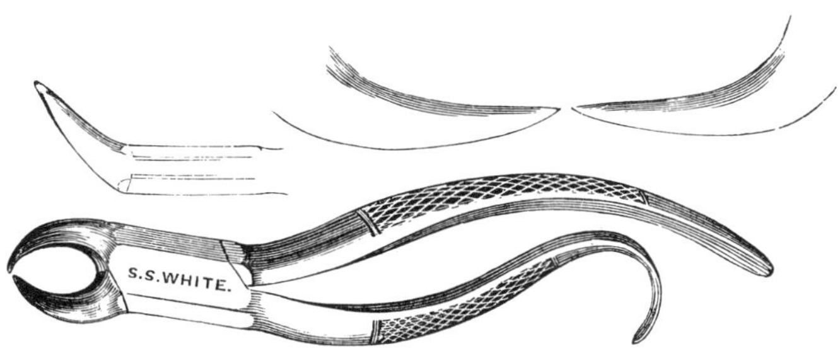

No. 56—Molar, Lower, cow horn, left side. This pair of Forceps, with the No. 55 for the right side, makes a very efficient set for Lower Molars.

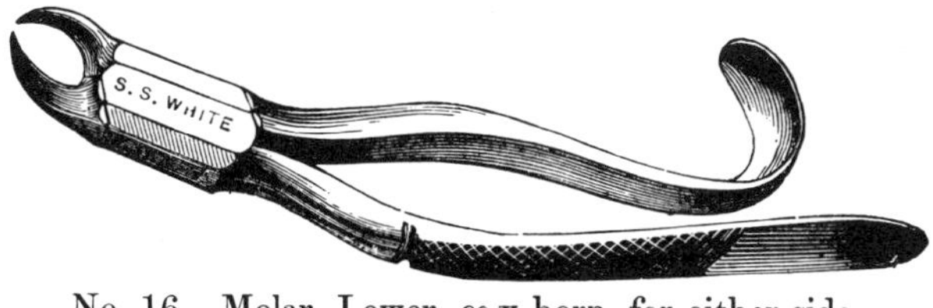

No. 16—Molar, Lower, cow horn, for either side.

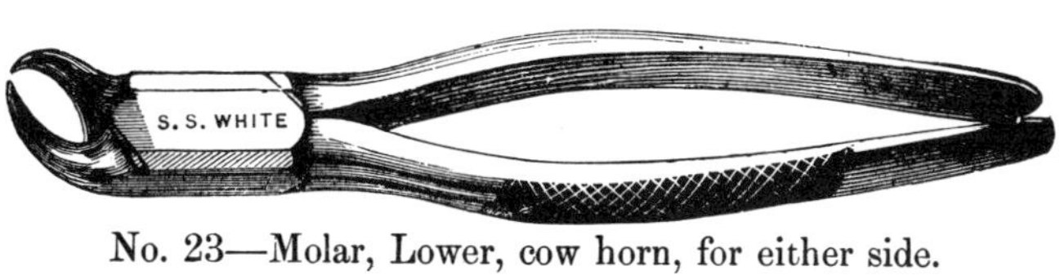

No. 23—Molar, Lower, cow horn, for either side.

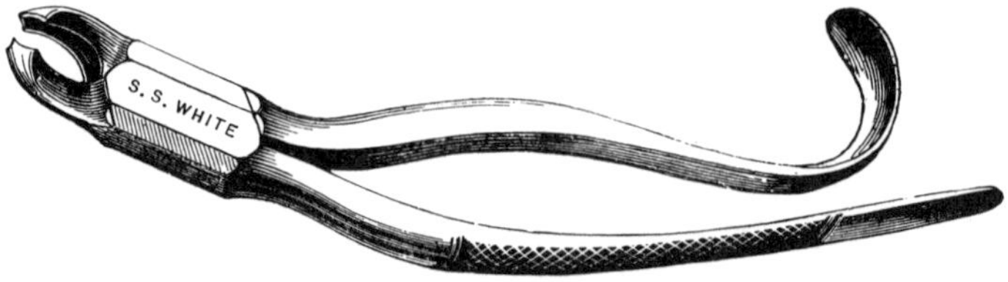

No. 15—Molar, Lower, for either side (Harris's).

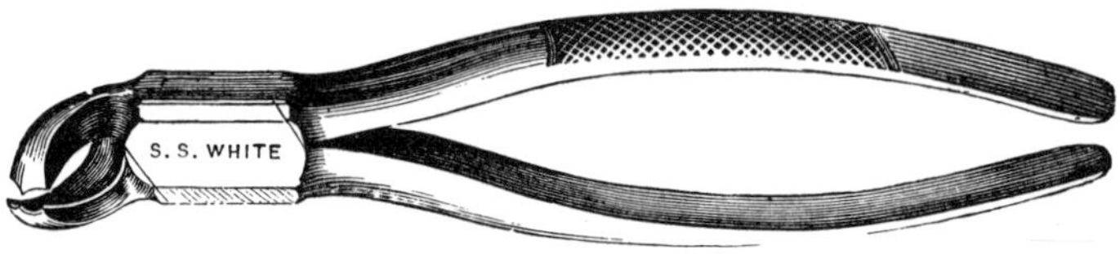

No. 17—Molar, Lower, pointed beak, for either side.

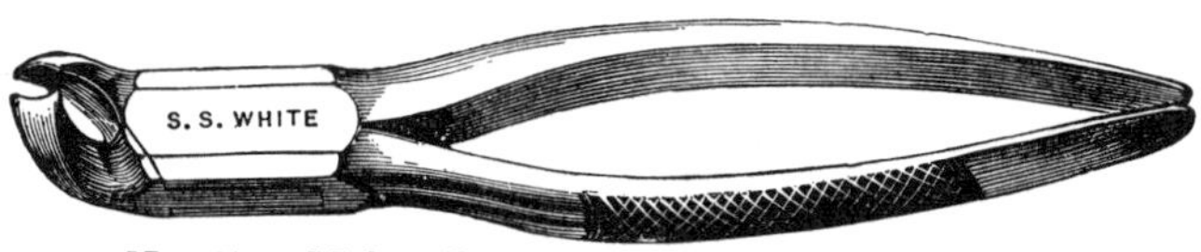

No. 27—Molar, Lower, plain beak, for either side.

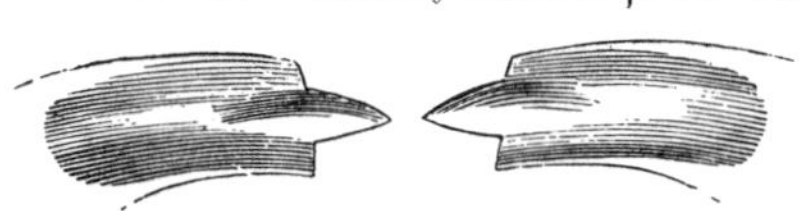

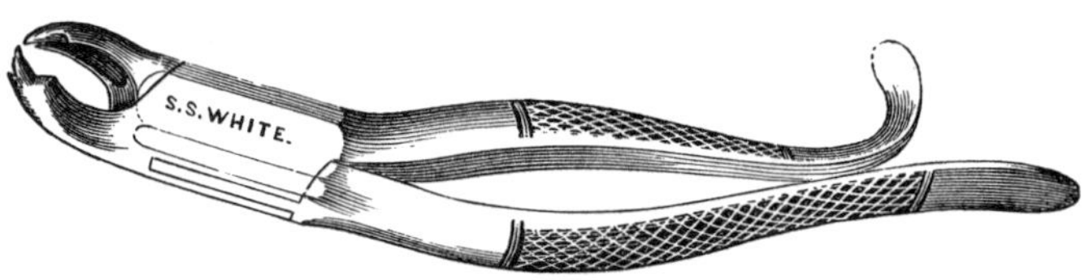

No. 60—Molar, Lower, for either side (Wolverton's).

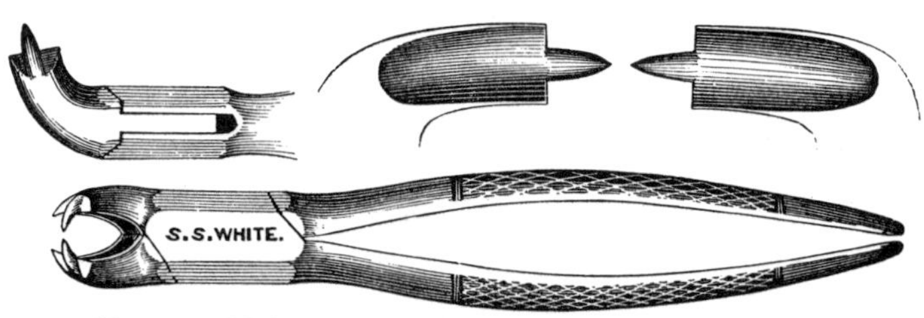

No. 51—Molar, Lower, for either side (Wolverton's).

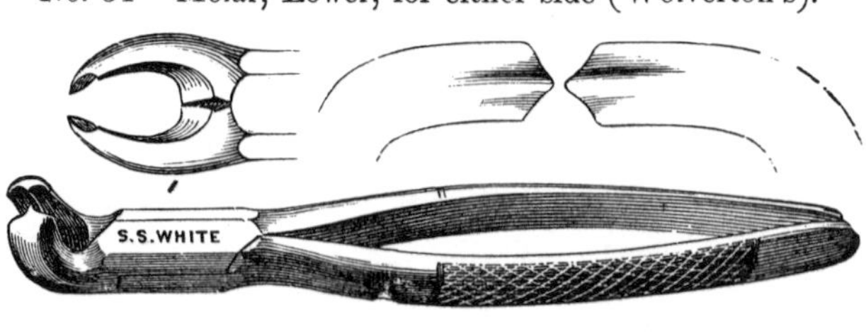

No. 47—Molar, Lower, for either side (Hutchinson's).

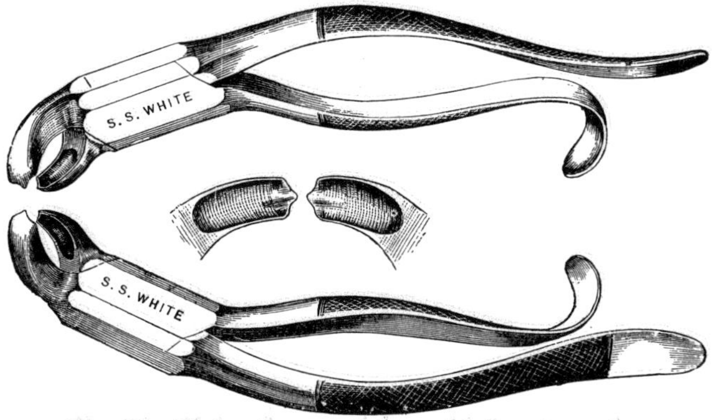

No. 28—Molar, Lower, right and left,—two pairs.

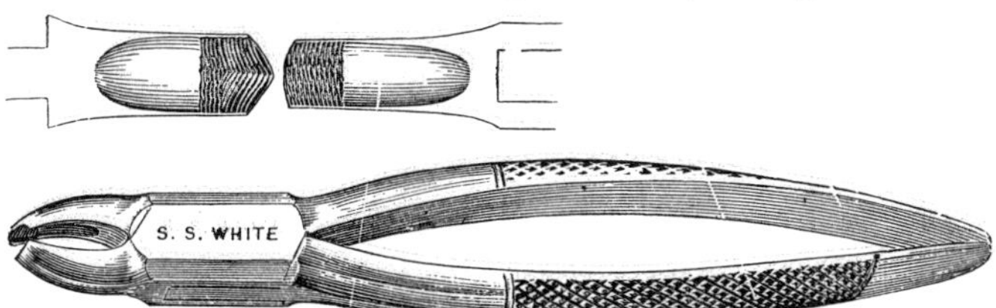

No. 68—Molar, Upper, straight, for either side (Stellwagen's).

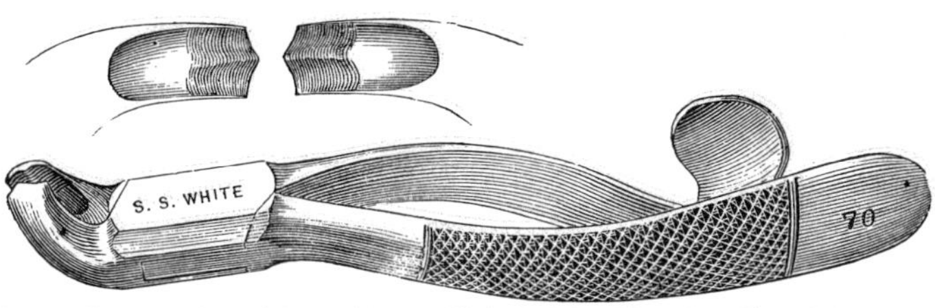

No. 70—Molar, Lower, for either side. This is like No. 15 (Harris's), except that the handles are bent upwards so as to avoid striking the upper incisors.

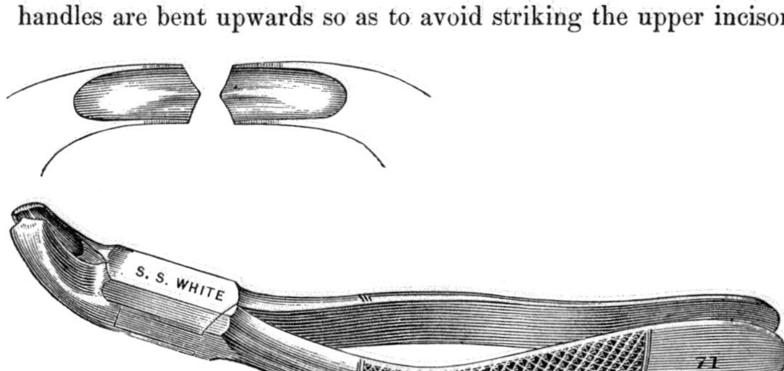

No. 71—Molar, Lower, for either side. It is curved in the handles, the reverse of No. 70, so as to bow over the lower incisors. The advantage in this construction is, that all the force of the hand tends to draw the tooth out of its socket without a separate lifting action. The inner faces of the beaks are smooth, except on the edges.

SS HC

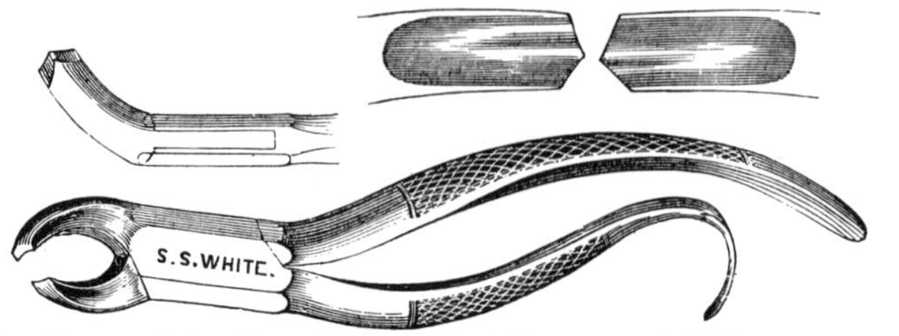

No. 54—Molar, Lower, left side. This pair of Forceps, with No. 28 for the right side, makes a very efficient set for Lower Molars.

DENTES SAPIENTIÆ FORCEPS.

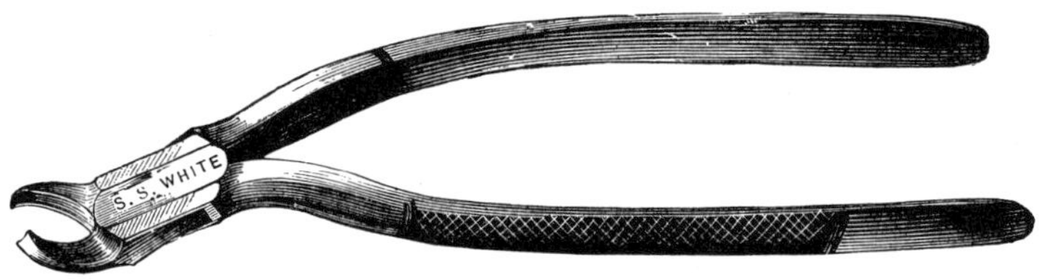

No. 8—Dentes Sapientiæ, Upper, for either side.

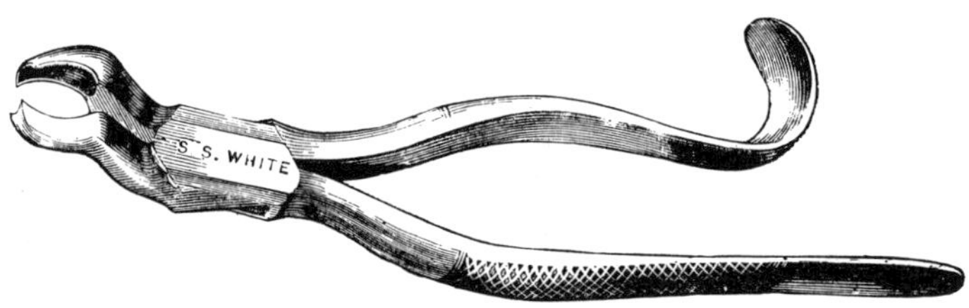

No. 10—Dentes Sapientiæ, Upper, for either side, with or without hook on handle.

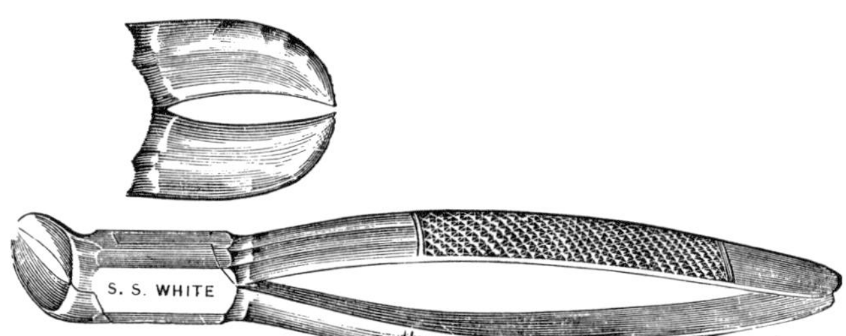

No. 5—Dentes Sapientiæ, Lower, for either side (Physick's).

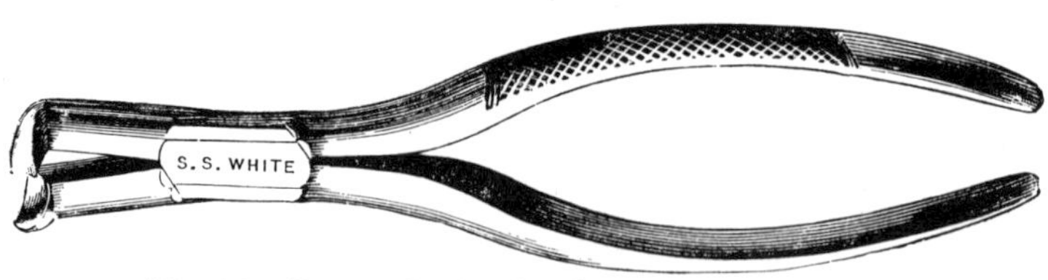

No. 22—Dentes Sapientiæ, Lower, for either side.

SEPARATING AND EXCISING FORCEPS.

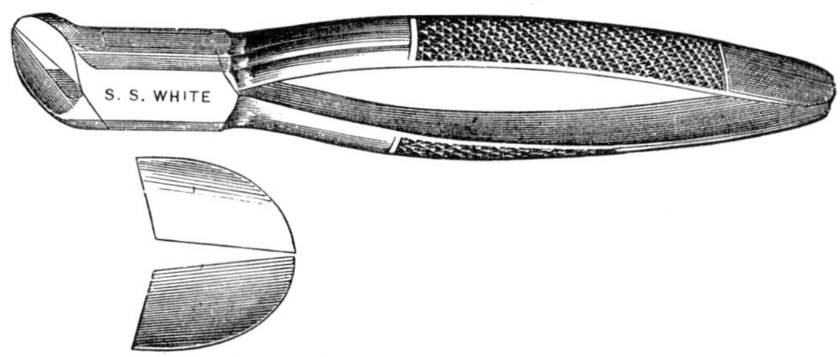

No. 6—Separating or Splitting.

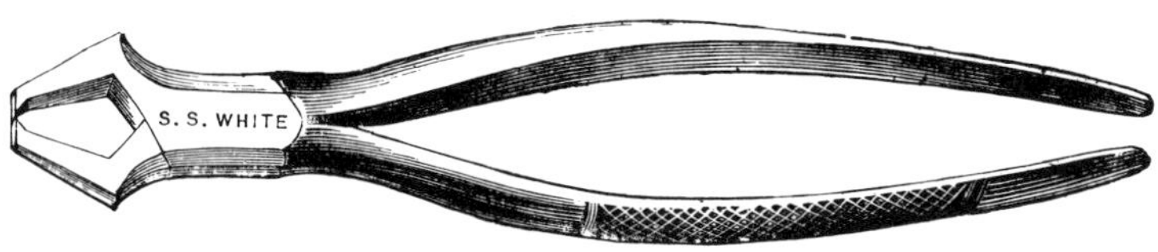

No. 12—Excising, Upper, straight beaks.

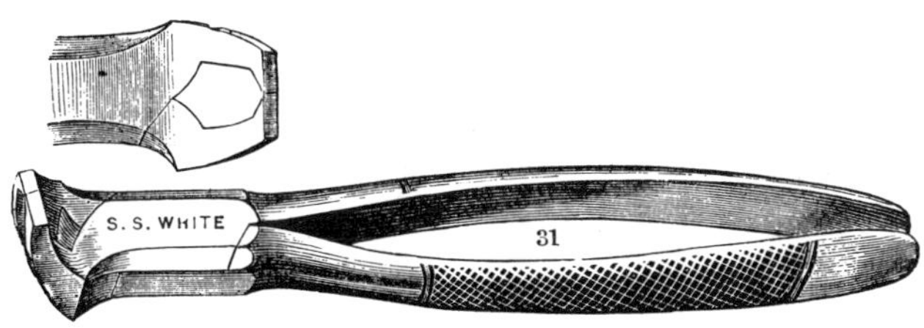

No. 31—Excising, Lower, curved beaks.

SEPARATING AND ELEVATING FORCEPS.

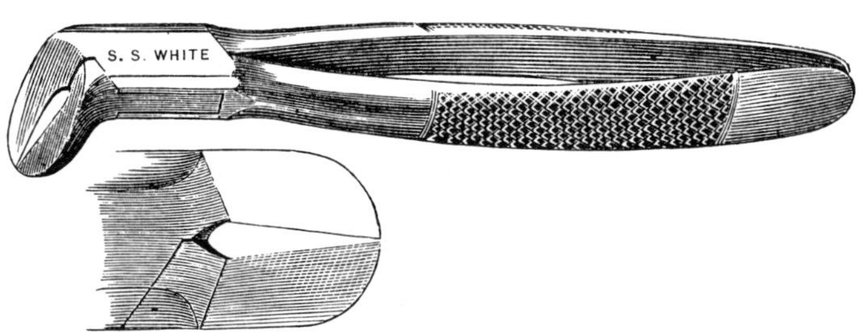

No. 66—Combined Root, Incising, Separating, and Elevating, Inferior (Stellwagen's).

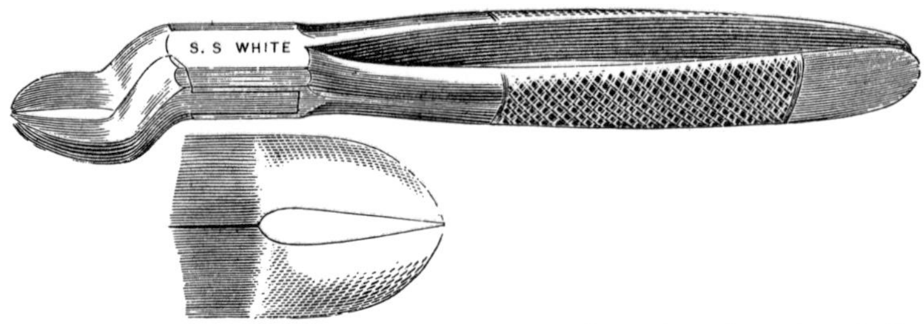

No. 67—Combined Root, Incising, Separating, and Elevating, Superior (Stellwagen's).

CHILDREN'S FORCEPS.

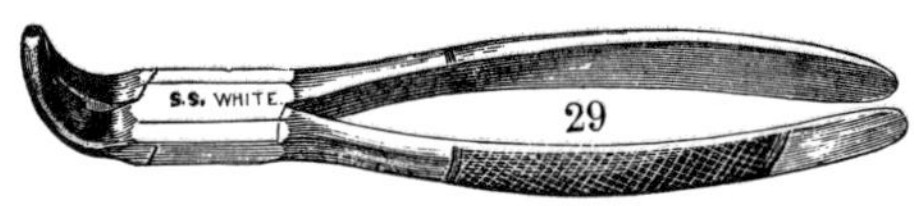

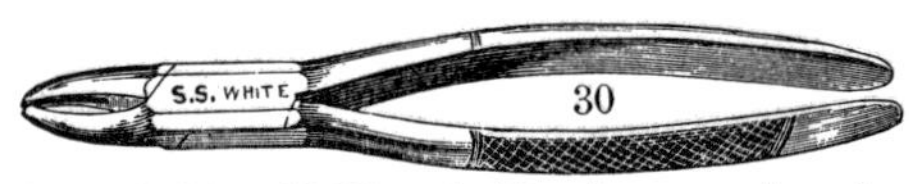

Nos. 29 and 30—Children's Teeth, curved and straight.

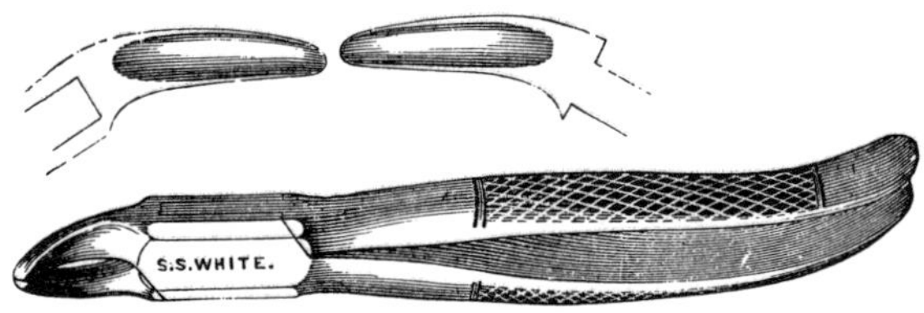

No. 62—Children's, and Universal Root.

Plain Line Forceps.

We make a Plain Line of Forceps, with Crocus-polished Octagon Joints, which in material, form, and all useful qualities and properties, are the same as our best Forceps. In style, finish, and durability these are equal to the best of any other make on sale in this country.

This line is now extended until it includes all the numbers, sizes, and varieties of every kind of Extracting, Excising, and Splitting Forceps which we make; and it is our intention to keep it full.

Price per pair (except Nos. 29, 30, 62, 66, 67) .	$2.60.	Nickel-Plated .	$3.00
" " Nos. 29, 30, 62	2.40.	" .	2.80
" " " 66, 67	3.00.	" .	3.50

DUBS'S SCREW FORCEPS.

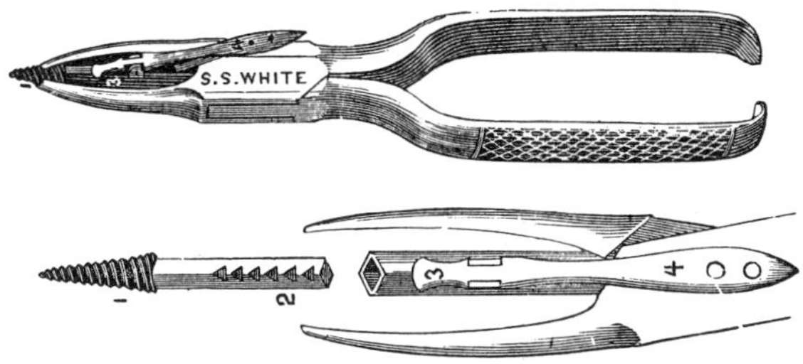

DESCRIPTION OF CUT.

1. Conical Screw with square Ratchet Shaft. 2 Beaks of Forceps, grooved inside. 3. Socket with square hole to receive Shaft. 4. Spring Trigger by which the Screw can be detached at pleasure, at any given point.

Price, Octagon Joint	per pair	$5.50
" " " Nickel-Plated	"	6.00

HULLIHEN'S SCREW FORCEPS

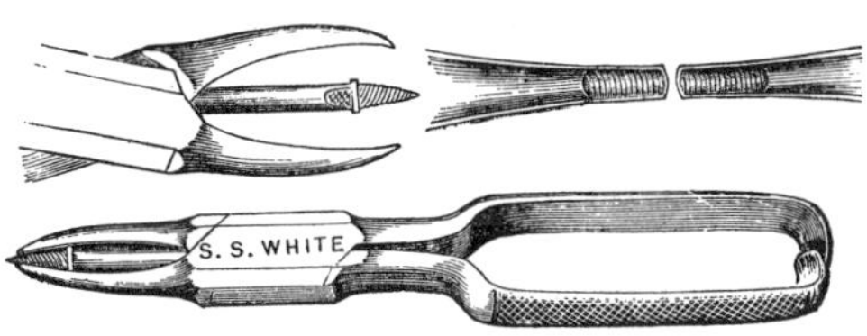

Price, Octagon Joint	per pair	$4.00
" " " Nickel-Plated	"	4.50

TURNKEYS.

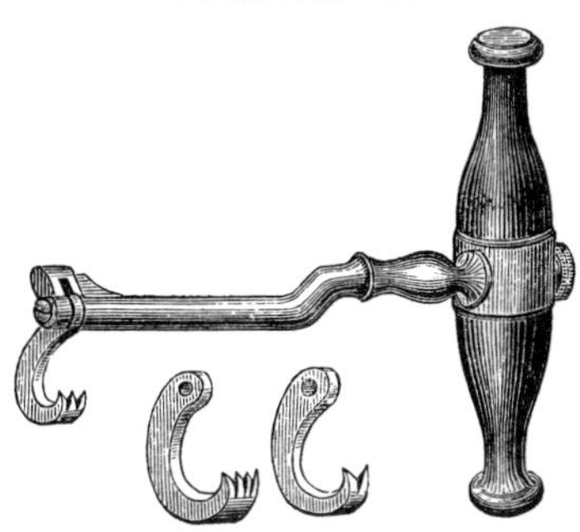

Price, Ebony Handle	each	$2.50
" Ivory "	"	3.00

STUMP EXTRACTORS.

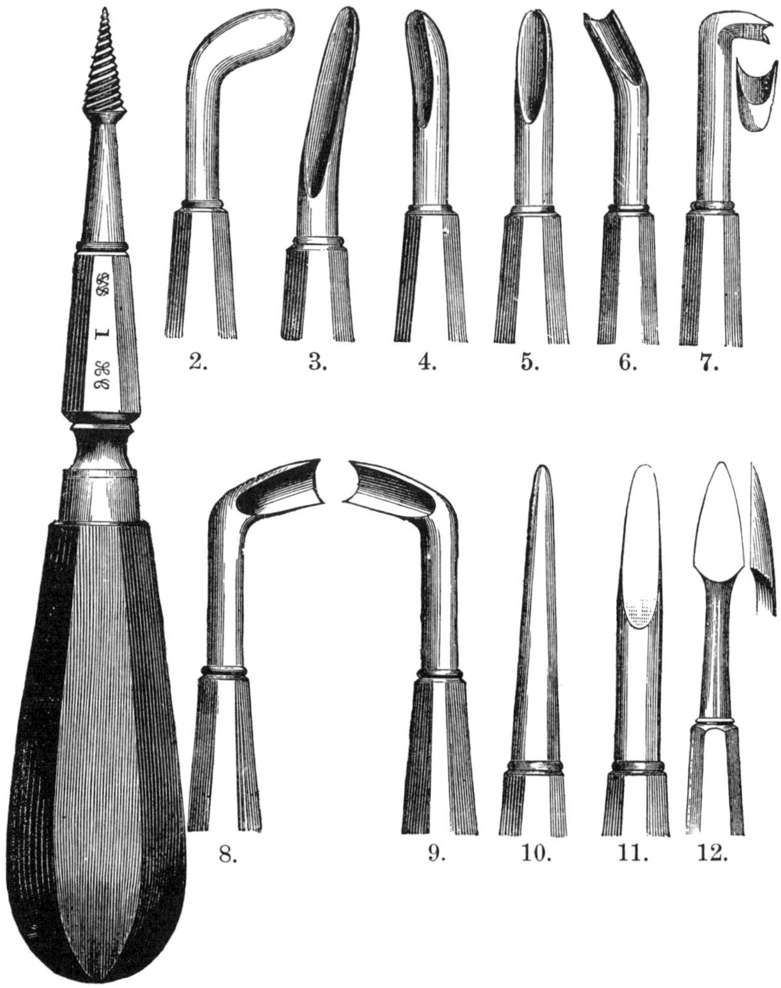

Screws, Punches, Hooks, and Elevators:

Round, with large round Ebony Handles		each	$0.75
Octagon, " octagon " "	as per cut	"	1.50
" " round Ivory Handles		"	2.00
" " octagon " "		"	2.50
" " " Cameo Handles, Gold Ferrules		"	4.00
" " " Pearl " " "		"	6.00

Other styles made to order.

Lancets.

FIXED BLADES.

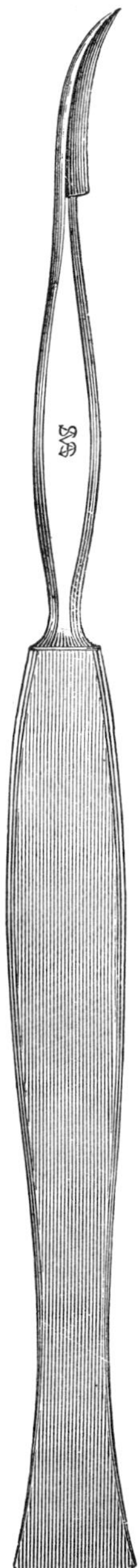

1.

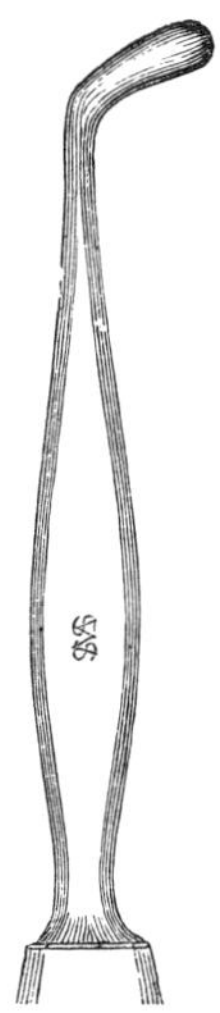

2.

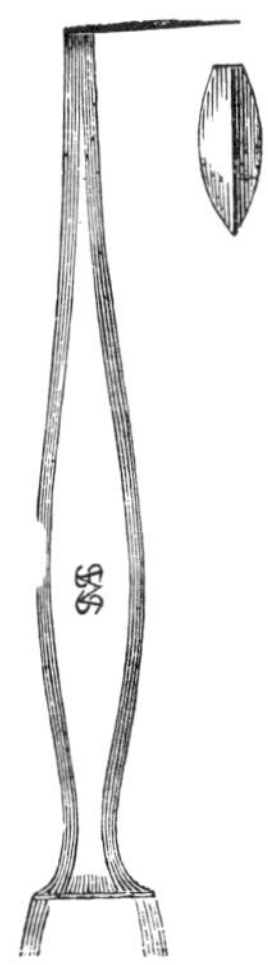

3.

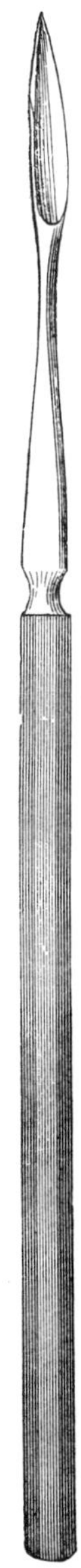

4.

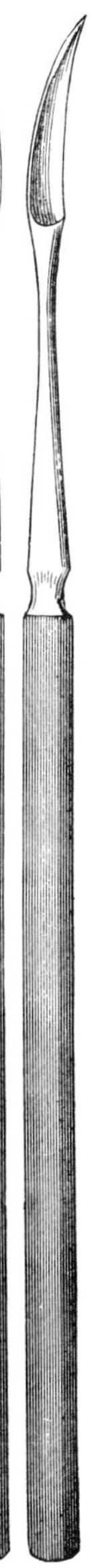

5.

PRICES.

Ivory	Handle	(Nos. 1, 2, and 3) . . .	each	$0.75
"	"	The best (Nos. 1, 2, and 3) .	"	1.00
Ebony	"	(Nos. 1, 2, and 3)	"	.60
Steel	"	File-cut (Nos. 1, 2, and 3) .	"	.60
"	"	Abscess (Nos. 4 and 5) .	per pair	.75
Pearl	"	Star Pattern, two Rosettes .	each	3.00
"	"	Shell Pattern, single Rosette .	"	2.75
"	"	Dolphin Pattern, single Rosette	"	2.75
"	"	" " without Rosette	"	2.50
"	"	Plain, Silver Ferrule . .	"	1.75
"	"	Fish Pattern	"	2.50

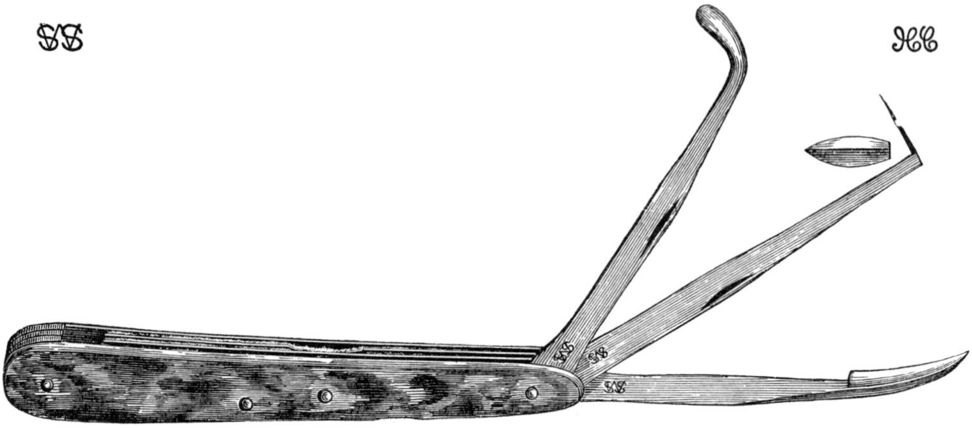

THREE-BLADE POCKET LANCET.

POCKET LANCETS.

Shell Handle,	one	Blade,	without Spring	. . . .	$1.00
"	"	"	" with Spring	. . . .	2.00
"	"	"	" with Stop	. . . .	2.00
"	"	two	" with Spring	. . . .	3.00
"	"	three	" " "	. . . .	5.00
"	"	two	" one in each end, with Stop	. . . . . .	3.00

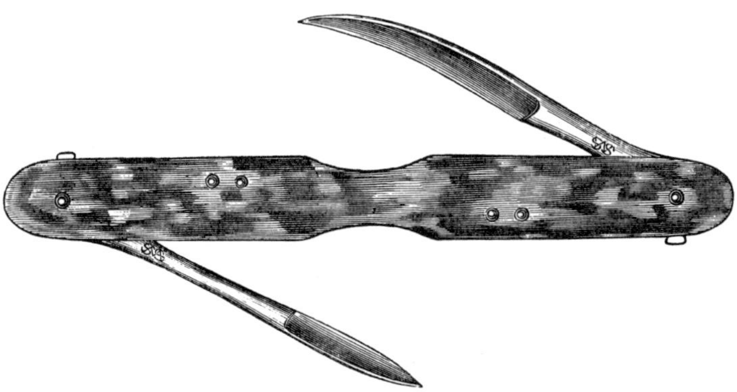

Curved Bistoury and Tenotome Knife, Shell Handle $3.50

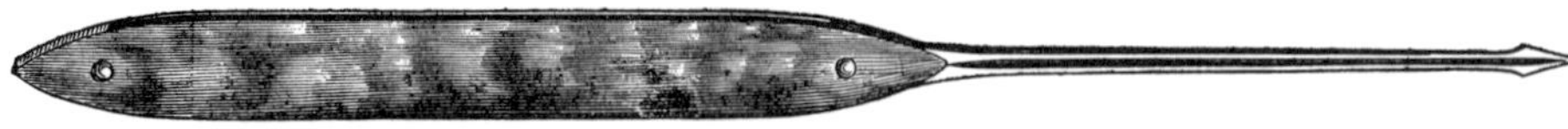

Abscess Exploring Needle, Shell Handle, Dr. W. H. Atkinson's $1.00

Excavators.

Made, shaped, polished, and bronzed, as our first-class instruments are, it is impossible to furnish them at the price which other manufacturers charge for inferior instruments. Ours not only *cost* more, but are abundantly worth the difference charged, to any operator who appreciates their elegance of form and high finish. Other manufacturers admit that merely to polish their instruments as ours are would necessitate an increase of price or loss of all profit. The fine bronzing we put on will, even when worn almost off, prevent the steel handles from soiling the fingers of the operator. High polish has great value in steel surfaces exposed to saliva, blood, and the excretions of the skin, which cause great trouble to clean from rough instruments.

Plain Octagon Steel Handles, Bronzed	per doz.	$2.70
Octagon Steel Handles, File-cut, "	"	3.60
" " " Tapering, Blued	"	3.00
" " " Plain line. The variety consists of Hatchets, Hoes, Rights and Lefts, not numbered, nor sold by numbers, but assorted in small, medium, and large sizes (see description, page 69) . . .	per doz.	2.30
Excavators for Socket	"	2.30

(Made with Round Steel, Ivory, Pearl, and Cameo Handles to order.)

The 142 Points are illustrations of our Plain Octagon Bronzed Handle Instruments.

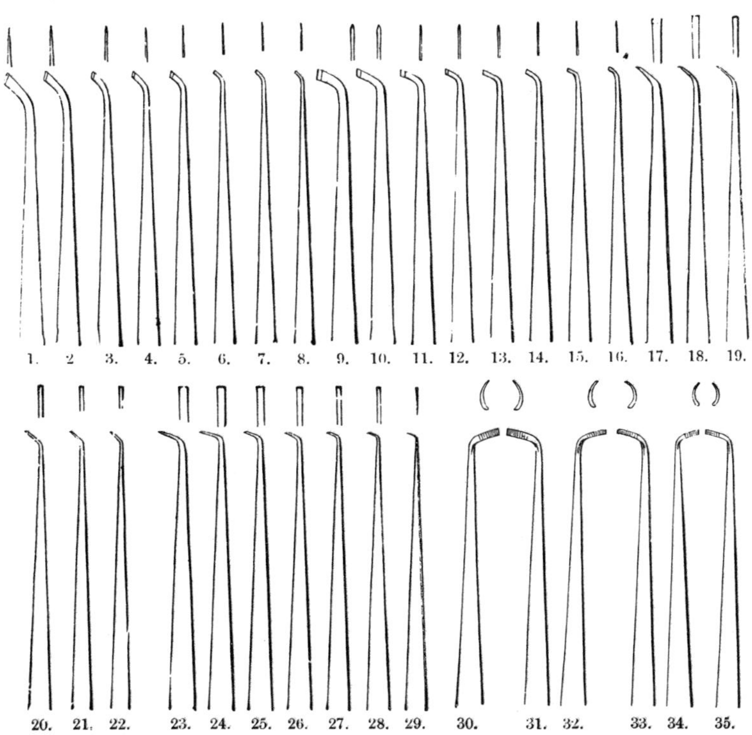

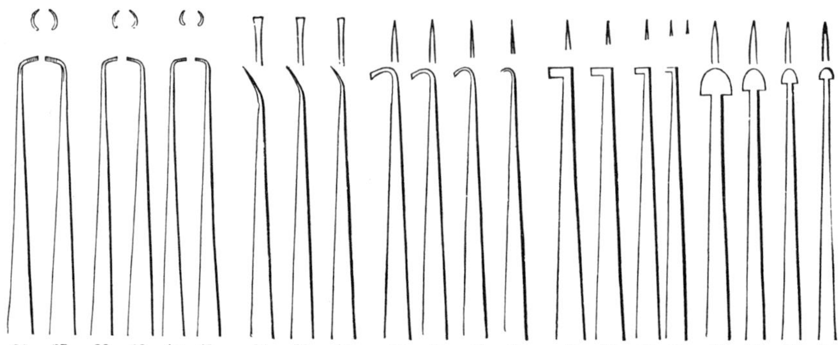

36. 37. 38. 39. 40. 41. 42. 43. 44. 45. 46. 47. 48. 49. 50. 51. 52. 53. 54. 55. 56.

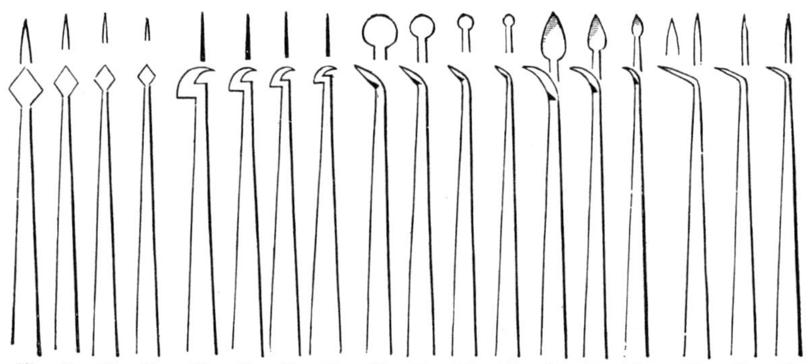

57. 58. 59. 60. 61. 62. 63. 64. 65. 66. 67. 68. 69. 70. 71. 72. 73. 74.

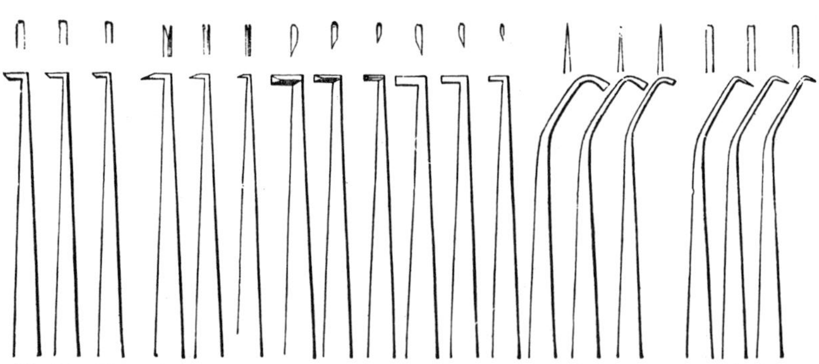

75. 76. 77. 78. 79. 80. 82. 84. 86. 81. 83. 85. 87. 88. 89. 90. 91. 92.

SS HC

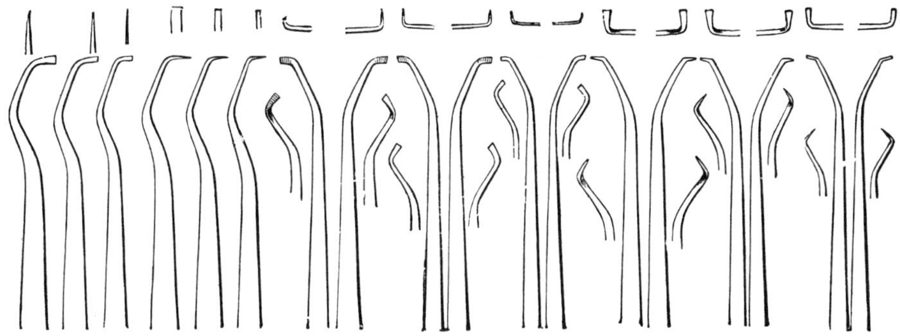

93. 94. 95. 96. 97. 98. 99. 100. 101. 102. 103. 104. 105. 106. 107. 108. 109. 110.

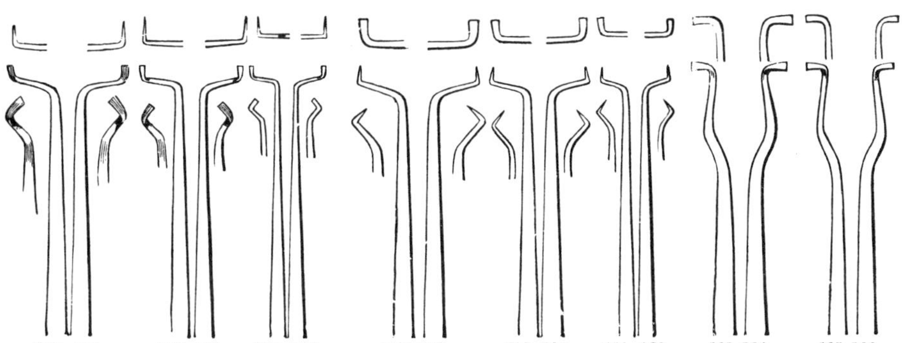

111. 112. 113. 114. 115. 116. 117. 118. 119. 120. 121. 122. 123. 124. 125. 126.

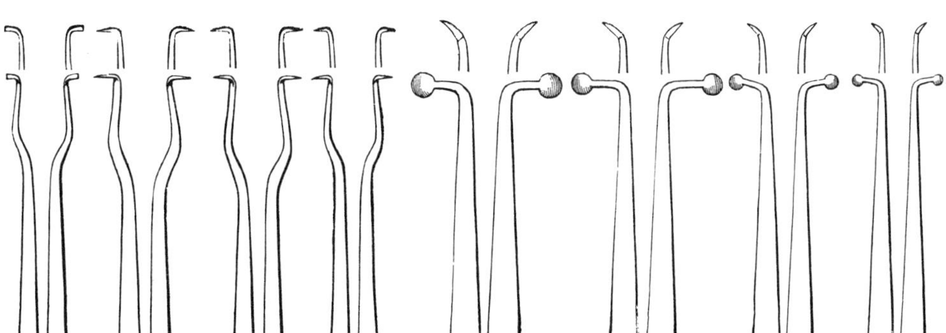

127. 128. 129. 130. 131. 132. 133. 134. 135. 136. 137. 138. 139. 140. 141. 142.

DR. W. C. HEAD'S SET OF EXCAVATORS.

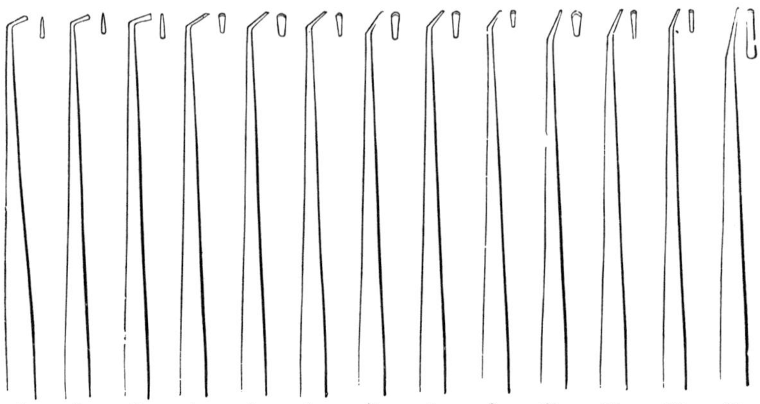

1. 2. 3. 4. 5. 6. 7. 8. 9. 10. 11. 12. 13.

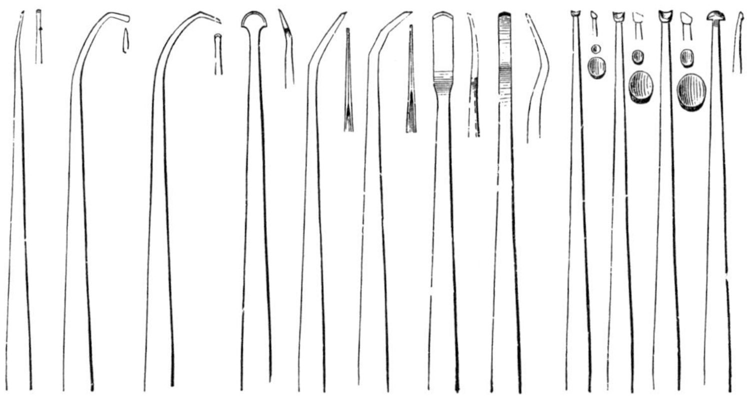

14. 15. 16. 17. 18. 19. 20. 21. 22. 23. 24. 25.

These Cuts represent twenty-five of the most approved Points.

Nos. 1 to 3 are ordinary Hatchet shape. Nos. 4 to 12 are Hoes for scraping or draw-cutting, which gives less pain than the direct or push-cut, and is equally expeditious. Nos. 13 and 14 are Chisel form. No. 15 Hatchet, and No. 16 Hoe, for posterior surfaces of molar teeth. Nos. 17, 20, and 21, Enamel Chisels. Nos. 18 and 19, for trimming between the teeth. Nos. 22 to 24 are useful in opening crown cavities and rounding the angles of sulci in lower molars. No. 25 is a Burnisher for approximal surfaces. These instruments, being extremely hard, will cut with less than the usual pressure. Care, however, should be used, in sharpening, not to diminish the angle of the edges, or they will be liable to chip. They are of the best quality, and warranted in every particular; made of $\frac{3}{16}$ inch octagon cast steel, 6 inches in length, bronzed handles.

Price	per doz.	$3.60
"	per set	7.50

SS DR. WETHERBEE'S CHISEL AND SPOON EXCAVATORS. HC

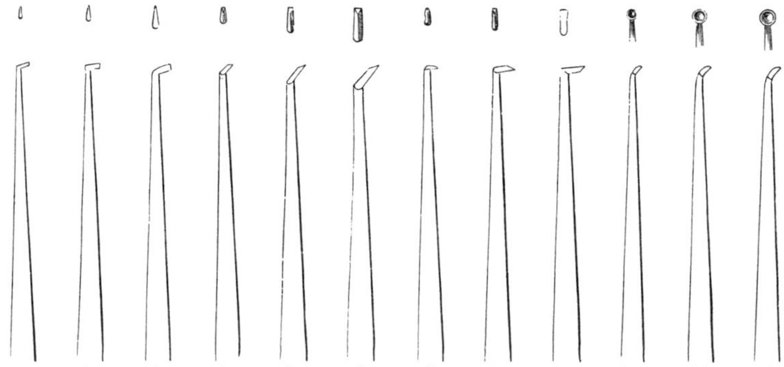

1. 2. 3. 4. 5. 6. 7. 8. 9. 10. 11. 12.

Set 12, $\frac{3}{16}$ inch Octagon Bronzed Handles . . . . . per doz. $3.60

A Plain Line of Burs, Drills, and Excavators.

To satisfy a demand and demonstrate our ability and willingness to furnish our customers with articles as good for the money as any other manufacturer, we make a *Plain Line* of these instruments. They are of the same external form and finish as the regular stock of any other manufacturer; and, in all respects, equal to our first-class instruments, except the polish.

The variety of Excavators consists of Hatchets, Hoes, Rights and Lefts.

The Trade-marks stand thus, SS——HC, the line between the two occupying the place of a number on the first quality instruments.

They are not numbered, nor are they sold by numbers, but are assorted in small, medium, and large sizes.

The Burs and Drills do not exceed No. 10 Bur Gauge in size; they are not sold by numbers, but are assorted in small and medium sizes.

Burs and Drills.

Plain Octagon Steel Handles, Bronzed	per doz.	$2.70
Octagon Steel Handles, File-cut, Bronzed	"	3.60
" " " Plain line. These do not exceed No. 10 Bur Gauge in size; they are not sold by numbers, but assorted, in small and medium sizes (see description, page 69)	per doz.	2.30
Octagon Steel Handles, Bronzed, Burs fine cut, Nos. 1 to 6 inclusive .	"	3.20
" " " " " " " 7 to 10 " .	"	3.60
" " " " Scranton Drills	"	3.00
Burs for Socket, Nos. 0 to 10	"	2.70
" " " 11 to 14	"	3.00
" " " 15 to 17	"	3.50
" " " 18 to 20	"	4.00
Drills for Socket	"	2.30

(Made with Round Steel, Ivory, Pearl, or Cameo Handles to order.)

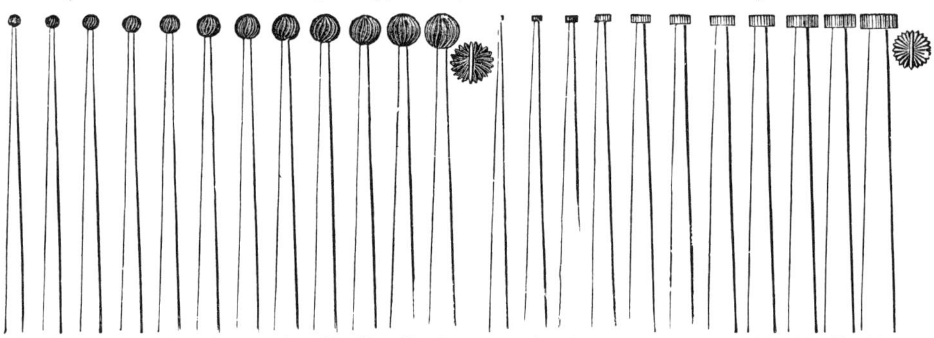

4. 6. 8. 10. 12. 14. 15. 16. 17. 18. 19. 20.
Round Burs.

2. 4. 6. 8. 10. 12. 14. 16. 18. 19. 20.
Wheel Burs.

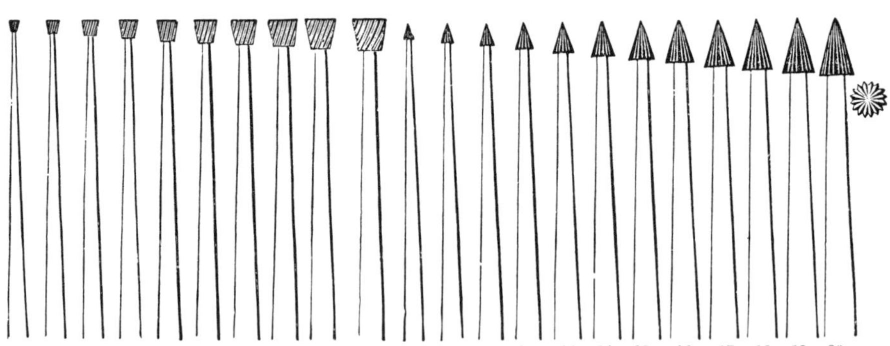

4. 6. 8. 10. 12. 14. 16. 18. 19. 20.
Inverted Cone Burs.

4. 6. 8. 10. 12. 14. 15. 16. 17. 18. 19. 20.
Cone Burs.

The above forms of coarse Burs are made in twenty-one sizes, from No. 0 to 20, bur gauge.

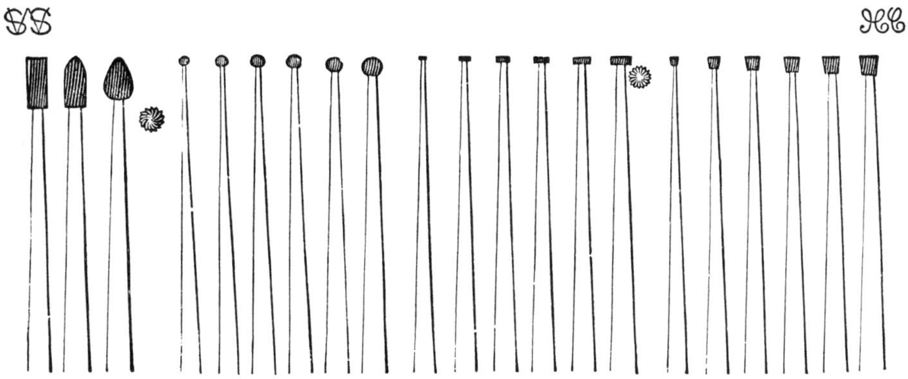

1. 3. 5. Odd. — 3. 4. 6. 7. 8. 10. Round, Fine Cut. — 3. 4. 6. 7. 8. 10. Wheel, Fine Cut. — 3. 4. 6. 7. 8. 10. Inverted Cone, Fine Cut.

Two sizes of each form. Cut shows largest size of each.

The above forms of fine-cut Burs are made in ten sizes, from No. 1 to 10, bur gauge.

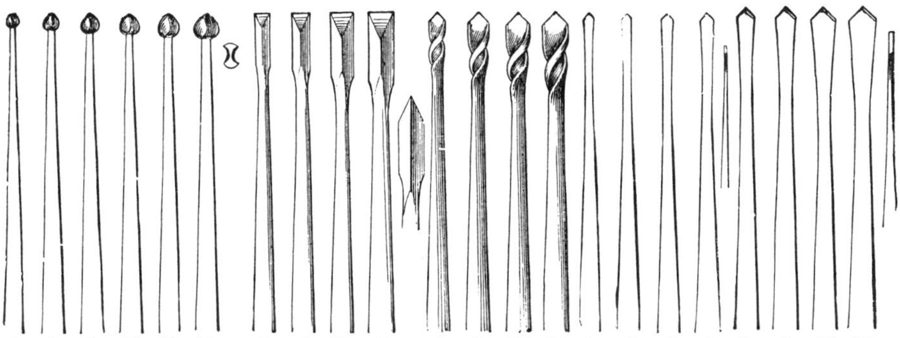

4. 6. 8. 10. 12. 14. Scranton Drills. — 6. 8. 12. 14. Square Drills. — 8. 10. 12. 14. Auger Drills. — 1. 2. 3. 4. Retaining-point Drills. — 6. 8. 12. 14. Flat Drills.

The above forms of Drills are made in eleven sizes, from No. 0 to 6, in regular gradations, and Nos. 8, 10, 12, and 14, bur gauge.

The Cuts of Excavators, Burs, and Drills represent the various and most improved forms of points in use. In some of the Cuts of Burs, etc., we have not given all the sizes; the differences being so slight that it was not thought necessary to illustrate each size. Enough, however, are given to enable the purchaser to judge of the smaller and intermediate sizes. In making out an order, give the number of the Cut and the Page, to insure obtaining what is wanted.

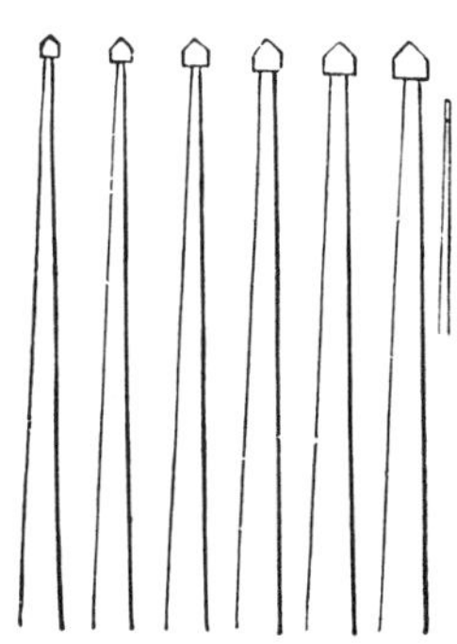

1. 2. 3. 4. 6. 8. Forbes's Drills.

Exploring Instruments.

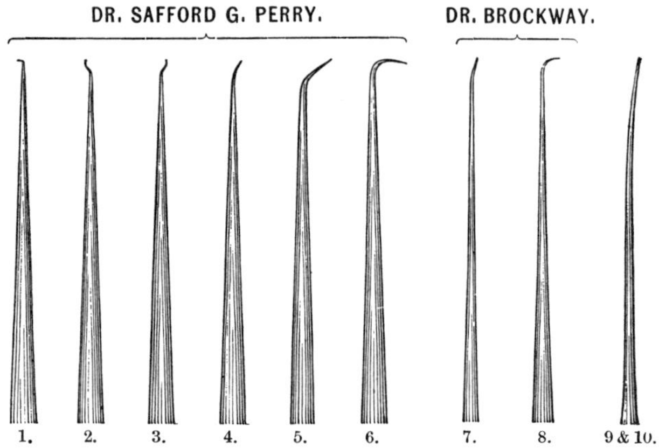

The above Cuts, from 1 to 6, show a set of instruments, the exact patterns of which were presented to us by Dr. S. G. Perry, after he had carefully proved the usefulness of each one in his practice. They have been accepted with approval by the Profession. Nos. 2 and 3 are right and left. Nos. 7 and 8 are from patterns furnished by Dr. Brockway. Nos. 9 and 10 are straight forms,—No. 10 a size larger than No. 9. They are tempered to permit bending into any desired shape with the fingers or pliers.

Price, Plain Octagon Steel Handles, Bronzed . . . . per doz. $2.70

THE S. S. WHITE DENTAL ENGINE.

THE FIRST PREMIUM, A SILVER MEDAL,

WAS AWARDED TO THE

S. S. WHITE DENTAL ENGINE"

AT THE

FRANKLIN INSTITUTE EXHIBITION,

PHILADELPHIA, 1874

ALSO, A

"SPECIAL AWARD"

(A MEDAL,)

AT THE

AMERICAN INSTITUTE EXHIBITION,

NEW YORK, 1874.

(*Extract from the Judges' Report, Forty-third Exhibition of the American Institute, October*, 1874.)

"No. 42.—DENTAL BURRING ENGINE.

"This ingenious machine is specially designed for the Dental Practitioner, and is probably the most complete instrument or machine ever made for this purpose. Its flexible shaft and tube, together with its spring pitman, is a very great improvement *over all others*, and is, as a whole, a long step forward in the application of machinery to Dental operations, and is deserving of *special award* as the best of its kind."

A medal was awarded.

We append a few testimonials from the large number received, showing the estimate in which the Dental Engine is held by prominent members of the Profession.

TESTIMONIALS.

In reply to your request to state my best advice to those contemplating the purchase of a Dental Engine, I would say, for facility, efficiency, and varied adaptability to direct, reverse and reciprocal motions, I cannot afford to be without the "S. S. White Dental Engine;" the direct and back-action hand-pieces for drills and burs, the reciprocal motion hand-piece for files, polishing slips, etc., etc., and the steady hand-piece for corundum wheels and disks, with adjustable attachment, giving ample range to meet the requirements of the entire dental arch in separating between the teeth, cutting out lingual and buccal fissures, and finishing fillings and rough surfaces. This I say after close and severe testing of the former much-admired instruments by alternate use of each. I will not say advance is impossible, but it looks quite improbable.

WM. H. ATKINSON, New York.

After several years' experience in the use of the various Dental Engines which have been introduced, I take great pleasure in recommending the "S. S. W." Dental Engine as far superior to any I have tried. It is very steady in all its movements, never gets out of order, and can always be depended upon to perform its work with nicety and precision.

A. L. NORTHROP, New York.

I have no hesitation in stating that in my judgment the S. S. White Dental Engine is the best Engine yet offered to the Dental Profession, for the following reasons:

1. There is less machinery about it, consequently it is less liable to get out of order, and the friction is much less when it is in use.

2. The facility with which your right-angle attachment is adjusted and removed is an improvement which every Dentist will readily appreciate, and can hardly be overestimated in the saving of time, etc.

FRANK ABBOTT, New York.

I *must thank* you for the hand-piece you sent me; the flexible tube, cable, and hand-piece are *perfect*. The new features are real improvements, and make the Engine a wonder in *power, adaptability*, and *completeness*.

O. E. HILL, Brooklyn.

The S. S. White Engine has arrived safely, and I am much delighted with it in every respect. I have used it to the exclusion of all others. (I have the Suspension Engine as well as the Morrison.) The new hand-piece fastening appears to me not only in itself very perfect, but likely to wear well.

CHARLES S. TOMES, London, England.

I have delayed acknowledging the receipt of the S. S. White Engine in order that I might have time to ascertain its merits or demerits. I have used it every business day since it came, and am thoroughly satisfied with it. On everything new I think I can usually suggest some improvement, but your Engine has taxed my ingenuity to its utmost, and I believe it is as near perfect as it can be made.

GEO. B. STEEL, Richmond, Va.

The Engine is a perfect "God-send." I like it better by far than the Morrison that I have been using.

THOS T. MOORE, Columbia, S. C.

I like the Engine *very much*,—yes, *love it*.

F. SEARLE, Springfield, Mass.

I am pleased to inform you that I have had the S. S. White Dental Engine in daily use in my practice since August last, and, after a most thorough test of its capacity for work, I am prepared to pronounce it a success. The ready adaptation of the machine to the variety of cases that present, and the steadiness and security with which the burs are run by it, may be noted as marked qualities of this Engine.

H. A. SMITH, CINCINNATI.

I have satisfied myself that the S S. White Engine justly deserves the title of *the very best*, as far at least as all others are known to me.

I have put up my old engine for sale.

* * * * * * * * * * * *

F. H. REHWINKEL, CHILLICOTHE, OHIO.

The S. S. White Dental Engine is worth its weight in gold.

S. C. SAWYER, LITTLETON, N. H.

It affords me pleasure to say that after using your Dental Engine for two months, I find it practically superior to any other I ever employed.

JOHN M. COMEGYS, ST. ALBANS, VT.

The Engine of your manufacture that I have had in use has more than satisfied me. It is the perfection of steadiness in motion, and accomplishes all that I desire in an instrument of this character. JAMES TRUMAN, PHILADELPHIA.

The dental engine known as the "S. S. White Engine" is everything that can be desired. Every day strengthens my admiration for it. C. N. PEIRCE, PHILADELPHIA.

I have been rather tardy in adopting any of the many innovations recently pressing upon the attention of the dental operator; yet a three months' experience with your new Engine has so impressed me with its value as a time- and labor-saving appliance, that I should feel it a great misfortune to be deprived of the advantages afforded by it. In the finishing of fillings it saves much tedious and tiresome manipulation; in the separation of approximal faces it effects, in the majority of cases, by the use of the disk, an opening of better shape and truer surface than can be obtained with the file or chisel, and renders easy the perfect finish of the parts denuded of enamel, which is so difficult to obtain from the inequalities generally following the use of the latter instruments; it enables one to easily and rapidly perform such uninteresting and time-consuming operations as opening up cavities, drilling teeth for treatment, removing gold or amalgam fillings, etc.; and, lastly, what is of major importance, it receives the commendation of almost all patients who have experienced its benefits.

While I am not sufficiently enthusiastic to say "I desire nothing better," I am so impressed with its manifold merits that I shall *rest content* until the "something better" offers, be it early or late. GEO. W. ELLIS, PHILADELPHIA.

Please allow me now to say a word in commendation of your Engine. I have used it about two months, and the more I use it the better I like it. The perfect range of movement without numerous joints and arms is a great end attained. I would particularly commend it, however, for the absolute lack of vibration in the hand-piece, allowing of a delicate use of the bur,—*touching* here and there,—which was next to impossible with my Morrison, where steadiness could only be secured by a more or less strong grip. I send you also the last of my Morrison points, to be changed to the S. S. W.

CHAS. F. ALLAN, NEWBURGH, N. Y.

The S. S. White Dental Engine I ordered from you when at the association at Niagara Falls, gives perfect satisfaction. I would not take one thousand dollars for it, if I could not get another one of the same kind. I want the Plugger for it next.

J. A. BROWN, PORT HOPE, CANADA

After a fair and unprejudiced trial, I have no hesitation in saying that I consider your Dental Engine, in simplicity of construction and efficiency of movement, decidedly superior to anything of the kind which has yet been given to the public, and I take pleasure in expressing my preference for it, and earnestly recommending its general use.

R B. WINDER, BALTIMORE, MD.

After two years' experience in the use of other dental engines, I purchased one of the S. S. White Engines, and have been using it constantly for more than a year past with the most perfect satisfaction. I consider it by far the best dental engine in use.

R. B. DONALDSON, WASHINGTON, D. C.

I am delighted with the execution of the S. S. White Dental Engine, and am sure it is ahead of any other I have ever used or seen. The spring-tempered rod in connection with the stationary treadle is a great improvement over the old rod and movable treadle, working with greater ease and steadiness; the flexible arm for driving burs, drills, and disks is still a greater improvement over all others, there being very little or no jar or vibration when running the corundum disk in separating the teeth; and the coil-spring lock in the hand-piece renders it impossible for an instrument to get out of place, making the use of the disks perfectly practicable, when separating teeth, in pulling towards you or pushing from you, —a perfection that no other hand-piece that I have ever used possesses. In a nut-shell, I think the Engine far surpasses any other now made, as I think it will be very hard to excel.

G. B. McDONNELD, CONNEAUTVILLE, PA.

The S S. White Engine is in daily use, and I like it more and *more;* think it has necessary power and practical *steadiness.* C. R. BUTLER, CLEVELAND, O.

After using Green's Pneumàtic and the Morrison Engines, alternately, through a period of three years, I think myself capable of comparing the S. S. White machine with them, and I do not hesitate to pronounce it far superior to either. I believe it superior to any machine of the kind now in the market. L. G. NOEL, NASHVILLE, TENN.

It gives me pleasure to state that the S. S. White Burring Engine, purchased from you some weeks since, has given entire satisfaction. For steadiness of motion in the hand-piece, ease and noiselessness with which it is operated, absence of liability to get out of order, and elegance of construction and finish, combined with the mechanical principles upon which it depends, and in which it differs from others, in my opinion it has not its equal.

E. R. PETTIT, PHILADELPHIA.

I bought one of your Dental Engines, and I would not be without it for five hundred dollars a year. It is the most perfect instrument for the purpose for which it is designed that I have ever seen or handled, and I think the Profession owes you a debt of gratitude for it.

E. L. PERRY, MILAN, O.

Let me in this connection express my appreciation of the excellences of your Engine. It has stood for some months beside my chair with the other engine. During the first few weeks it was used but little; I found myself decidedly preferring my old one. After the improved cable was attached I found myself using it more and more, until now I use it constantly. Actions speak louder than words, so I send you the record of my actions, together with my thanks for your perseverance in perfecting so admirable an instrument.

E. A. BOGUE, NEW YORK.

I wish to thank you for the Dental Engine. I have used it since last May, fell in love with it at once, and have not ceased to love it since. No one who has not used it can have any idea how pleasant it is to fill teeth with it, and what an immense amount of old-fashioned labor—real hard work—it relieves us of. It is always ready, does not easily get out of order, never refuses to perform its work, and never gets tired. I call it my Pet.

A. NEWTON, HARTFORD, CT.

The S. S. White Dental Engine.

PRICES.

Engine complete, nine and one-half inch Driving-Wheel, with 14 instruments, all the bright steel parts of the Engine nickel-plated	$50.00
Engine complete, twelve and one-half inch Driving-Wheel, with 14 instruments, all the bright steel parts of the Engine nickel-plated	55.00
Boxing	1.00

We are now supplying a Foot-Power Dental Engine which combines all the recent improvements, which cannot fail to commend themselves to every experienced operator. It is put upon the market as a Complete Engine, and has been found far superior to any combination of it in part with others; the novel *plate-spring* pitman, and the larger and *heavier* driving-wheel, giving to the foot-power advantages no less conspicuous than those found in the upper works of the Engine.

We offer in these machines immunity from royalties or license fees, and take pleasure in announcing to our customers that, by the purchase of governing patents, or of rights thereunder, we have acquired the control of this class of engines, embracing the following devices and combinations:

1. The use of a flexible wire shaft in a Dental Engine.
2. The combination of a flexible wire shaft and a flexible sheath.
3. The combination of the base or stand with the upper works.
4. A device for operating the power from either side of the chair.
5. A hand-piece, with hardened steel bearings, and tool mutually locking; the tool, easily placed or removed, remains undisturbed in its security by the pulling-cut, or by the swiftest revolution without pressure.

The opinion of one who is well versed in mechanism thus aptly describes this Engine: "A machine, which for simplicity, ease in movement, and adaptation, excels anything I have ever seen."

We have spared no pains or expense to perfect this Engine in all its details. It is believed to be the best ever put upon the market, and it will be in every way to the advantage of those who contemplate the exchange of old engines, or the purchase of new ones (in order to avoid litigation threatened or apprehended), to examine this new Engine.

Aside from its intrinsic excellences and its superiority to any engine heretofore made, purchasers of the old engines or their new attachments will still be liable for the future use of the patents controlled by us on machines of other manufacturers.

Our purpose, however, is not to oppress the Profession by claims for past infringements, but to assert our rights in the future against manufacturers and others who attempt to infringe them after due warning to desist, or who attempt to interfere with our trade or annoy our customers.

DESCRIPTION OF THE ENGINE.

CUT NO. 1.

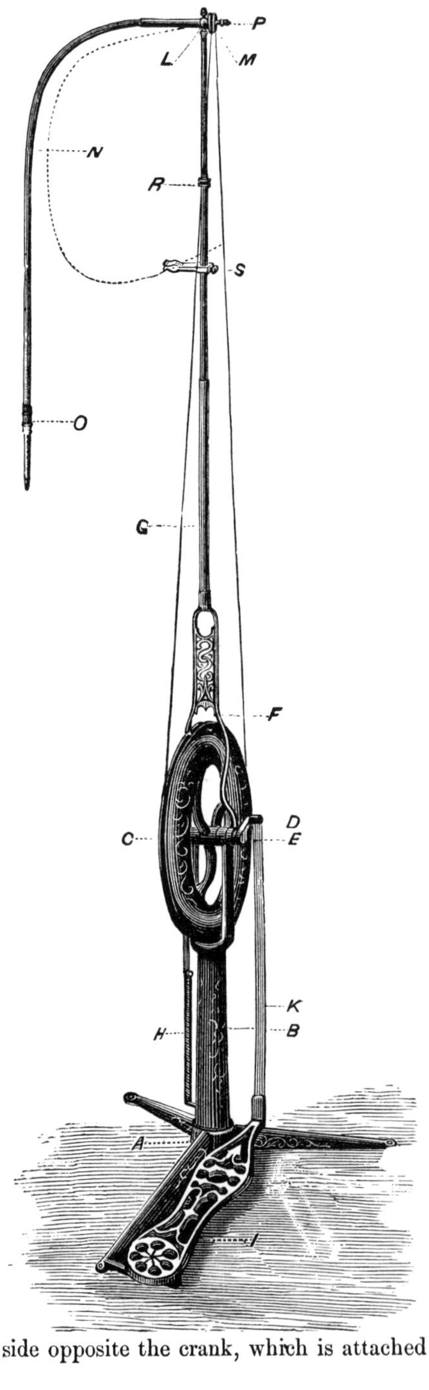

The base (A) is divided radially into three feet, which form, with the weight upon it, makes it steady and firm on the floor. One foot is prolonged and has a spur on which the heel of the fixed pedal (I) is hinged.

The post (B) planted in the center of the base is about fifteen inches high, and is forked to pass the driving-wheel and form the bearings for its axle-shaft and support the uprights.

The wheel (C) is 9½ inches in diameter, weighs 10½ pounds, and is grooved on the edge for the band, or belt.

The axle-shaft (D) of the driving-wheel is prolonged so as to pass through the journal-bosses (E) of the yoke of the upright, and has also a crank (D) to which the upper end of the pitman (K) is connected. The shaft and crank (D) are steel, and made in one piece, and so fastened to the wheel as to avoid the possibility of loosening or misplacement.

The pedal (I) has the pitman (K) screwed to it at the toe. The upper end of the pitman is pivoted on the crank. The pitman is a flat steel spring, set at such an angle as always to keep the crank off the dead center, and is so adjusted as to throw the crank above its center, giving the operator greater length of turn in starting the Engine. The spring pitman is a novel invention, and gives to the crank when on the down center an upward motion (or as the inventor calls it, "a live motion"), allowing the operator to run the machine with perfect ease.

The upright is composed of two parts, a yoke (F) and post (G). The yoke is forked to pass the upper half of the driving-wheel and hinges on the journal-bosses (E); thus constituting it, with the post, a rocking arm. It constant return to the upright position is secured by a prolongation of the yoke on the side opposite the crank, which is attached to a spiral spring (H).

This rocking motion is among the important features comprised in the patents exclusively owned by us, and is invaluable to the operator, not only by the greater extent and increased freedom of motion with which it endows the flexible working arm of the Engine, but also because it practically eradicates the tremor inseparable from the rigid post engines, which is conveyed in the stiff upright engines not only to the working arm, hand-piece, and tool, but also to the hand of the operator.

Seven inches above the top of the yoke, the upright post (or rocking arm) consists of a slender cylinder, provided at R with a screwed extension joint and jam-nut (unscrewing this lengthens the post), by which the belt may be tightened. When the extension joint is unscrewed, the jam-nut should be run down until it touches the post; this will hold it steady.

A spring catch (S), sliding on the post and secured by a set-screw, is provided for holding the hand-piece out of the way when not in use.

A right-angled head-piece (L) is pivoted on top of the upright rocking arm. (See full-size Cut No. 2.)

CUT NO. 2.

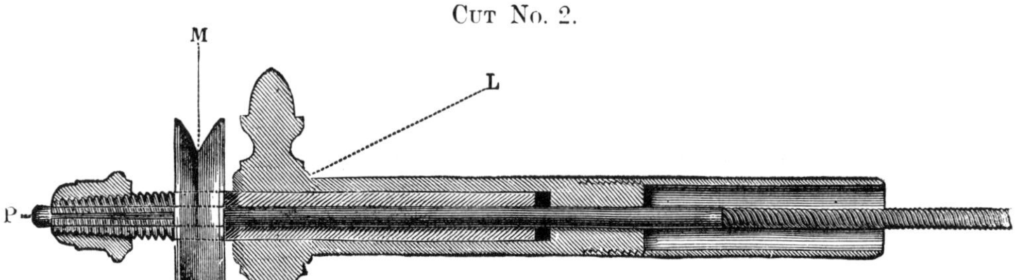

This head-piece has free motion horizontally, and is the coupling between the upright and the working arm, the horizontal part of it being drilled to receive a stem (P), upon which the driven pulley (M) is fastened by a squeeze-nut upon a conical screw. This much is external to the cross-piece. The end of the stem inside is connected to the rotating shaft of the flexible arm, which thus transmits the power to the mandrel of the hand-piece, which is attached to the extreme end of the rotating shaft. This rotating shaft passes through and is covered by the flexible sheath (N, Cut No. 1), which is attached to the head-piece (L) and does not rotate.

The sheath (N) and driven shaft passing through it compose the *flexible working arm of this Engine*, which is one of its characteristic and peculiar parts. The shaft joins the stem, which passes through the head-piece (L) and carries the driven pulley (M), and at the other end is joined to the mandrel of the hand-piece, the extreme end of which is formed into the socket, chuck, or tool-holder. The sheath joins the head-piece (L) exteriorly, and at the other end is secured to the hand-piece (O, Cut No. 1), which covers or incases the tool-holder.

The peculiar construction of this working arm, sheath, and shaft is such that besides having free horizontal motion by the pivoted head-piece (L), it is flexible at nearly every portion of its length, 26 inches, while in all other engines the flexibility is limited to a few inches of spiral spring between a stiff rod and the hand-piece.

THE HAND-PIECE AND TOOL

combine several novel and effective devices, as shown (full size) in Cut No. 3. The tool or bit (A), at the end of its shank, is reduced to a wedge-shape on one side to the extent of one-fourth of an inch from the end, terminating in a lateral groove embracing one-third the circumference of the shank. The tool-holder or chuck has a pin (B) inserted tangentially across the bore at the proper distance to interlock with the lateral groove of the tool; beneath the pin a wedge (C), corresponding to the wedged end of the bit, is held in position by a spiral spring (D); this wedge is fastened through a slot in the

Cut No. 3.

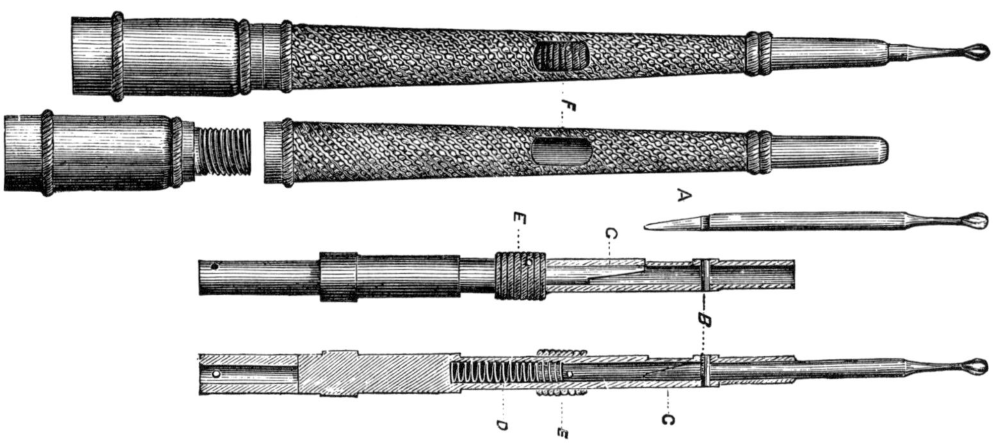

chuck to a cylindrical grooved collar or ring (E) working longitudinally upon the outside. The outer case of the hand-piece has an oval aperture (F) exposing the grooved collar, which may thus be worked by the thumb-nail. In order to secure the tool in the holder, it is only necessary to insert the shank, turn it until its wedge-face clears the pin, and push it into the socket; this pressure also forces down the wedge and spring inside; then a slight turn of the tool locks its lateral groove on the pin and removes the pressure from the wedge, which is then forced up by the spring and secures the tool in its place (G), so that it cannot possibly pull out when in use, or fly out when run without being pressed upon.

To remove the tool, simply push back the grooved collar, and reverse the turn by which the bit was locked on the pin.

In this hand-piece the tool is not dependent upon the external case for its bearing, as in other hand-pieces, but passes into the socket far enough to be held securely, and to revolve with the chuck.

A NEW HAND-PIECE.

CUT NO. 4.

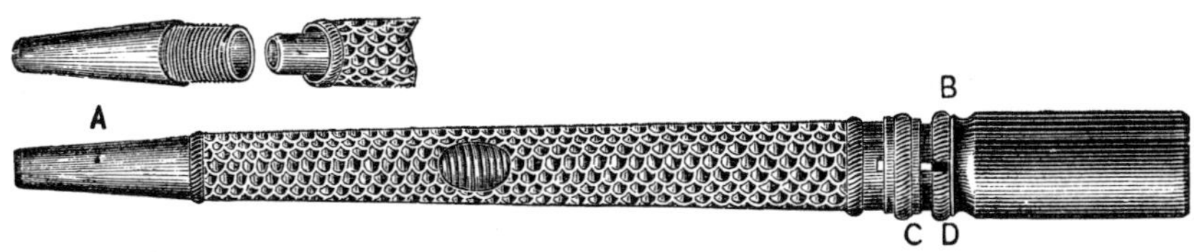

Although the hand-piece formerly sold with the Engine was equal, if not superior, to any other in the market, we were dissatisfied with it because it wore too rapidly, especially when the operator allowed polishing powders to work into the socket of the point. After persistent and patient endeavor to improve wherever improvement seemed desirable or possible, we now offer a new and very superior hand-piece, illustrated by the Cut.

The bearings of the shaft or tool-holder, A B, are made of hardened steel.

The hand-piece case is provided with a notch, into which a screw ferrule (C) carries (through the slot D in the screw) a small pin which effectually locks it.

By turning the screw ferrule C to the left, it will carry the pin out of the notch in the case; then by revolving the case to the right, the spindle can be removed. The blued steel point can be removed, if it is desired to replace it, by unscrewing it to the left.

Price $10.00

A

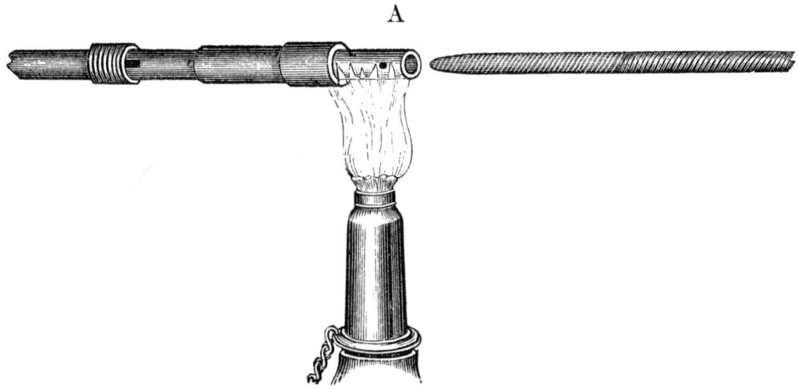

Fig. A illustrates a method by which those who cannot return the parts to us can attach a cable to the spindle of the hand-piece themselves. The cable, as obtained from us, has the end to be inserted in the spindle *tinned*, ready for soldering. Place a single drop of muriate of zinc (made by dissolving zinc in muriatic acid to saturation) in the hole in the end of the spindle; then a piece of soft solder not larger than a canary-seed; then hold the end of the *spindle* over a spirit-lamp, as shown in Cut, and when the solder flows, insert the tinned end of the cable and hold it in position until it chills, being careful not to overheat the cable, so as to draw the temper of the wire. The flame should not come in contact with the *cable.*

B

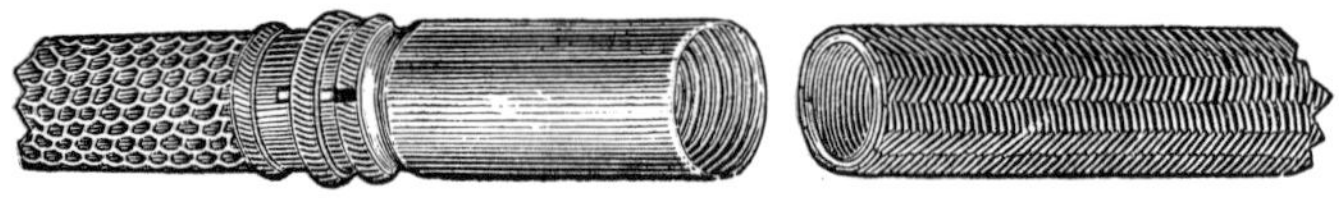

Fig. B shows the end of the sleeve or sheath of the cable, and the screw end of the hand-piece. The sleeve is screwed into the hand-piece and retained without any cement, and can be unscrewed at pleasure.

We are now manufacturing an Engine having a larger driving-wheel, twelve and one-half inches in diameter, and weighing twelve pounds, giving greater speed to the bit by the same movement of the treadle.

OUR COMPOUND OR EXTENSION TREADLE

Cut No. 5.

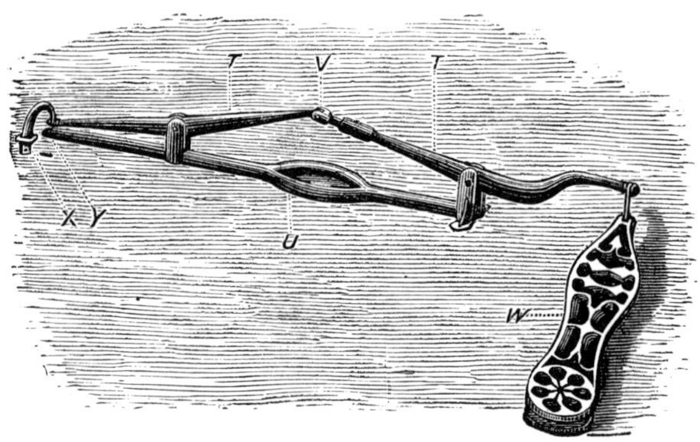

is composed of two levers (TT), pivoted on two upright posts of a base-piece (U), their inner ends connected by a socket and knuckle-joint (V), their outer ends having loosely attached—to one a treadle (W), to the other a goose-neck or crane (X), with a lug and pin-hole for attaching to the stationary treadle of the Engine (I, Cut No. 1). The end of the base-piece under the crane is provided with a screw-hole (Y) for pivoting to the floor at that point, thus enabling the operator to swing the treadle at the other end in a full circle, and to stand in any desired position. This admirable device gives the choice of a treadle on either side of the chair without moving the Engine. The diagrams (Cut No. 6) suggest the positions which have been found the most convenient for the Engine and compound treadle.

Price $5.00

CUT No. 6.

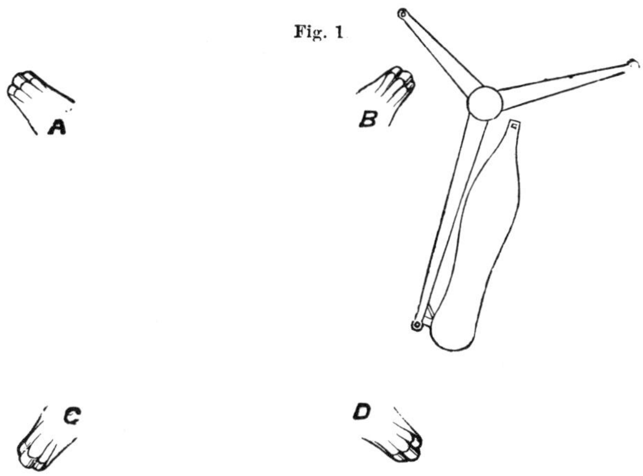

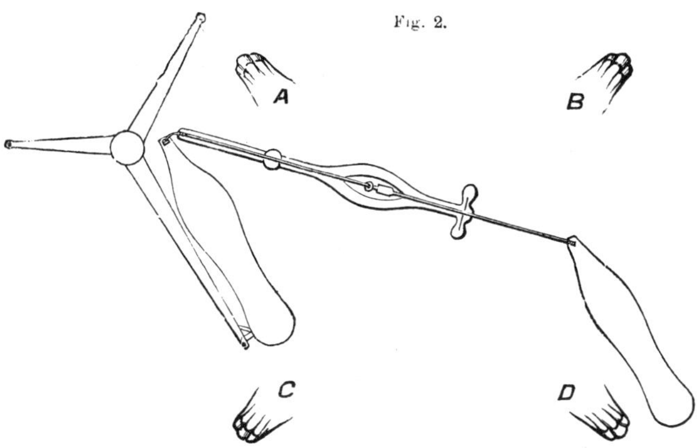

Fig. 1 shows the Engine on the right side of the chair; Fig. 2, the Engine on the left side worked by the compound treadle from the right side, the letters A B representing the front feet, and C D the rear feet, of a Harris chair. The positions designated for the Engine are considered important, in order to obtain the full benefit of the rocking arm, and as bringing the treadle directly under the foot of the operator.

The foregoing description of the Engine, and detailed explanation of its separate parts and their construction, will enable its merits to be understood, which merits justify us in offering the following conclusive

SIX REASONS FOR PURCHASING THE S. S. WHITE DENTAL ENGINE IN PREFERENCE TO ANY OTHER.

1. The flat spring pitman always holding the crank off the center when at rest, and the pedal always in place for a forward motion of the Engine on foot-pressure; besides which it is noiseless. This pitman cannot be obtained with any other engine. No. 1 is an *exclusive* feature.

2. The larger and heavier fly-wheel, insuring a steadier movement at slower speed, affording increased speed with equal pedal action; and what is of the greatest consequence and relief to many operators, communicating high speed to the tool without such excessively rapid pedal action as some engines require. Add to this, that we are also enabled to give to the driven pulley an increase in size which, though very little in measure, adds greatly to the steady cutting power of the tool. These combined advantages are of decided value to the operator. No. 2 is a comparative feature, and we invite the comparison.

3. The pivoted upright with its return spring always recovering the perpendicular when freed, and to one who studies placing the Engine properly, always yielding freely to any extra call on the working arm, avoiding the tremor inseparable from a stiff upright, and, in conjunction with the free horizontal movement of the head-piece, making the whole Engine from the crank-shaft up entirely responsive to the hand and wrist motions of the operator. No. 3 is exclusive and comparative. Its use and value are well known to hundreds from several years' experience. It can hereafter be obtained only with the S. S. White Engine.

4. The flexible working arm, composed of a shaft and sheath; bending, curving, and yielding to every motion; an exclusive and peculiar feature, which a dentist who has used the rigid arm can appreciate at a touch. We claim as the *special distinctive* feature of our Engine, in which it differs from all others, and which, to the extent of this difference, makes it superior to all others, this flexible arm, with the pivoted upright and its return spring.

5. The wedgelock hand-piece and tool, described and explained by the text and cuts. These are intrinsically good and convenient, possessing valuable features not presented in any other hand-piece. The tool, easily placed and removed, is as secure in the hand-piece with the *pull-* as with the *push*-cut; nor can it fly out at the highest speed when not pressed upon. No. 5 is exclusive with this Engine.

6. The price of the S. S. White Engine is extremely low for a machine combining so many excellences in device and workmanship, and including license under so many valuable patents.

INSTRUCTIONS.

In attaching the driving-cord to the Engine, place it around the driving-wheel and pulley and cut to proper length; then bring the two ends together without overlapping, running a threaded needle through and down the cord, passing it out through one end and into the other, so as to avoid forming a knot at the splice. To place the cord on the Engine so as to turn the bit or tool to the right, stand in front of the Engine as if to start it by the treadle; take the cord in the right hand, and with the left hand place the pulley-head into the upright or extension post, then place the cord on the small pulley-wheel.

Care should be taken to *oil daily* the *mandrel* in the *hand-piece* and the *shaft* in the *pulley-head;* also the shaft of the driving-wheel.

In adjusting the pulley in the head-piece after oiling, leave the pulley one-fourth of an inch play outside the head-piece, in order to allow for the curving of the shaft and case.

The Engine may be conveniently lifted by inserting the finger in the upper part of the yoke, above the monogram "S. S. W."

EQUIPMENTS

FOR THE

S. S. White Dental Engine.

EXCAVATING BURS.

Round.

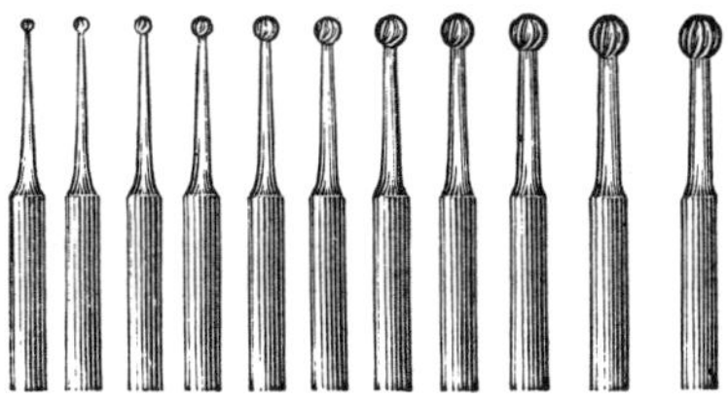

1. 2. 3. 4. 5. 6. 7. 8. 9. 10. 11.

1–8: 25 cents each. 9–11: 35 cents each.

Wheel.

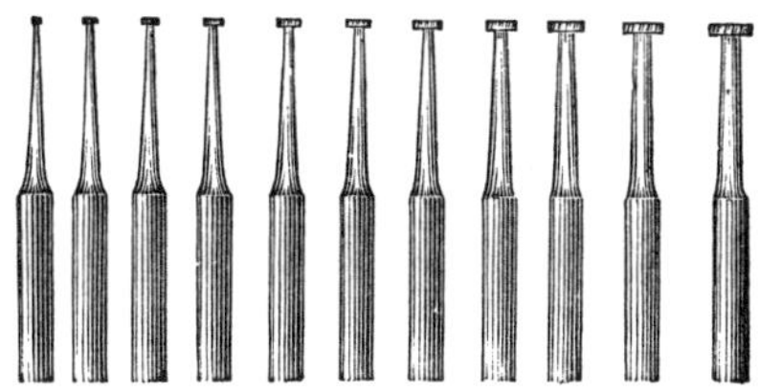

12. 13. 14. 15. 16. 17. 18. 19. 20. 21. 22.

12–19: 25 cents each. 20–22: 35 cents each.

Cone.

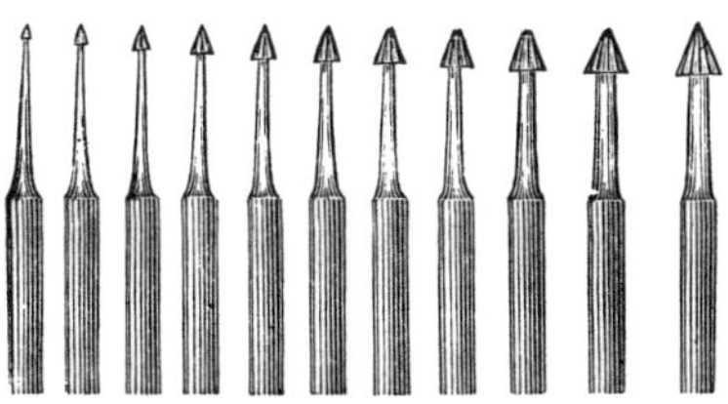

23. 24. 25. 26. 27. 28. 29. 30. 31. 32. 33.

23–30: 25 cents each. 31–33: 35 cents each.

Inverted Cone.

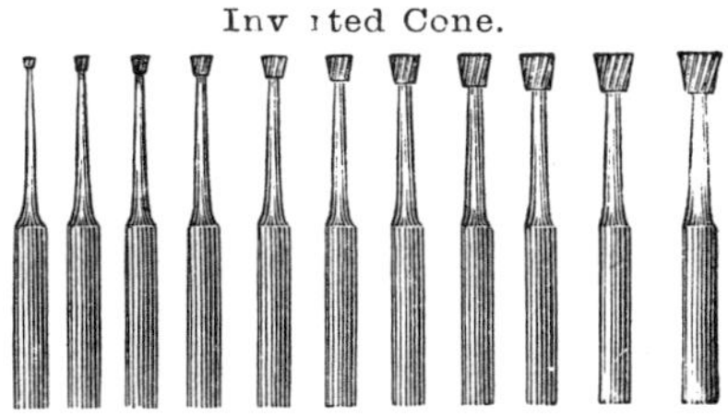

34. 35. 36. 37. 38. 39. 40. 41. 42. 43. 44.

34–41: 25 cents each. 42–44: 35 cents each.

Bud.

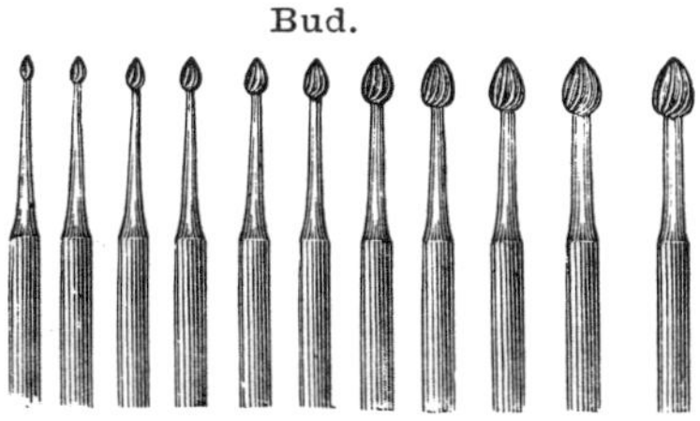

45. 46. 47. 48. 49. 50. 51. 52. 53. 54. 55.

45–52: 25 cents each. 53–55: 35 cents each.

Fissure, Square End.

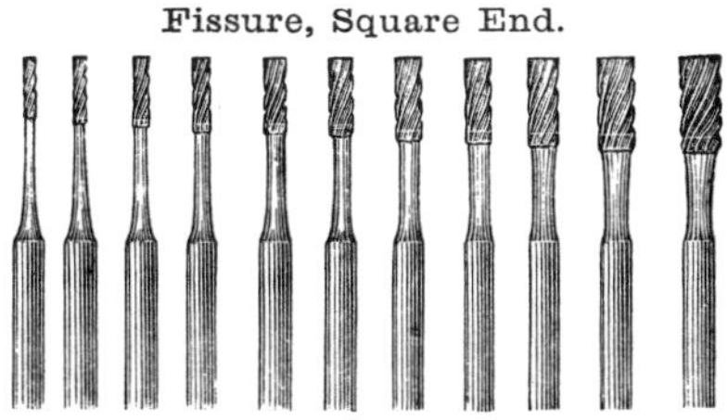

56. 57. 58. 59. 60. 61. 62. 63. 64. 65. 66.

56–63: 25 cents each. 64–66: 35 cents each.

Fissure, Pointed.

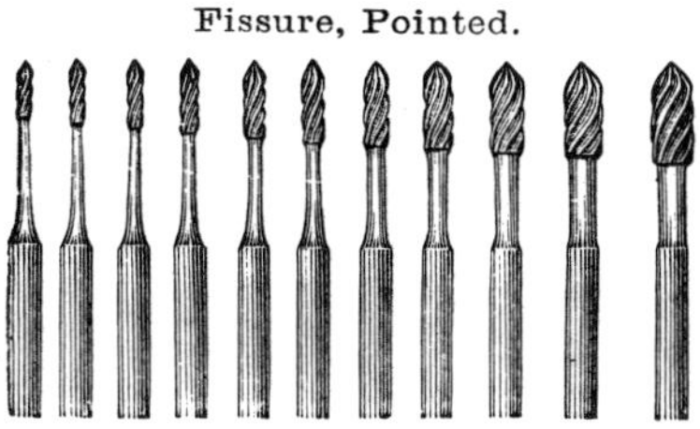

67. 68. 69. 70. 71. 72. 73. 74. 75. 76. 77.

67–74: 25 cents each. 75–77: 35 cents each.

Oval.

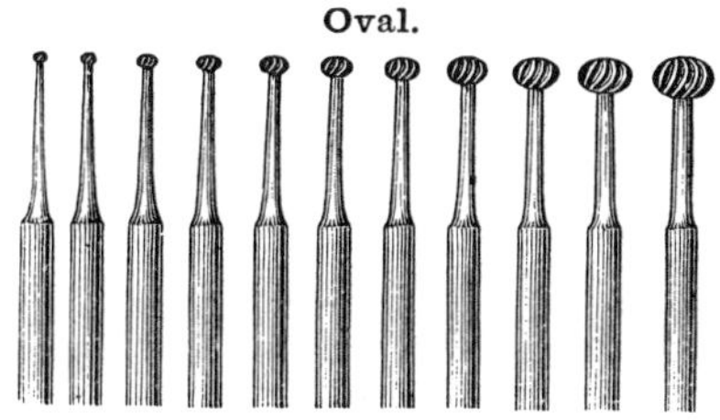

89. 90. 91. 92. 93. 94. 95. 96. 97. 98. 99.

89–96: 25 cents each. 97–99: 35 cents each.

DRILLS.

Flat, Spear Point. **Square.** **Flat, Square Point.** **Spade.**

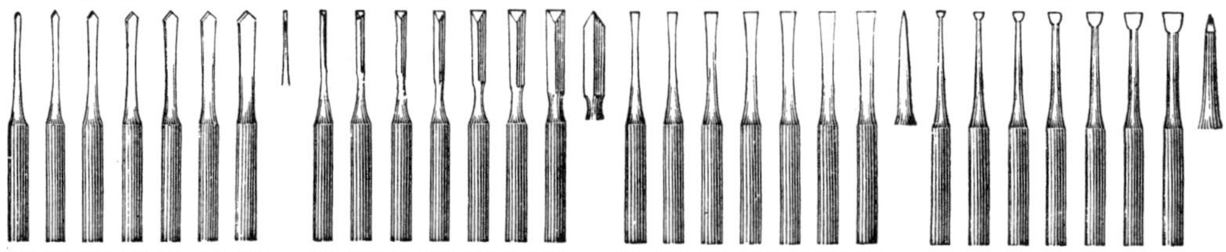

100. 101. 102. 103. 104. 105. 106. 107. 108. 109. 110. 111. 112. 113. 114. 115. 116. 117. 118. 119. 120. 121. 122. 123. 124. 125. 126. 127.

25 cents each.

Forbes's. **Round.** **Five-Sided.**

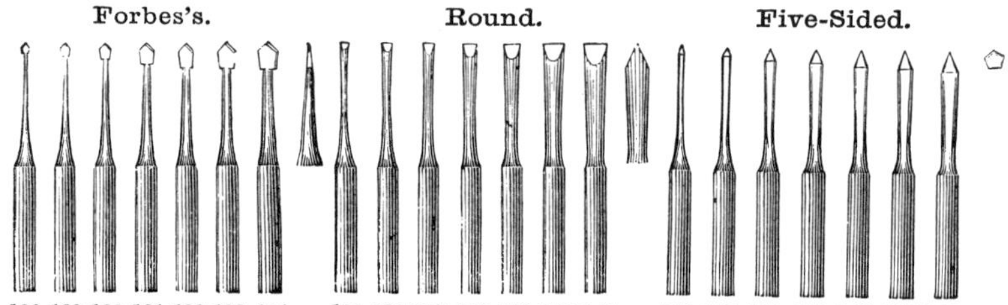

128. 129. 130. 131. 132. 133. 134. 135. 136. 137. 138. 139. 140. 141. 142. 143. 144. 145. 146. 147. 148.

25 cents each.

Twist Drills.

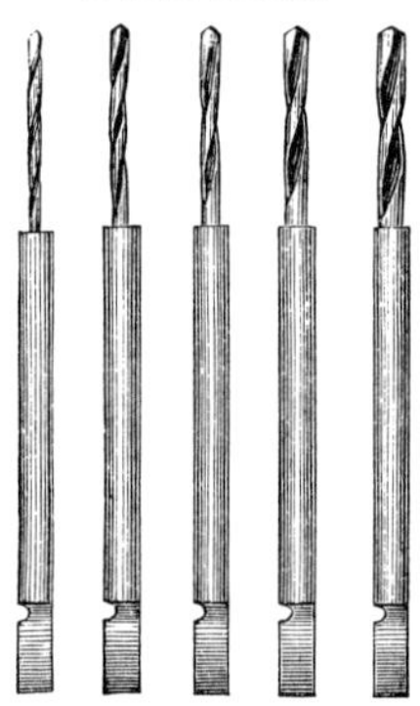

150. 151. 152. 153. 154.

40 cents each.

"Flexible" Burs and Drills.

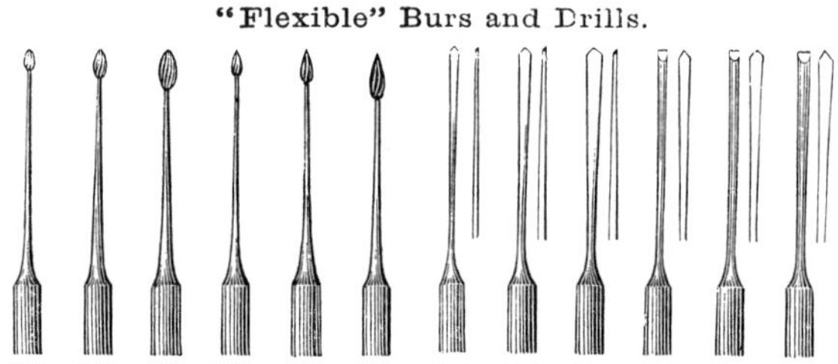

155. 156. 157. 158. 159. 160. 161. 162. 163. 164. 165. 166.

40 cents each.

Trephines.

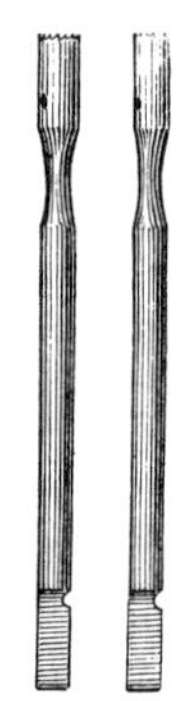

75 cents each.

Plate Saws.

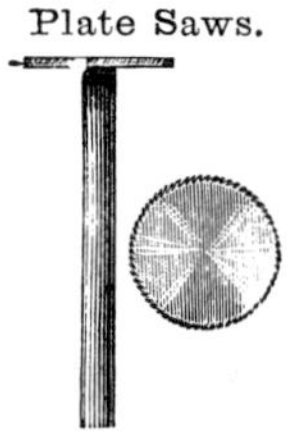

$1.00 each.

"FLEXIBLE" BURS AND DRILLS.

FOR OPENING AND PREPARING NERVE CANALS.

These have spring-tempered stems, longer than regular stock. The bur-heads are formed like those of Dr. Gates and the Gates-Glidden burs, so as to guide easily in the canal; and they are cut to adapt them for Engine work, of a medium fineness between cavity and finishing burs.

BURNISHERS.

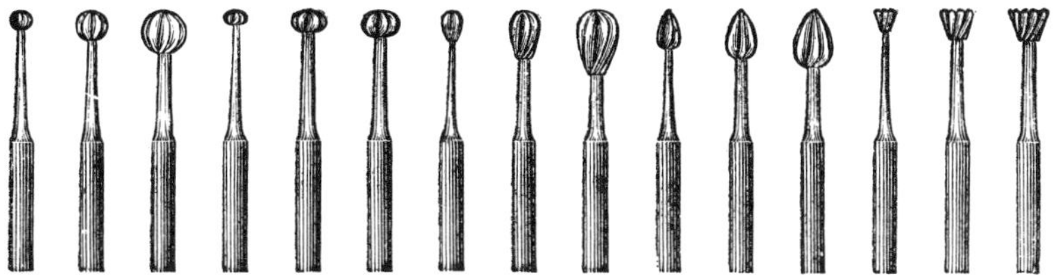

A. B. C. D. E. F. G. H. J. K. L. M. N. O. P.

CORRUGATED, as shown in Cut, 75 cents each.

With SMOOTH HEADS (greatly preferred by some operators), 50 cents each.

PLUG-FINISHING BURS.

Round. Wheel. Inverted Cone.

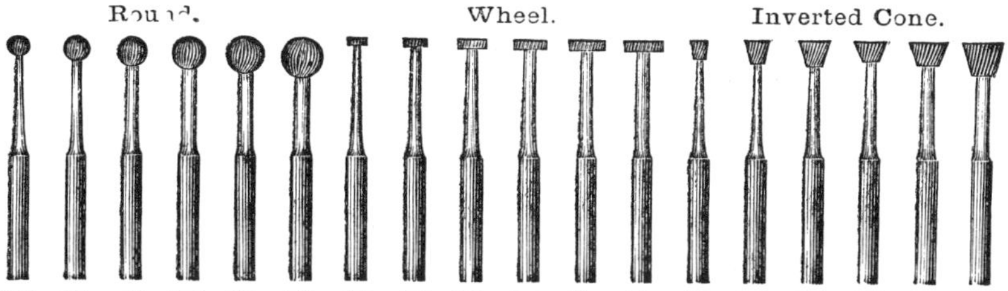

200. 201. 202. 203. 204. — 50 cents each. 205. — 60 cents. 206. 207. 208. 209. 210. — 50 cents each. 211. — 60 cents. 212. 213. 214. 215. 216. — 50 cents each. 217. — 60 cents.

Oval. Bud. Pear.

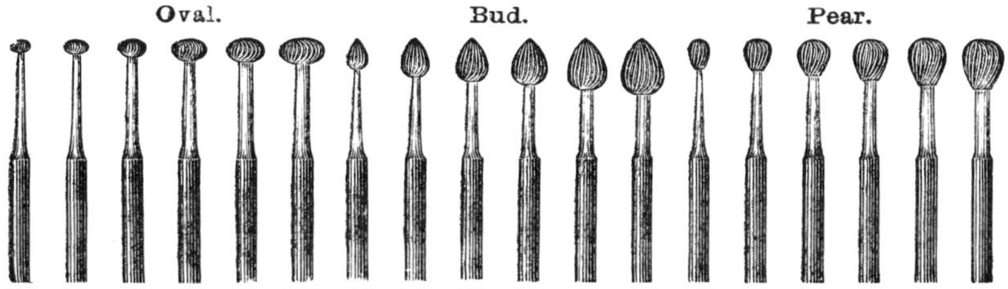

218. 219. 220. 221. 222. — 50 cents each. 223. — 60 cents. 224. 225. 226. 227. 228. — 50 cents each. 229. — 60 cents. 230. 231. 232. 233. 234. — 50 cents each. 235. — 60 cents.

Barrel. Sugar Loaf. Knife Edge.

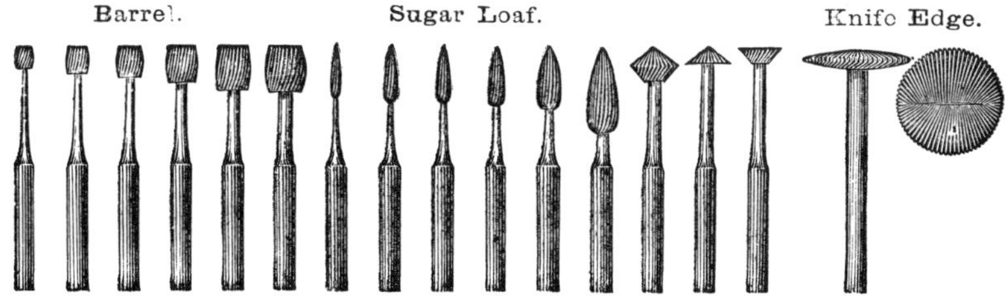

236. 237. 238. 239. 240. — 50 cents each. 241. — 60 cents. 242. 243. 244. 245. 246. — 50 cents each. 247. 248. 249. 250. — 60 cents each.

Price, $1.25.

STONED BURS.

Every leaf stoned sharp like a lancet blade. Originated with us in steel-handled burs, seven years ago. A supply of them in suitable shapes and sizes in stock at the following prices:

Stoned Cavity Burs, from No. 0 to 7, bur gauge	each	$0.50
" Fissure " " " "	"	75
" Finishing Burs, from No. 6 to 14, bur gauge	"	1.00

Extra sizes at proportional prices.

SUPER BURS.

This assortment of Burs for the Engine includes round, wheel, cone, inverted-cone, and bud shapes, of extremely small sizes and extra quality. We distinguish these as the "Super" Burs. They are superior in workmanship, the divisions extremely regular, with very fine and sharp edges,—as good as can be made with the file. These Burs receive a second dressing with a very fine file, which makes them keen and durable. We do not gauge them, but supply this "Super" sort in the various forms as small as burs can be made.

Price . . . . 34 cents each, or $4.00 per dozen.

Screw-Head Mandrel
Invention of Dr. Robert Huey.

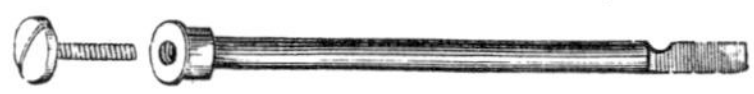

30 cents each.

Parting-Nut Mandrel.

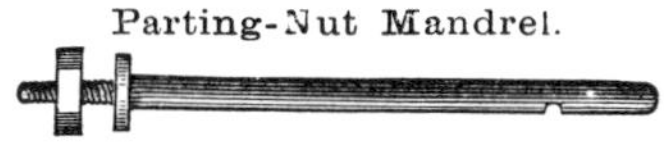

German-Silver Nut.	Right Hand .	. 30 cents each.
Nickel-Plated	" " .	. 40 " "
"	Left " .	. 40 " "

Screw Mandrel, with Shoulder

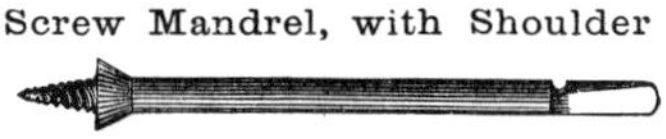

25 cents each.

Screw Mandrel, without Shoulder.

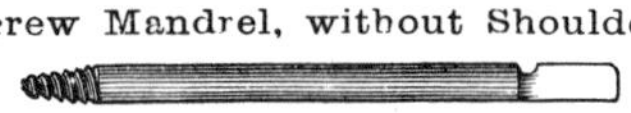

13 cents each.

Screw-Clamp Porte Polisher.
Invention of Dr. G. W. Klump.

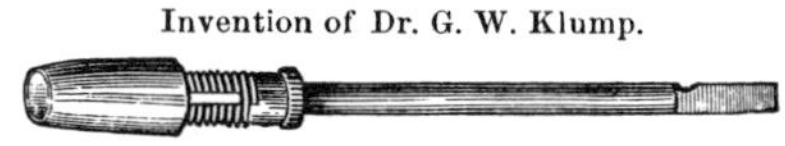

35 cents each.

Porte Polisher, Plain Socket.

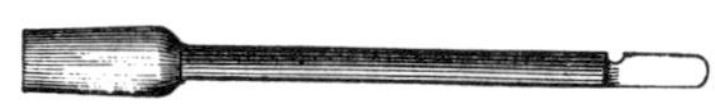

25 cents each.

Porte Polisher, Screw Socket, Nickel-Plated.

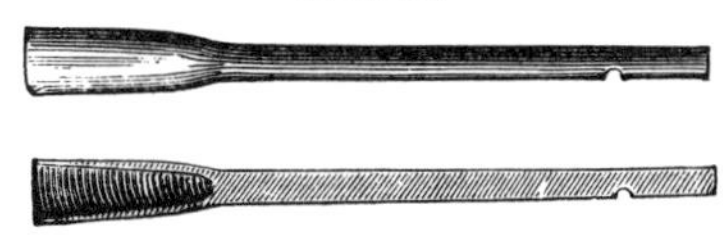

35 cents each.

CORUNDUM POINTS, SET OF 12.

FROM FORMS FURNISHED BY DR. A. L. NORTHROP

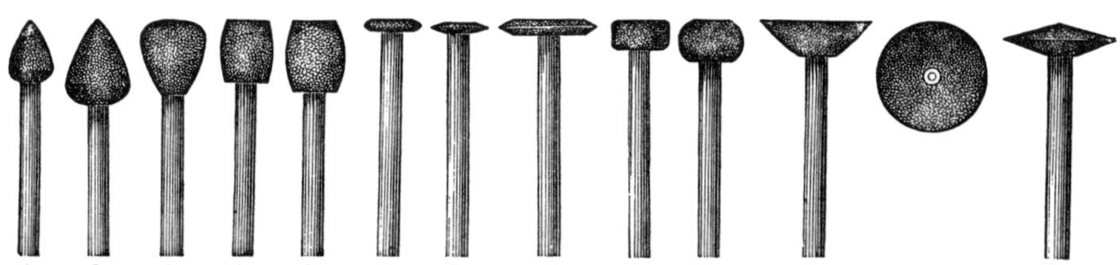

1. 2. 3. 4. 5. 6. 7. 8. 9. 10. 11. 12.

Points, not mounted . . . . per doz. $0.75
Mounted on Mandrels . . . . " 1.50

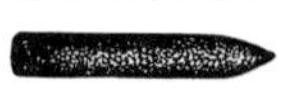 Butler's Corundum Points for Porte Polisher . . " .75

"STUMP" CORUNDUM WHEELS.

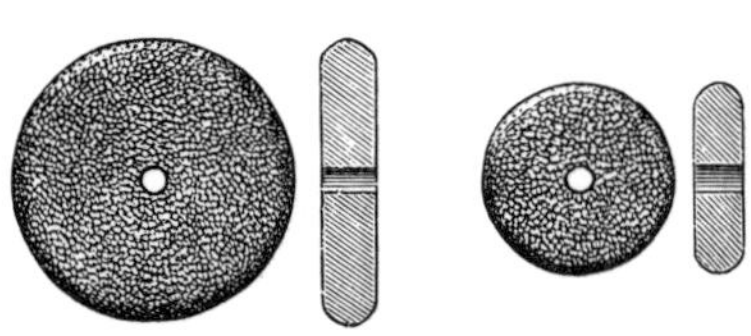

The Cuts illustrate the forms of two new styles of Corundum Wheels, one-half and three-quarters of an inch in diameter, one-eighth of an inch thick. They are intended for use with the Dental Engine in the preparation of roots for pivoting and for cutting off projections of natural teeth.

Price . . . . 13 cents each, or $1.40 per dozen.

ARKANSAS, HINDOSTAN, AND SCOTCH STONES.

These illustrations show a selection of the forms made. We do not conform exactly to these sizes, but have an approximate variety. It is necessary to mount these on mandrels before turning them into shape. They cannot therefore be supplied unmounted.

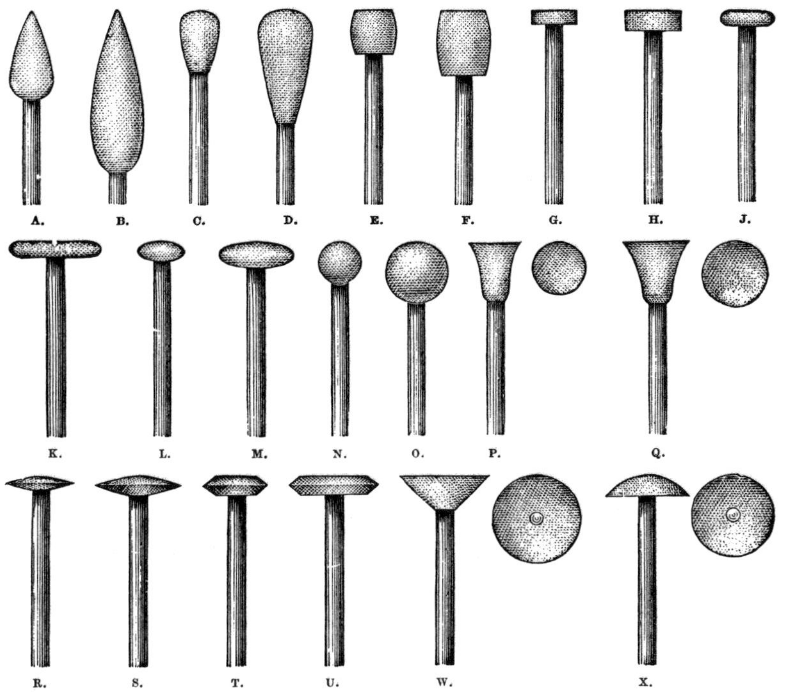

Arkansas Stone, $1.00 each. Hindostan Stone, 50 cents each. Scotch Stone, 30 cents each.

BOXWOOD DISKS.

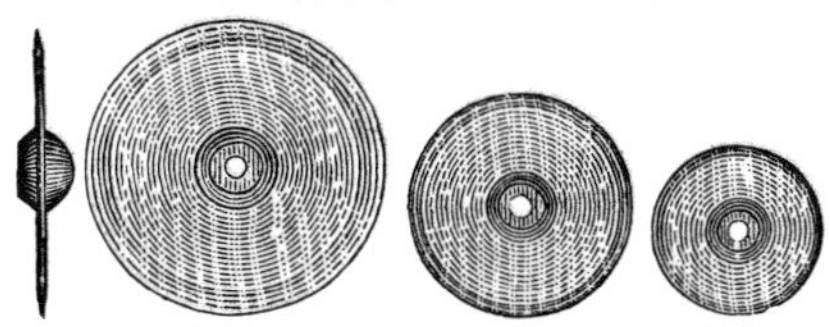

$\frac{3}{4}$ in. $\frac{9}{16}$ in. $\frac{7}{16}$ in.

5 sizes, from $\frac{7}{16}$ to $\frac{3}{4}$ inch. $\frac{3}{4}$ inch, per doz., $1.50. Other sizes, per doz., 60 cents.

WOOD POLISHING POINTS.

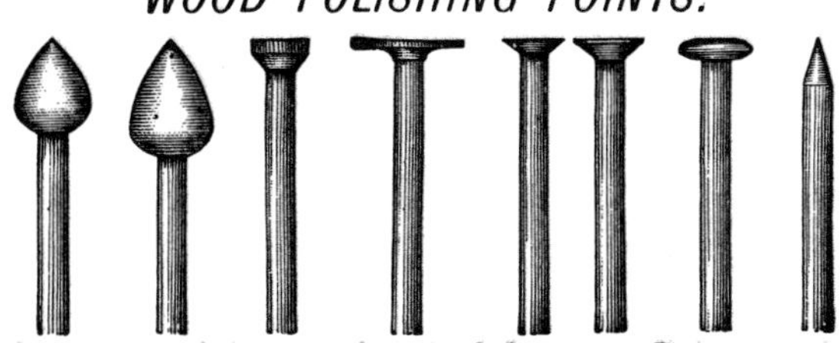

Put up in boxes containing one hundred Points. Price, per box, $1.25.

RUBBER DISKS AND POINTS.

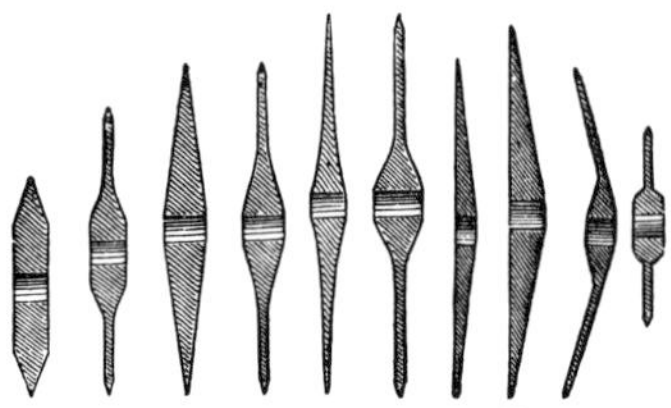

A. B. C. D. E. F. G. H. I. K.

These Disks are of Hard or Soft Rubber, for carrying powders for polishing the natural teeth and finishing fillings. The Cuts illustrate the forms and sizes.

Price of the Hard Rubber . .	each 10 cents.
Mounted	" 20 "
Price of the Soft Rubber, used with the Parting-Nut Mandrel . .	" 10 "

SOFT RUBBER POINTS.

FOR MOUNTING ON SCREW MANDRELS.

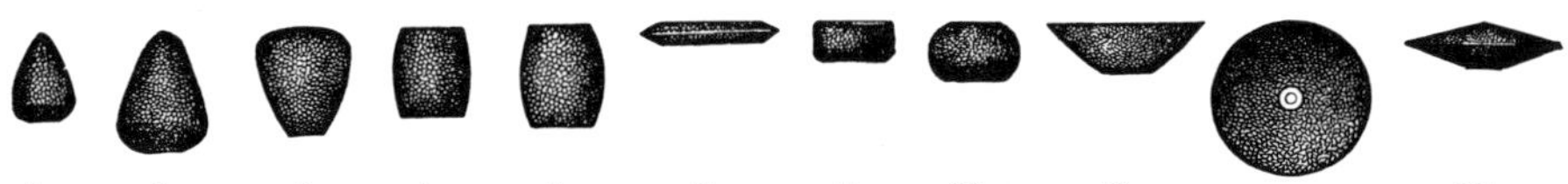

1. 2. 3. 4. 5. 8. 9. 10. 11. 12.

Price, per doz. $0.75

SHELLAC FOR MOUNTING.

For the convenience of operators in mounting Disks and Points, we have had Shellac prepared in Sticks, ¼ inch diameter, 3 inches long, put up in boxes of one dozen. Prepared also in Powder, for the same purpose.

Price, per box, in Sticks	25 cents.
" " Powder	10 "

POLISHING POWDERS.

We have prepared several additional Powders for polishing and finishing purposes, and the variety now offered will probably meet all preferences. These Powders are intended for use with felt and leather buffs, wood points and disks, hard rubber disks, and will be found particularly useful with the soft rubber disks.

Hindostan Stone Powder	per box, 12 cents.
Arkansas " "	" 25 "
Pumice " " (per lb. 15 cents)	" 10 "
Emery Powder (per lb. 25 cents)	" 10 "
Buck-horn Powder, small boxes	" 12 "
" " large "	" 38 "
Corundum Flour	" 25 "
" " Extra Fine	" 25 "
Rouge	" 20 "

Corundum is, without doubt, a more rapid polisher than anything hitherto offered for the above uses. Highly recommended by those who have tried it.

There are two grades, one EXTRA FINE.

DR. R. ARTHUR'S DISKS.

FOR PERMANENTLY SEPARATING AND POLISHING THE TEETH.

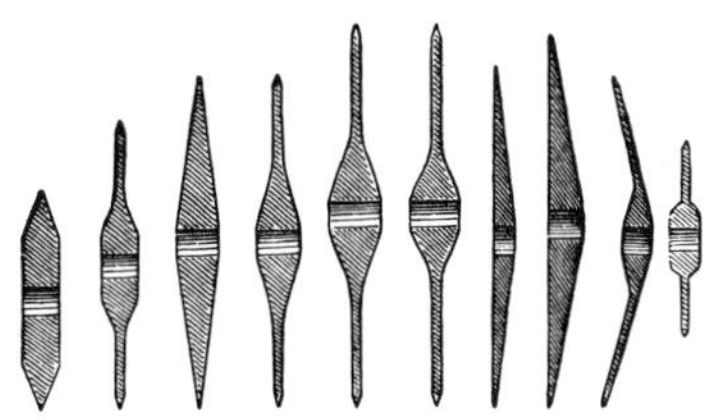

A. B. C. D. E. F. G. H. I. K.

A and K, not mounted, each 13 cents; per doz.	. . . . . .	$1.40
All others, " " " 25 " "	. . . . . .	2.75
A and K, mounted, " 23 " "	. . . . . .	2.50
All others, " " 35 " "	. . . . . .	3.75
Not mounted, per Set—6, A to F	. . . . . .	1.25
Mounted, " 6, A to F	. . . . . .	1.75
Not mounted, " 10, A to K	. . . . . .	2.00
Mounted, " 10, A to K	. . . . . .	2.90

Every dentist has encountered the great difficulties attendant upon the permanent separation of the teeth, especially the bicuspids and molars, whether for the arrest of incipient caries, the prevention of caries, or as a preliminary step to the filling of proximate surfaces. The removal of the excess of gold of proximate fillings is equally difficult and laborious.

The object of these Disks is to overcome the difficulties and disadvantages of the file and chisel for the purpose in view. This it is claimed they do in the most effectual manner.

The advantages claimed for them over any other means now known for the purpose are:

1st. By their use the requisite separations are made in a manner far less disagreeable and painful to the patient, and in much shorter time.

2d. The separated surfaces can be polished very quickly and more perfectly than by any other means.

3d. The separations are made with great rapidity, as the Disks readily grind away the hardest enamel.

4th. No operator who has once used these Disks will be able to dispense with them, and no patient who has had teeth separated with them will afterwards willingly consent to the use of the file or chisel for the purpose.

They are made of *carefully selected crystals of corundum*, approaching in *cutting quality* very nearly to diamond powder.

STANDS FOR ENGINE BITS.

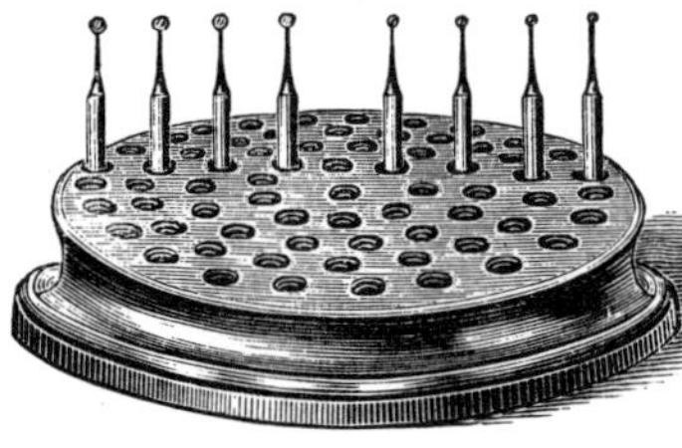

1.

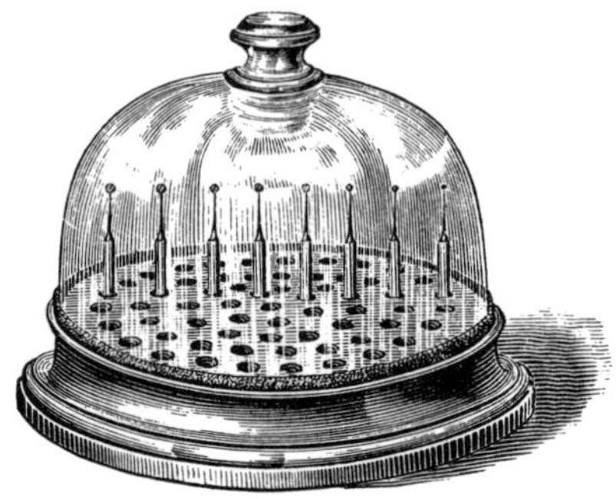

2.

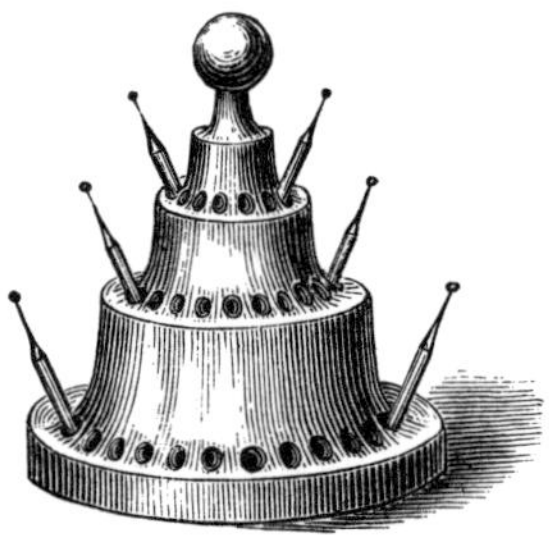

3.

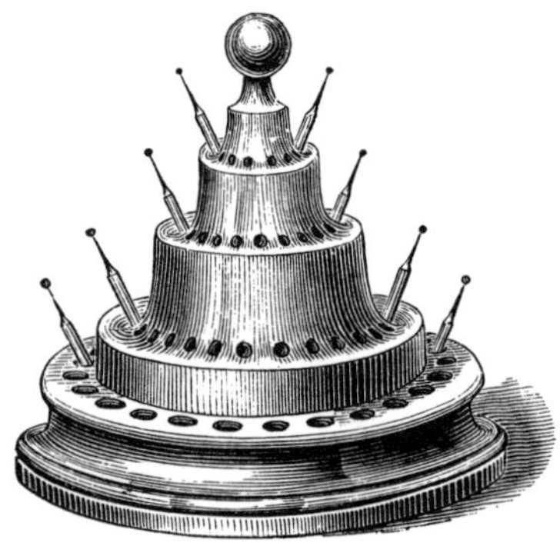

4.

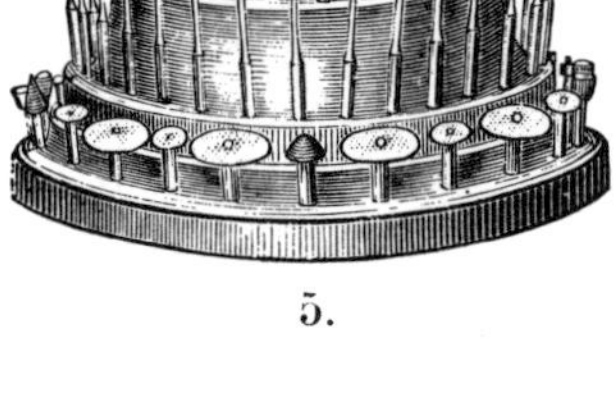

5.

Nos. 3, 4, and 5 Patented March 2d, 1875.

The Cuts illustrate five varieties of Stands for the convenient keeping of Engine Bits.

No. 1 is of polished maple, 5 inches in diameter, 1 inch high, containing 72 holes.

No. 2, same, with glass cover, but contains only 60 holes.

No. 3 is of either polished maple or walnut; $3\frac{1}{4}$ inches in diameter, $3\frac{1}{2}$ inches high, containing 48 holes.

No. 4 is of either polished maple or walnut; $4\frac{3}{4}$ inches in diameter, $4\frac{1}{2}$ inches high, containing 78 holes.

No. 5 is a Revolving Stand, of polished maple, 7 inches in diameter, $7\frac{1}{2}$ inches high, containing 120 holes.

No. 1	$1.00
No. 2	1.50
No. 3	1.00
No. 4	1.50
No. 5	3.00

TOOTH-BRUSH WHEELS.

FOR USE WITH THE DENTAL ENGINE IN CLEANING TEETH AND POLISHING FILLINGS.

They are made with bone center and stem, for use with Klump's porte polisher. No. 2 is also made with a wood center and without stem, to use on screw mandrel.

No. 1, Cup-shaped, one row bristles . 25 cents.
No. 2, Straight, two rows bristles . . 35 "

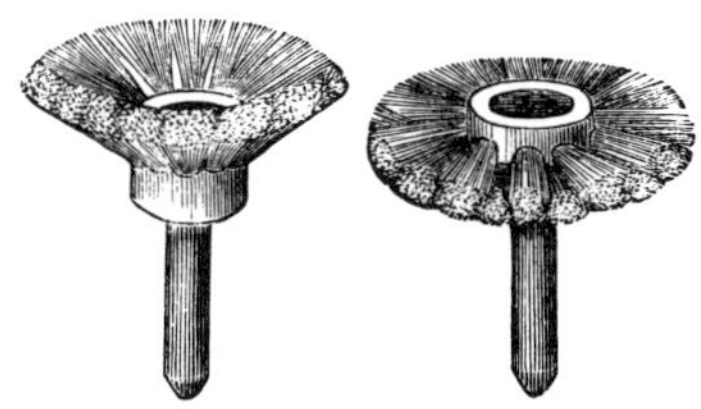

No. 1. No. 2.

STEEL WIRE WHEEL BRUSH.

FOR CLEANING ENGINE TOOLS (BURS) AND FILES.

For use with the screw mandrel of the S. S. W. Engine.

1 inch diameter, two rows . . . . . . 50 cents each.

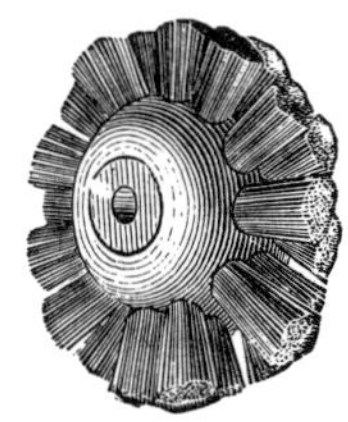

No. 1.

LOCK-BIT ATTACHMENTS.

Patented June 2d and December 29th, 1874.

RIGHT-ANGLE.

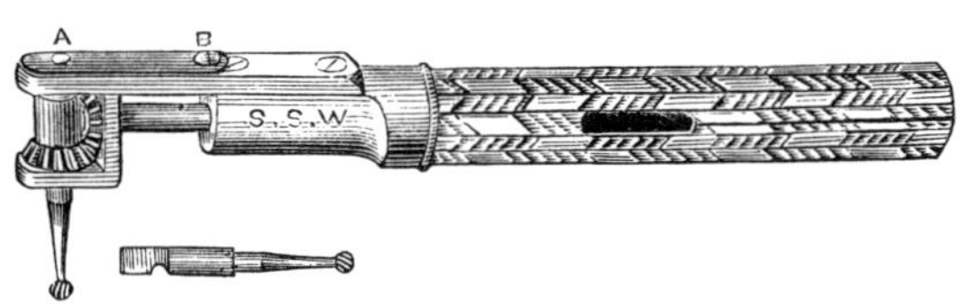

ACUTE-ANGLE.

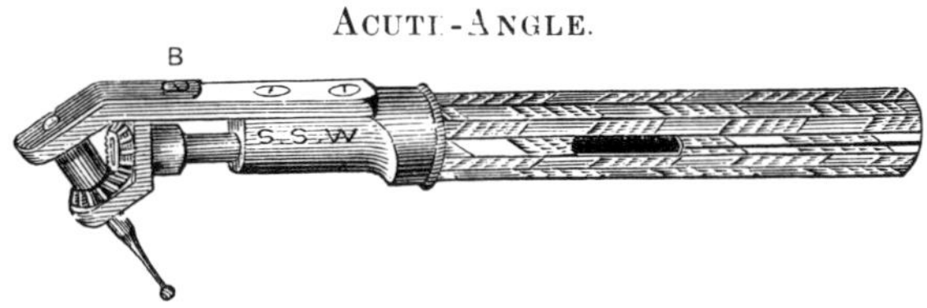

Price of either $5.00

The advantage of these Attachments is that the bit is *securely locked in the socket*, on the same principle as that by which the hand-piece bit is held. To attach the bit, place it in the socket and gently force it, turning it at the same time, which securely locks it; to remove it, place the finger-nail under the end of the spring at A, and lift it slightly; with the other hand turn the bit and withdraw it from the socket. The spring is held by a screw at B, which can be removed when worn out and a new one substituted. The journals of the tool-socket are made of hardened steel, to prevent wear. In these Attachments, the distance from the head at A to the point of the bur is nearly a quarter of an inch shorter than in those previously made.

The tube is split so that it may be sprung over the hand-piece and turned at the will of the operator, for use in any part of the mouth.

DR. F. HICKMAN'S DISK CARRIER.

Patented April 7th, 1874, and January 5th, 1875.

IMPROVED. OLD STYLE.

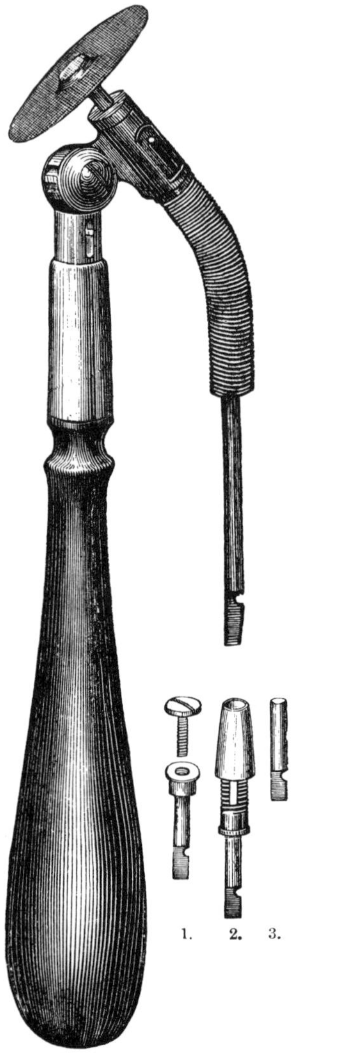

1. 2. 3.

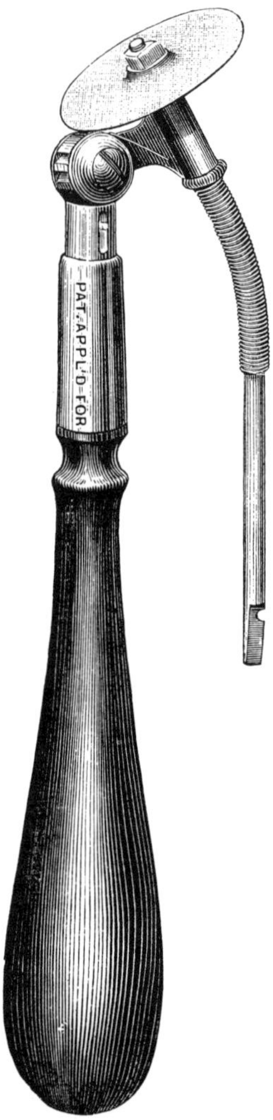

Attention is called to a recent improvement in this Instrument, in the substitution of a LOCK-BIT in the shaft (the same as in the Hand-Piece of the Dental Engine).

By the use of Blank Mandrels Disks of different sizes may be used and changed with facility. A Screw-Clamp Porte Polisher, a Screw-Head Mandrel, and a Plain Mandrel (as shown in the Cut) are adapted to be used with the Carrier.

In the above appliance, the Disk has an independent holder attached by a short flexible shaft to the driving-bit, which is secured in the hand-piece of the Engine like the ordinary bit; the ratchet-wheel in the head of the Carrier is controlled by the pin which emerges from the slot below, enabling the operator to adjust and guide the Disk in the mouth **parallel with the handle,** or at any desired angle, and giving ample range to meet the requirements of the entire dental arch in separating the teeth, cutting out lingual and buccal fissures, and finishing fillings and rough surfaces.

Price of Carrier, either style	each	$5.00
" Screw-Head Mandrel, 1	"	30
" Porte Polisher, 2	"	35
" Plain Mandrel, 3	"	7

CHANGEABLE-ANGLE DISK CARRIER.

INVENTION OF DR. GEO. H. CUSHING.

(Patented November 2d, 1875.)

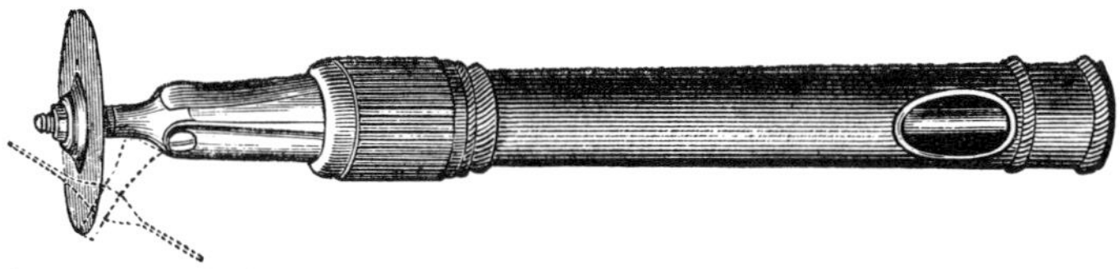

The advantages of this Carrier are manifest in the facility with which it may be attached to and removed from the Dental Engine hand-piece, in the same manner as the right-angle attachment; in the *absolute steadiness of motion attained;* and in the omission of the external driving-spring. The *angular range* of the Disk, indicated by the dotted lines, has been found sufficient to meet all the requirements for separating teeth in both the upper and lower jaws. A slight turn of the *milled collar* will lock the Disk at any desired angle. The Disk is attached to the spindle by a nut, on the principle of the parting-nut mandrel. This appliance is made and finished in the best manner, is convenient in size, and without rough surfaces to chafe the mouth or fingers while in use.

Price $10.00

FIXED-ANGLE DISK-CARRIER, WITH STOP-MOTION.

(Patented November 2d, 1875; April 4th, 1876.)

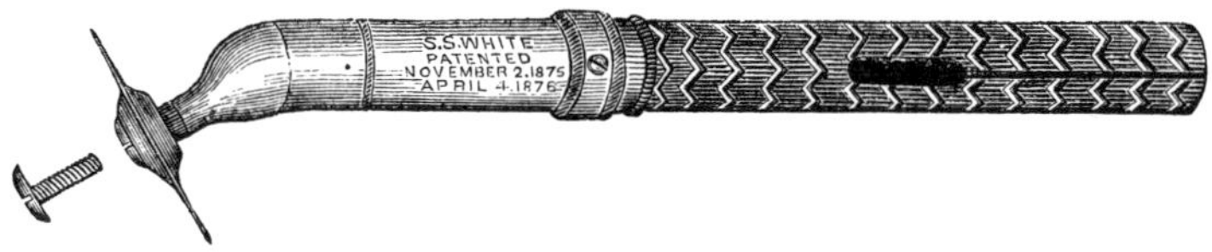

As some operators have suggested that the angle shown in the Cut will meet most of the requirements in separating teeth, we have made a Disk-Carrier having this fixed angle, and with the driving parts protected by an extension of the tubular casing. It is attached to the hand-piece in the same manner as the above. The Disk is secured to the spindle in the same manner as in the screw-head mandrel. The revolution of the Disk can be stopped at pleasure, without slackening the speed of the Engine, by a simple pressure of the fore-finger upon the collar; the removal of the finger allowing it to again revolve.

Price $6.00

DR. F. HICKMAN'S DROP-TUBE AND SPONGE-HOLDER.

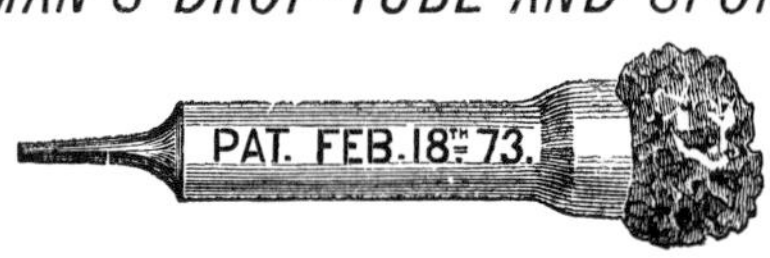

The Cut represents an appliance designed to accompany the Dental Engine when disks are used. The nozzle is of metal, nickel-plated, and the whole length, including the sponge, is about 4¼ inches. It is simple, neat, cleanly, and indestructible. The sponge attachment makes it useful either to wet or clean the disk.

Price . . . . 35 cents.

FOUNTAIN MOUTH PROTECTOR.

(Patented January 26th, 1875.)

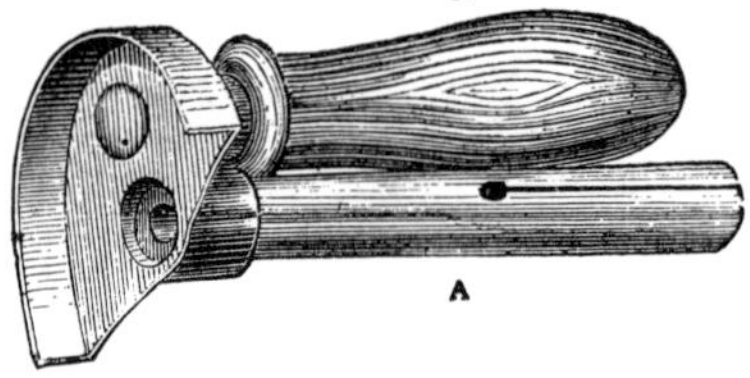

The Cut illustrates an admirable little device, which serves the double purpose of protecting the tongue and cheek from injury by the disk, and at the same time supplies water to keep the disk wet while in motion. In the Cut "A" is a tube, slit so that it may be sprung over the hand-piece of the Engine, and turned at the will of the operator, for use in any part of the mouth. "B' is a small rubber bulb communicating by a minute aperture with the Protector, as shown in the Cut. When compressed with the finger and thumb, and immersed in water, it will fill readily, and carry water enough to keep the disk wet for a considerable time, the supply being kept up by a touch of the operator's finger on the rubber bulb. When slipped off the hand-piece, if the rubber bulb is compressed and the Protector dropped into a tumbler of water, it will fill again, and in this manner may be kept always ready for use.

Price $1.00

DR. F. HICKMAN'S AIR INJECTOR, OR AUTOMATIC CHIP BLOWER.

(Patented March 31st, 1874.)

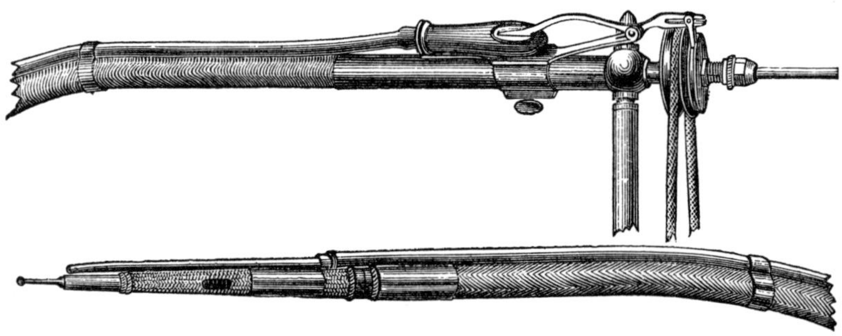

The invention here illustrated is designed for use with the Dental Engine. A rubber bulb or bellows is compressed automatically by means of a simple mechanism which is connected with and worked by the driven pulley. The air is forced from the bulb through the connecting rubber tube to a fixed nozzle at the hand-piece, whence it is thrown into the cavity of the tooth. The air thus driven out of the bulb leaves a vacuum which is instantly filled again with air. This alternate exhaustion and supply is kept up so rapidly, even at the ordinary speed of the Engine, that the air is injected in a continuous stream into the cavity. This appliance operates to keep the cavity clear of bur-dust and cuttings, and also to keep the bur cool while in use.

Full instructions accompany the Injector.

Price $5.00

FOUNTAIN DRIP-POINT.

SUGGESTED BY DR. F. HERRICK.

Covered by Patent January 2[illegible]th, 1875.

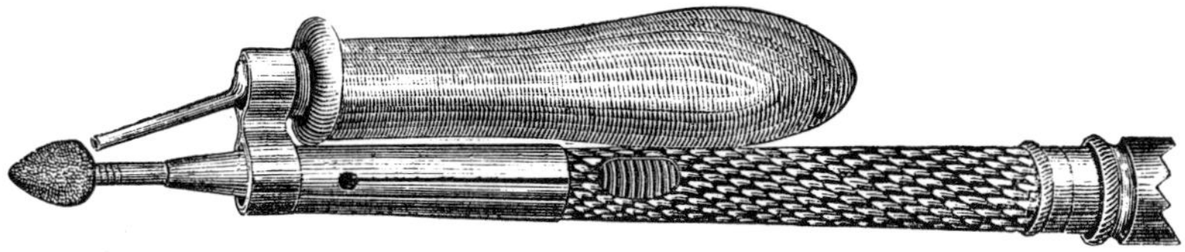

The device illustrated in Cut is intended for use with the Northrop set of corundum points. The rubber bulb being compressed with the finger and thumb, and immersed in water, will fill in a little while, and carry water enough to keep the point wet for a considerable time, the supply being kept up by a touch of the operator's finger on the bulb.

Price . . . . 75 cents.

POLISHER AND FILE CARRIER,

FOR USE WITH THE DENTAL ENGINE.

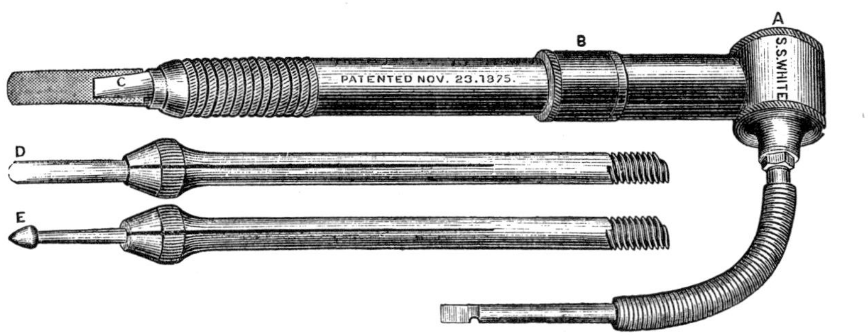

The Cut illustrates an instrument designed for use with the Dental Engine, for polishing, burnishing, or filing.

A is the cap of the head-piece, which has a milled edge, and can be removed by unscrewing with the thumb and finger. The removal of this cap exposes the disk, having two holes at different distances from the center, giving opportunity, by changing the screw, to lengthen or shorten the stroke of the plunger.

B is a shoulder-joint, allowing free rotary motion of the lower end of the case when in use.

C is a flat porte polisher, adapted to carrying files.

D is a carrier for wood or corundum points.

E is a carrier for engine burnishers.

With this set a file can be used for separating teeth or dressing down fillings; a corundum point, or a wood point for carrying powders for removing tartar, etc., or a burnisher for polishing fillings.

As will be seen by the Cut, the holders may be changed by simply unscrewing one and screwing in another at pleasure.

Price of the instrument, with three Carriers $8.00

Automatic Plugger for Engine.

INVENTION OF DR. T. L. BUCKINGHAM.

Patented August 26th, 1873.

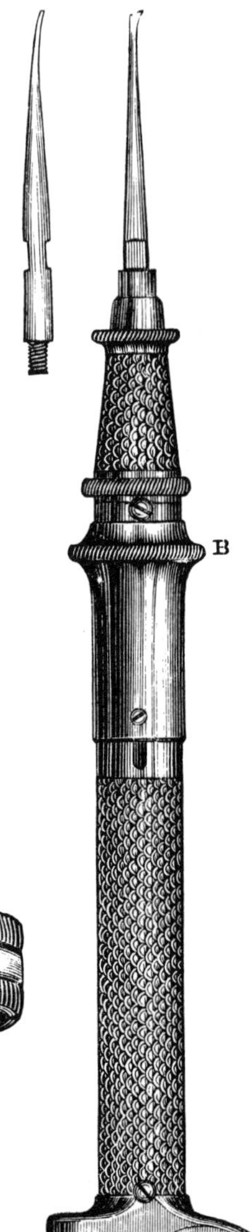

After a protracted effort, including the trial of a variety of devices, we were enabled to offer to the Profession an Automatic Plugger adapted to the Engine, which has proved to be an indispensable assistant to the operator. It is in use in the offices of many prominent practitioners, and receives their unqualified indorsement.

It is claimed that this instrument possesses all the qualities needed in such an appliance.

The force of the blow is entirely under control, being determined by the set-screw A, which, if turned to the right, increases the force, and if turned to the left lessens it. The force can also be kept constantly under control by the collar B on the hand-piece. By an almost automatic or instinctive movement of the thumb of the operator, the collar is moved up or down, according to the force desired in the blow.

In the same manner the blow can be suspended altogether, at any instant, without interfering with the rhythmical movement of the foot propelling the Engine, as when picking up a pellet of gold, or when it is desirable, for any reason, to use the instrument temporarily as a hand-plugger.

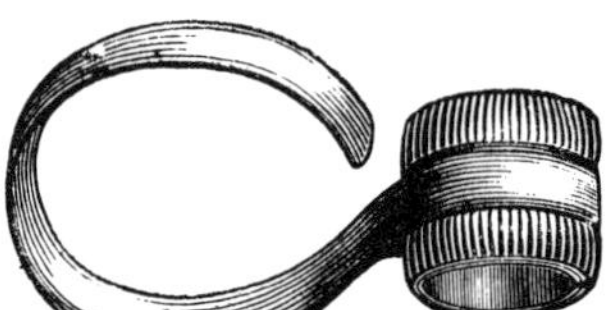

The force and effect of the blow may also be accurately regulated by the distance at which the point is held from the filling,—being heavier according to its proximity to the surface to be condensed. Thus, where very delicate and careful manipulation is necessary, as at the edges of a cavity in a frail tooth, the operator may determine the precise force by the distance at which the point is held.

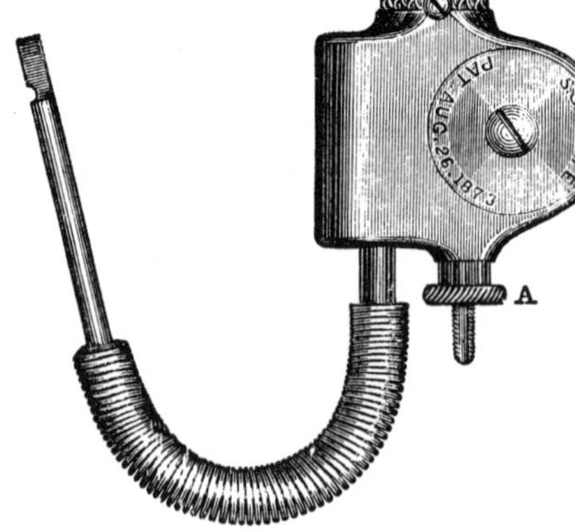

The bit-holder has a small spiral spring at its inner end, which, after each blow, draws it back instantly to receive the next blow of the plunger.

When the Engine is run at moderate speed, the Plugger will give about 1800 blows per minute; but, if desired, the number can be reduced one-half, by removing two of the spuds in the cog-wheel in the head of the Plugger. Then, by slowing the speed of the Engine, single and distinct blows as low as 75 or 100 per minute can be given.

Most of the points for standard automatic pluggers may be used in this Plugger, though many of the points made for these instruments will be found to have deeper serrations than are desirable for use with such rapid motion as is given by the Engine. Very fine and shallow serrations or smooth points will be found best adapted to produce solidity of a filling; the coarser kinds being liable to chop up the gold and so make it porous.

Any one having valuable points which he desires to use in this mallet, can be supplied, on order, with a mallet and socket adapted to them.

The Plugger is very neatly made; the workmanship is first-class, and the parts are interchangeable. Its movements are simple, and therefore it is not likely to get out of order. It can be adapted to any engine by a modification of the connecting-bit at the end of the driving-spring.

The Plugger is complete without the ring; but some very much prefer its use with the ring. It is readily slipped on the case by removing the head of the Plugger, and can be held at any point desired. The forefinger being passed through the ring, supports the weight of the Plugger, and gives the operator a better command of its movements.

Price of Plugger	$20.00
" Finger-Ring	1.00

TESTIMONIALS

IN FAVOR OF

THE S. S. WHITE ENGINE PLUGGER.

Below we give a few of the many testimonials received from the Profession:

The Automatic Plugger adapted to the S. S. White Engine, which I received from you some weeks ago, I have had in daily use since. Your prophetic remark that you "believe it will prove to be an indispensable assistant to the operator," has been more than realized in my experience. This little instrument, impelled so noiselessly and easily that the movement of the foot upon the treadle becomes as automatic as if the motive-power was from some foreign source, will undoubtedly commend itself to all who can appreciate freedom from annoyances and efficiency of work in such an instrument. Its condensing power is unsurpassed, while the accurate and complete control which the operator has over the blow is surprising, as well as especially gratifying in its results.

C. N. PEIRCE, PHILADELPHIA.

I regard the S. S. White Engine Plugger a valuable auxiliary. It condenses well and rapidly, and is often commended by patients for absence of unpleasant sensations.

D. D. SMITH, PHILADELPHIA.

It affords me much pleasure to give my testimony in behalf of the S. S. White Engine Plugger; after a thorough trial of it I feel prepared to say that it is *the* appliance of them all next to rubber dam and the S. S. W. Burring Engine. I find that with it I can pack gold faster and *better* than with my hand-mallet, thus effecting a saving of considerable time, and making a denser plug than *can* be made in the old way, besides doing the work with much more comfort both to myself and patient. I am delighted with it, and would not be without it for any consideration.

C. F. WHEELER, ALBANY, N. Y.

It affords me pleasure to give my testimony in favor of an instrument so valuable to the dentist as the S. S. White Engine Plugger, which is destined to come into general use.

Besides possessing all the valuable qualities claimed for it, there is one feature that I have not seen noticed and find of great advantage, viz., the certainty and ease with which enamel can be cut by the use of chisels fitting the socket the same as the plugger points. These are especially applicable in either approximal or crown cavities in bicuspids or molars, where there is overhanging enamel to be cut away, which is chipped off with ease; while there is no danger of the instrument slipping, it being more easily and perfectly controlled than a hand-chisel, hand-mallet, or the ordinary automatic.

G. W. KLUMP, WILLIAMSPORT, PA.

I to-day filled a central incisor which took over a half-book of gold foil, malleting the gold with the S. S. White Engine Plugger, and I am constrained to say that the Plugger more than meets my expectation. The first filling I put in with it, it seemed all the time I was at work as if it did not condense the gold, the blows being so very delicate; but when I was through and came to finish it up, to my utter surprise I found it a perfectly condensed filling. It received a beautiful finish.

Having made a fair trial of the Engine Plugger, I can cordially recommend it to all who desire to fill teeth with ease to themselves and their patients. As for myself, I could not do without it.

J. H. SMITH, NEW HAVEN, CONN.

Later he says: I wish you could have seen me build up a tooth to-day with your Plugger; it works like a charm. I am more and more pleased with it every day.

I have been using the Buckingham Automatic Plugger attached to your Engine for about four months, and to say that I am delighted with its execution is stating a simple fact.

I can pack four times the amount of gold, in a given length of time, with it that I can either by the use of the ordinary automatic or by the use of the hand-mallet and an assistant; in fact, it does away with the need of an assistant, and should be called the dentist's ready assistant.

Its advantages may be summed up as follows:

1st. It strikes a lighter and more uniform blow than either the hand or automatic mallet, thereby enabling patients to endure the fatigues of plugging with greater ease and comfort.

2d. It facilitates packing three or four times as much gold in the same time as by the before-mentioned processes.

3d. Its extreme cheapness,—twenty-one dollars,—and its easy attachment to the Engine, being as quickly done as the attachment of a drill or bur.

I can only say, in conclusion, I think it will pay any dentist using an engine to give it a trial. I am perfectly satisfied that it will come into general use by the Profession.

G. B. McDONNELD, CONNEAUTVILLE, PA.

I have used the S. S. White Engine Plugger with so much satisfaction that I would not be without it, and for medium-sized fillings I prefer it to the Electric.

J. H. JOHNSTON, SHAMOKIN, PA.

I consider the S. S. White Engine Plugger a great success, and indispensable to easy, rapid, and perfect filling. The ease with which it can be made to do its work, and not being liable to get out of repair, renders it always reliable. It relieves the patient of much of the tedium of protracted dental operations, and all of the unpleasantness incident to the use of the hand mallet. It strikes a blow so effective, yet so delicate and painless, as to be beyond reach of imitation by nerve and muscle. I have used this Plugger daily, and almost hourly, for six months, with the greatest satisfaction to self and patients.

I could as easily dispense with my engine as with my mallet. In no other way have I ever been able to obtain such perfect adaptation to cavity walls, such solidity and finish, with such rapidity and comfort to patients, as with the S. S. White Engine Plugger. To praise it would be as faint a tribute to its true merits as to say of rubber dam that it is a good thing.

J. W. DENNIS, PEKIN, ILL.

It affords me pleasure to say that I am well pleased with the S S. White Engine Plugger attached to the S. S. White Engine, it being much more pleasant to my patients than any other automatic plugger I have ever seen or tried. It gives a light and quick blow, which is essential to welding the layers of gold, condenses perfectly and uniformly throughout. Any operator who follows the printed directions with it will be highly pleased with its work.

J. T. LEET, HOLLIDAYSBURG, PA.

I am much pleased with your Engine Mallet. Extended experience proves that it is most valuable. If used in its proper place it fills a void that has long been felt. It is labor-saving, and condenses every variety of foil most admirably. I prefer to use it with smooth points.

J. BELISARIO, SYDNEY, N. S. W.

We must not fail to state that, after trying the S. S. White Engine Plugger, we consider it the most complete and serviceable mallet known for plugging teeth. It has no equal. Being accustomed to condense the gold so thoroughly and with such care with the other kind of mallet, we are surprised to find how thoroughly and rapidly the gold becomes consolidated with less than half the labor. The work is the same as that done by the Electric Mallet, but with the advantage that it is not unwieldy like the Electric, and is *always in working order*. In other words, one *can depend upon it*. Patients will not allow us to use any other mallet after having had it once used upon them; neither will either of us use any other while it is in use by the other. For that reason we order another for ourselves, and one for Dr. E.

SHRIGLEY & HAY, VALPARAISO, S. A.

I am using the S. S. White Engine Plugger from six to eight hours daily, and in justice due, must say that it surpasses my most sanguine expectations. It is far more pleasant to the patients than any other, so much so that they all admire it, and give their approbation. It does about twice the amount of work that a hand automatic plugger will do, with little or no labor; is under *perfect control* of the operator in so many different ways in regard to the *force* of blow and picking up the gold; *condenses thoroughly* without shocking the patient by pain; is so simple in construction that it is never out of order, and is always ready to work at your will. In short, it becomes a pleasure and pastime to fill teeth with the S. S. White Engine Plugger.

WM. H. HERTZ, HAZLETON, PA.

It gives me pleasure to say that I am wonderfully pleased with the working of the S. S. White Engine Plugger. I have been doing my work with it since July, with more satisfaction than at any other time in twelve years' practice.

J. W. ISENBERG, ALTOONA, PA.

I am free to say that your Engine Plugger is a perfect little clipper, the most pert and complete chatterbox imaginable; a gem of work and duty not to be dispensed with in any well-ordered dental outfit; liked by the gentlemen, petted by the ladies, and endeared to the little patients by its agreeable manners and thorough work.

M. D. L. DODSON, TOWANDA, PA.

A SET OF PLUGGER POINTS FOR THE S. S. WHITE ENGINE AUTOMATIC PLUGGER.

The Set of Points for our Engine Plugger (illustrated on opposite page) has been carefully chosen, arranged, and modified. The modifications are in size and facial angles, adapting them to reach cavities easily; and in fineness of serrations, to fit them for packing gold safely under the rapid blows of the Engine Plugger. They are, as a set, serrated finer and shallower than any ever before offered to the Profession. The beauty, fineness, and perfect workmanship of these instruments can only be appreciated by using them, or by an examination with a magnifying-glass.

The small side Cuts show the size and shape of each face. The magnified ones are added to display the exact count and style of serrations. Parties at a distance, by noting these carefully, can order about as safely as they could select from a pattern set.

Nos. 1 and 2 are curved along the whole shaft, which enables the operator to hold the Plugger with more ease, and to apply it with more freedom, than if they were straight.

Nos. 3 and 4 are slightly curved.

Nos. 7 and 8 and 13 are plain Rounds of different angles.

Nos. 9 and 10, and 11 and 12 are, by the combined curve and face angles, adapted in many cavities to pack, contour, and condense the whole filling.

No. 14 is a very peculiar curved point, having the range and use of a pair of Rights and Lefts. Face concave, with lipped edges. We also make this point with serrated face. It is adapted for under-filling incisors, buccal cavities, etc.

Nos. 19 to 24, inclusive, are smooth Pluggers and Burnishers. No. 23 is slightly modified, and resembles the No. 13 Varney.

[The blanks between 14 and 19 are reserved for approved additional points.]

Nos. 5 and 6, 29 and 30, 33 and 34 are pairs of Rights and Lefts—round, flat, and square faces.

Nos. 38 and 39 are Foot-shaped, right and left, very thin instep. The lateral curve cannot be shown in Cut.

Nos. 40 and 41 are Universal Pluggers, serrated on the end and back of curve. They differ only in size, and may be used to pack, margin, contour, and condense.

Nos. 31 and 32, and 42 and 43 are two sizes of the same shape. The Abbott have single, and the Butler, double, rows of serrations. This form has place in every fine set of Mallet Pluggers,—for fissures, margins, and to build up in proximals.

No. 37, and Nos. 44 to 48, inclusive, are choice selections of Foot and Condenser points of various curves, insteps, face-angles and face-shapes, which are well shown in the Cuts.

The prices of these Plugger Points are for stock made of uniform sizes on large orders. No special orders can be filled at these rates, either for single Points, varying from these, for this Plugger, or for these Points, made otherwise than as we keep them in stock.

The black spots on the bright part of the Engine Plugger Points are intended to indicate prices. 3 spots denote 37½ cents each. 2 spots denote 50 cents each. 1 spot denotes 60 cents each.

SS HC

Round. Oval. CURVED SHAFT. 2 Sizes. Dr. Varney. Flat. Round Points. Right & Left. Round, Plain. Short Angles. Inside Slants. 2 Sizes. Back Slants. 2 Sizes. Round Plain. Long Angle. Dr. Atkinson. Concave Face.

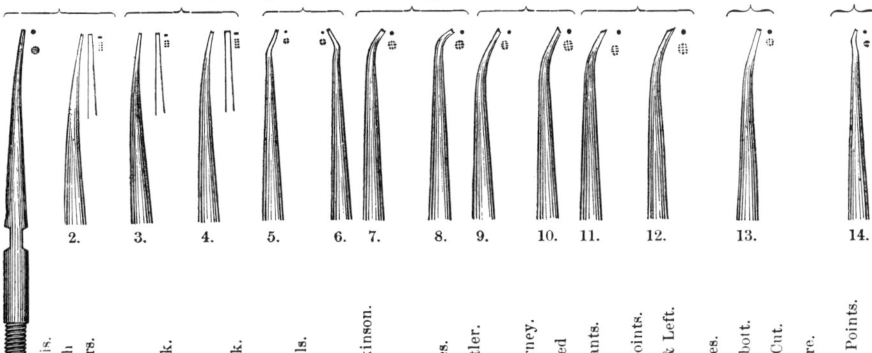

1. 2. 3. 4. 5. 6. 7. 8. 9. 10. 11. 12. 13. 14.

Dr. Mills. Smooth Pluggers. Dr. Jack. Dr. Jack. Dr. Mills. Dr. Atkinson. BURNISHERS. 2 Sizes. Dr. Butler. Dr. Varney. Curved Side Slants. Flat Points. Right & Left. 2 Sizes. Dr. Abbott. Single Cut. Fissure. Square Points. Right & Left.

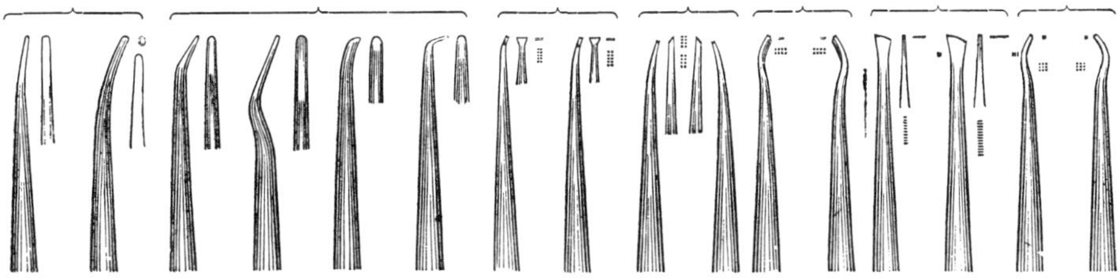

19. 20. 21. 22. 23. 24. 25. 26. 27. 28. 29. 30. 31. 32. 33. 34.

Square Point. Bayonets. Flat Point. Foot Shape. Dr. North. R. & L. Foot. 2 Sizes. Dr. C. Palmer. 2 Sizes. Dr. Butler. Dr. Atkinson. Dr. Varney. Dr. Pugh. Dr. Jack. Dr. Pugh.

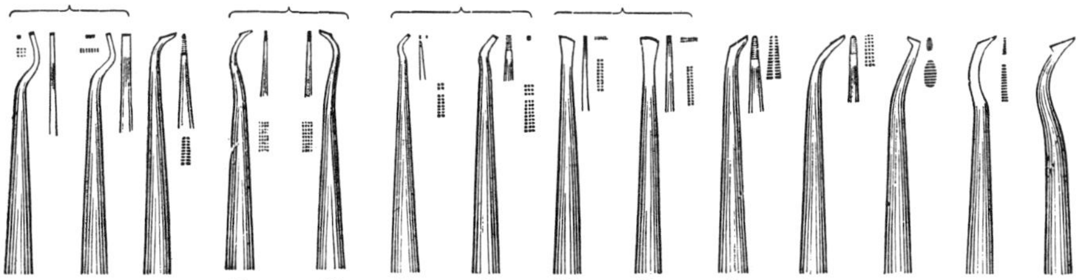

35. 36. 37. 38. 39. 40. 41. 42. 43. 44. 45. 46. 47. 48.

Prices from 1 to 24, inclusive	. . . .	37½ cents each.
" " 25 to 37, "	. . . .	50 " "
" " 38 to 48, "	. . . .	60 " "
Price, complete set of 44 Points	. . . .	$20.50

Dental Engine and Equipment.

RECAPITULATION.

Engine complete, nine and one-half inch Driving-Wheel, with fourteen instruments, all the bright steel parts Nickel-Plated	$50.00
Engine complete, twelve and one-half inch Driving-Wheel, with fourteen instruments, all the bright steel parts Nickel-Plated	55.00
Boxing	1.00

Appliances.

Extension Treadle	5.00
Lock-Bit, Right-Angle Attachment	5.00
Lock-Bit, Acute Angle "	5.00
Disk Carrier, Lock-Bit, Hickman's	5.00
" " Changeable Angle, Cushing's	10.00
" " Fixed Angle, With Stop Motion	6.00
Rotary File Carrier and Porte Polisher	8.00
New Hand-Piece, with Steel Bearings	10.00
Air Injector	5.00
Balance Spring for Engine	.50
Mouth Protector, Fountain, for Disks	1.00
Drop-Tube and Sponge-Holder	.35
Drip-Point, Fountain	.75
Cord, for Driving Engine	.10
Automatic Plugger for Engine	20.00
Finger-Ring for same, extra	1.00
Plugger Points for same, from 37½ to 60 cts. each.	

Tools, etc.

Burs, Cavity, of any form, from 0 to 7, bur gauge	each	.25
" " " " " 8 " 11, "	"	.35
" " " " " 12 " 14, "	"	.40
" " " " " 15 " 20, "	"	.50
" Fissure, Square, and Pointed Ends, from 0 to 7, bur gauge	"	.25
" Cavity, "Super," Round, Wheel, Cone, Inverted Cone, and Bud Shapes, extremely small, and extra quality, per doz., $4.00	"	.34
" Flexible, for opening and preparing Nerve-Canals	"	.40
". and Drills, Cavity, for Right and Acute Angle Attachments, from 0 to 6, bur gauge (not made in larger sizes)	"	.25
" Cavity, Stoned, from 0 to 7, bur gauge	"	.50
" Fissure, " " 0 " 7, "	"	.75
" Plug-Finishing, Stoned, from 6 to 14, bur gauge	"	1.00

BURS, STONED, extra sizes, proportional prices.		
" PLUG-FINISHING, from 6 to 14, bur gauge	each	$0.50
" " " " 15 " 18, "	"	.60
" " " " 19 and 20, "	"	.70
" " " Large Knife-Edge Wheel	"	1.25
Burnishers, Smooth	"	.50
" Corrugated	"	.75
Buffs, Leather, No. 1, not mounted	per doz.	1.00
" " " 2, "	"	.50
" " " 1, mounted	"	2.00
" Felt, assorted shapes, not mounted	"	.50
DRILLS, Cavity, from 0 to 6, Bur Gauge	"	.25
" Twist, from 1 to 5, Bur Gauge	"	.40
" Flexible, for opening and preparing Nerve-Canals	"	.40
Diamond Reamer	"	20.00
DISKS, Corundum, Arthur's:		
" A and K, not mounted	each 13 cts.; per doz.	1.40
" All others, not mounted	" 25 " "	2.75
" A and K, mounted	" 23 " "	2.50
" All others, mounted	" 35 " "	3.75
" Not mounted, per Set—6, A to F		1.25
" Mounted, " 6, A to F		1.75
" Not mounted, " 10, A to K		2.00
" Mounted, " 10, A to K		2.90
" Arkansas Stone, mounted	each	2.00
" Hindostan " "	"	.75
" Boxwood, five sizes, from $\frac{7}{16}$ to $\frac{3}{4}$ in. diameter;	$\frac{3}{4}$ in., per doz.	1.50
other sizes	"	.60
" Rubber, Hard and Soft	each	.10
" " " mounted on Mandrels	"	.20
MANDRELS, Blank	per doz. $0.75 "	.07
" Screw, without Shoulder	" .75 "	.07
" " with Shoulder	" 3.00 "	.25
" Screw-Head, Huey's	"	.30
" Parting-Nut, Right Hand, German-Silver Nuts	"	.30
" " " Nickel-Plated	"	.40
" " Left Hand, "	"	.40
Nerve Instruments, or Flexible Burs and Drills	"	.40
PORTE POLISHERS, German-Silver, Plain Socket	"	.25
" Nickel-Plated, Screw Socket	"	.35
" Screw Clamp, Klump's	"	.35
POINTS, Corundum (Set 12), Northrop's	per doz.	.75
" " " " mounted on Mandrels	"	1.50
" " for Porte Polisher, Butler's	"	.75
" Wood-Polishing, put up in boxes of 100 Points	per box	1.25
" Rubber, Soft, Wheels, Cones, etc., for dressing down fillings	per doz.	.75

POINTS, Arkansas Stone, mounted on Mandrels, a large variety of forms	each	$1.00
" Hindostan " " " " " "	"	.50
" Scotch " " " " " "	"	.30
Plate Saws	"	1.00
Shellac Sticks for mounting Disks, etc.	per box	.25
Shellac Powder for mounting Disks, etc.	"	.10
STANDS for Engine Bits, No. 1, 5 in. diameter, 1 in. high, 72 holes	each	1.00
" " " " " 2, same size as No. 1, Glass Cover, 60 holes	"	1.50
" " " " " 3, Pyramid, 3¼ in. diam., 3½ in. high, 48 "	"	1.00
" " " " " 4, " 4¾ " 4½ " 78 "	"	1.50
" " " " " 5, Pyramid, Revolving, 7 in. diameter, 7½ in. high, 120 holes	"	3.00
TREPHINES	"	.75
WHEELS, BRUSH, Bone Center, Cup-Shape, 1 Row	"	.25
" " " Straight, 2 Rows	"	.35
" Corundum "Stump," ½ in. diameter, ⅛ in. thick, Round Edge, per doz., $1.40	each	.13
" Corundum "Stump," ¾ in. diameter, ⅛ in. thick, Round Edge, per doz., $1.40	each	.13
" WIRE, STEEL, 1 in. diameter, 2 rows	"	.50

POLISHING POWDERS:

Hindostan Stone Powder	per box	.12
Arkansas " "	"	.25
Pumice " " (per lb. 15 cts.)	"	.10
Emery " " 25 "	"	.10
Buck Horn "	small "	.12
" "	large "	.38
Corundum Flour	"	.25
" " Extra Fine	"	.25
Rouge	"	.20

DISCOUNT.

On orders for Engine Tools of not less than Twenty-five Dollars, *accompanied by the Cash*, we will allow a discount of 10 per cent. from the foregoing prices.

Instruments of other hand-pieces altered to suit ours for 25 cts. per doz.

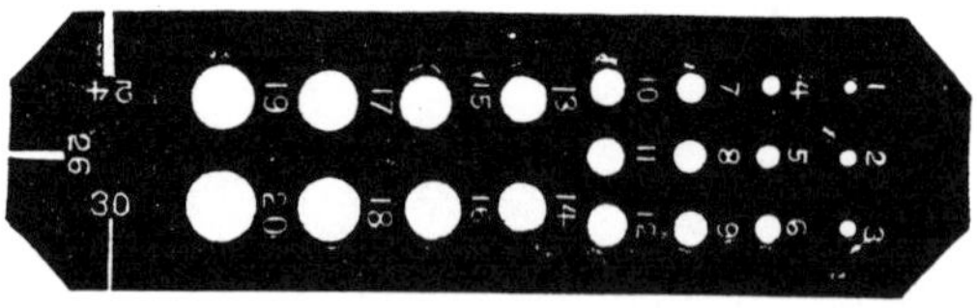

BUR GAUGE, by which burs and drills can be ordered by number.

German-Silver	$0.75
Steel	1.00

The Electro-Magnetic Burring-Engine.

Patented January 26th, 1875; August 17th, 1875; December 14th, 1875; February 1st, 1876.

This efficient little Engine is still regarded by a few gentlemen of the Dental Profession as the most desirable among all that have been offered for sale.

As it can be used with satisfaction only by those who understand a little about electricity, and who exercise daily care to maintain the electrical connections, it has not won favor with the majority of Dentists equally with the mechanical machines, which require no special knowledge or care to use efficiently. But from the well-settled judgment of those who have used the Electric Engine for a long time, and their continued testimony to its intrinsic and comparative merits, we are confirmed in our purpose to keep it before the Profession, believing that there is a growing class of operators who will cheerfully devote some study and care to escape the tyranny of the treadle.

Many improvements have recently been made in the construction of this Engine, making it much more compact and convenient in form; and it has also been adapted to receive the same instruments which we make for the S. S. White Dental Engine.

We therefore feel no hesitation in continuing to recommend the Electric Engine to operators who are willing to acquire the slight knowledge necessary to understand its working, and to devote a little extra care to maintain the conditions of success.

A distinguished practitioner, of national reputation, who has used this Engine in his daily practice for years, thus writes, unsolicited, in regard to it: "My Electric Engines are working most admirably. I have a feeling of commiseration for the men who remain obstinately blind to the immense advantage of these splendid implements."

Price (Battery extra) $65.00

The Electro-Magnetic Dental Plugger.

Patented January 26th, 1875; December 14th, 1875 (four patents); February 15th, 1876. Others pending.

A few Electric Pluggers that have been in use during the last year or two have given satisfaction to those who used them intelligently, and this class of instrument promises a greater efficiency when manufactured properly, and with the latest improvements.

We are preparing to manufacture an Electro-Magnetic Plugger which will have manifest improvements in construction, being lighter, and more compact and convenient, than any other of this kind heretofore offered for sale. It is the result of much study and experience, and we have every reason to believe that it will meet the desires of those who are willing, by extra care, to secure superior advantages in such an instrument.

This Plugger will be manufactured under numerous patents (issued and pending), covering, broadly and in detail, the entire field of the invention and improvements.

We have already a number of orders on file for these Pluggers, and shall have some completed and on sale at as early a date as is consistent with thorough workmanship and prolonged testing; but we cannot, at present, indicate the time more definitely, nor can we name the price until some of the instruments are completed.

Nerve Cavity Instruments.

FOR EXTRACTING NERVES, EXCAVATING AND FILLING NERVE CAVITIES.

GATES'S NERVE AND BUR DRILL.

(Patented October, 1868.)

The invention of this Drill marked a new era in fang filling, while it also furnished an improved Bur. It combines the essential properties of a pulp-canal reamer, drill, bur, and compound excavator. It clears itself in operating, cuts instead of scraping, and can be sharpened with a stone until consumed. When used in the flat pulp-canals, its round form shields it from breaking, its guide-point confines it to the canal in ordinary deviations from a straight course, and (of paramount importance), by its perfect manner of clearing itself, it avoids the pneumatic effect of other forms for cleansing, which, piston-like, injure by exhaustion or *by forcing the deteriorated fluids and air through the foramen*, thereby creating or aggravating disease in the periosteum. By enlarging the canal it also prevents like effects from the subsequent process of filling. Differing essentially from any other in use, this Bur Drill is as efficient in starting and penetrating through solid material as when employed to enlarge cavities.

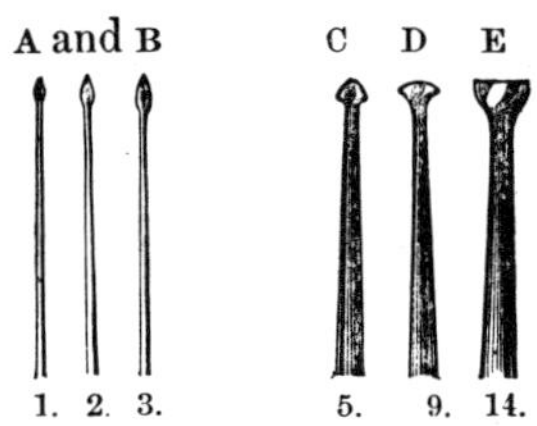

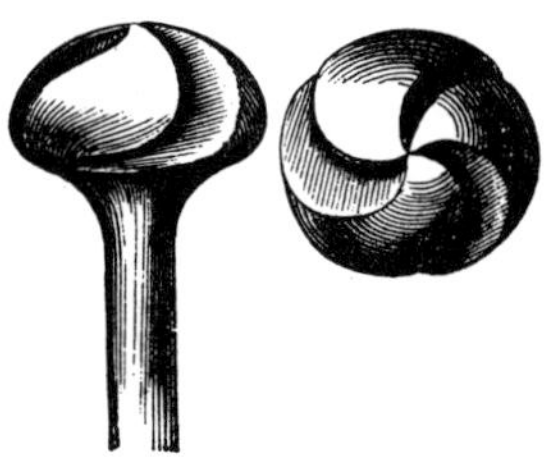

The large Cuts are given to show the form of the head C.

The set consists of five varieties, A, B, C, D, E. A and B represent the Pulp-Canal Reamers.

There are three sizes, as shown in Cut, Nos. 1, 2, and 3.

A indicates a Flexible Stem, B an Inflexible Stem.

C represents the Round Bur Drill, 12 sizes, Cut showing No. 5.

D represents the Excavating Bur Drill, 12 sizes, Cut showing No. 9.

E represents the Undercutting Bur Drill, 12 sizes, Cut showing No. 14.

C, D, and E are designated by letters and numbers as above, viz., C 1 to 12; D 1 to 10 and 12 and 14; E 1 to 10 and 12 and 14.

C, D, and E have only Inflexible Stems.

Price . . . . per doz. $3.00
Case of Turkey Morocco, with knife-edge Arkansas stone, each 4.00

GATES-GLIDDEN DRILLS.

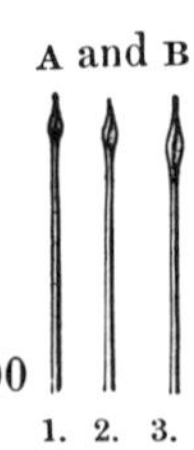

The set consists of two varieties, A and B.

A indicates a Flexible Stem, B an Inflexible Stem.

There are three sizes of each, as shown in Cut, Nos. 1, 2, and 3.

Price . . . . per doz. $6.00

BARBED NERVE EXTRACTORS

These Extractors are very delicately and beautifully barbed; the triangular forms tapering from the barbed end.

The Cuts illustrate three varieties of these instruments. Size of each shown by the Cut.

Fig. 1 shows an Ivory Handle Broach Holder with Ring Slide.

Price $1.00

Extractors put up in packages of one dozen, assorted sizes, soft and half soft 75

Fig. 2 shows Extractors with Steel Shank of proper length to serve for a handle. Sold in packages of one dozen, soft and half soft.

Price per package $1.50

Fig. 3 represents a Steel Handle Broach Holder with Ring Slide.

Price $0.75

Triangular Extractors, in packages of one dozen, assorted sizes, soft and half soft 75

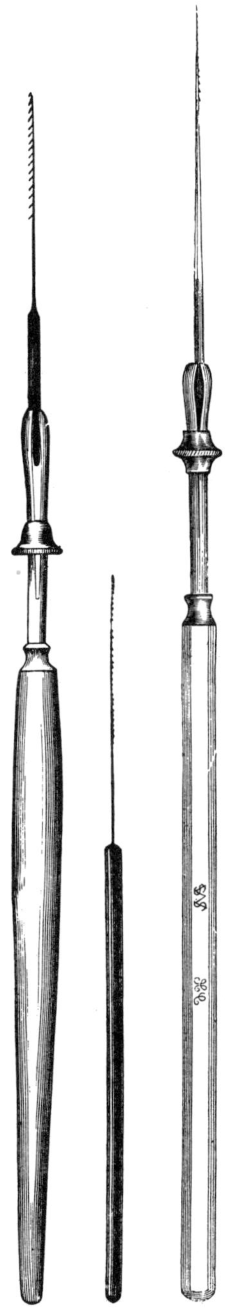

FIG. 1. FIG. 2. FIG. 3.

DR. CORYDON PALMER'S NERVE INSTRUMENTS.

PATTERNS FURNISHED BY DR. PALMER.

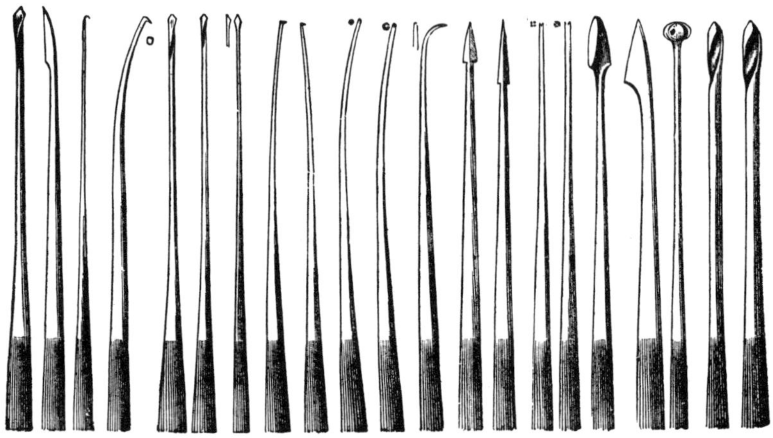

The set consists of 21 Instruments, made of the best quality of steel, finished and tempered in the best manner.

Price, per set of 21 . . . . $8.00
" " 21, in case 9.00

Or separately as follows: Nos. 4, 5,—60 cts. Nos. 6, 7,—50 cts. Nos. 1, 2, 3,—45 cts. Nos. 8, 9, 10, 14, 16,—40 cts. Nos. 12, 13, 15, 17,—30 cts. Nos. 11, 18, 19, 20, 21,—25 cts.

DR. HUNTER'S NERVE-CANAL PLUGGERS.

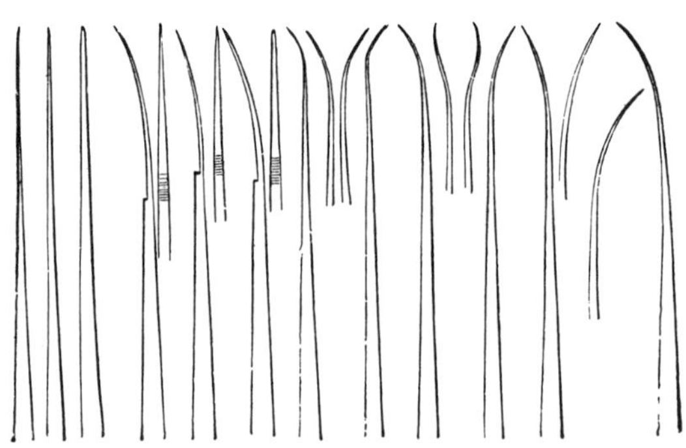

The set consists of 12 Instruments, carefully made, and tempered in the best manner.

Price, per set of 12 . . . . $3 60

DR. ARRINGTON'S NERVE EXTRACTORS AND ROOT FILLERS.

Drawn and Spring Temper.

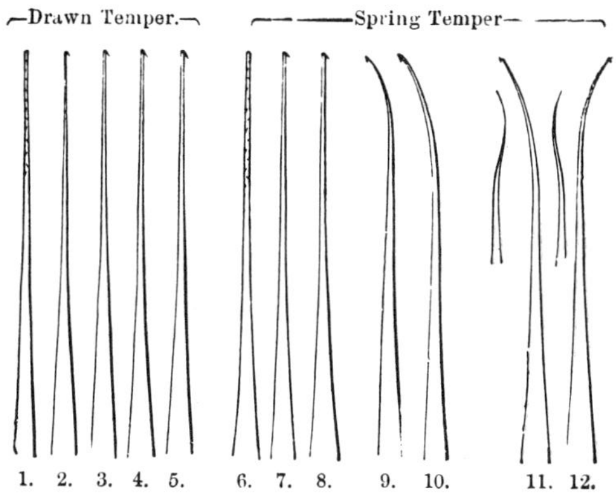

Nerve Extractors.

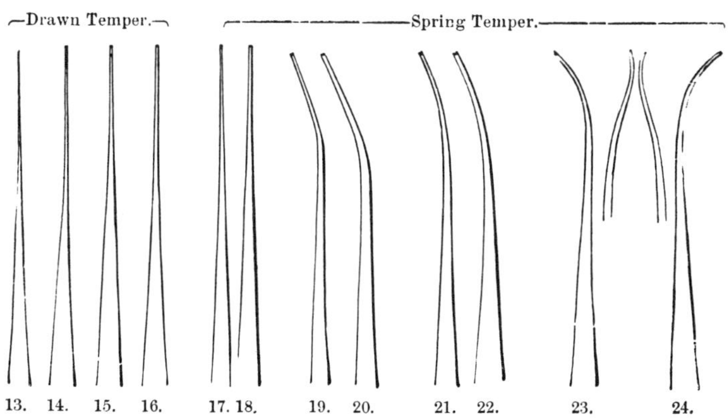

Nerve Cavity Pluggers.

The set consists of 24 Instruments, best quality of steel, made and finished in the best manner.

Price, per set of 24		$6.00
Nerve Instruments, Probes, Square and Octagon Handles . .	per doz.	2.00
Nerve Extractors, Barbed and Hook	"	2.70
Nerve Cavity Pluggers (Bits)	"	.75

Instruments.

Steel Handle, Octagon, Plain	per doz.	$4.00
" " " Taper	"	4.80
" " " File-cut Taper	"	6.00
" " " 1/4 inch, File-cut	"	7.20
" " " 3/8 " "	"	9.00
Plugger Bits for Socket, ordinary points	"	4.00
*Ivory Handle, German-Silver Ferrules, 3/8 inch, Octagon, Taper . .	"	16.50
* " " " " " 1/2 " " " . .	"	20.00
* " " " " " 5/8 " " " . .	"	24.00
Bleached Bone, 1/2 inch, Fluted	"	9.00
" " 5/8 " "	"	12.00
Ebony Handle, 3/8 " Octagon, Taper	"	7.50
" " 1/2 " "	"	10.00
" " 5/8 " "	"	12.00
Walrus Handles, 1/2 inch, Octagon, German-Silver Ferrules	"	10.00
" " 5/8 " " " " "	"	12.00
Buffalo Handles, 1/2 " " " " "	"	10.00
" " 5/8 " " " " "	"	12.00
Cameo Handles, 1/2 " " Gold Mounted	"	30.00
" " 5/8 " " " "	"	35.00
Pearl Handles, 1/2 " " " "	"	40.00
" " 5/8 " " " "	"	55.00
Burgos Handles, 1/2 " " " "	"	35.00
" " 5/8 " " " "	"	50.00

Note.—All our Gold-Plated Ferrules are warranted 16 carat gold, and are one-fourth gold in *thickness*. The trade rule is usually one-tenth in *weight* only, which is very little better than good gilding.

Coin Silver Ferrules add $2.00, $2.50, and $3.00 per dozen to the above prices.

---

* The figures adopted by manufacturers do not generally express the real size of the Handle. In most cases they are at least 1/8 inch less than described. The sizes here enumerated for Ivory Handles are warranted to be correct, a fact to be remembered when comparing prices.

HAND-PRESSURE PLUGGING INSTRUMENTS.

S. S. WHITE'S SET OF SIXTY PLUGGERS.

These are ¼ inch File-cut Handles, Turned Shanks and Ball Ends. Sixty Points are given. They can be adapted to any style of Handles.

Price, per dozen $7.20

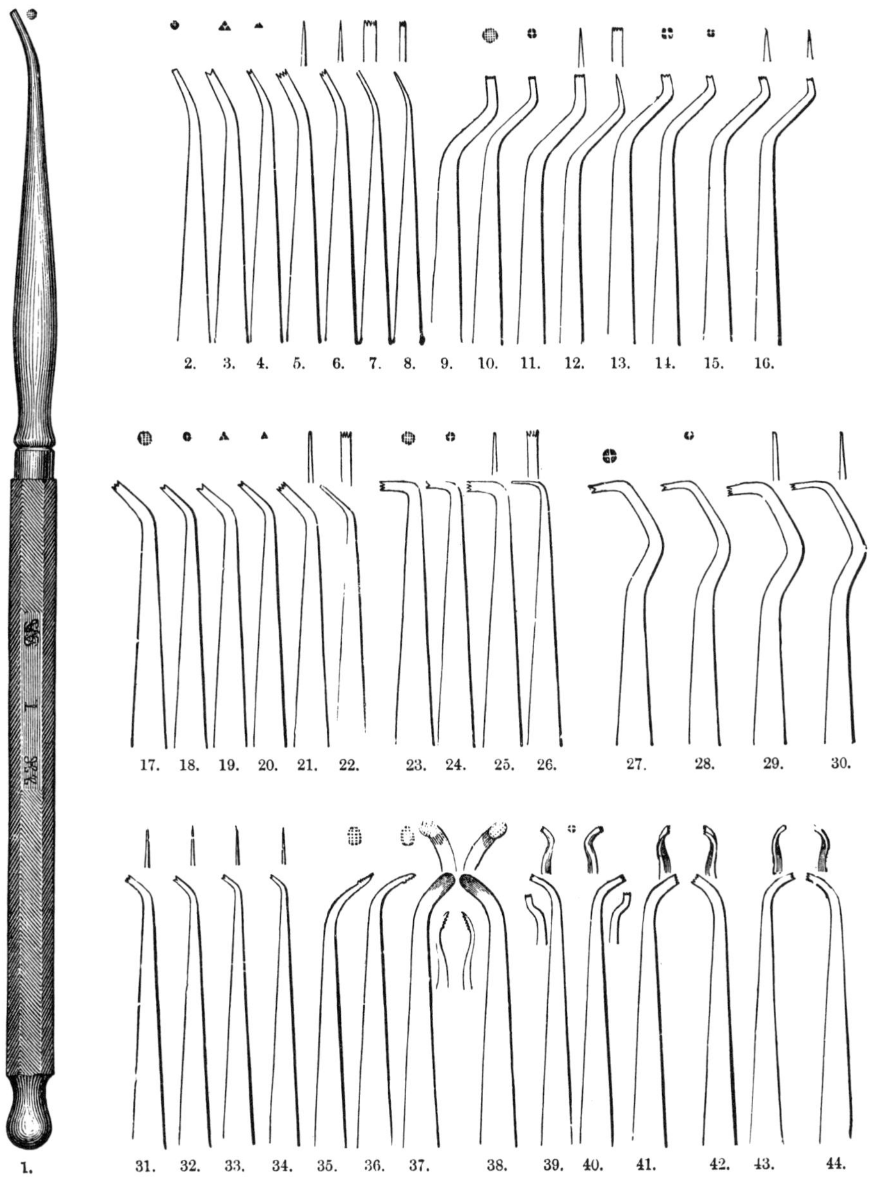

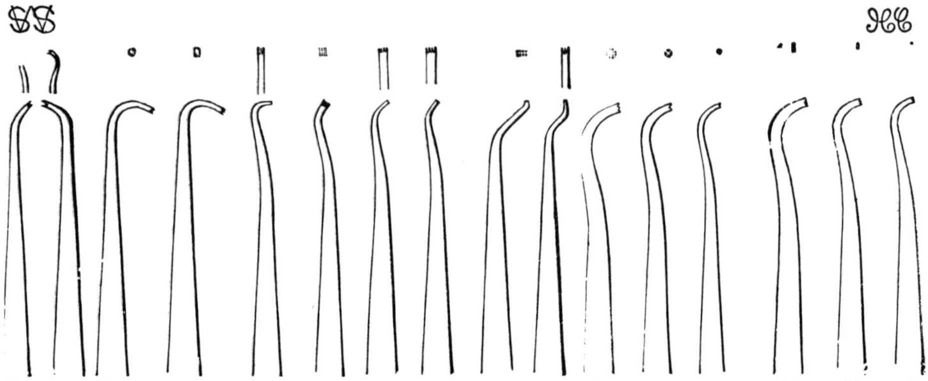

45. 46. 47. 48. 49. 50. 51. 52. 53. 54. 55. 56. 57. 58. 59. 60.

The Cuts of Pluggers, Burnishers, Scalers, and Chisels represent the various and most approved forms in use. In making out an order, give the number of the Cut and the Page, to insure obtaining what is wanted.

SMALL PLUGGERS.

Set of 72,—22 forms, from 3 to 4 sizes of each. Cuts represent a medium size. The numbers run from large to small.

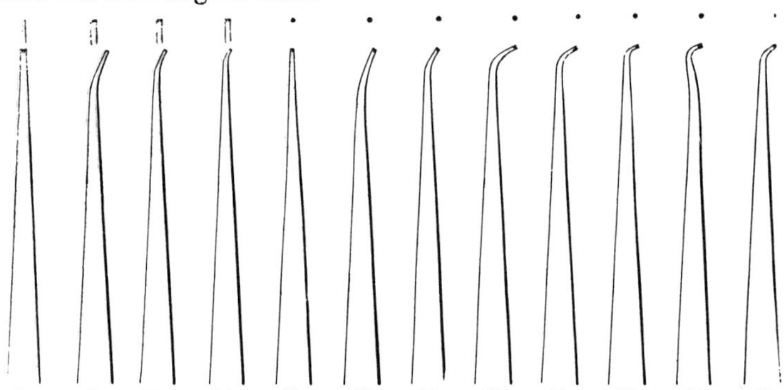

2. 6. 10. 14. 18. 21. 24. 27. 30. 33. 36. 39.

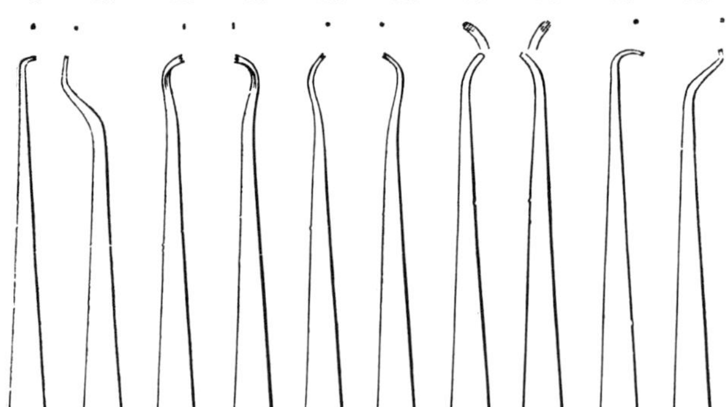

43. 47. 51. 52. 59. 60. 63. 64. 68. 71.

Steel Handles,	Octagon,	Plain	. . . .	per doz.	$4.00
"	"	" Taper	. . . .	"	4.80
"	"	" File-cut	. . . .	"	6.00

"NEW YORK" PLUGGERS.

A SELECTION OF 144 OF THE FINEST HAND PLUGGERS.

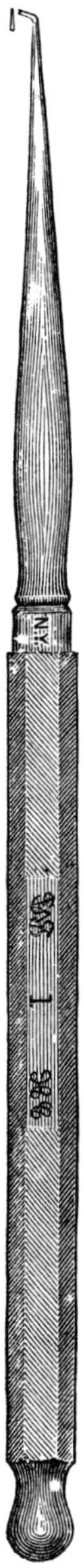

The patterns for this series of Points for Hand Pluggers have been selected with great care. The object was to furnish a set of Points from which the most advanced Practitioners could choose instruments adapted to every situation or size of cavity, without the trouble of pattern-making, or the delay of having them made to order.

Seven years' experience has demonstrated the wisdom of the selection. The Pluggers for all our Dental Cases are selected from this "New York" set.

"New York" Pluggers may be known from all others, of the same numbers, by the initials "N. Y." stamped upon the bright rim between the handle and the shaft.

An examination of these Points is recommended to Dentists about to buy Hand Pluggers. The set includes graded sizes of all the most useful Points, so that the desired size can be selected. Buyers can rely upon getting their orders filled exactly true to number in size and bend.

We make these Pluggers to order with every style of handle, from plain octagon steel to cameo and pearl, with solid gold ferrules; also, for all the sockets and the various Automatic Pluggers.

Price, with ¼ in. File-cut Handles . . . . each 60 cents.

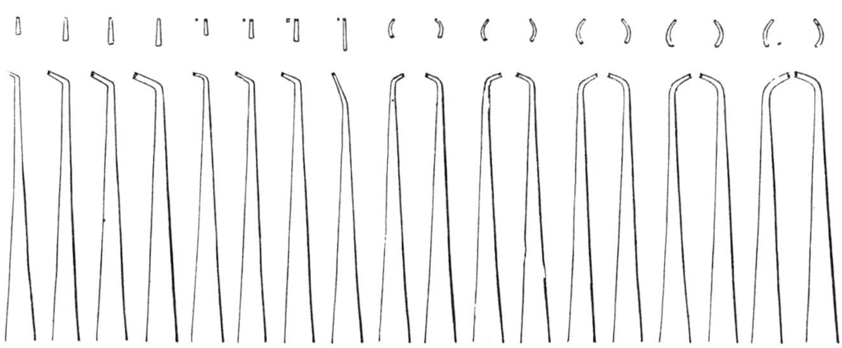

1. 2. 3. 4. 5. 6. 7. 8. 9. 10. 11. 12. 13. 14. 15. 16. 17. 18. 19.

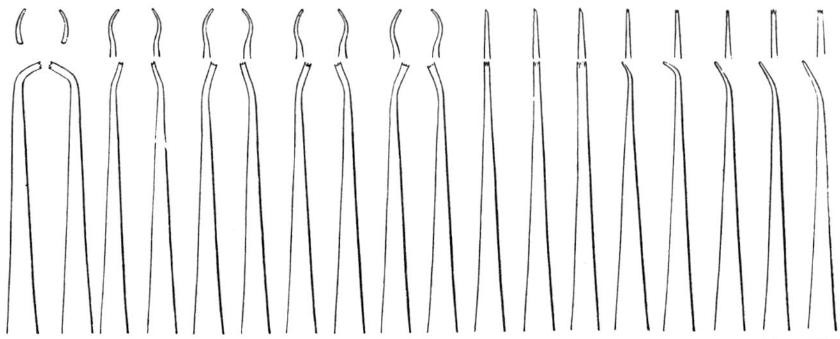

20. 21. 22. 23. 24. 25. 26. 27. 28. 29. 30. 31. 32. 33. 34. 35. 36. 37.

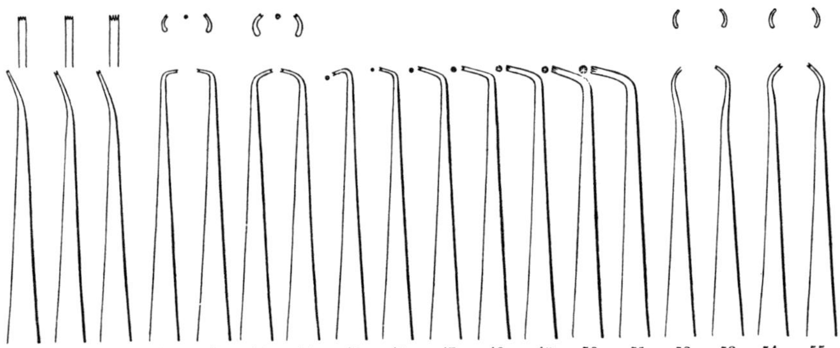

38. 39. 40. 41. 42. 43. 44. 45. 46. 47. 48. 49. 50. 51. 52. 53. 54. 55.

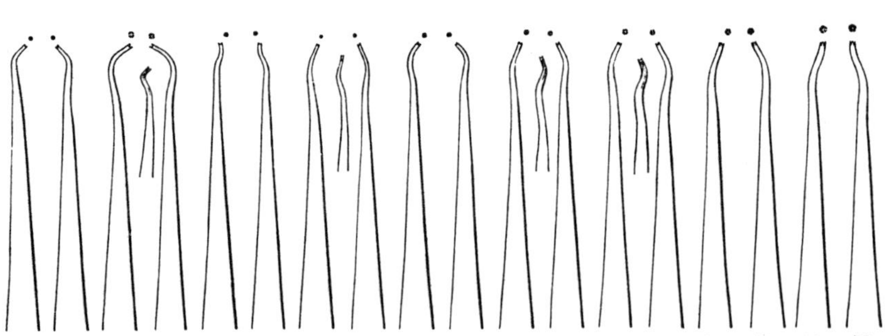

56. 57. 58. 59. 60. 61. 62. 63. 64. 65. 66. 67. 68. 69. 70. 71. 72. 73.

SS HC

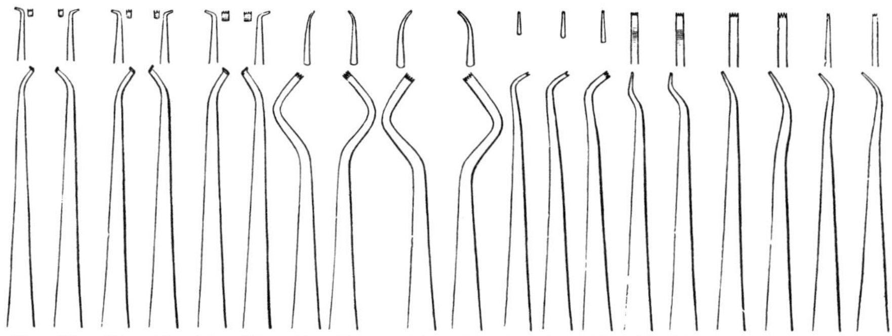

74. 75. 76. 77. 78. 79. 80. 81. 82. 83. 84. 85. 86. 87. 88. 89. 90. 91. 92.

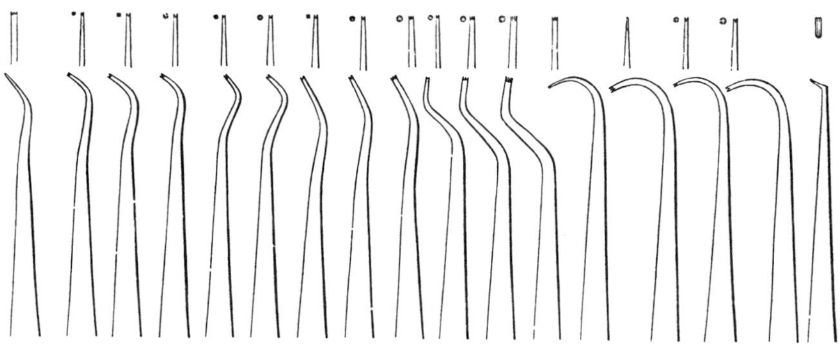

93. 94. 95. 96. 97. 98. 99. 100. 101. 102. 103. 104. 105. 106. 107. 108. 109.

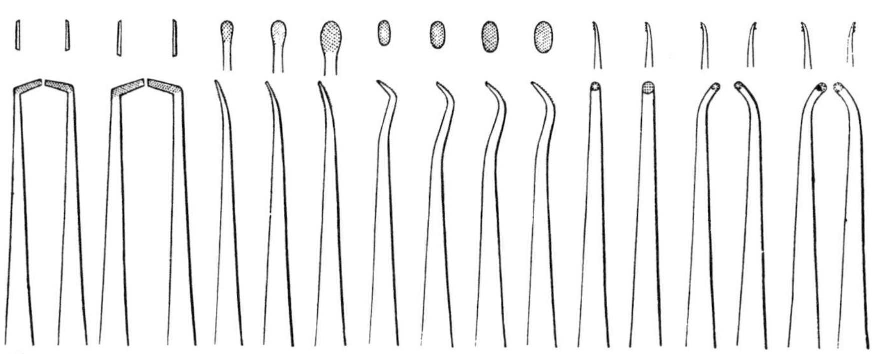

110. 111. 112. 113. 114. 115. 116. 117. 118. 119. 120. 121. 122. 123. 124. 125. 126.

SS HC

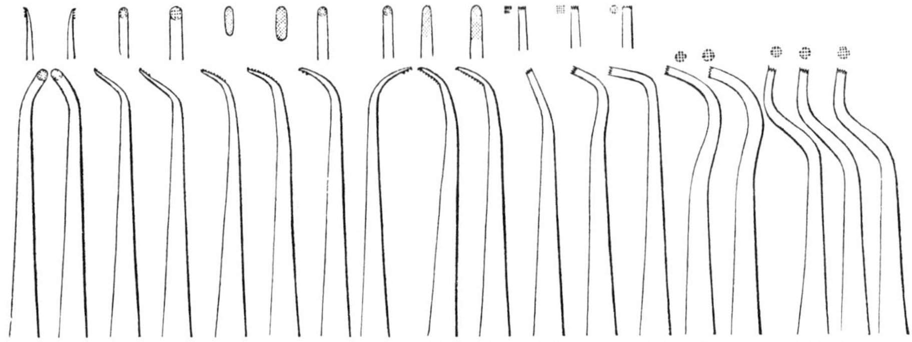

127. 128. 129. 130. 131. 132. 133. 134. 135. 136. 137. 138 139. 140. 141. 142. 143. 144.

DR. GEO. W. ELLIS'S SET OF PLASTIC GOLD PLUGGERS.

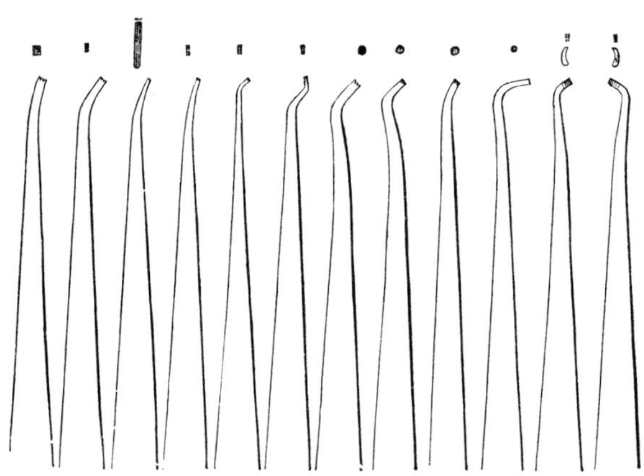

1. 2. 3. 4. 5. 6. 7. 8. 9. 10. 11. 12.

These Cuts represent twelve of the most approved Points.

Octagon Cast Steel, Bronzed Handles, $\frac{7}{32}$ inch	per set	$5.00
File-cut Handles, Ball Ends, ¼ inch	"	7.20
File-cut Handles, ⅜ inch	"	9.00

DR. F. ABBOTT'S SET OF PLUGGERS.

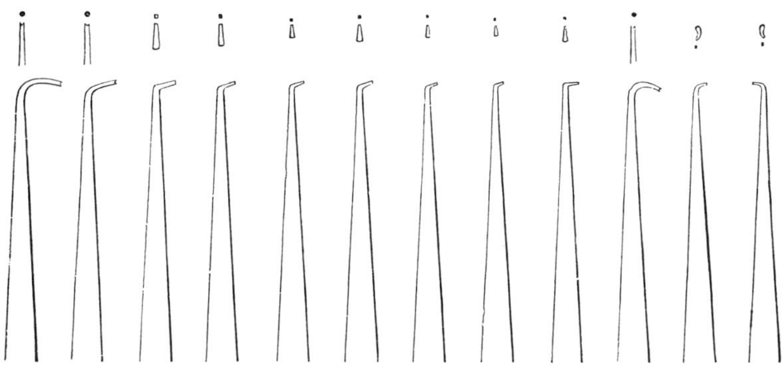

1. 2. 3. 4. 5. 6. 7. 8. 9. 10. 11. 12.

The above set of 12 Hand Pluggers is made from patterns furnished and revised expressly for us.

Plain Octagon Handle, $\frac{3}{16}$ inch, Black or Bronzed . . . . . per set $4.00

DR. W. C. HEAD'S SET OF PLUGGERS.

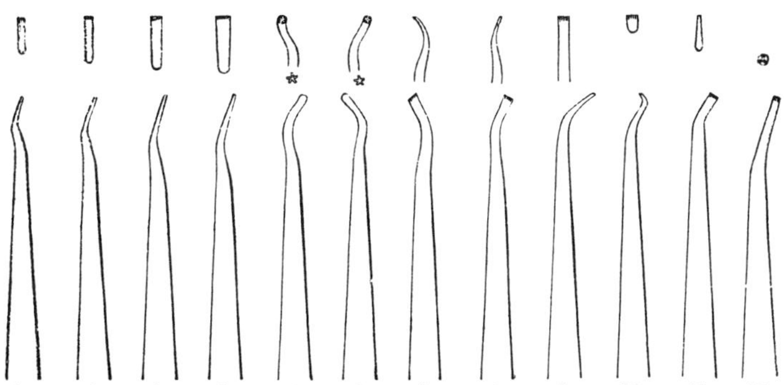

1. 2. 3. 4. 5. 6. 7. 8. 9. 10. 11. 12.

Dr. Head describes them as follows:

"These Pluggers are best suited for filling with gold foil prepared in mats or ribbons folded in short pieces, but will be found useful with gold prepared in any other manner. By their peculiar serration they carry the gold through small places without cutting through it.

"Nos. 4 to 9 are also well adapted to the use of sponge or plastic gold and tin foil.

"These instruments are serrated, tempered, and finished with great care, and are satisfactory in every respect."

Octagon Cast Steel,	Plain Taper Handle,	$\frac{3}{16}$ in.,	6 in.	long,	Bronzed	per set	$4.80
"	" File-cut	" $\frac{3}{16}$ "	6	"	"	"	6.00

DR. W. G. REDMAN'S SET OF PLUGGERS.

FOR CYLINDER FILLINGS.

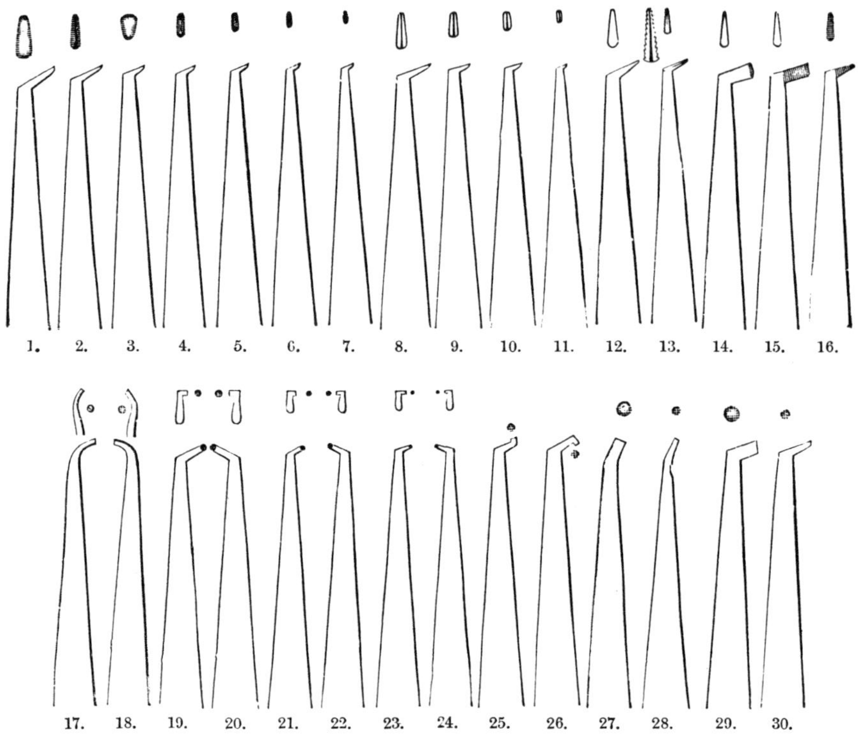

These Cuts represent thirty of the most approved Points. They are made with handles to suit the purchaser. Dr. Redman recommends a half-inch Ivory or Ebony Handle. Nos. 1 to 7 (serrated foot instruments) are lateral Condensers for all Cavities. Nos. 8 to 11 (smooth foot instruments) are used in the same Cavities and in the same manner, but not until the Cavities are nearly full. Nos. 12 to 24 are all Approximal Condensers. No. 25 is for Anterior Approximal Cavities, Molars, and Bicuspids. No. 26 is for Posterior Approximal Cavities, Molars, and Bicuspids. Nos. 27 and 28 are for Crown Cavities, Upper Molars, and Bicuspids. Nos. 29 and 30 are for Crown Cavities, Lower Molars, and Bicuspids.

Ivory Handles, $\frac{5}{8}$ inch	per set of thirty	$64.50
Ivory Handles, $\frac{1}{2}$ inch	" "	54.50
Ebony Handles, $\frac{5}{8}$ inch	" "	34.50
Ebony Handles, $\frac{1}{2}$ inch	" "	29.50
Octagon File-cut Steel Handles, $\frac{3}{8}$ inch	" "	27.00
Octagon File-cut Steel Handles, $\frac{1}{4}$ inch	" "	22.50

Or at the same rates per dozen.

DR. B. J. BING'S SET OF SOFT GOLD OR TAPE PLUGGERS.

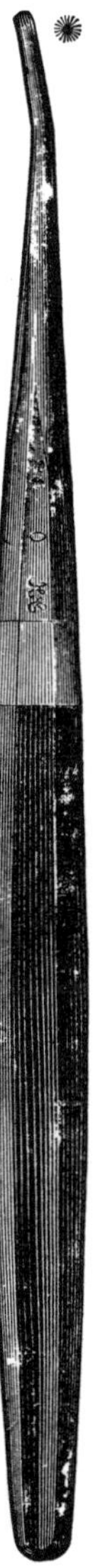

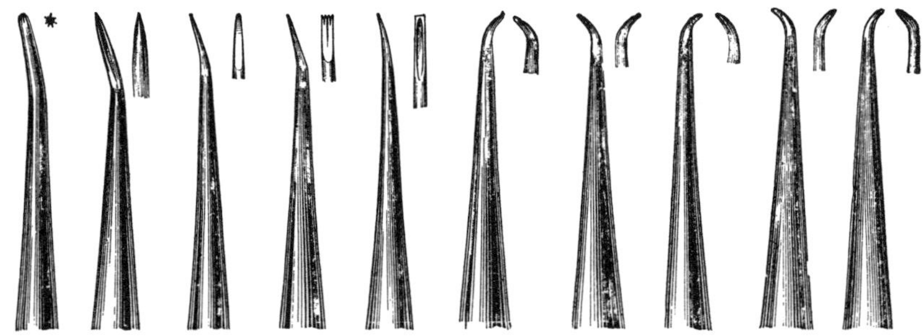

1. 2. 3. 4. 5. 6. 7. 8. 9. 10.

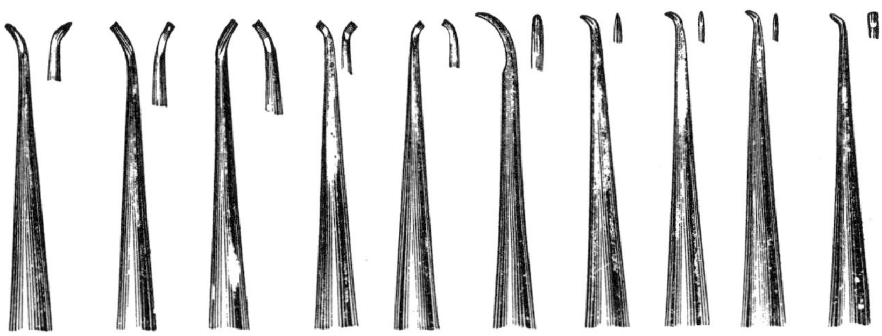

11. 12. 13. 14. 15. 16. 17. 18. 19. 20.

0.

S. S. WHITE. 11 RUE CAUMARTIN, January 13th.

DEAR SIR,—I find the set of Soft Gold or *Tape* Pluggers to be everything that can be desired, and are just as those used in my office.

I am, dear sir, yours truly, B. J. BING.

These Pluggers are intended for use with Tape Gold, and have nothing in common with our ordinary serrated Points, being instead Fillers, Packers, and Condensers, with points, sides, ends, and corrugations, carefully designed to accomplish these modes of inserting the gold.

These Points have immense popularity in Paris (where Dr. Bing resides), London, and many other European cities. For many purposes they will be found to have merit, and for their own special uses they are unique and superior to any other set.

The handles are of Ebony, and are graded to correspond with the size and use of point.

No. 0	each $1.25
Nos. 1, 2, 16	" 1.00
" 4, 6, 7, 8, 9, 10, 11, 12, 13, 14, 15	" .90
" 3, 5, 17, 18, 19, 20	" .75
Set of 21	per set 18.50

DR. E. T. DARBY'S PLUGGERS AND BURNISHERS.

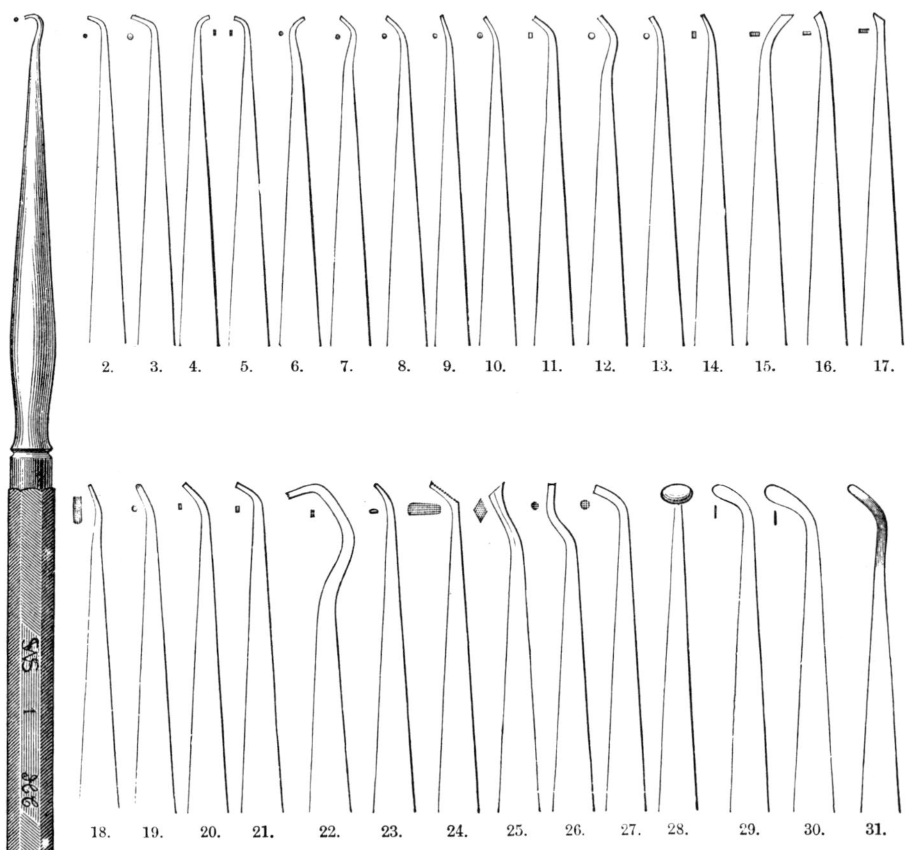

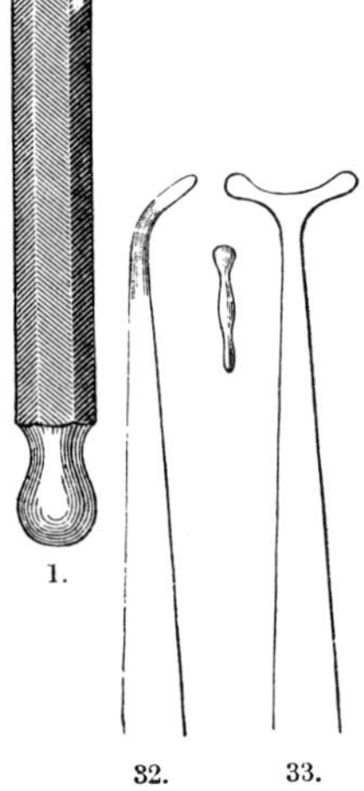

This set comprises 33 Points, six of which are Burnishers.

These instruments are of the finest quality, with File-cut Handles, Turned Shanks, and Ball Ends. Each instrument is numbered, and can be duplicated by number.

Price per doz. (except No. 33)	$7.20
" No. 33, each	.75
" per set of 33, inclosed in a Morocco Case . .	21.00

PLASTIC AND CRYSTALLINE GOLD PLUGGERS AND CONDENSERS.

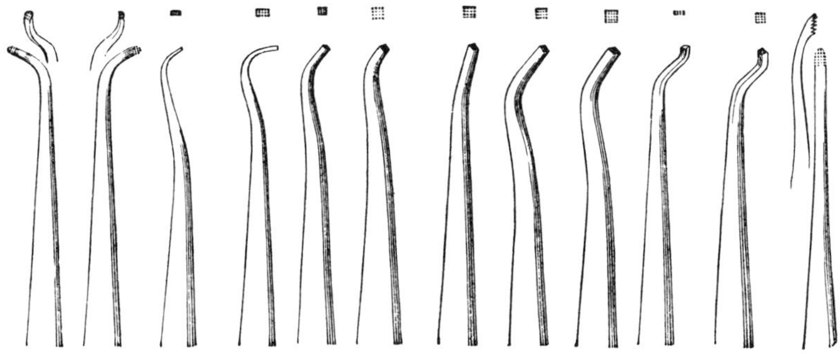

1. 2. 3. 4. 5. 6. 7. 8. 9. 10. 11. 12.

These Points as now made are one-third smaller than represented in Cut.
Steel, File-cut Handles, $\frac{3}{8}$ inch, Bronzed . . . . per doz. $9.00

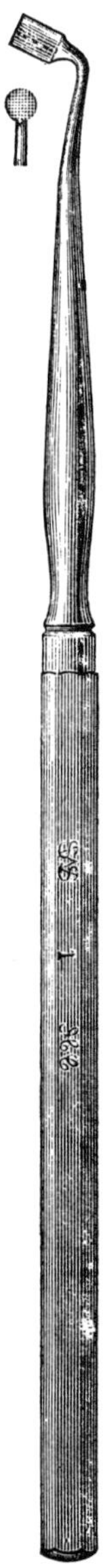

1.

DR. B. F. ARRINGTON'S AMALGAM PLUGGERS AND BURNISHERS.

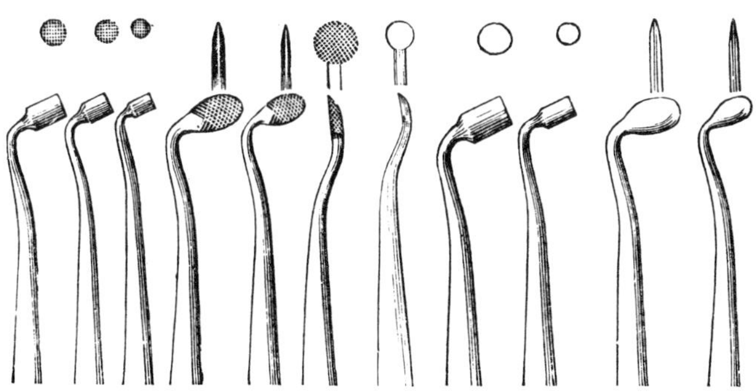

2. 3. 4. 5. 6. 7. 8. 9. 10. 11. 12.

These instruments are adapted to the use of Amalgam, Hill's Stopping, and Fusible Metal.

Octagon Cast Steel, $\frac{7}{32}$ in., Bronzed Handles	per set	$6.70
Pluggers, from No. 1 to 7, inclusive	each	.60
Burnishers, from No. 8 to 12, inclusive	"	.50
File-cut Handles, $\frac{1}{4}$ in., Ball Ends, Bronzed	per set	7.90
Pluggers, from No. 1 to 7, inclusive	each	.70
Burnishers, from No. 8 to 12, inclusive	"	.60

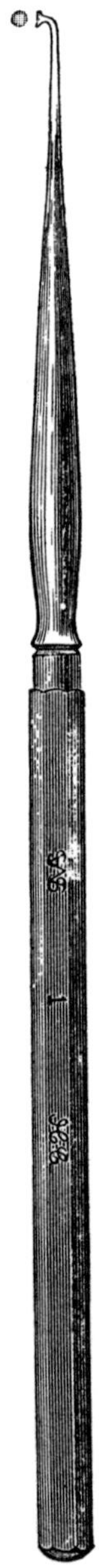

1.

WESTON'S AMALGAM PLUGGERS.

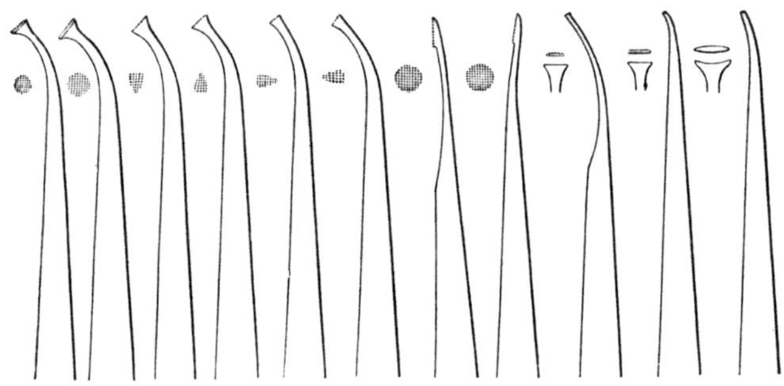

2. 3. 4. 5. 6. 7. 8. 9. 10. 11. 12.

The faces of these instruments are intended to be like those of finely serrated Pluggers which have been well worn.

No. 1.—For filling undercuts generally.

Nos. 2 and 3.—For crown and buccal cavities in upper and lower molars.

Nos. 4 and 5.—V-shaped fissure Pluggers for filling anterior and posterior V-shaped fissures in molars and bicuspids.

Nos. 6 and 7.—Right and left V-shaped fissure Pluggers for right and left V-shaped cavities in molars and bicuspids.

Nos. 8 and 9.—Adapted for working in anterior and posterior approximal cavities, and specially useful in removing excess of amalgam when finishing.

No. 10.—For commencing a filling in the cervical portion of an approximal cavity.

Nos. 11 and 12.—New Burnishers, applicable to a great variety of cases.

Octagon Cast Steel, $\frac{7}{32}$ in., 6 in. long, Blued Handles . .	per set	$7.00
Nos. 1 to 10, inclusive, Serrated	each	.60
Nos. 11 and 12, Plain	"	.50

ATKINSON'S OXYCHLORIDE CEMENT PLUGGERS.

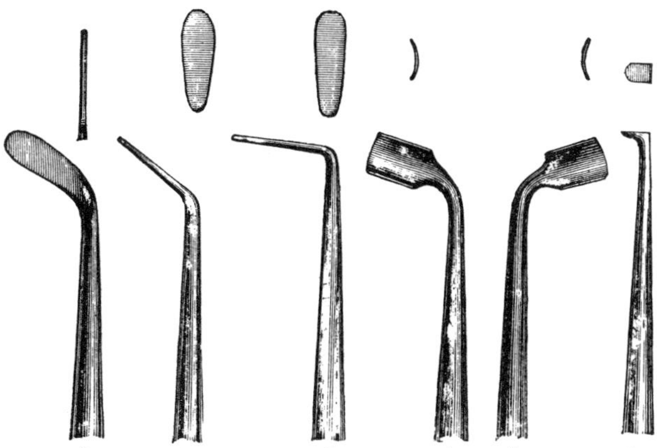

1. 2. 3. 4. 5. 6.

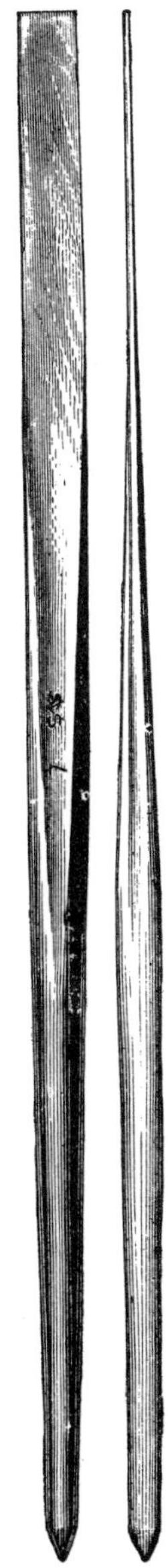

7.

Nos. 1; 2, 3, 4, 5, and 6 are of $\frac{7}{32}$ in. Octagon Cast Steel, Blued Handles.

No. 7, Bright Steel, size and shape shown in Cut.

Price, per set of 7		$5.75
" Nos. 1, 2, 3, 6, and 7	each	.75
" Nos. 4 and 5	"	1.00

DR. HOUGHTON'S SPATULA

FOR OS-ARTIFICIEL AND OTHER PLASTIC FILLINGS.

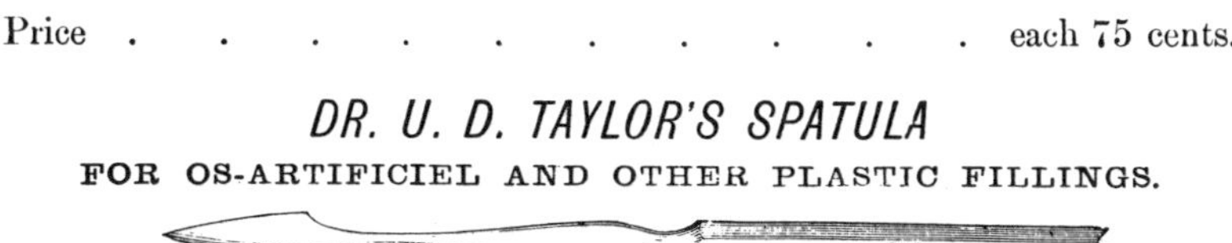

The Cut represents an instrument for the manipulation of Plastic Fillings. Made of best quality steel, double end, thin blades, spring temper.

Price . . . . each 75 cents.

DR. U. D. TAYLOR'S SPATULA

FOR OS-ARTIFICIEL AND OTHER PLASTIC FILLINGS.

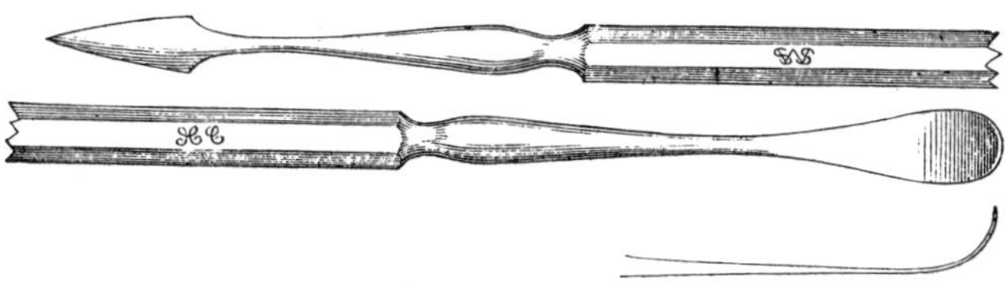

An instrument for the manipulation of Plastic Fillings. Best quality.

Price . . . . each 75 cents.

PLUGGING FORCEPS.

Many Forceps have been sold, purporting to be made according to Dr. Flagg's patterns, which have not been correct in shape; some of them so badly constructed as to be entirely useless. Those of our manufacture have received Dr. Flagg's approval.

These Forceps combine ease of adaptation, lightness, delicacy of form, and strength sufficient to compact a plug.

The set consists of three pairs.

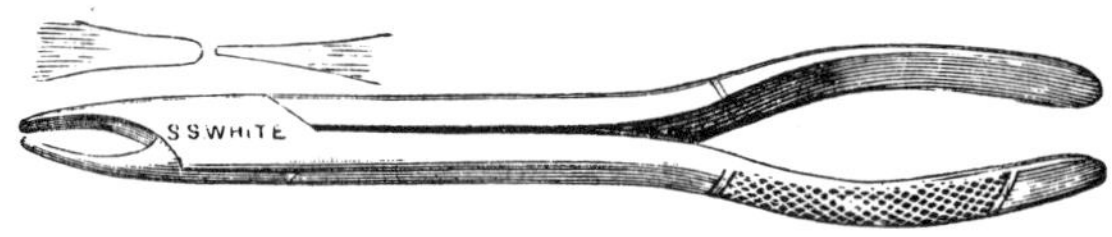

No. 1—Straight beaks, for condensing plugs between teeth, upon the mesial or lateral faces above or below, the plugs being located near the cutting edges of the incisors, the cusps of the cuspids or bicuspids, and the buccal *edges* of the *approximating faces* of the molars.

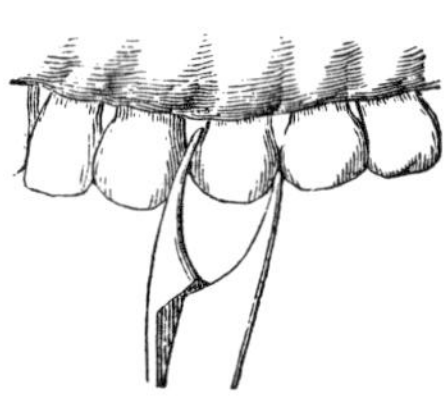

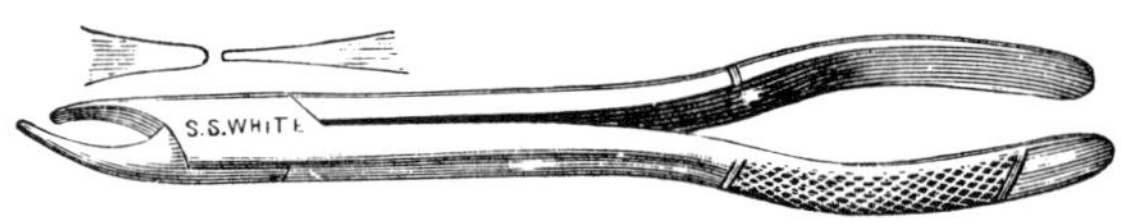

No. 2—For condensing such plugs or parts of plugs as are located between upper incisors, cuspids, and bicuspids, near their necks, and the lingual or palatine *edges* of the approximal plugs of superior or inferior teeth.

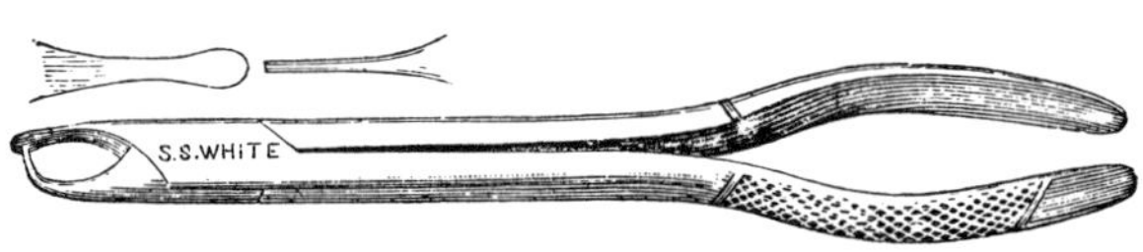

No. 3—For condensing plugs upon the labial, palatine, and lingual faces of incisors and cuspids above and below; also upon the buccal, palatine, and lingual faces of bicuspids and molars above and below, right and left sides.

Price	per pair	$2.75
Dr. J. D. White's set of 7 Plugging Forceps	"	2.75
Nickel-Plated	"	3.25

Mallet Pluggers.

DR. WM. H. ATKINSON'S SET OF PLUGGERS AND BURNISHERS.

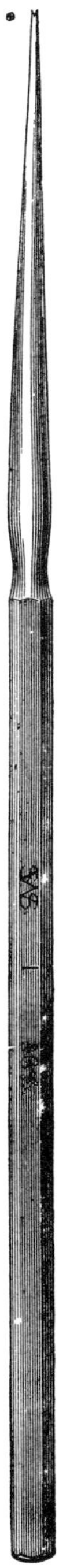

1.

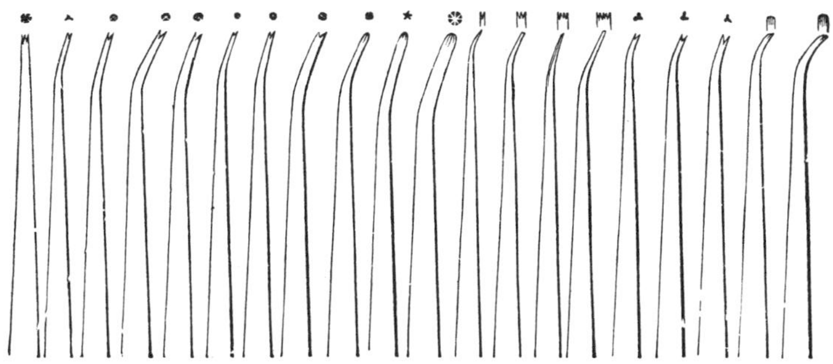

2. 3. 4. 5. 6. 7. 8. 9. 10. 11. 12. 13. 14. 15. 16. 17. 18. 19. 20. 21.

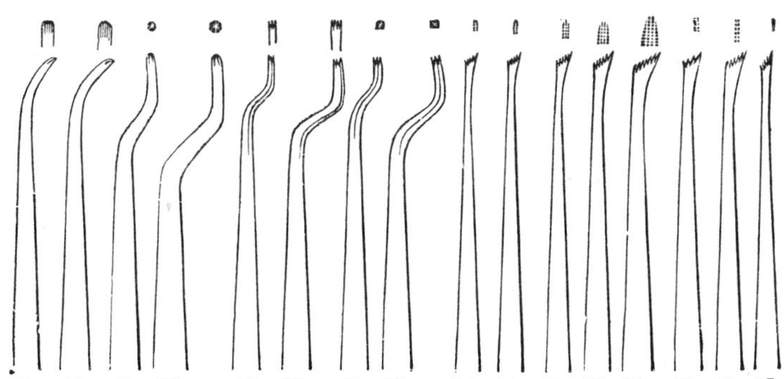

22. 23. 24. 25. 26. 27. 28. 29. 30. 31. 32. 33. 34. 35. 36. 37.

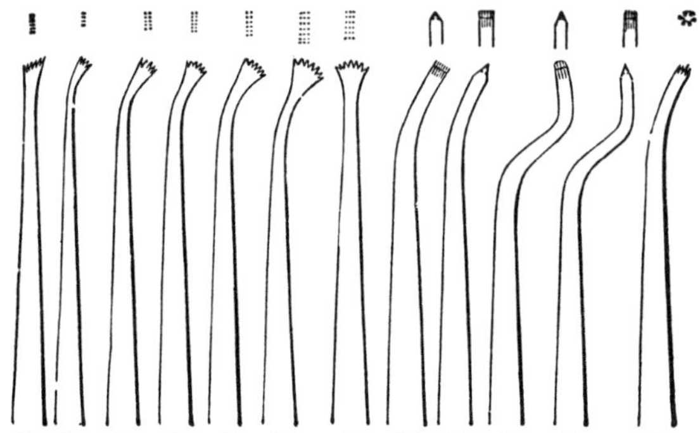

38. 49. 50. 51. 52. 53. 54. 55. 56. 57. 58. 59.

DR. WM H. ATKINSON'S SET OF BURNISHERS.

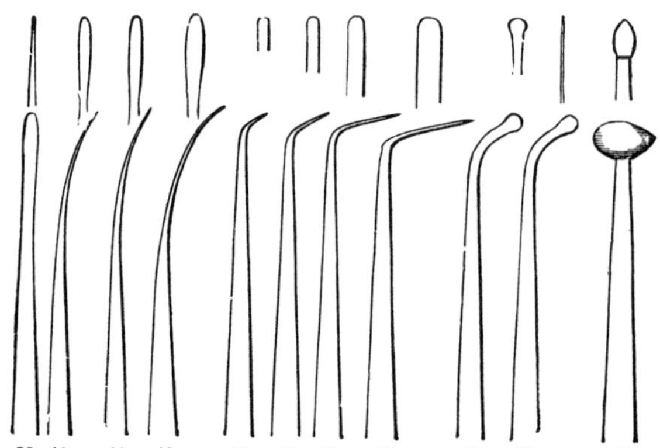

39. 40. 41. 42. 43. 44. 45. 46. 47. 48. 60.

These instruments are designed to be used with the Mallet, and are adapted for that purpose. The Serrations are well defined and the Points nicely finished.

☞ There are many instruments sold, bearing Dr. Atkinson's name, which are not correct copies of his Points, and not adapted to the style of work for which they are intended. Those here offered have been approved by the inventor.

Price, per set of 60	$27.00
" per dozen	5.40

DR. F. ABBOTT'S SET OF PLUGGERS.

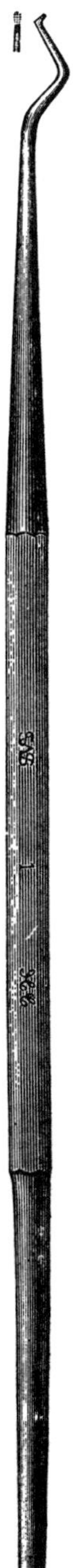

1.

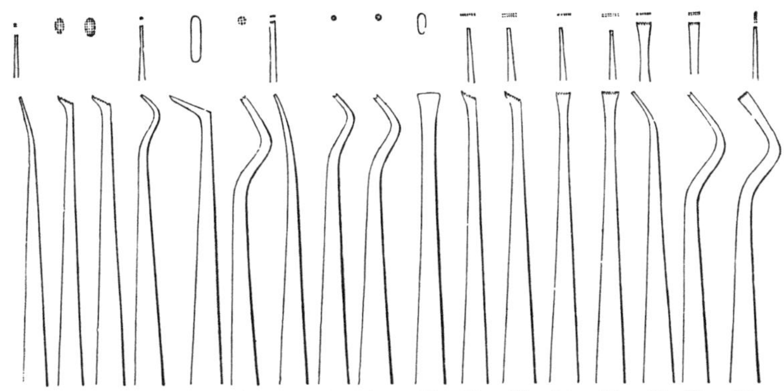

2. 3. 4. 5. 6. 7. 8. 9. 10. 11. 12. 13. 14. 15. 16. 17. 18.

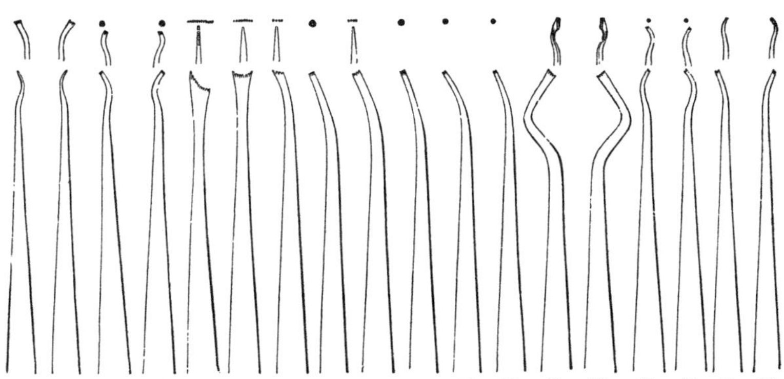

19. 20. 21. 22. 23. 24. 25. 26. 27. 28. 29. 30. 31. 32. 33. 34. 35. 36.

This is a very complete set of Mallet Pluggers, highly approved by the Profession, and of our best quality of manufacture, our pattern set having been examined and approved by Dr. Abbott.

The instruments are 7 inches long, of $\frac{7}{32}$ Octagon Steel, with the Mallet end tapered and polished one and three-quarter inches.

Price, per set of 36	$18.00
" per dozen	6.00
Morocco Case, extra	1.00

DR. R. W. VARNEY'S SET OF PLUGGERS.

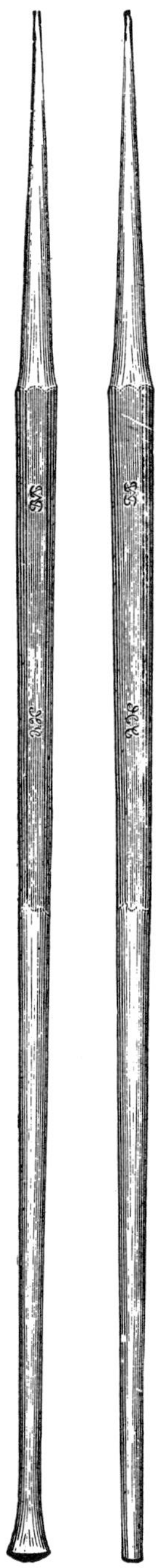

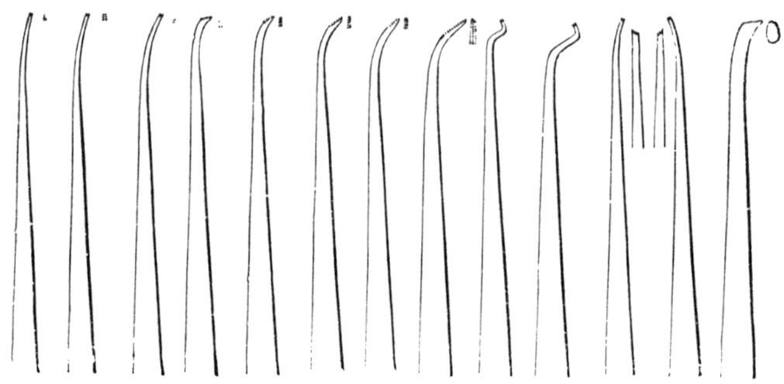

1. 2. 3. 4. 5. 6. 7. 8. 9. 10 11. 12. 13.

Our working patterns of these exquisite instruments were copied from the original set which Dr. Varney himself used. Permission to name them as his could only be obtained on the guarantee that every Plugger should be as perfectly made as though it were for his own use.

The full-length Cuts represent the exact sizes. The swell-end is Dr. V.'s own pattern; the *taper-end* differs from it in that respect only. Made of the finest steel, with extreme care in forming and serrating. Tempered all over. Octagon shaft lacquered fire-gray. Both ends crocus polished. The Cuts show the size and bends, but the serrations are too fine for illustration.

Another variety, somewhat heavier in handle, and with every other side of the Octagon part of the handle File-cut, is preferred by some; we make them to order at the same price.

Dr. Varney's suggestions for the application of each instrument accompany each set.

Price, per set of 13 . . . . $20.00

Or separately as follows:

No. 13 (the Burnisher)		$1.00
Nos. 1, 2, and 3	each	1.25
Nos. 11 and 12	"	1.50
Nos. 4, 5, 6, 7, 9, and 10	"	1.75
No. 8	"	2.00

Morocco Case, holding each instrument in position and open at the end, to throw light on Serrations, extra . . . . . each $2.00

DR. C. R. BUTLER'S SET OF PLUGGERS.

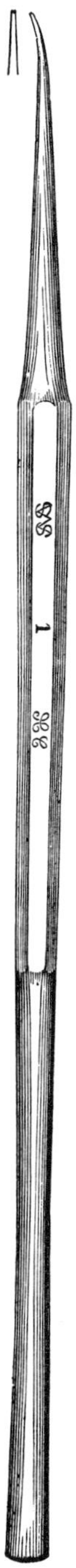

1.

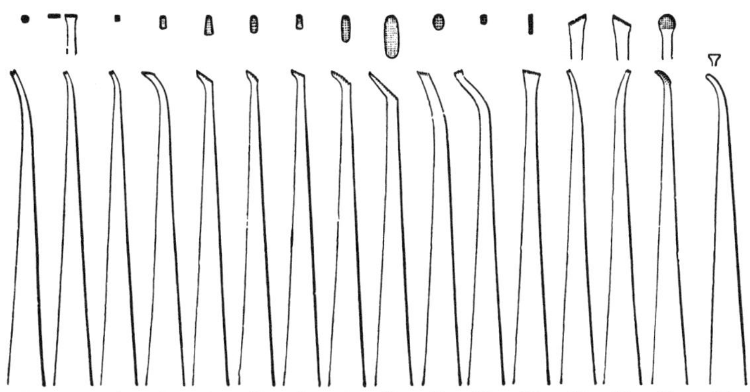

2. 3. 4. 5. 6. 7. 8. 9. 10. 11. 12. 13. 14. 15. 16. 17.

This set of Dr. Butler's Pluggers realizes his highest conception in practice, and fills the wants of a large class of careful operators.

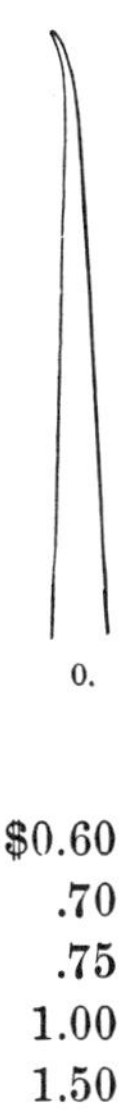

0.

By request, Dr. Butler has furnished, as an adjunct to his set, an instrument—marked 0—designed to be used as a "Holder," or "Left-hand Assistant," in starting the gold in the points of anchorage, and also to hold pieces of gold in position while building up. Made of round $\frac{3}{16}$ inch steel, it will be easily distinguished among the other instruments. The point is fine, without serration. We have not numbered it in the set,—it being an instrument for general use. Sold singly for 30 cents.

Also, a Burnisher, same style of handle as in illustration, and numbered 17.

Price, per set of 18 . . . . $14.80

Or separately, as follows:

Nos. 1, 2, 4	each	$0.60
No. 11	"	.70
Nos. 3, 6, 8, 13, 14, 15	"	.75
Nos. 5, 7, 9, 10, and 12	"	1.00
No. 16	"	1.50
No. 17	"	1.00

These are in stock, bronzed handles. May be ordered lacquered fire-gray, without extra charge.

Morocco Case, holding each instrument in position and open at the end, to show Points, extra . . . . each $2.50

DR. CHARLES R. BUTLER'S SET OF BEVELED PLUGGERS, AND DR. H. L. AMBLER'S PLUGGING ASSISTANT.

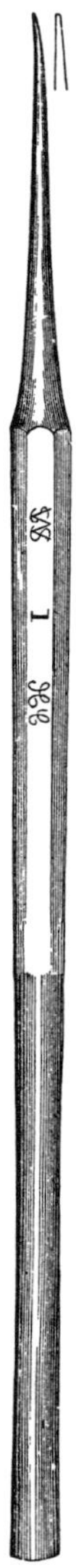

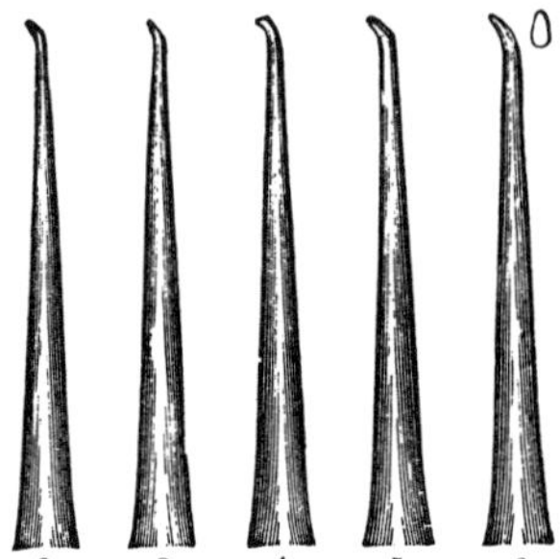

2. 3. 4. 5. 6.

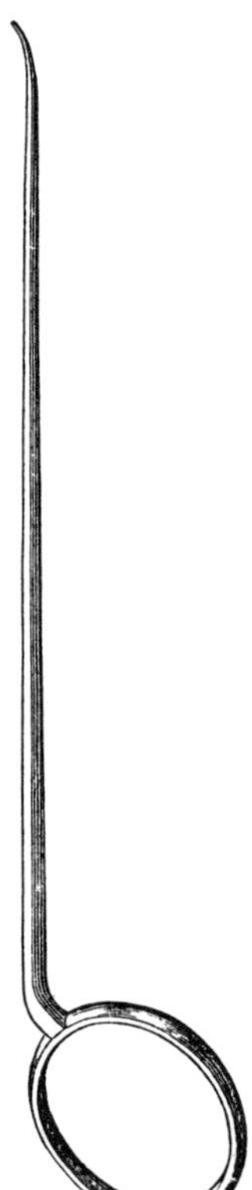

1. 7.

These instruments are wrought and polished all over; bright burnished; tapered, with a very slight swell end. The Cut of No. 1 properly represents the style of shaft in all, but the other numbers vary a little from it in length and weight.

In the following description Dr. Butler's language is given in italics.

No. 1 is a very fine, delicately tapered point. Slightly curved. Not serrated. *For fine pits and slots, also for tacking the gold after commencing.*

Nos. 2 and 3 are combined Foot and Point Pluggers, with beveled edges. Serrated on points and top edge of foot. The serrations being single valleys with a division on the foot of both; single on point of No. 2, and crossed on point of No. 3. *Well adapted for proximal cavities by turning the point toward the angle, pit or groove. They work as a Point or Foot, and also as a Curve, by applying directing force with the stroke of the mallet. No. 3 may be used without the mallet to carry gold under a margin.*

No. 4 is a Foot instrument with curved neck and beveled faces. Single valleys across the top face, which is made at right angles with the axis of the shaft. *Capable of use in narrow spaces and fine slots.*

No. 5 is shaped like No. 3, but larger, stronger, and not serrated. Beveled faces. Combined Foot and Point. *Can be used in any part of packing, especially along margins and where strength of point is needed.*

No. 6 is shaped like an apple-seed, small end up. Dead smooth. *Used as a surface condenser, or to burnish.*

No. 7. Dr. Ambler's "Assistant." Designed to be used (by slipping the second finger of left hand through the ring, shaft inside) while starting the filling.

Price, No. 1	each	$1.00
" Nos. 2 and 3	"	2.00
" No. 4	"	1.50
" Nos. 5 and 6	"	1.25
Price, per set of 7, including the "Assistant"		10.00

The "Assistant" will also be sold separately.

Nickel-Plated	Price $1.00	Fire-Gray Lacquered	Price $0.60
Crocus-Polished	" .80	Plain	" .50

DR. LOUIS JACK'S "MATRIX" PLUGGERS.

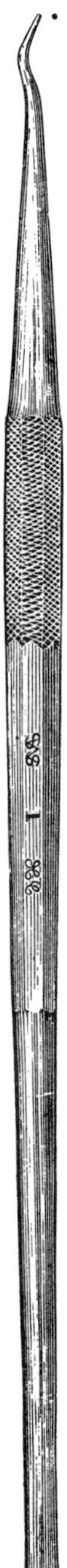

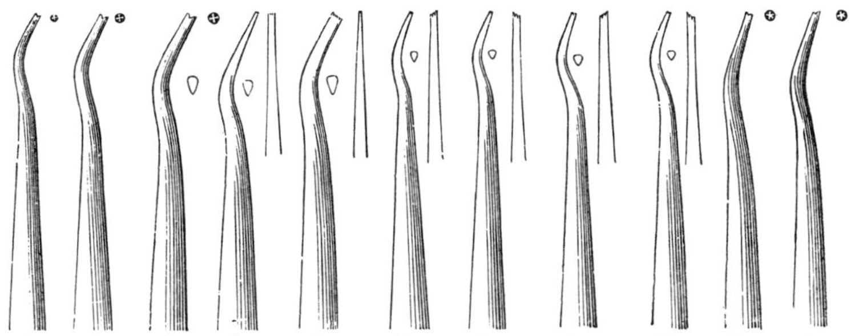

2. 3. 4. 5. 6. 7. 8. 9. 10. 11. 12.

Designed and fashioned expressly for use in Filling Approximal Cavities, with the aid of a "Matrix," as described in Dental Cosmos for April, 1871.

The perusal of this article will show that these Pluggers were adapted by Dr. Jack to be used with either mallet or hand-pressure; for adhesive or soft gold,—his own practice including both in the same cavity. They had, therefore, deep serrations. This was objected to by those who mallet exclusively, and use adhesive gold throughout. To accommodate the demand, we now make all the stock supply of these Pluggers with serrations of the same fineness as the latest style of Butler's.

We are indebted to Dr. Jack for the following description of the uses of his Pluggers by number:

"Nos. 1, 2, 3, 4, 5 are intended for fixing the mats of gold in the cavity in the positions they are to occupy. Selection of number to be used will be governed by the size of cavity.

"Nos. 7, 8, 9, 10 are for consolidation of the gold,—to be used with the mallet, as special'y directed in April number, page 175, vol. xiii., of the DENTAL COSMOS. To save the trouble of reference, we quote the passages:

FIG. 5.

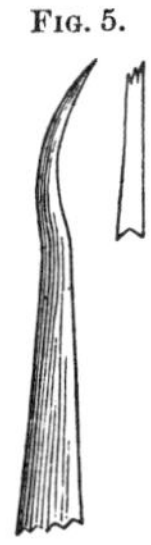

"'The important modifications needed are some pairs of mated pluggers, formed as at Fig. 5, in which one side of the edge is considerably longer than the other, which longer side, in malleting, is constantly kept against the matrix; this effects the greatest pressure upon the margins, and secures with positiveness the perfect fullness and the proper consolidation of the gold at these parts. Several sizes and varied curves of this point are required.'

"No. 6, for consolidation of first layers along cervical wall of very large distal cavities of superior molars.

"No. 11, for consolidation of very large distal molar; and No. 12, of large mesial superior molar cavities."

The Cuts illustrate the length, style, and form of the shaft, also shape of each point and bend; but the instruments are one-third less in size than the Cuts exhibit and really *fine* Pluggers, but of great firmness by reason of the ovoid shape shown in the tiny sectional diagrams, which exhibit in Nos. 4, 5, 6, 7, 8, 9, and 10 quite truly the shape and size of each at the bend opposite to which it is placed.

1.

Price, per set of 12, with Fine Serrations $15.00

DR. WM. H. ATKINSON'S "OMEGA" PLUGGERS.

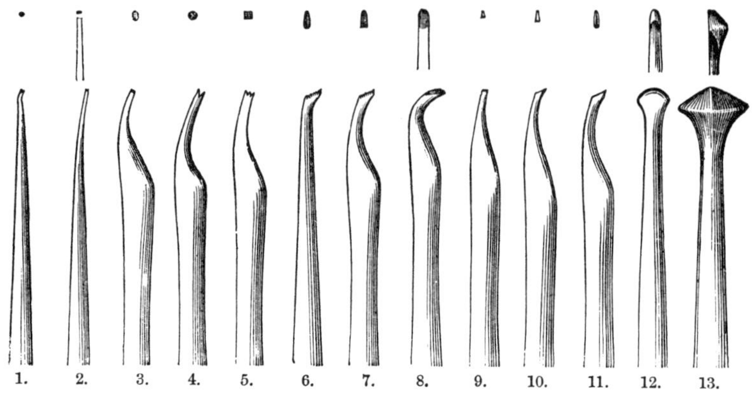

This illustration represents the last improvements in Pluggers by Dr. Atkinson. The points are very peculiar, several of them having very delicate serrations. Our pattern set has been carefully revised by Dr. A. He recognizes no other make.

Each one of this set, in addition to our trade-marks and the regular number figure, is stamped "A. ω."

These instruments are $7\frac{1}{2}$ inches long, of $\frac{7}{32}$ Octagon Steel, Black.

Price	per set	$13.00
Or separately as follows:		
Nos. 1, 2, and 12	each	.60
Nos. 3, 4, 5, 6, 9, 10, 11, 13	"	1.00
No. 7	"	1.50
No. 8	"	1.75

PLUGGERS FOR SPONGE OR PLASTIC GOLD.

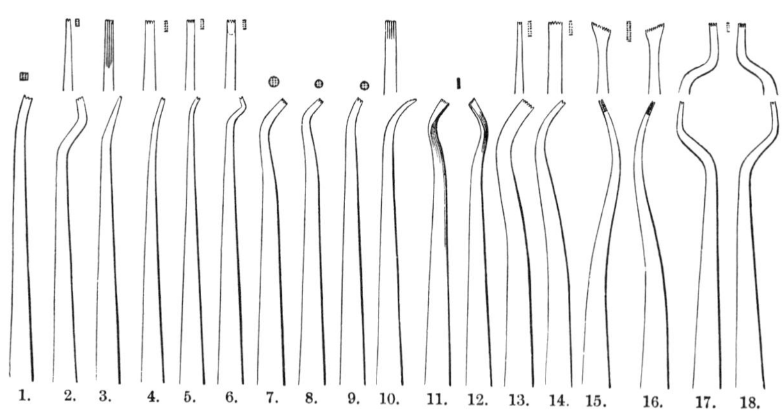

The above Cut represents a set of 18 Pluggers, for the use their name indicates. There are many Dentists, with whom the practice of malleting every filling is the rule,

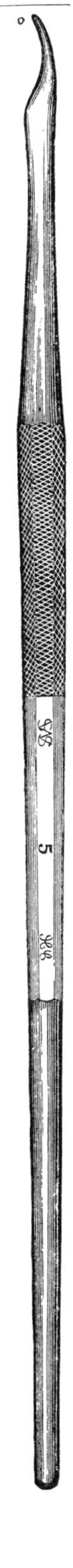

who desire at times to use Sponge or Plastic Gold. Changing the position of the patient and operator to suit hand-plugging is inconvenient. This is especially so in the numerous cases where it is desired to fill only a part of the cavity in this way. To meet these wants this set of Pluggers has been selected and modified.

They are from Ellis's, Head's, and Forbes's sets, the bends and facial angles of the points being altered, where necessary, to bring the serrations in place when held as in malleting. All of the points except those for margins and crevices have two or more rows of fine, shallow serrations, so formed and finished that they will not drag, cut, or powder the gold.

They are in stock as 7-inch Taper ends only. Made to order, with plain shaft, like those of Atkinson's set of 60.

Price, either style, per set of 18 . . . . $9.00

DR. GEO. A. MILLS'S "SMOOTH CONVEX SURFACE FILLERS."

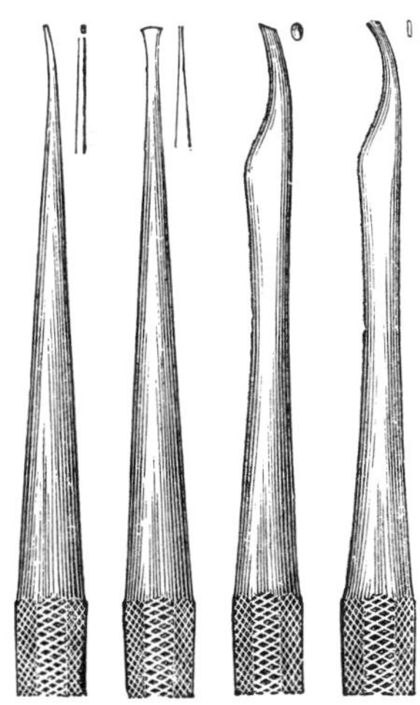

1. 2. 3. 4.

A set of 5 instruments, so well represented by the Cuts as scarcely to need description. In all their features, they are illustrated exactly. They are designed to be used with the mallet, especially for heavy foil. The faces are all convex, and finished as smooth and fine as burnishers. The set which we now have as patterns were used by Dr. Mills for three years, and he was able with them to fill any case occurring in his practice. The following description includes Dr. Mills's notes of their separate intentions and uses:

No. 1 is a thin, flat, slightly curved Point, used for small proximal surfaces or cavities.

No. 2 is perfectly straight, spread at the end, about double the width of No. 1. It is applicable for fissures and slots, and in beating gold to the margins.

No. 3 is a Foot shape, ovoid face.

No. 4 is a "Foot," with extremely narrow face, adapted to the uses of No. 2.

Nos. 3 and 4 are used in driving and packing.

No. 5 has a round end, small; generally useful.

All the faces are convex. The gold welds beautifully under them, and success has attended their use with block and sponge gold, as well as with foils.

Made in our best style and quality of workmanship and material. Crocus polished. Octagon portion fire-gray lacquered.

Price, per set $5.00

DR. ISAIAH FORBES'S RIGHT AND LEFT PLUGGERS.

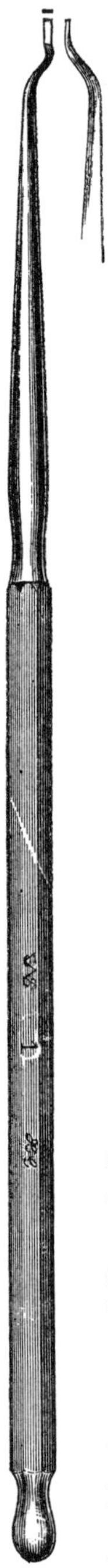

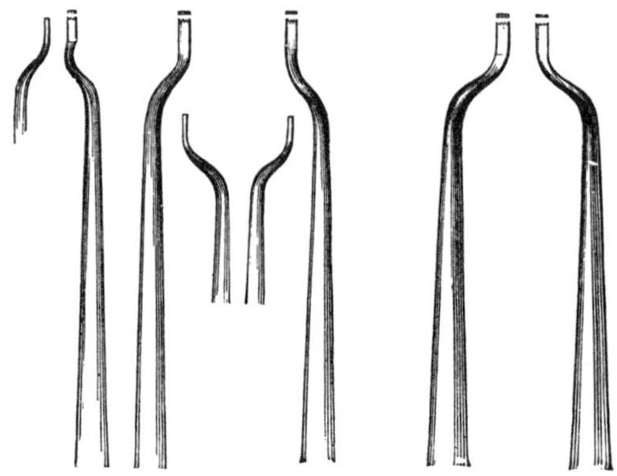

2. 3. 4. 5. 6.

This set consists of three pairs of instruments of different sizes.

Plain Octagon, $\frac{3}{16}$ inch Ball End, 7 inches long . . per set $3.60

DR. GEO. A. WILSON'S SMOOTH-FACED PLUGGERS.

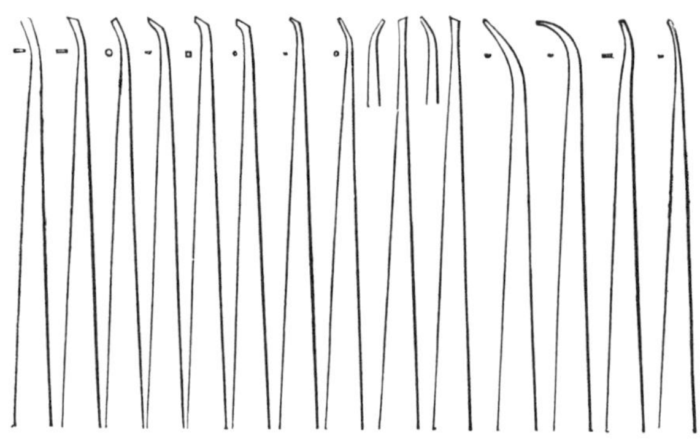

2. 3. 4. 5. 6. 7. 8. 9. 10. 11. 12. 13. 14. 15.

Although absolutely without serrations, these faces are very carefully made. so that they take hold perfectly; and this finish, combined with the curve and angle, insures perfect immunity from slipping.

They are Mallet-Pluggers, the shafts being of the style, finish, and general form of the well-known Varney Pluggers,—hardened, tempered, and polished all over.

Recognizing that the forms of these Pluggers have considerable merit, we will furnish them to order, with serrations similar to those of Dr. Varney's, charging for them according to that No. of Varney's which they most nearly resemble.

Price, set of 15, Points after patterns of Dr. Wilson, with Varney style of Shafts, 7 of the same size, and 8 one-quarter larger, smooth. $20.00

With Plain Octagon Handles, 7 inches 15.00

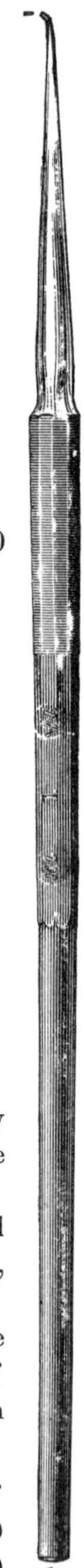

1.

PLUGGER POINTS FOR AUTOMATIC MALLETS.

Our stock of Points for all kinds of Automatic Mallets is, in quality, variety, and extent, the best that can be found.

Beside the selections illustrated we have in stock, always, full lines of Atkinson (set of 60), Butler, Varney, and a large and choice selection of other Points.

The Plugger Points of named sets are, in material, workmanship, and finish, equal always to the regular sets—with handles—to which they belong, perfect in form and serrations.

We make to order also what any customer desires; but of late such orders are generally filled from stock, at stock prices.

Those which rule higher in price are stamped with abbreviation of the name, as ATK., BUT., VAR., etc. The abbreviations are on the shank which enters the socket. Varney Points are charged by number at $\frac{3}{4}$ the price of instruments with full handles; Butler's at $\frac{2}{3}$ price, Atkinson's "Omega" at $\frac{3}{4}$ price, and others at prices which allow a full deduction for the cost of handle.

Selection No. 1.

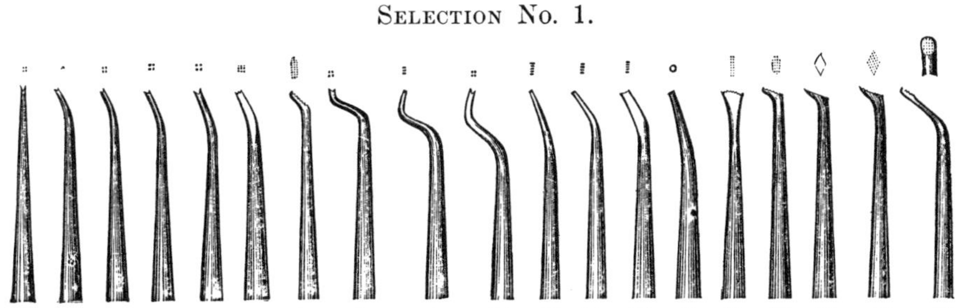

1. 2. 3. 4. 5. 6. 7. 8. 9. 10. 11. 12. 13. 14. 15. 16. 17. 17. 18.
Smooth. Serrated.

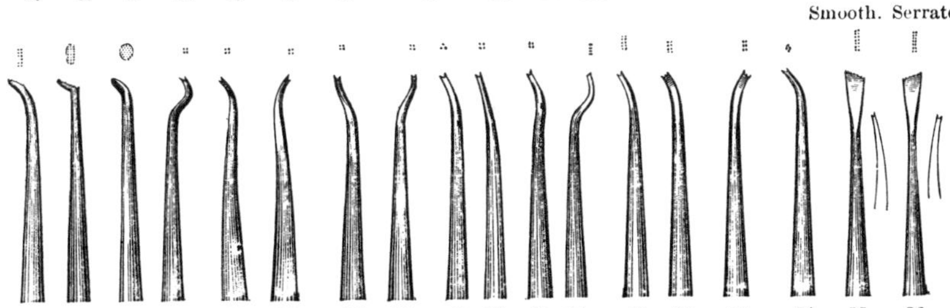

19. 20. 21. 22. 23. 24. 25. 26. 27. 28. 29. 30. 31. 32. 33. 34. 35. 36.

Price . . . . per doz. $4.50

Selection No. 2.

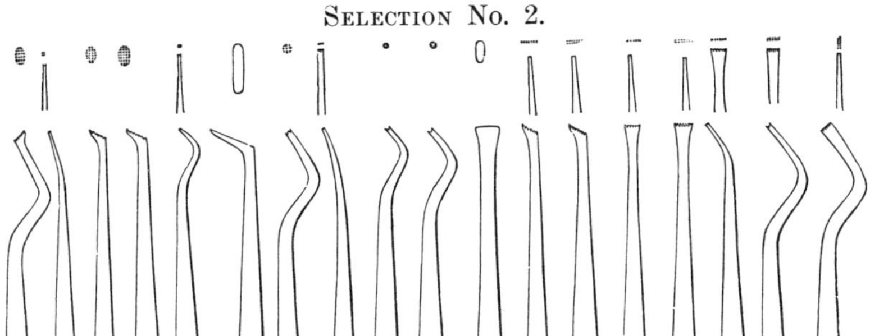

1. 2. 3. 4. 5. 6. 7. 8. 9. 10. 11. 12. 13. 14. 15. 16. 17. 18.

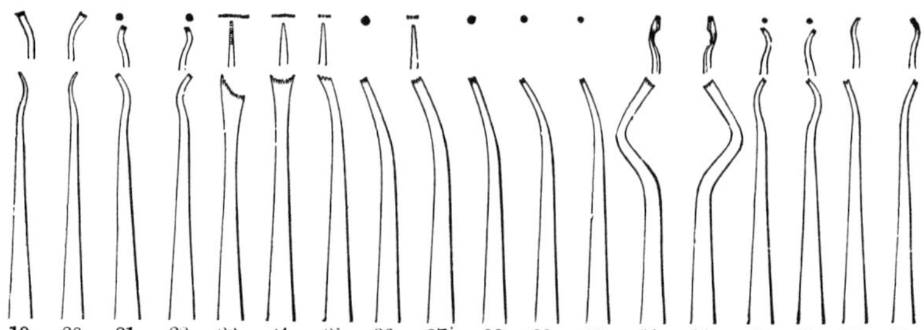

19. 20. 21. 22. 23. 24. 25. 26. 27. 28. 29. 30. 31. 32. 33. 34. 35. 36.

Price, except No. 1 . . . . per doz. $4.50
No. 1 . . . . each .50

Selection No. 3.

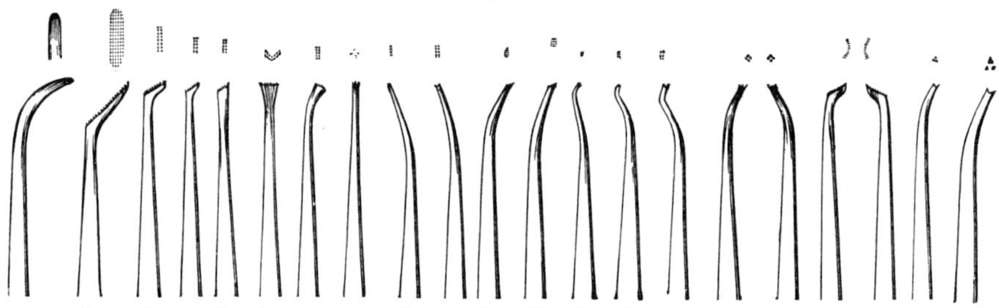

1. 2. 3. 4. 5. 6. 7. 8. 9. 10. 11. 12. 13. 14. 15. 16. 17. 18. 19. 20. 21.
Cork Screw.

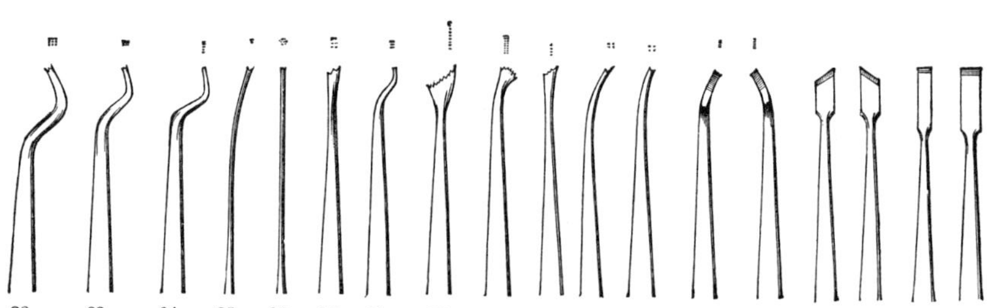

22. 23. 24. 25. 26. 27. 28. 29. 30. 31. 32. 33. 34. 35. A. B. C. D.

Price, except No. 2 . . . . per doz. $4.50
No. 2 . . . . each .60

The above are made to fit any of the Automatic Pluggers in use. In ordering please state "*Selection*," *Numbers of Instruments*, and make of Automatic Plugger they are desired to fit.

SALMON'S NEW AUTOMATIC MALLET.

Under Patents bearing the following dates: July 11th, 1865; September 25th, 1866; February 26th, 1867; and August 3d, 1875; also, Reissues dated February 8th, 1870; October 21st, 1873.

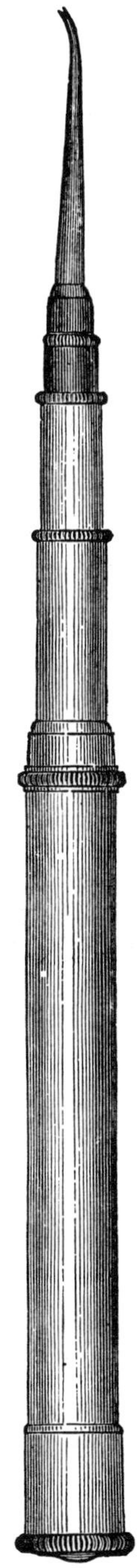

PRICES REDUCED.

More than nine years' test had proved the "Salmon Automatic Mallet" to be a superior instrument of its kind. Still, there was room for improvement, and the inventor has made such important changes in its construction as to give the new Mallet the following advantages over the old one:

1. The hammer is centered by the spindle, which *prevents friction* against the case.

2. The steel spring (which in the old Mallet pressed the hammer against the case) is dispensed with, and a catch plate attached to the end of the hammer which engages with the spindle, and is operated by a fine wire spring, making it a very much smoother-working instrument, and much less liable to get out of order.

3. The hammer can be *loaded with lead*, thereby giving a blow like that produced by the lead-mallet.

The Back-Action Automatic is more indispensable when needed than the direct action. With this the difficulties heretofore experienced in filling distal or posterior cavities are overcome without sacrificing so much sound tooth-substance. The point being curved, is hooked over beyond the gold in a posterior cavity, and by a pull (instead of a push) the hammer is caused to strike toward the operator.

The new works are applied to both instruments.

A case, of French goat-skin, containing a rack to accommodate 24 or 30 Points, if desired, will be furnished, to hold one or both Mallets.

PRICES.

Direct-Action Mallet, Nickel-Plated (not loaded)		$10.00
" " " (loaded)		12.00
" " with extra finished working parts (extra)		2.00
Back-Action Mallet, Nickel-Plated		15.00
" " " extra finished		18.00
Direct-Action Points	per doz.	4.50
" " *long*, for molars	"	4.50
Back-Action Points, for molars	"	6.00
Case for one Mallet, with rack to hold 24 Points		6.00
" two Mallets " " 24 "		6.50
" one Mallet " " 30 "		7.00
" two Mallets " " 30 "		7.50
Wide racks, without cases, to hold 30 long Points		3.00

A large variety of Points constantly in stock (See List, pages 137-138). Any not in the list, made to order.

THE SNOW & LEWIS AUTOMATIC PLUGGER.

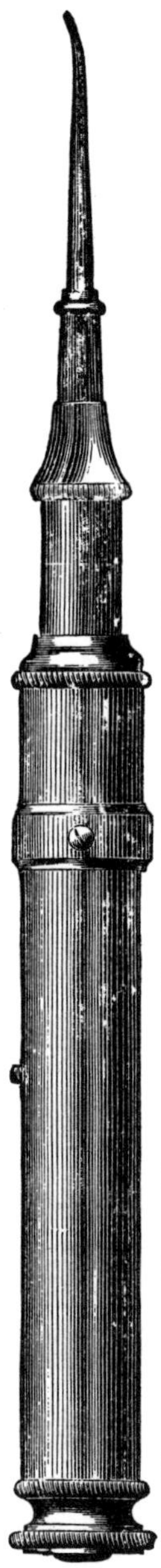

The manufacturers say, "From this date (July 1st, 1873) we will manufacture an Improved Automatic Plugger, with the wearing surfaces of steel, and a finer quality of workmanship than heretofore, in all its parts. The new Plugger will combine the qualities of the Snow & Lewis Nos. 1 and 2, and save dealers the necessity of keeping double stock on hand.

"This instrument has a series of Two Distinct Grades of Blows, regulated by the tension knob on the top of the instrument and by the extension of the socket piece, allowing the hammer to descend through a greater space. When at its shortest stroke the socket recedes but an eighth of an inch, and one-fourth of an inch at the longest stroke. The different degrees of blows are obtained by means of the milled head on the top of the case, which, upon being turned, carries a screw follower down upon the spring. All Pluggers will, hereafter, have this arrangement for compressing the spring and regulating the blow.

"The Plugger can be locked by the ring on the handle, and used as a hand instrument."

PRICES.

Automatic Plugger, Triple Gilt, No. 1 or 2		$16.00
" " Silver or Nickel-Plated		12.00
Points, per dozen . . . S S W Manufacture		4.50
Varney's Points, per set of 13 . " "		15.00
Varney's Points, Separately, " "		
Nos. 1, 2, 3,	each	.94
" 4, 5, 6, 7, 9, 10	"	1.32
" 8	"	1.50
" 11, 12	"	1.13
" 13	"	.67
Butler's Points, per set of 17		9.50
Butler's Points, Separately, S S W Manufacture.		
Nos. 1, 2, 4		.40
" 3, 6, 8, 13, 14, 15		.50
" 5, 7, 9, 10, 12, 17		.67
" 11		.47
" 16		1.00
Morocco Case, with Snow & Lewis's Rack for 18 Points		3.50
" " " Foote's Rack for 24 Points, and space for loose Points, superior finish		6.00

Points of any desired pattern furnished to order. All styles of Atkinson's, Butler's, and Abbott's Points constantly on hand.

SOCKET HANDLES.

CUTS REPRESENT THE FULL SIZE.

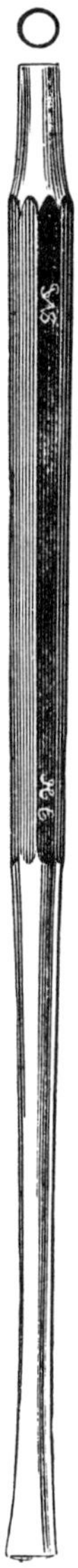

A.

"A," Butler's Sockets for Automatic Points	each	$1.00
¼ in. File-cut " " "	"	.60
"B" { Ivory Revolving Head Sockets	"	2.25
"B" { Pearl " " "	"	6.00
"C" { Ivory Adjustable " "	"	3 00
"C" { Ebony " " "	"	1.50

SOCKETS FOR EXCAVATORS, BURS, DRILLS, ETC.

Ivory Handle, ⅝ inch Sockets	each	$2.00
" " ½ " "	"	1.75
" " ⅜ " "	"	1.38
" " 5/16 " "	"	1.15
Ebony " ⅝ " "	"	1 00
" " ½ " "	"	.84
" " ⅜ " "	"	.63
Bone " ⅝ " "	"	1.00
" " ½ " "	"	.75
Steel " ¼ " File-cut Sockets	"	.60
" " Octagon " "	"	.50

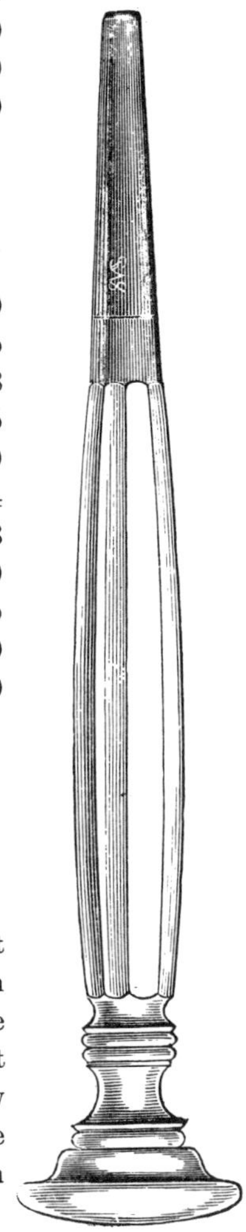

B.

SHORT REVOLVING HEAD SOCKETS "D."

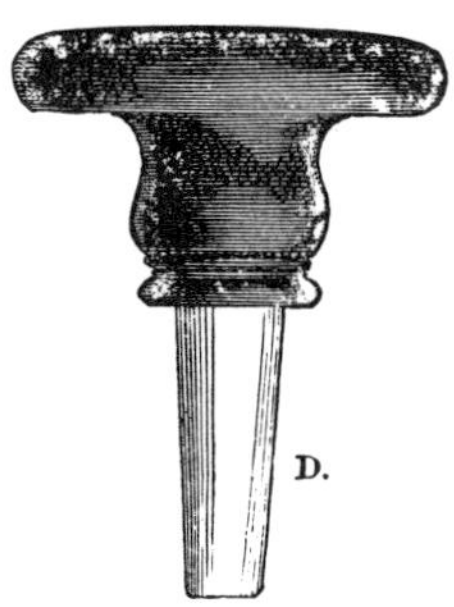

D.

The Cut "D" represents a short Revolving Head Socket for the palm of the hand, by means of which the *ordinary* drill can be rotated without chafing the hand. It is preferred by many to the bur thimble, and has the advantage over the *long* drill stock, in that bits are dispensed with.

Ebony Head	$0.60
Ivory "	.80

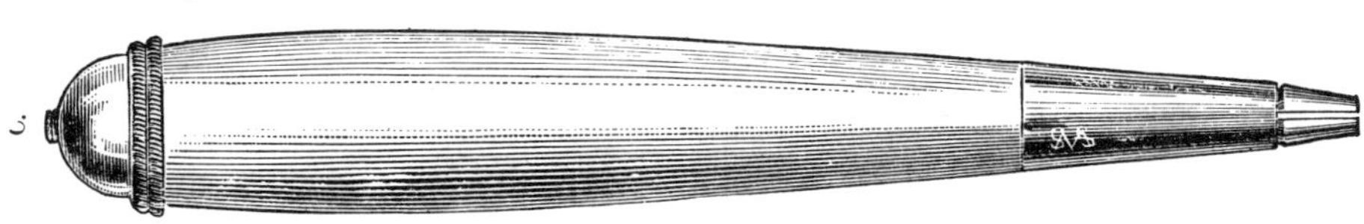

PLUG-FINISHING BURS.

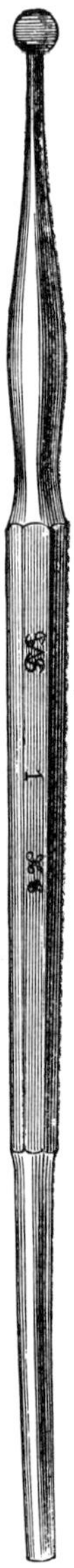

1.

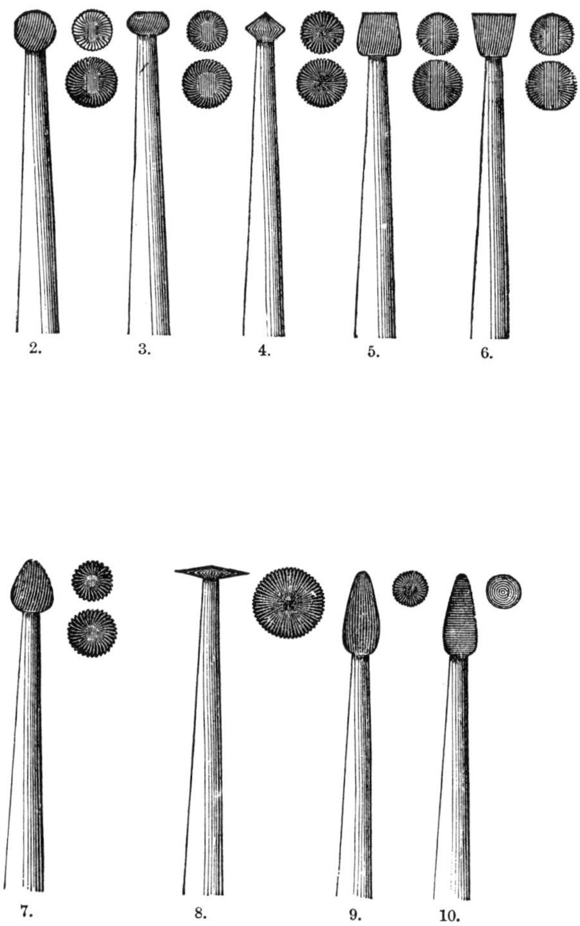

These Burs are made of first quality steel, extra fine cut, and finished in the best manner. Numbers 1 to 7 are made of two sizes, as shown in Cut. Numbers 8, 9, and 10 are of one size only.

Each . . . . 75 cents.

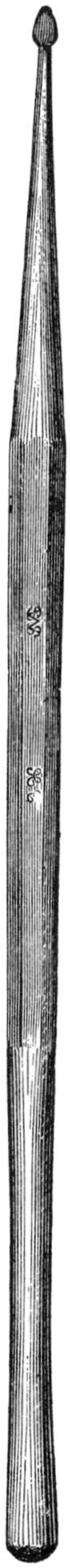

1.

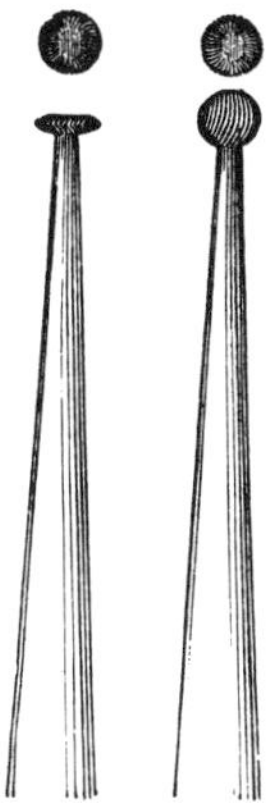

2. 3.

DR. C. R. BUTLER'S PLUG-FINISHING BURS.

The accompanying Cuts exhibit a set of 3 Plug-Finishing Burs which Dr Butler designed and uses.

Their peculiarity lies in the *end* of the handle being large, rounded, and smooth, making their use easy on the hand, and the execution much more rapid—as held by him—than with taper ends.

We will furnish any of our standard forms of Plug-Finishing Burs to order, with this handle and finish, at the same price as these.

Price . . . . each **$1.00**

DR. F. ABBOTT'S PLUG-FINISHING BURS.

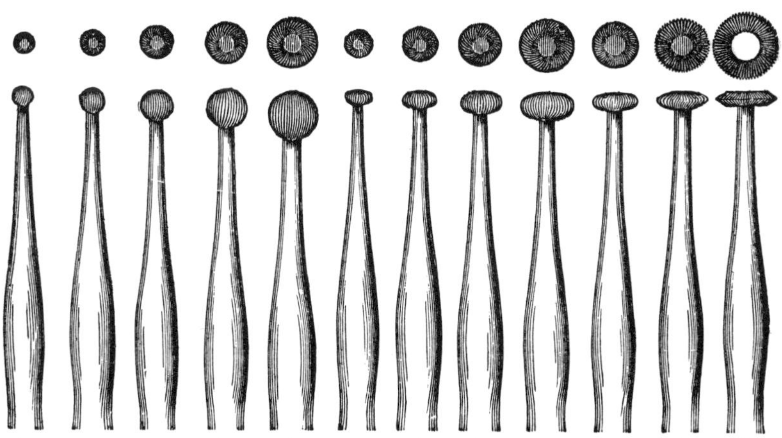

1. 2. 3. 4. 5. 6. 7. 8. 9. 10. 11. 12.

This Cut shows a selection, made by Dr. F. Abbott, of 12 Plug-Finishing Burs. They are extra fine cut, and finished in the best manner, Handles Bronzed, same size and style as our regular Plug-Finishing Burs.

Price . . . . **each 75 cents.**

PLUG-TRIMMERS AND PLUG-FINISHING FILES.

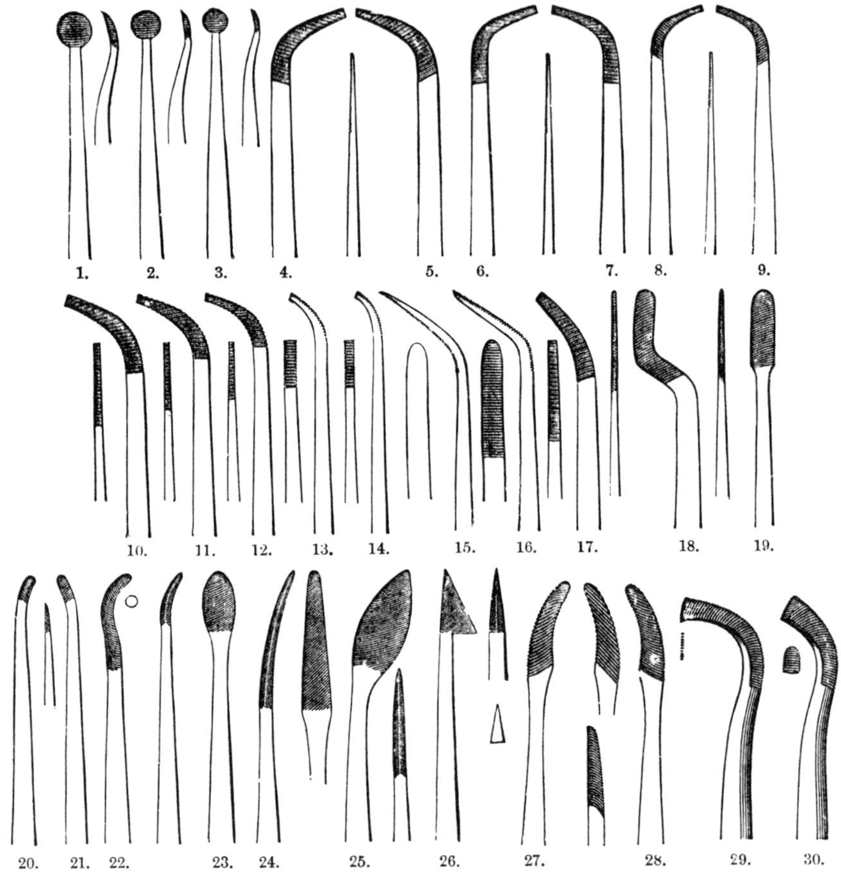

The above Cuts represent a line of Tools introduced by us. The series to No. 19, also 27, 28, 29, and 30, are float-cut. Nos. 6, 7, 11, 15, 16, 17, 29, and 30, are Dr. F. Searle's set. Nos. 1, 2, 3, 18, and 19 are also made fine file-cut, for finishing up fillings. The series from No. 20 to 26 inclusive is made from a selection by Dr. Jack. These are fine file-cut only. Nos. 1 to 9, and 13, 14, 15, 16, 20, and 21, are cut only on one side. The other Nos. are always cut on more than one side.

We make them all as Socket Bits, and also as 5-inch Octagon Handle Instruments.

PRICES.

Socket Bits, Per Dozen.

Cut only on one side (except Nos. 27, 28, 29, 30)			$3.00
Cut on more than one side (except Nos. 27, 28, 29, 30)			4.00
Nos. 27 and 28	$5.00	Nos. 29 and 30	8.00

Octagon Handles, Bronzed, Per Dozen.

Cut only on one side (except Nos. 27, 28, 29, 30)			3.50
Cut on more than one side (except Nos. 27, 28, 29, 30)			4.50
Nos. 27 and 28	$6.00	Nos. 29 and 30	9.00

Burnishers.

S. S. WHITE'S SET OF BURNISHERS.

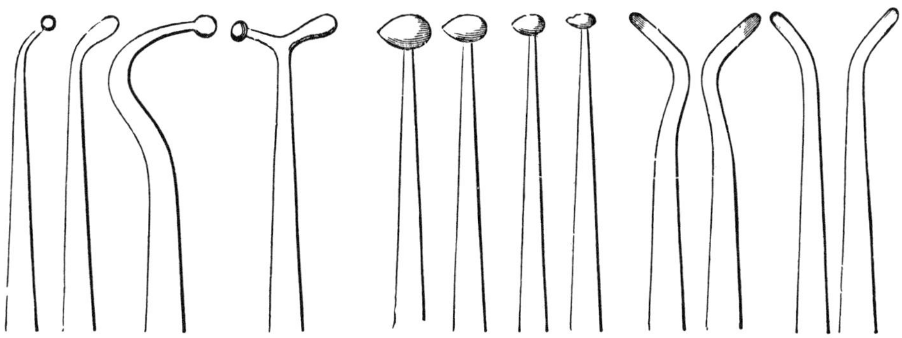

1. 2. 3. 4. 5. 6. 7. 8. 9. 10. 11. 12.

These are ¼ inch File-cut Handles, turned Shanks, Ball ends.
Can be made with any other style of handle desired.

Nos. 1 to 3, and 5 to 12	each 60 cents.
No. 4, Double end	" 75 "

A, B, C, BURNISHERS.

A is a Burnisher designed by Dr. Atkinson. It is of great value as a Mallet Burnisher. B is a reverse of A, giving the ball or larger end on the top of the bend.

C is a Hand Burnisher. Its especial use is shown by the rims on either end, which are finished to burnish on their edges, and furnish the best form for crevice fillings in any position. The faces are slightly rounded for use on crown fillings.

They are used on each end, and on each side; are suitable for crown, crevice, labial, or approximal surfaces.

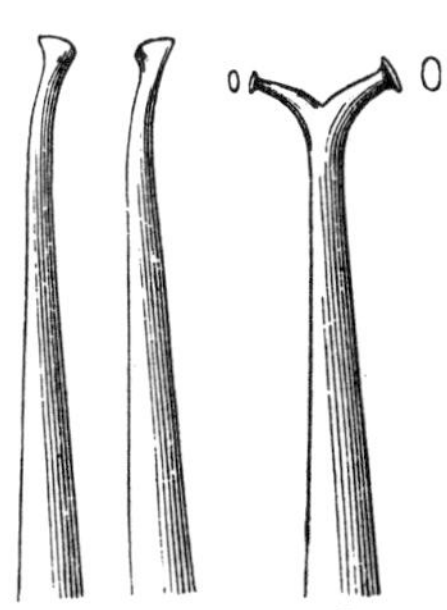

A. B. C.

We will supply the A and B Burnishers in styles of all our fine Mallet Pluggers, and also of Hand Pluggers, at the following prices:

Atkinson's Plain 7-inch Handle	each $0.50
Abbott's 7-inch Taper Handle	" .50
Varney's, Butler's, Wilson's, or Jack's Handle	" 1.00
¼-inch File-cut Handles, 6-inch	" .60
C Burnisher, Steel, ¼-inch File-cut	" .75

Other styles of Handles at proportionate prices.

DR. E. T. DARBY'S SET OF BURNISHERS.

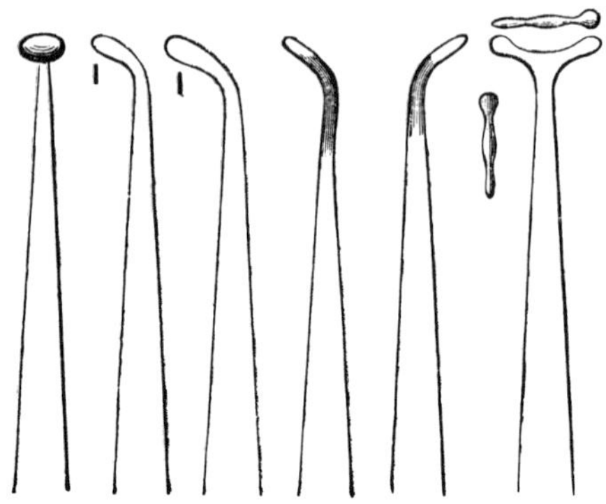

28. 29. 30. 31. 32. 33.

$\frac{1}{4}$ inch File-cut Handles, turned Shanks, Ball ends.

Nos. 28 to 32	each 60 cents.
No. 33, Double-end	" 75 "

DR. WM. H. ATKINSON'S SET OF MALLET BURNISHERS.

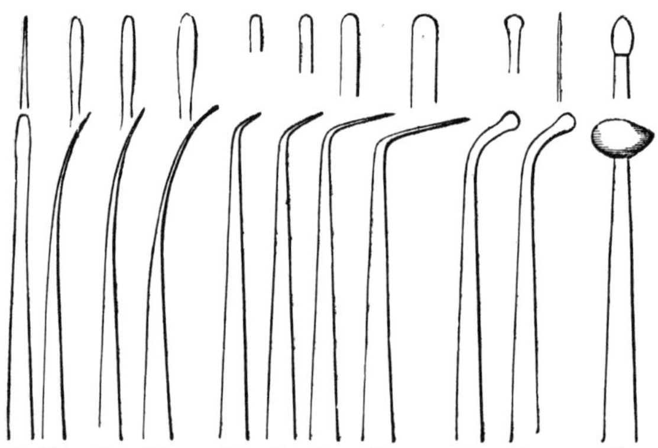

39. 40. 41. 42. 43. 44. 45. 46. 47. 48. 60.

$\frac{7}{32}$ inch Plain Octagon Bronzed Handles, seven inches long . . . per doz. $5.40

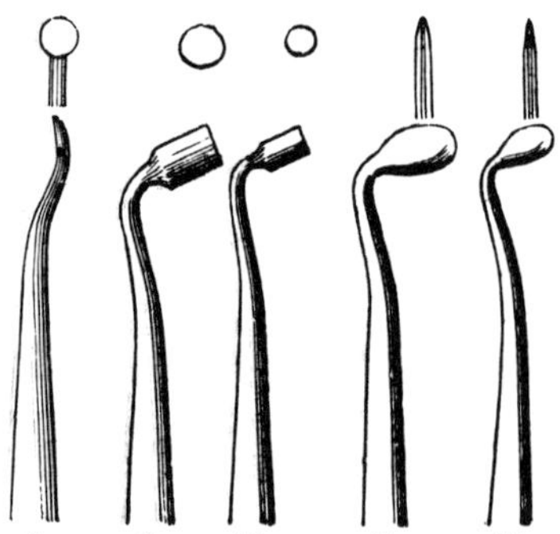

8. 9. 10. 11. 12.

DR. B. F. ARRINGTON'S SET OF AMALGAM BURNISHERS.

These Instruments are adapted to the use of Amalgam, Hill's Stopping, and Fusible Metal.

$\frac{1}{4}$ inch File-cut Handles, Ball ends . each 60 cents.

$\frac{7}{32}$ inch Octagon Cast Steel, six inches long, Bronzed Handles . . . . . each 50 cents.

Chisels.

S. S. WHITE'S SET OF CHISELS.

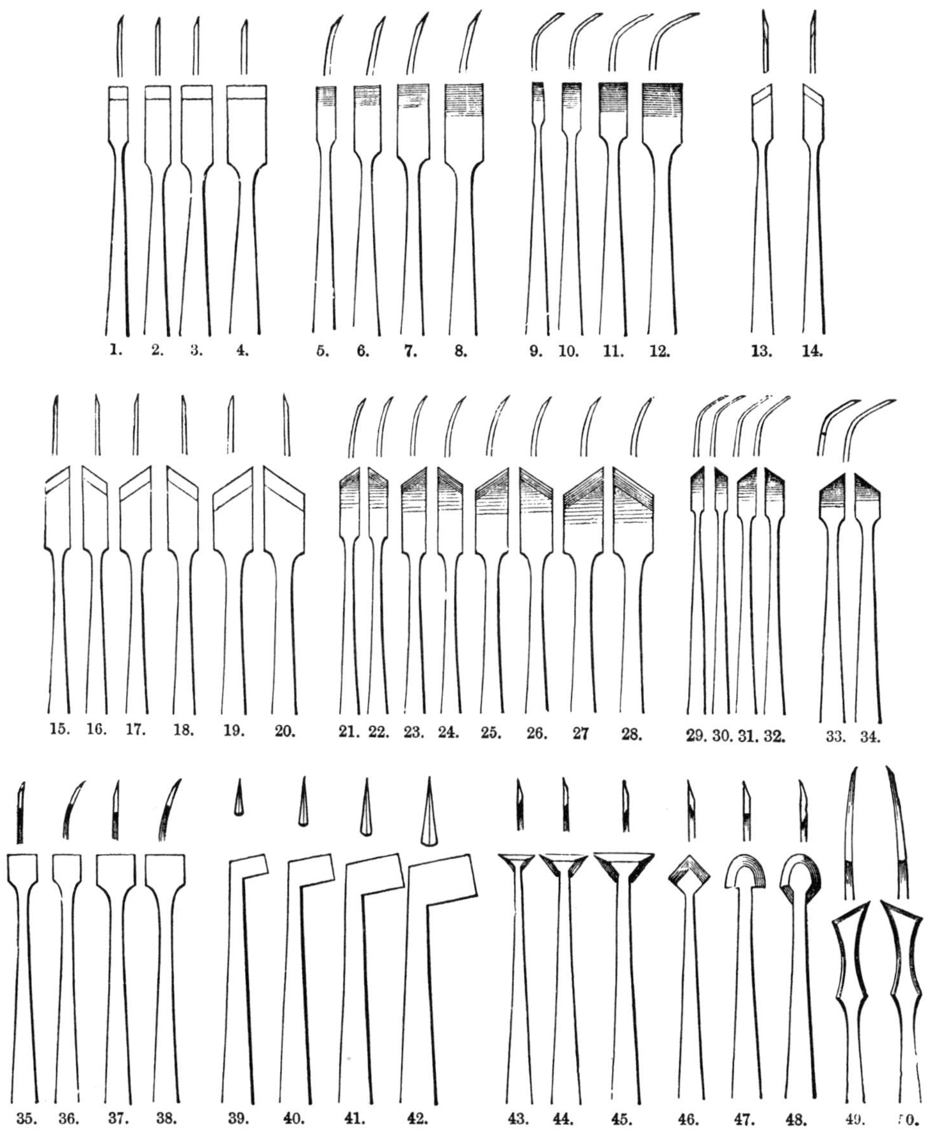

¼ inch File-cut Handles, turned Shanks, Ball ends.

Per dozen $7.20

DR. F. ABBOTT'S SET OF CHISELS.

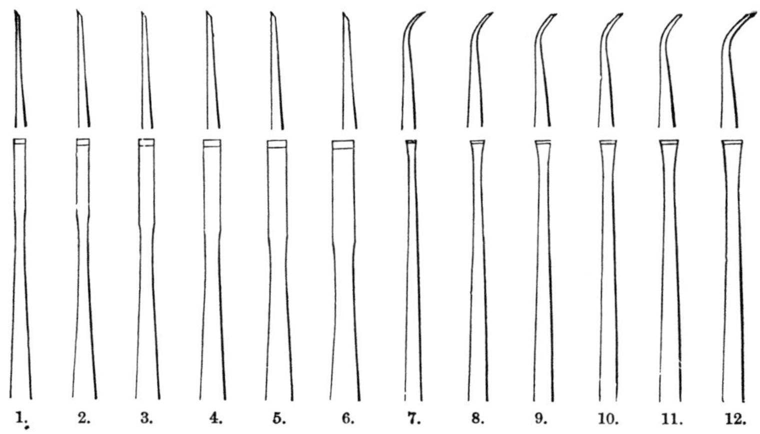

The above Cuts represent a set of 12 straight and curved Enamel and Excavating Chisels. Six of each. From Dr. Abbott's patterns, and expressly approved by him.

¼ inch File-cut Handle	per set	$7.20
$\frac{3}{16}$ " Octagon "	"	4.00
½ " Ivory "	"	20.00
½ " Ebony "	"	10.00

DR. D. H. GOODWILLIE'S SET OF CHISELS AND EXCAVATORS.

Complete set of Chisels and Excavators, 40 Instruments.

8 ¼ inch File-cut Chisels	each	$0.60
32 $\frac{3}{16}$ inch Excavators	per doz.	4.50
Set complete		16.80

Also, similarly arranged for traveling Dentists:

Socket Bits, set of 25	per doz.	$4.50

DR. LOUIS JACK'S DOUBLE-END ENAMEL CHISELS.

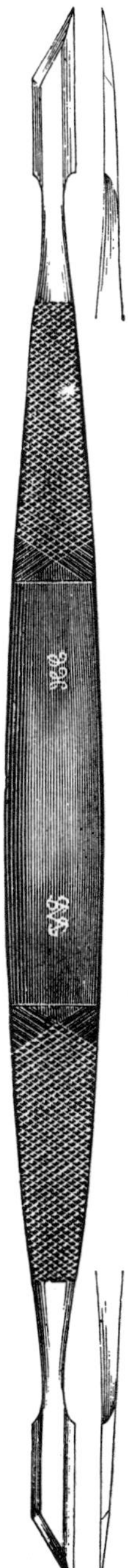

1.

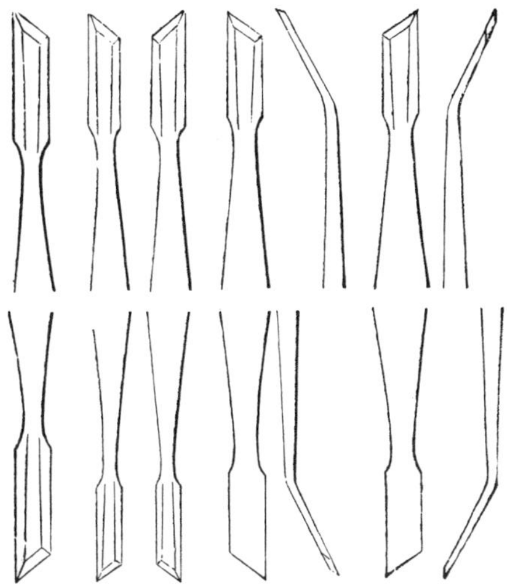

2. 3. 4. 5. 6.

The pattern of the handle, so formed as to give security in use, and the points, are exclusively the invention of Dr. Jack, the "double-end" constituting each tool a pair of Right and Left instruments for the same cut.

The set of 6 is designed to furnish all the forms needed for freely cutting the enamel in separating the teeth.

No. 5 is more particularly intended for cutting down the inner distal surfaces of the molars.

No. 6 is for the same purpose on the inner mesial surfaces of the same class of teeth.

In tempering, we make them as near to the hardness Dr. Jack prescribes as we judge possible or safe in work.

The immediate edge should be removed at an angle of seventy or eighty degrees after each dressing on the grinding stone.

Price, per set of 6 . . . . $12.00

CAVITY CHISELS—SELECTED POINTS.

Comprising about one dozen Points.

Blued Taper Handles . . . . . . per doz. $4.00

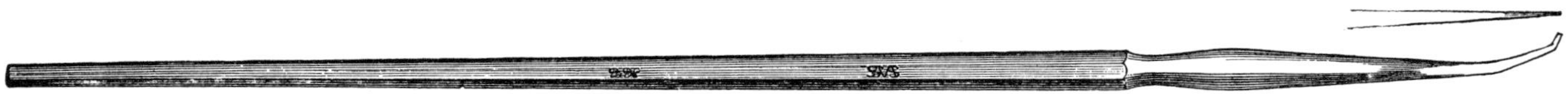

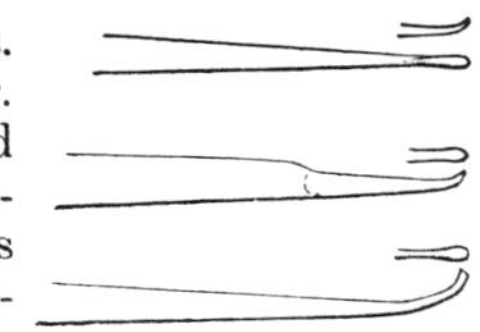

Our full-size Cut represents the shape and general size of our whole line of Blued Taper Handle Excavators. These are in stock of all the desirable forms. Blued Taper Cavity Chisels include the whole sets of Dr. Head's Excavators, Dr. Weatherbee's Excavators, Dr. Goodwillie's smaller Chisels, any of which may be ordered with these elegant handles; and a few special forms, 4 of which are shown in our Cuts. These are very desirable new shapes. We make three sizes of each. The term Cavity Chisels refers to thick-edged instruments formed suitably for excavating and cutting soft dentine, as distinguished from those straight or thick-edged instruments, which are only convenient for cutting enamel.

DR. ARRINGTON'S HEAVY MOLAR AND BICUSPID CHISELS

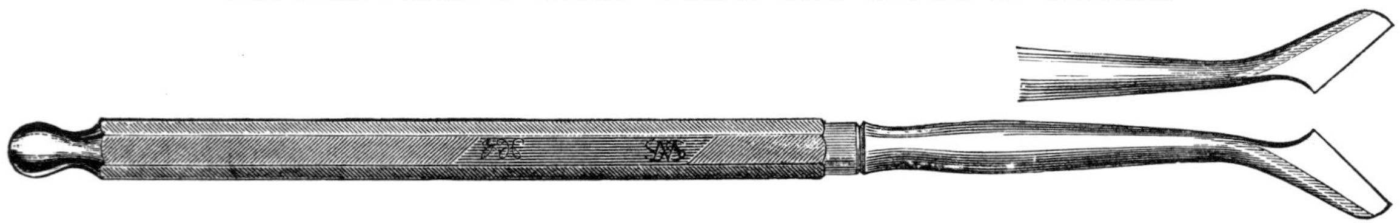

Are especially adapted for opening and edging approximal cavities. Their form, with Right and Left Slopes, is such that they can be used to dress mesial and distal surfaces with a shearing cut very rapidly and with less discomfort to the patient than the separating file causes. Price, ¼ inch File-cut . . . . . per pair $1.50

DR. A. M. HOLMES'S SHOULDER CHISELS.

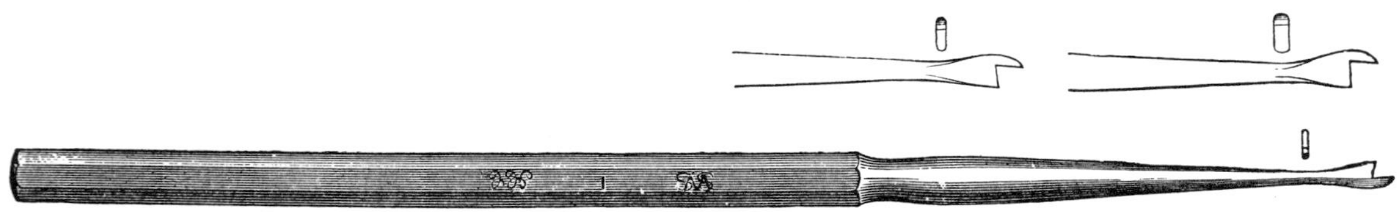

Are for cutting down enamel to open cavities; the small end forming a strong short Chisel, easily sharpened, while the shoulder stops it from entering to a dangerous depth. Rapid and safe work can be done with these.

Price, $\frac{7}{32}$ inch Octagon Handle, Blued . . . . each 75 cents.

DR. JACK'S PARABOLOID AND DR. FORBES'S GOUGE CHISELS.

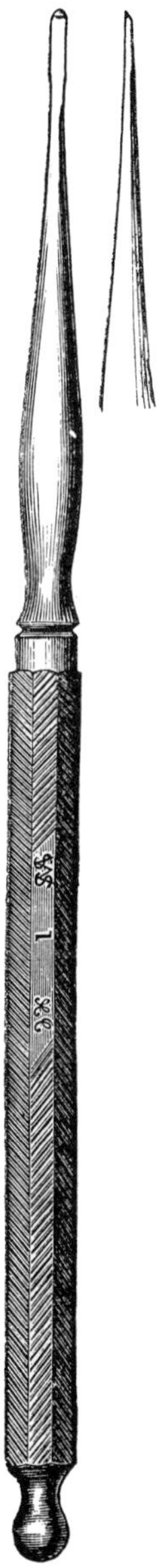

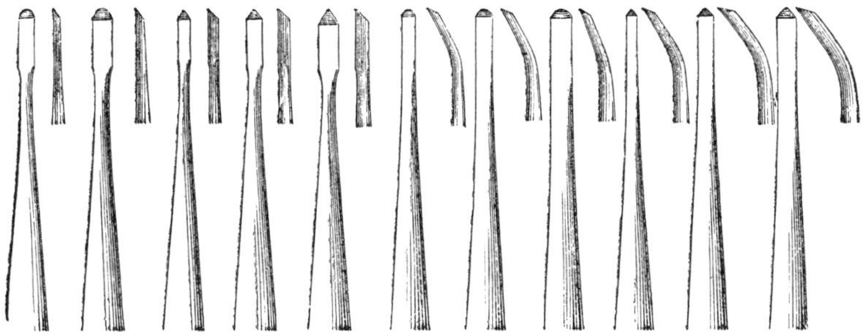

2. 3. 4. 5. 6. 7. 8. 9. 10. 11. 12.

The accompanying Cuts represent the Chisels recommended on page 170 of the DENTAL COSMOS for April, 1871. Nos. 1, 2, 3, 7, 8, and 9 show the Forbes Gouge; and Nos. 4, 5, 6, 10, 11, and 12 illustrate Dr. Jack's Paraboloid Chisels, which are intended for opening fissures, cutting retaining-grooves in large cavities, and for enamel-cutting wherever applicable.

To fit them for cutting enamel easily, these Chisels are made very hard, which necessitates some care in their use. The angle of sharpening should not be acute.

We add below outline drawings, showing exact sizes and forms of two Excavators supplementary to this set of Chisels. Their use is so connected in practice with that of the Chisels, that we have decided this to be their natural place, and have numbered them 13 and 14. The Chisels, 1 to 12, are made with $\frac{1}{4}$ inch File-cut Handles, Ball Ends, Bronzed. Nos. 13 and 14 are plain $\frac{3}{16}$ inch Handles, Blued or Bronzed.

These last are extremely useful Excavators. With them every part of an approximal cavity can be reached to excise it by the direct cut. They have this great range of applicability in addition to their special use in grooving small cavities and thin edges preparatory to matrix fillings.

13.

14.

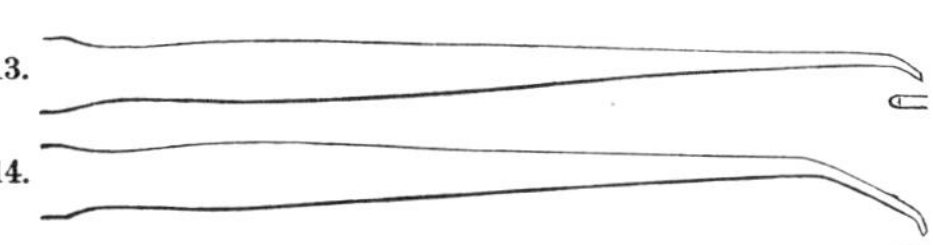

In addition to the above, we have a set of Paraboloid and Gouge Chisels, extra quality, or best, with two additional Points, making the set 14, independent of the supplementaries. All the foregoing are tempered extremely hard.

1.

PRICES.

Chisels, Nos. 1 to 12	per set	$12.00
Nos. 13 and 14	each	.30
Best quality, $\frac{15}{64}$ inch Plain Octagon Handles, Blued, per set of 14		17.50

DR. CHAS. R. BUTLER'S SET OF ENAMEL CHISELS.

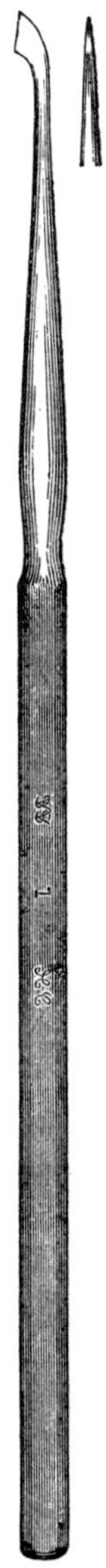

1.

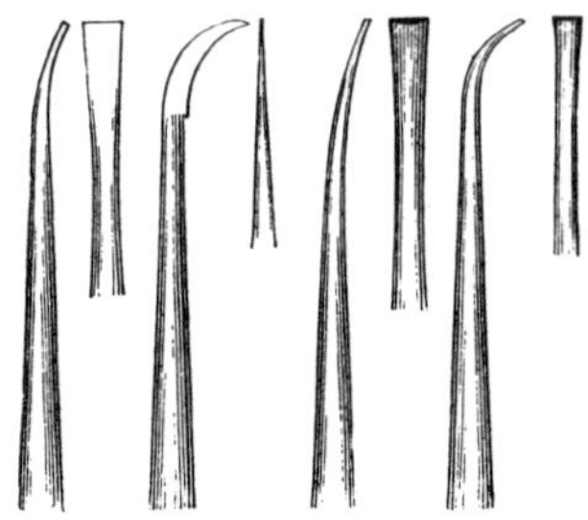

2. 3. 4. 5.

The forms of these Chisels will explain and commend themselves to Dentists, who will see that they have distinctive and peculiar shapes.

These shapes must be examined in connection with the edges in order to a full understanding of the originality and nicety of adaptation of each instrument for its special and relative use.

Dr. Butler describes them as intended "for separating back teeth for filling or preservation, by trimming palatal and proximal surfaces from the inside; the Sickle-shaped No. 3 being also used to scrape and finish surfaces before polishing."

"These Chisels should be held with the hand-grasp, with the thumb resting on some tooth as guard or fulcrum."

They are tempered very hard, made of the finest steel, with Polished Fire-gray Lacquered Handles. Crocus-polished Points.

Price, per set of 5 . . . . $2.00

DR. E. T. DARBY'S SET OF CHISELS.

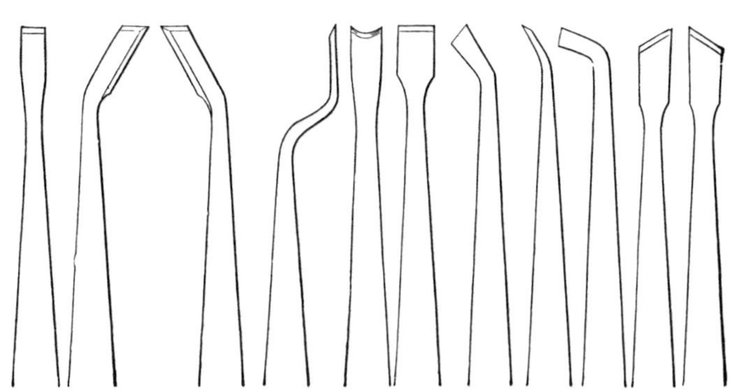

2. 3. 4. 5. 6. 7. 8. 9. 10 11. 12.

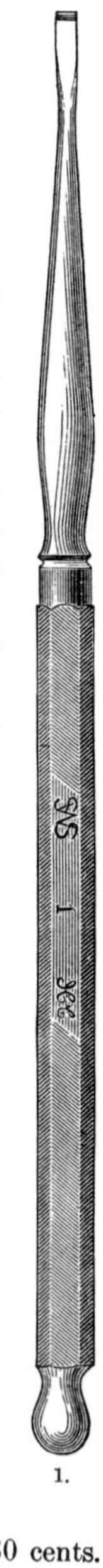

1.

¼ inch File-cut Handles . . . . each 60 cents.

HARD BITS.

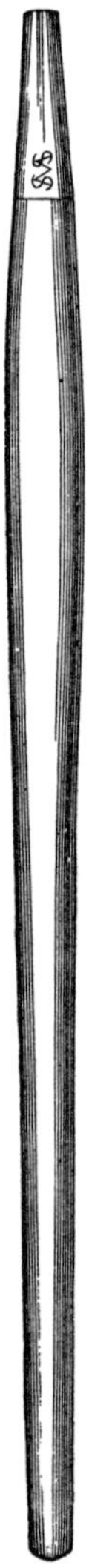

A.

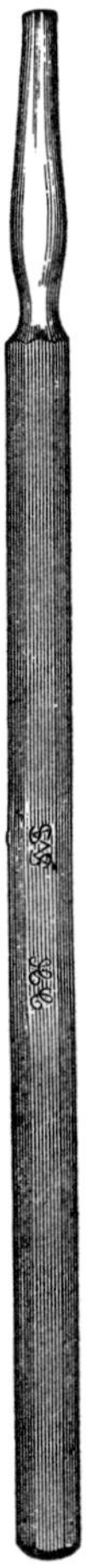

B.

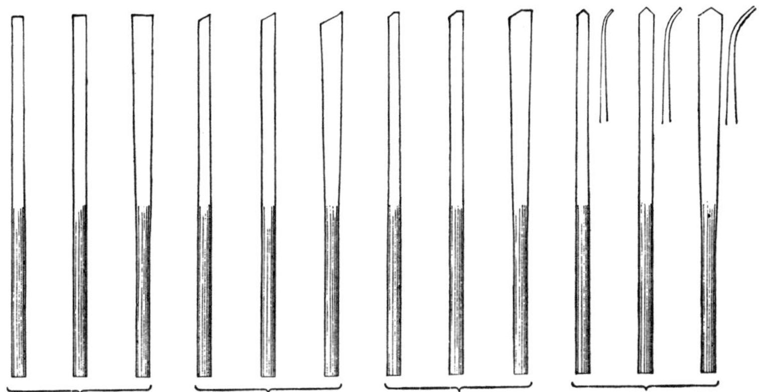

1. 2. 3. 4. 5. 6. 7. 8. 9. 10. 11. 12.

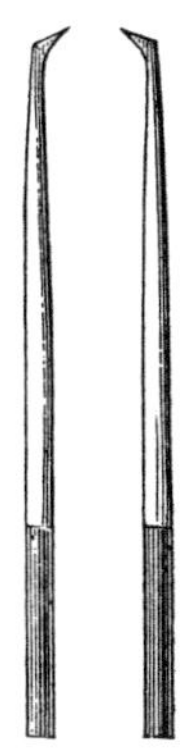

13. 14.

The Cuts are full size, and represent the Bits and Handles truly. The first 12 Instruments comprise four groups; each containing three Instruments. Each group differs in end-form. Each of the three in a group differs from the other considerably in width, and very little in thickness.

The drawings show the exact sizes and forms; and the sectional drawing, which shows the curved ends of the last group, shows also the thicknesses of the three sizes in all.

The first group having plain, square ends, and the second group slant ends, are more especially designed for paring off superficial decay. The third group has its ends formed for opening fissures. The fourth is for paring down the enamel edges of cavities. All of them are used, also, to excavate hard dentine and for separating. The edges of all are plain right angles, square with the flat sides. They are to be sharpened by stoning square on the edge. In use, being set in the socket, and held as a pen in writing, the square, sharp edge is worked rapidly against the part to be removed so as to powder it away.

The size and style of these Bits as fixed by us and shown in the drawings, we do not propose to alter. We cannot procure steel of which to make them with handles; and if we could it would be undesirable, as we cannot re-work or make over tools of this hard temper. We therefore adapt them to a Socket-handle (shown in illustration), and to meet the wants of those who, instead of changing, wish a handle for each Bit. The round part of the Bit is straight, not coned. The size will be maintained by us for these Bits and Sockets with exactness. Should they wear loose, they may be set with shellac.

Price for Bits	each	$0.30
" Octagon Steel Handles, B	"	.20
" Ebony Handles, A	"	1.00
" Ivory " A	"	1.50

DR. B. F. ARRINGTON'S SET OF ENAMEL CHISELS AND SMALL SCALERS.

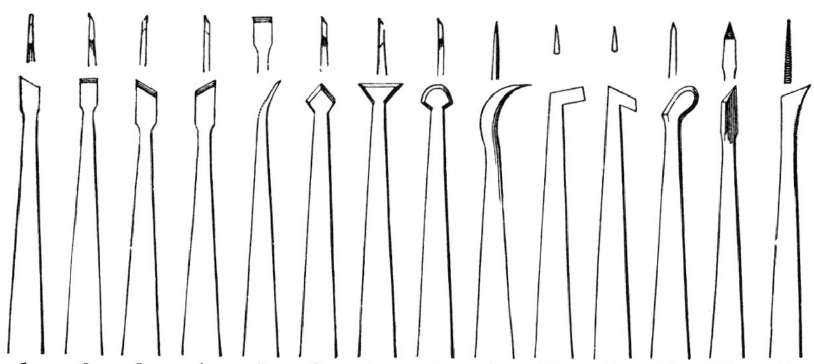

1. 2. 3. 4. 5. 6. 7. 8. 9. 10. 11. 12. 13. 14.

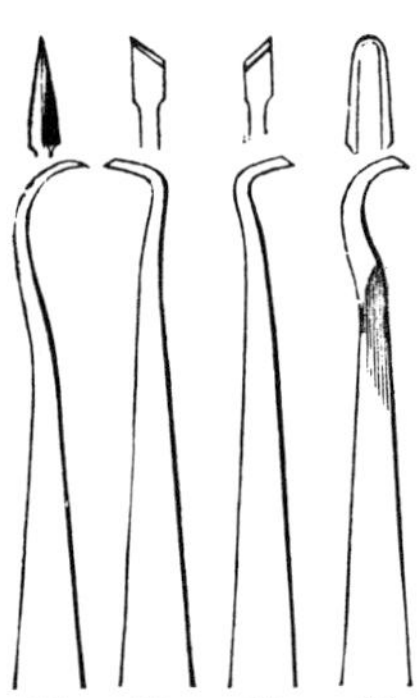

15. 16. 17. 18.

They are of the very best quality and warranted in every particular. Made of $\frac{7}{32}$ inch Octagon Cast Steel, $6\frac{1}{2}$ inches in length, Bronzed Handles.

Price, per doz. $4.00
" " set of 18 . . . . 6.00

Scalers.

DR. HERBERT S. BAYLIS'S SET OF SCALERS.

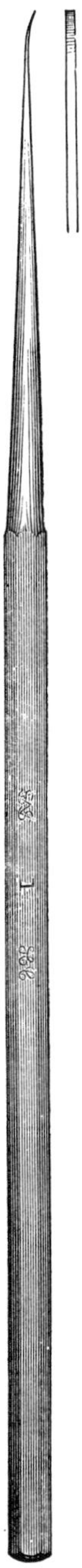

1.

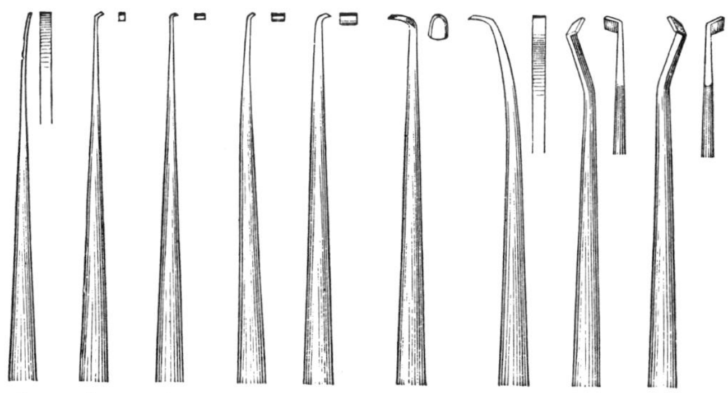

2. 3. 4. 5. 6. 7. 8. 9. 10.

Especially shaped and designed for removing deposits of salivary calculus from the necks and interspaces of the teeth.

This set of Instruments was shown at a meeting of the New York Odontological Society, and received high commendation from several eminent practitioners, for special adaptation of the angles, edges, and bends, for reaching and removing tartar.

Price, $\frac{3}{16}$ inch Bronzed Octagon Handles, Plain	per set	$4.00
" Extra quality, Crocus-polished, Handles Finished and Fire-gray Lacquered	"	6.00

S. S. WHITE'S SET OF SCALERS.

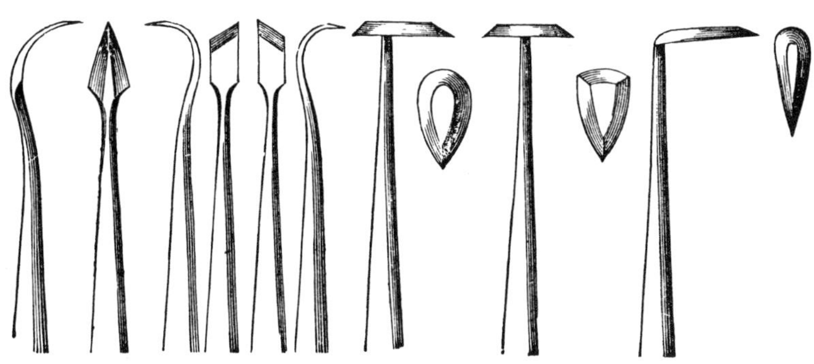

1. 2. 3. 4. 5. 6.

SS HC

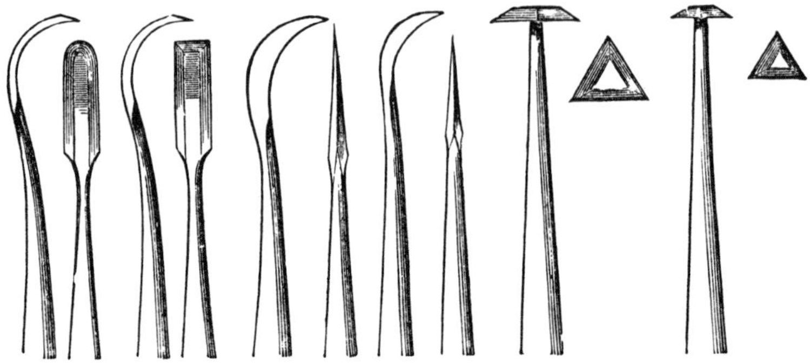

7. 8. 9. 10. 11. 12.

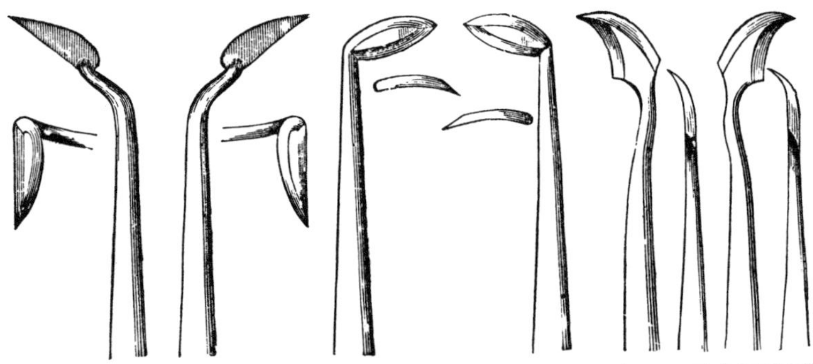

13. 14. 15. 16. 17. 18.

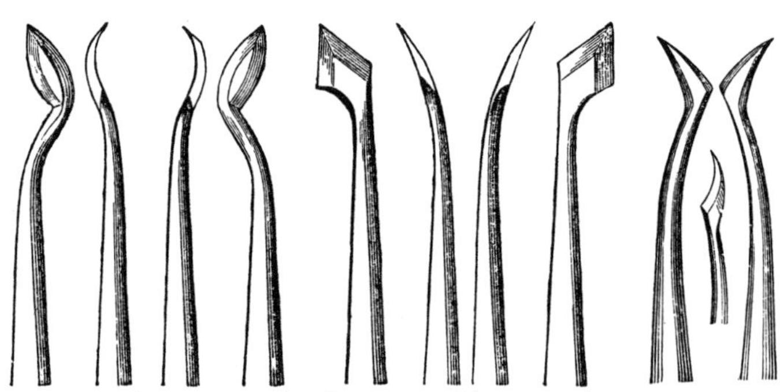

19. 20. 21. 22. 23. 24.

¼ inch File-cut Handles, Turned Shanks, Ball Ends. Any other style of Handles made to order.

Price . . . . per doz. $7.20

SS HC

SMALL SCALERS.

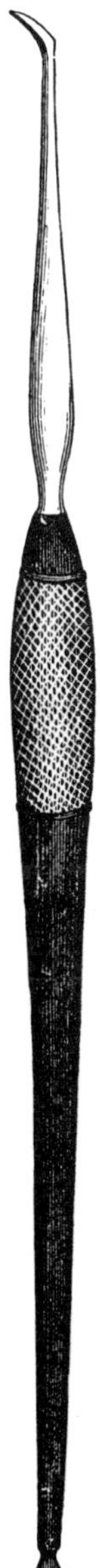

1.

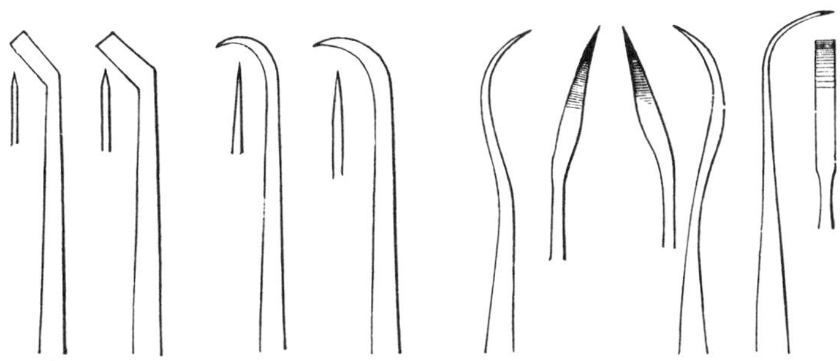

2. 3. 4. 5. 6. 7. 8.

Ivory Handles,	each $1.25
Ebony Handles, as per Cut,	" .50
Plain Octagon Steel Handles	per doz. 4.00

DR. F. ABBOTT'S SET OF SMALL SCALERS.

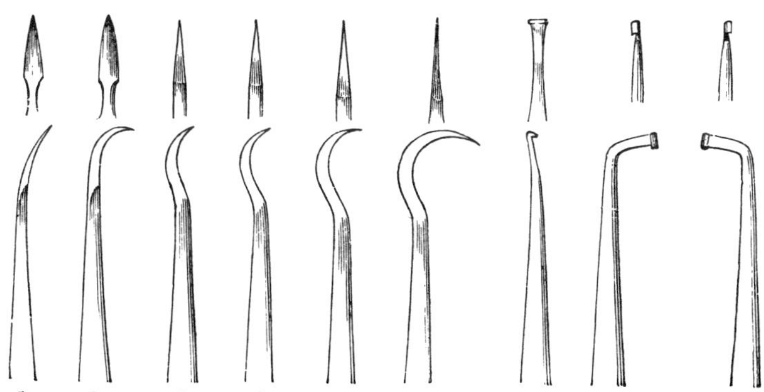

1. 2. 3. 4. 5. 6. 7. 8. 9.

This Cut represents a set of 9 small Scalers, the patterns for which were selected by Dr. Abbott.

They are constructed with the extremest nicety in curve and edges.

Octagon Steel Handles, $\frac{3}{16}$ inch, Bronzed or Black	per doz. $4.00
Ivory Handles, $\frac{3}{8}$ inch	" 16.50
Ebony " $\frac{3}{8}$ "	" 7.50

DR. RIGGS'S SET OF SCALERS.

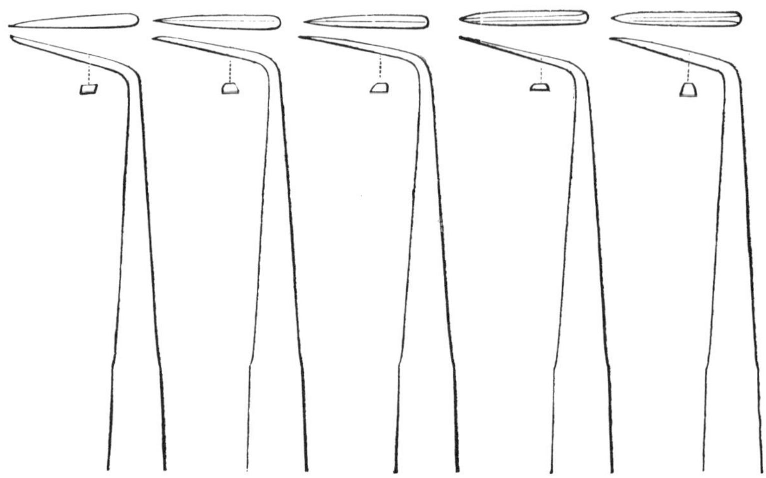

2. 3. 4. 5. 6.

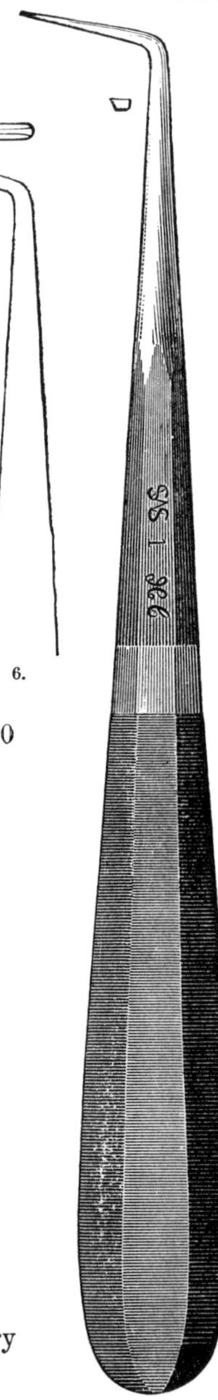

1.

Price, $\frac{5}{8}$ inch Ebony Handles . . . . . . each $1.50

DR. HOWE'S SET OF FINE SCALERS.

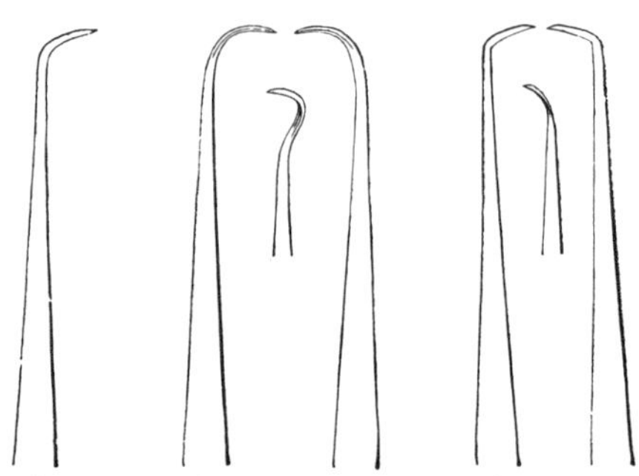

1. 2. 3. 4. 5.

Our Cuts represent in size and outline this set of supplementary Scalers.

They are curved and bent so as to adapt them perfectly for getting into narrow and difficult places, and between irregular teeth.

Small as these Scalers look, their shapes are so well studied,—the material being put in exactly the right place,—that they may be fully relied on to do the work for which they are designed.

Price, Plain $\frac{3}{16}$ inch Octagon Handles . . . . per doz. $4.00

DR. LORD'S GRADED SICKLE SCALERS AND TRIMMERS.

PATTERNS FURNISHED BY DR. BENJAMIN LORD, WITH SPECIAL INSTRUCTIONS AS TO TEMPER.

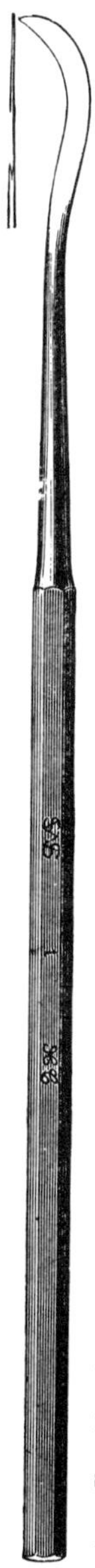

1.

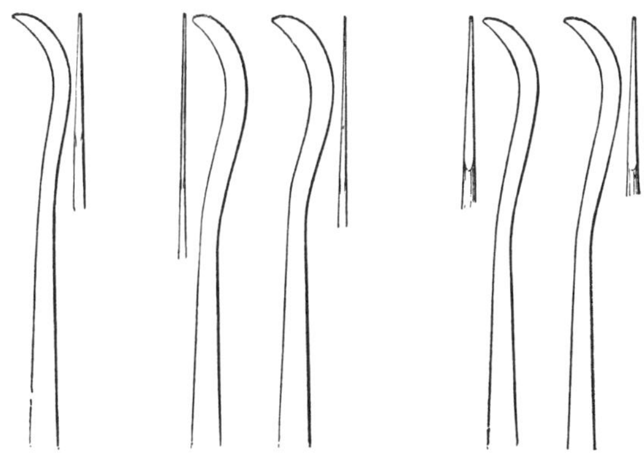

2. 3. 4. 5. 6.

These Scalers, as indicated by the placing of the Cuts, are grouped into 3 pairs, indicating temper as follows:

1 and 2, Full Spring. 3 and 4, Low Spring. 5 and 6, Very Hard.

Each one varies from its mate in thickness.

Dr. Lord describes these instruments as "well adapted for the removal of tartar, the separation of the incisors and canine teeth;" also for "trimming down of fillings, and the examination of proximate surfaces."

Nos. 5 and 6 are suitable for Enamel Chisels and Plug-Trimmers.

Nos 1, 2, 3, and 4 are designed to be used for "removing tartar from necks of teeth beneath the gums, and dressing edges of proximate fillings." These may be sharpened with a file, making an edge on them which is excellent for such uses, and the thickness can thus be adapted to the case.

Plain Octagon Handles, Bronzed or Blued, set of 6 . . . per set $2.00

DR. W. H. ATKINSON'S SET OF SCALERS.

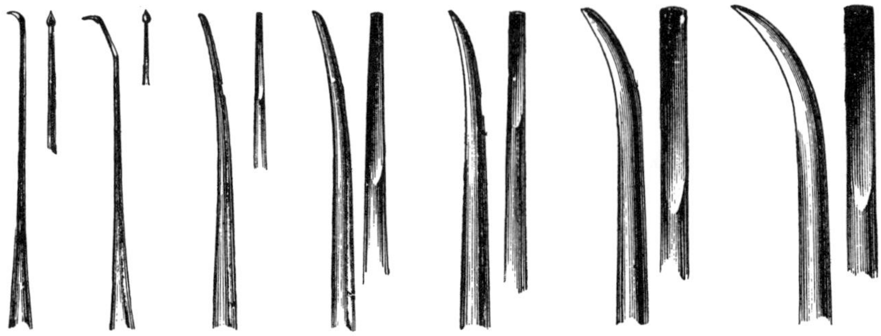

1. 2. 3. 4. 5. 6. 7.

Dr. Atkinson thus expresses himself in regard to the uses of these instruments:

"Calcareous concretions should always be started from the teeth, by placing the Scaler adapted to each against the margin of the deposit; then have an assistant give a blow sufficient to start the scale from its attachments in a mass or in fragments.

"Nos. 1 and 2 are slender Scrapers for removing loose calcareous granules from deep, narrow pockets about the roots of the teeth. Nos. 3, 4, 5, 6, and 7 are adapted to chip off deposits from the necks and roots of the various classes of teeth to whose roots they correspond in size."

Plain Octagon Handles, Blued.

Nos. 1, 2	each $0.50	Nos. 3, 4	each $0.75
" 5, 6, 7	" 1.00	Per set	5.50

REPAIRING AND POLISHING.

Repairing and Polishing Ordinary Excavators and Burs, Assorted	per doz.	$0.75
" " " " to Number or Pattern	"	1.00
" " Steel Handle Pluggers, Burnishers and Scalers	"	1.80
" " Fancy " " "	"	3.00
" " Nerve Instruments	"	1.80
" " Socket Plugger Bits	"	1.80
" " " Excavators, Assorted	"	.75
" " " " to Number or Pattern	"	1.00
" " Octagon and Oval Joint Forceps	each	.75 to 1.00
Polishing Octagon and Oval Joint Forceps	each	.50
" Gum Lancets	"	.25
" Foil Shears, Steel	each	.25 to .50
" " Fancy Handles	"	.50 to 1.50
" Pluggers, Burnishers, and Scalers, in Fancy Handles	per doz.	1.50
" File Carriers	each	.50
" Wedge Cutters	"	.50
Nickel-Plating Forceps to Order		.75 to 1.00

NOTE.—Special repairs charged for in accordance with the work done. Instruments made over into new forms, forged over, or wholly repointed, are considered "special." Making over, or changing the beaks of Forceps, is also "special."

BROWN'S DEPRESSED DENTAL RUBBER DAM.

Patented March 21st, 1876, in the United States, Canada, and Europe.

Fig. 1, Depressed Dam; Fig. 2, Sectional View.

HOWELLS' MIRROR COMBINATION WITH DEPRESSED DAM.

Patented April 4th, 1876, in the United States, Canada, and Europe.

Fig. 3, Stud Back Hinged Stem Mirror, German Silver, Nickel-Plated.

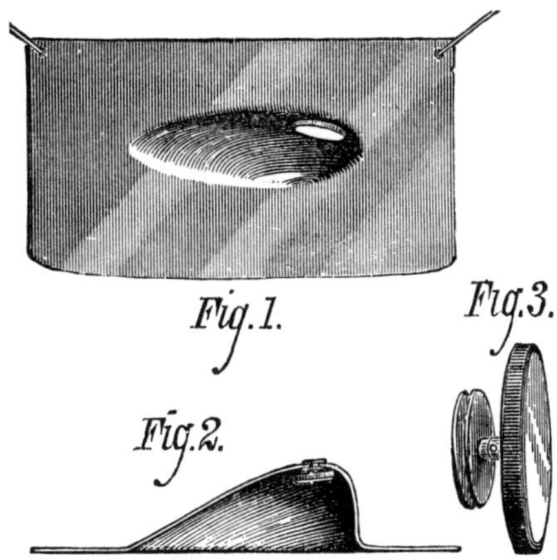

The advantages to be derived from the use of these improvements are obvious, to-wit:

The *Depressed* form saves the Practitioner much time in the labor of isolating the teeth to be operated on, while the smooth walls of the depression aid in the admission of light, and sustain in the desired position a Reflector, to concentrate it as needed.

No weights are required to keep the Dam in place; thus the comfort of the patient is greatly increased. Gold, that would otherwise be lost, is saved in the *depression*.

The form of the Dam causes, when in the mouth, involuntary effort by the patient to swallow, which prevents the accumulation of saliva.

The arched form of the Depression allows strain on the rubber in any direction, without interference with the security of its attachment to the isolated tooth.

The Dam can be used either side up, and becomes right or left, at pleasure.

DIRECTIONS.—Adjust the Dam in the mouth; take a soft pencil and mark it where perforations for teeth and mirror are desired; remove the Dam and make the perforations with a *punch*.

NEW YORK CITY, April 4th, 1876.

The "DEPRESSED DENTAL RUBBER DAM" is a vast improvement on the hitherto indispensable Sheet Rubber Dam, and in connection with the Mirror, under the Howells Patent, it cannot fail to obtain merited success.

W. H ATKINSON, M.D., 41 E. 9th St.
WM. M. REYNOLDS, M D, 62 W. 14th St.
CORYDON PALMER, M.D, 102 W. 38th St.
JOHN B. RICH, M.D., 35 E. 10th St.
WM. H. ALLEN, M.D., 18 W. 11th St.
O. A. JARVIS, M D.S., 119 W. 13th St.
WM. H. DWINELLE, M.D., 27 W. 34th St.

Perfect uniformity in the quality and strength of this Dam is guaranteed.

Put up in Assorted Sizes, 100 in a Box, price $12.50

A specimen Dam will be sent, postage paid, on receipt of 15 cents.

The Mirrors are made in three sizes, diameters $\frac{5}{8}$, $\frac{3}{4}$, and $\frac{7}{8}$ inch, both plane and concave, and are of excellent workmanship.

Price, German Silver, Nickel-Plated, Plane	each	$2.00
" " " " " Concave	"	2.25
Mounted Handsomely in Black Rubber, Plane	"	1.25
" " " " Concave	"	1.50

SAMUEL S. WHITE has been appointed Sole Agent for the United States.

Coffer Dam Rubber.

INTRODUCED BY DR. S. C. BARNUM.

After a number of experimental tests with various manufactures of Rubber Dam, we are prepared to recommend that which we offer as possessing in a great degree the necessary qualities of softness, elasticity, and strength.

For sale in quantities to suit purchasers. It should be well washed in warm water and soap before using, and exposed to the air, when the odor of the sulphur rapidly disappears.

PRICES.

Thin, per yard	$2.50
Medium, "	3.00
Thick, "	3.50

TRIPLEX RUBBER DAM PUNCH.

AN EXACT COPY OF THE ORIGINAL PATTERN FURNISHED US BY DR. DOLBEARE.

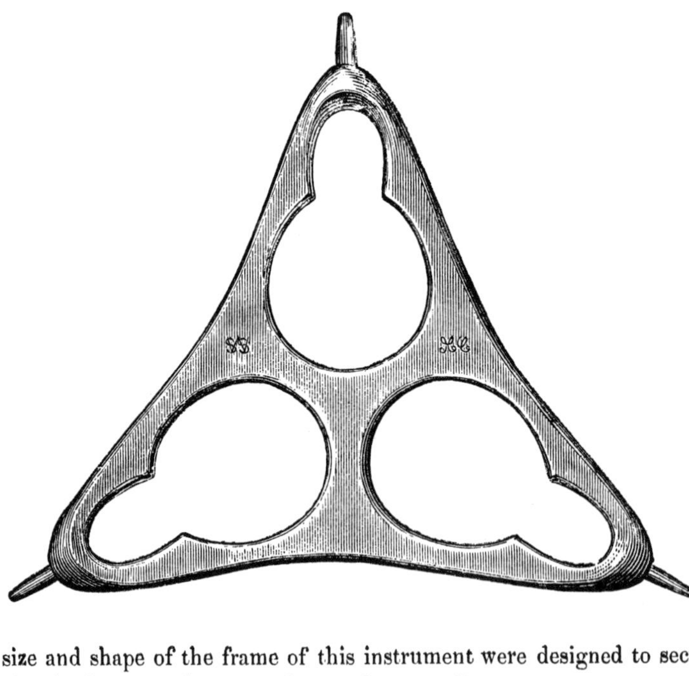

The size and shape of the frame of this instrument were designed to secure comfort in use, by Dr. Dolbeare, and presented to us for manufacture.

Price, Nickel-Plated . . . . each $1.50

RUBBER DAM PUNCHES.

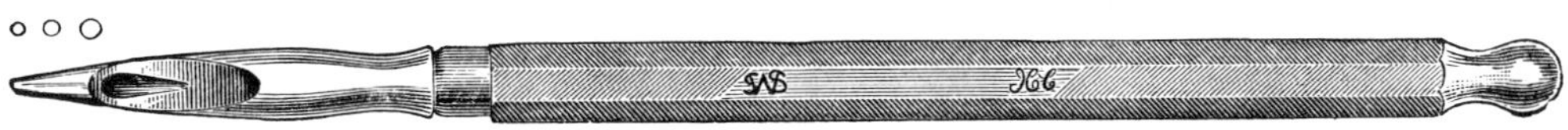

Octagon, Bronzed Handles . . . . each $0.40
¼ inch, File cut, Bronzed Handles . . . . " .60
⅝ " Bone Handles . . . . " 1.00
Dr. Corydon Palmer's Rubber Dam Punching Pliers . . . . per pair 3.25

RUBBER DAM HOLDER.

DESIGN OF DR. COGSWELL.

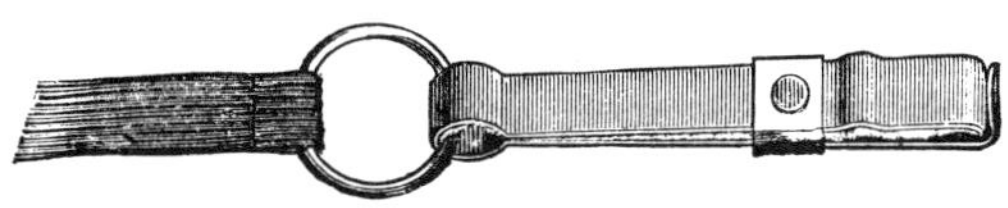

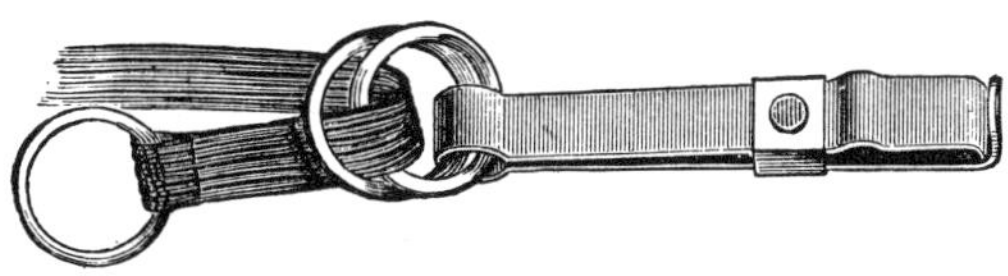

Our manufacture of this useful auxiliary appliance is of superior quality in every detail. The springs and slides are made and finished in the best style, and carefully adjusted so as to hold the Rubber firmly without cutting it. All the metal work is Polished fine and Nickel-Plated.

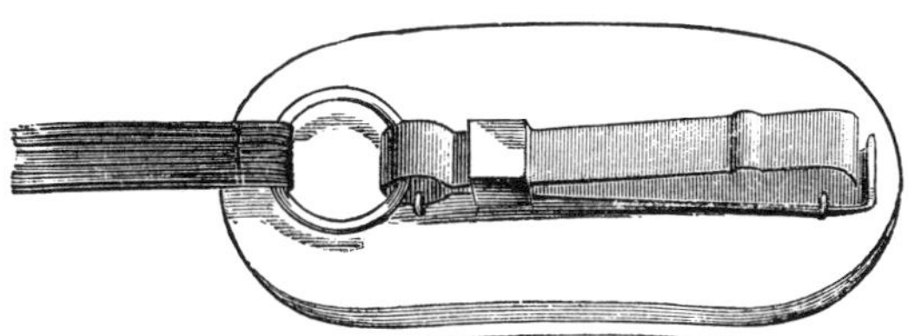

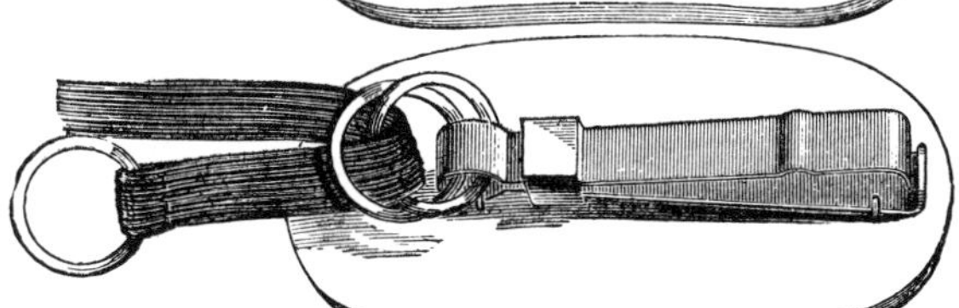

Plain . . . . each $0.60
With Buffalo Horn Guards . . . . " 1.00
" Ivory Guards (Silk Braid) . . . . " 1.50
Silk Gum Braid on the Plain or Buffalo Guard, to order, 10 cents extra.
Putting new Braid on Holder . . . . each 15 cents.
" " Silk Braid on Holder . . . . " 25 "

RUBBER DAM BUCKLE.

INVENTION OF DR. W. T. MAGILL, ROCK ISLAND, ILLINOIS.

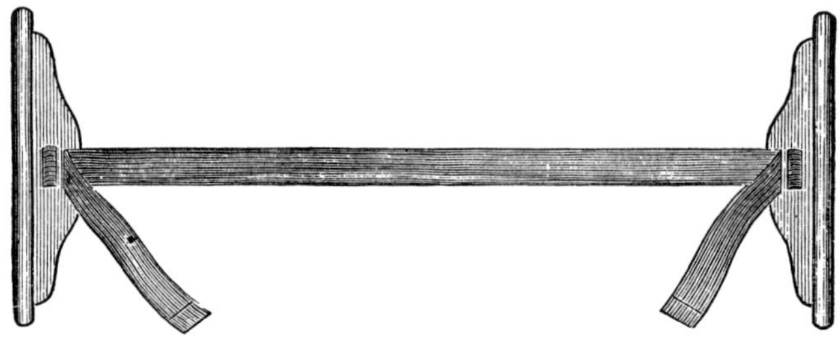

The Cut illustrates an ingenious little contrivance for holding the Rubber Dam in position while operating, dispensing with weights. The Rubber is simply stretched over the ends of the Buckles, and is securely held in place by its own contraction, without damage to its texture. By this arrangement, the Rubber is smoothly and tightly stretched over the patient's lips and cheeks, and is entirely out of the way of the operator. A silk braid passes from one Buckle to the other around the patient's head.

Price, per pair, Nickel-Plated . . . . 75 cents.

RUBBER DAM APPLIER.

PATTERN FURNISHED BY DR. FORBES.

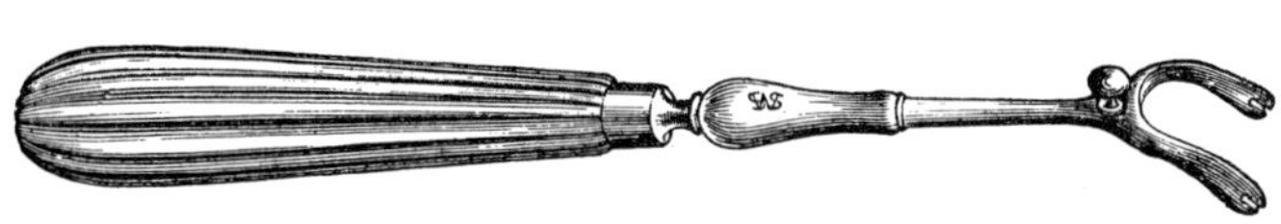

This tool is used with a cord across the ends to force the Rubber down between back teeth, evenly to the necks, without tearing it; and also to pass the tying cord around molars more pleasantly than can be done with the fingers. When a very high strain on the cord is needed, fix it in position with half a turn around the button, and tighten it while pressing the points of the fork between the thumb and finger.

Attention is requested to this tool, mounted with Buffalo Horn Handle and Aluminum Bronze Ferrule, as being a very elegant style.

They are in stock of three sizes of fork. The Cut represents the smallest at half size. The largest is about $\frac{1}{4}$ of an inch wider.

Price, with	$\frac{5}{8}$ inch	Ivory Handles,	German Silver Ferrules	$3.00
" "	$\frac{5}{8}$ "	Buffalo "	Aluminum Bronzed Ferrules . . .	2.50
" "	$\frac{5}{8}$ "	Walrus "	German Silver "	1.75
" "	$\frac{5}{8}$ "	Bleached Bone Handles,	German Silver Ferrules . . .	1.62
" "	$\frac{1}{4}$ "	File-cut Steel "	. . . .	1.25

RUBBER DAM WEIGHTS AND SPRINGS.

PATTERNS FURNISHED BY DR. W. M. REYNOLDS.

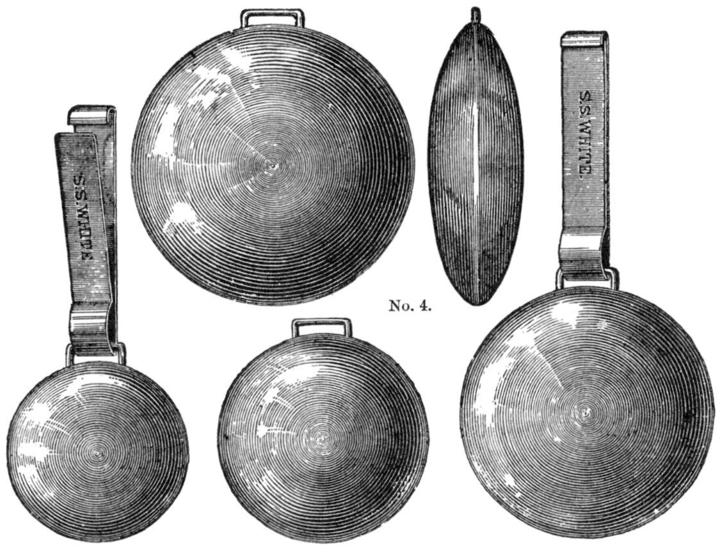

No. 4.

No. 1. No. 2. No. 3.

These Weights are intended to be suspended from the free ends or borders of the Dam when in use, thus keeping it out of the way of the operator. They are of metal, Nickel-Plated, and Polished. The Springs are of German Silver, Nickel-Plated. They are readily attached to and detached from the Rubber without injury to it.

There are four sizes.

No. 1 weighs 1 oz.; No. 2 weighs 1½ oz.; No. 3 weighs 2½ oz.; No. 4 weighs 3½ oz.

Price, with Spring . . . . each 50 cents.

RUBBER DAM CLAMPS.

SET OF 6, ORIGINAL ALLAN.

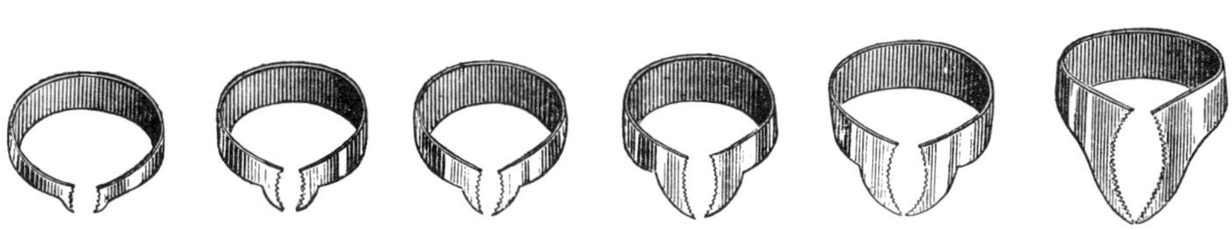

1. 2. 3. 4. 5. 6.

These are always kept in stock, plain and serrated.

Price . . . . each 60 cents.

NEW MOLAR CLAMPS.

PATTERNS FURNISHED BY DR. CHARLES F. ALLAN.

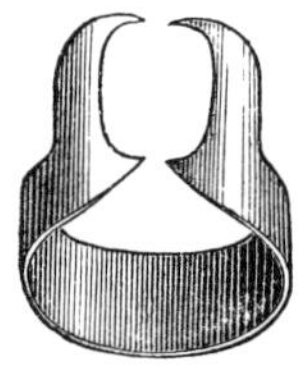

LARGE.

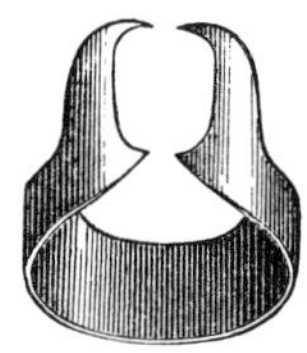

MEDIUM.

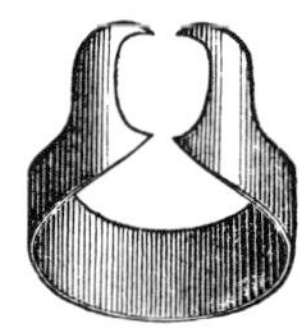

SMALL.

These Clamps are made from the patterns to which Dr. Allan now restricts the use of his name.

They are especially designed for use on lower molars,—the inside edges of the Clamp being shaped to conform to the necks of these teeth. They have great back-set, entirely clearing the tooth on which they clamp, and broad flanges to keep the Rubber spread. Our stock includes different thicknesses to suit those who wish light or heavy spring. They are not serrated.

Price, Nickel-Plated . . . . each 60 cents.

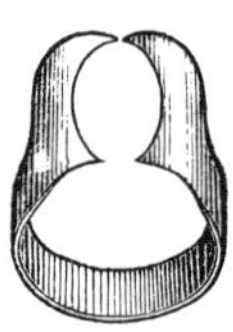

H. C.

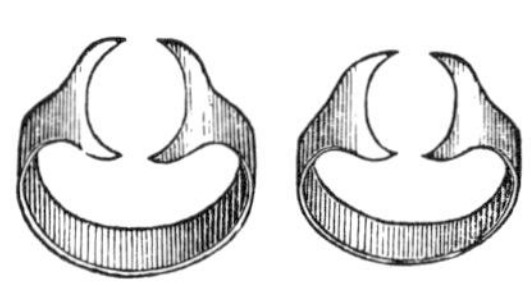

DR. HUEY'S.

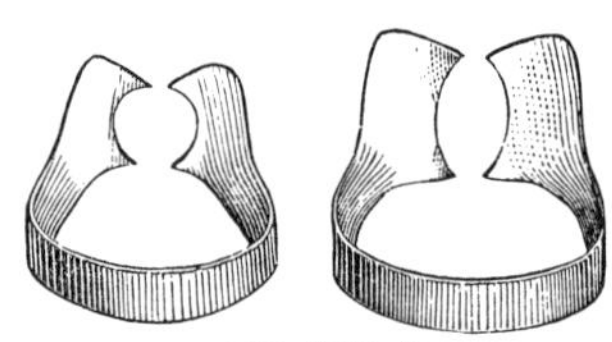

DR. TEES'S.

The H. C. Clamp for ladies' and children's molars. A light, small, very elastic Clamp. Never serrated. Modeled and designed to fill a place of great usefulness, for which other Clamps are not suited. It has good back-set and well-spread flanges, affording easy access to any cavity in the tooth it clamps on. It is a universal Clamp; and its small hoop allows an easy "open" to the patient, and enables a very light Clamp to hold the Dam down securely without pain.

Dr. Huey's Dens Sap. Clamp is represented in two sizes,—the largest and smallest. They are also in stock of various thicknesses. This Clamp has had a large and constant sale since it was introduced, meeting as it does a peculiar set of very difficult cases to which all other Clamps are inapplicable.

Dr. Tees's Clamps, for molar and bicuspid teeth, have very broad flanges, intended to spread the Dam wide. Our Cuts show straight lips; but we also make Dr. Tees's Clamps with curved lips which adapt them for deeply festooned gums.

Price, Nickel-Plated . . . . each 60 cents.

DR. F. HICKMAN'S PATENT DOUBLE LIPPED RUBBER DAM CLAMP.

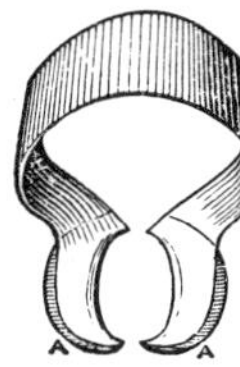

Fig. 1.

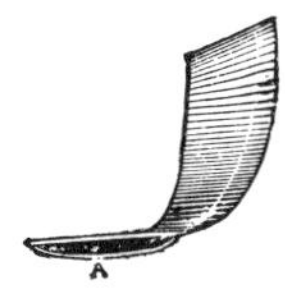

Fig. 2.

These Clamps are made with a Double Lip, forming a clear space for the Rubber to be lodged in before applying to the tooth.

When the Rubber is punched it is to be put on the Clamp by stretching it over the lip *A*, and allowing it to fall into the open space between *A* and the Clamp proper. Then apply the Clamp and Rubber, spreading both together; after which, stretch the Rubber out of the recess, or free space, and allow it to close on the neck of the tooth.

It is especially adapted for teeth which are spurred and jagged, or where they are broken down low on one side, so as to make it difficult to apply and retain a Dam on them.

Price, Nickel-Plated . . . . each $1.20

COMBINED RUBBER DAM CLAMP AND TONGUE HOLDER.

C. Bancroft's Patent. (No. 151,265, May 26th, 1874.)

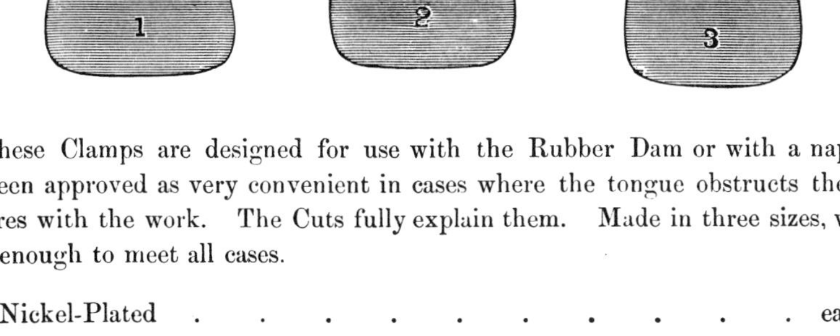

These Clamps are designed for use with the Rubber Dam or with a napkin, and have been approved as very convenient in cases where the tongue obstructs the sight or interferes with the work. The Cuts fully explain them. Made in three sizes, which are varied enough to meet all cases.

Price, Nickel-Plated . . . . each $1.50

IMPROVED RUBBER DAM CLAMPS,

FOR USE WITH RUBBER DAM CLAMP FORCEPS.

FROM PATTERNS OF DR. DELOS PALMER.

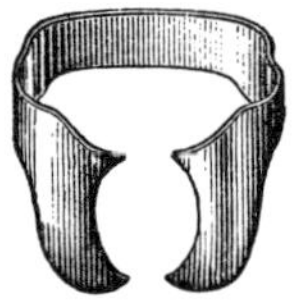
1.

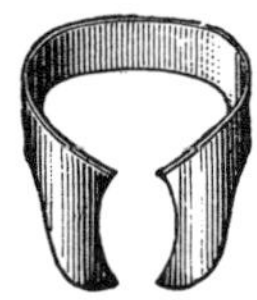
2.

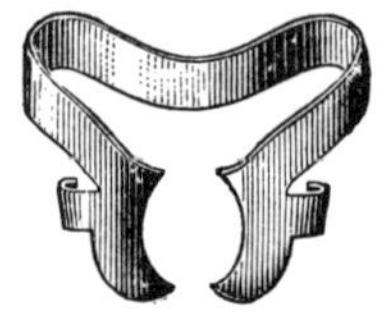
3.

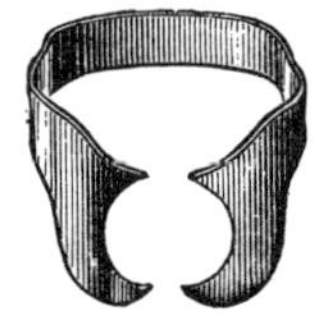
4.

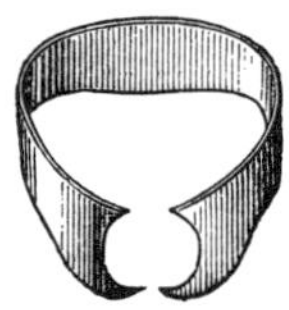
5.

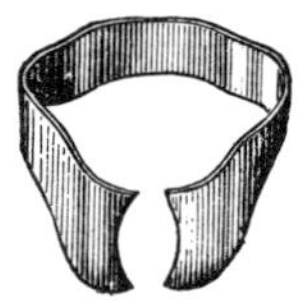
6.

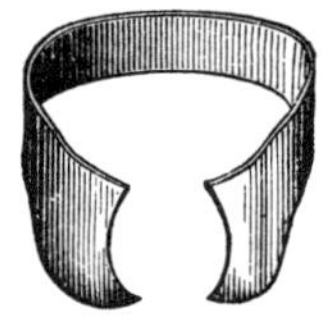
7.

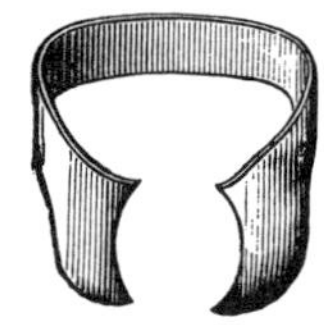
8.

These Clamps are intended to be placed on the tooth previous to the operation—the Rubber Dam to be subsequently passed over both tooth and clamp.

Nos. 1 and 2 are Universal Clamps for molars; No. 3 for posterior cavities in isolated molars; No. 4 for wisdom-teeth; No. 5 for bicuspids; No. 6 for incisors; Nos. 7 and 8—rights and lefts—for cervical cavities in the buccal or lingual faces of molars.

Price, Nickel-Plated . . . . each 60 cents.

DR. OLIVER'S WIRE SPRING CLAMPS.

INVENTION OF DR. THOS. O. OLIVER.

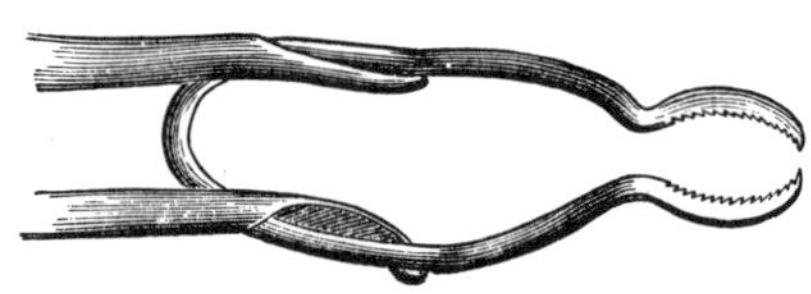

Three sizes, large, medium, and small. The Cut represents the medium size.

Price . . . . each 50 cents.

GILLING TWINE.

Adapted for ligatures for correcting irregularities; for holding Rubber Dam in position; also, for passing between teeth to discover imperfections in the enamel, and for cleansing and polishing. Two sizes, coarse and fine.

Put up in plaits, convenient for use, in lengths of twenty-four inches.

Price, per Plait	$0.10
" " ½ lb. Ball, Coarse	1.00
" " " " Fine	1.25

BOWMAN-ALLAN CLAMP FORCEPS.

Combination of Dr. Bowman's and Dr. Allan's Rubber Dam Clamp Applier, with H. Coy's Locking Slide-Ring. Known to the Profession and trade as the "Bowman-Allan" Clamp Forceps.

We have remodeled our pattern so as to make these Forceps combine every advantage in shape with superior workmanship and elegance of outlines.

The Cut illustrates these claims.

The Side-Cut shows the spread of the points when the Lock-Slide is slipped down to the Joint-Screw.

Price, Crocus-Polished . . $3.00

" Nickel-Plated . . 3.50

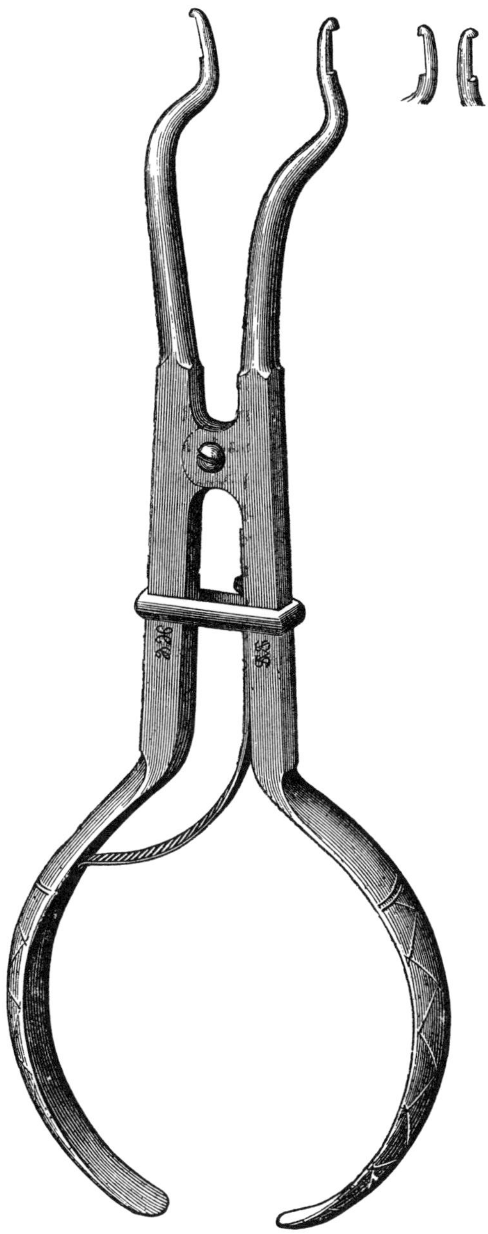

FISK'S AUTOMATIC SALIVA EJECTOR.

THE MOST SIMPLE AND EFFECTIVE SALIVA PUMP YET OFFERED TO THE DENTAL PROFESSION.

It is well known that a rapid jet of water, steam, or air will carry along with it another stream, if brought in contact in suitable tubes. The principle is as old as the junction of two rivers. It was first practically applied in what is known as the Giffard Injector, for filling steam-boilers with water by means of a jet of steam. The principle is here applied to the removal of the saliva from the mouth, by means of a jet of water.

The construction of the instrument will be readily seen by referring to the Cut. A is the Body, about six inches long; B, the Stop-Cock; C, Water Nozzle; D, Vacuum Chamber; E, Check-Valve; F, Saliva Tube and Mouth-Piece. The Arrows show the direction of the streams united.

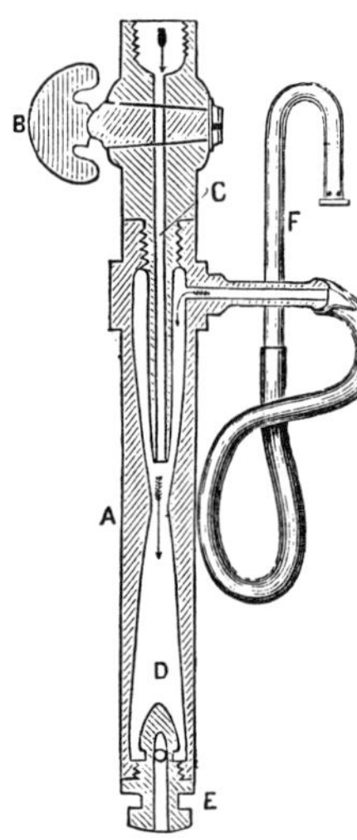

The jet of water through the narrow throat of the chamber drags along with it, by friction, air or any liquid body with great force; and the check-valve below sets the water back in such a manner as to close the throat to the external air, and produce a vacuum in the chamber above. A pressure of forty pounds to the square inch on the Water Nozzle will raise a column of mercury in the Saliva Tube twenty-eight inches,—showing almost a perfect vacuum. The instrument can be used, of course, only where there is a water pressure, and a pressure anywhere above *twelve* pounds to the square inch is sufficient to operate it successfully.

The Water Nozzle is very small,—only $\frac{1}{16}$ of an inch in diameter; consequently, it takes very little water to operate it. It is very durable,—there being no valves or springs to get out of order,—and will last a lifetime. It not only removes the saliva, but is constantly drawing into the mouth a supply of *fresh air*, which is very soothing to the patient, and allays much of the discomfort of protracted operations,—an important feature of its value. It is a great aid to the Rubber Dam, and in many cases it will obviate the necessity for the Dam altogether. It requires very little attention, either from the patient or operator, while in use.

The instrument is small and compact, and can be sent direct, with all its attachments, to any part of the country, either by mail or express. A liberal Discount to the Trade.

Price $15.00

S. S. WHITE has been appointed SOLE AGENT for the Sale of FISK'S SALIVA EJECTOR to the Dental Profession and Trade.

GLASS SALIVA PUMP.

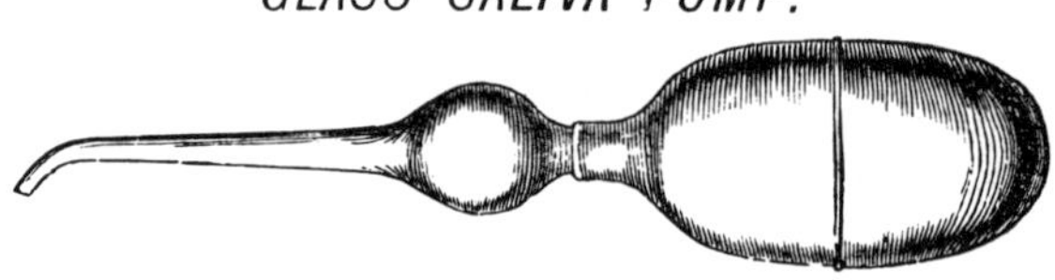

Glass Tube, Elastic Bulb, ... 75 cents.
Extra Glass Tube . . . . 38 "

DUCT OF STENO COMPRESSOR, AND FORCEPS TO APPLY IT.

PATTERN FURNISHED TO US BY DR. RICH.

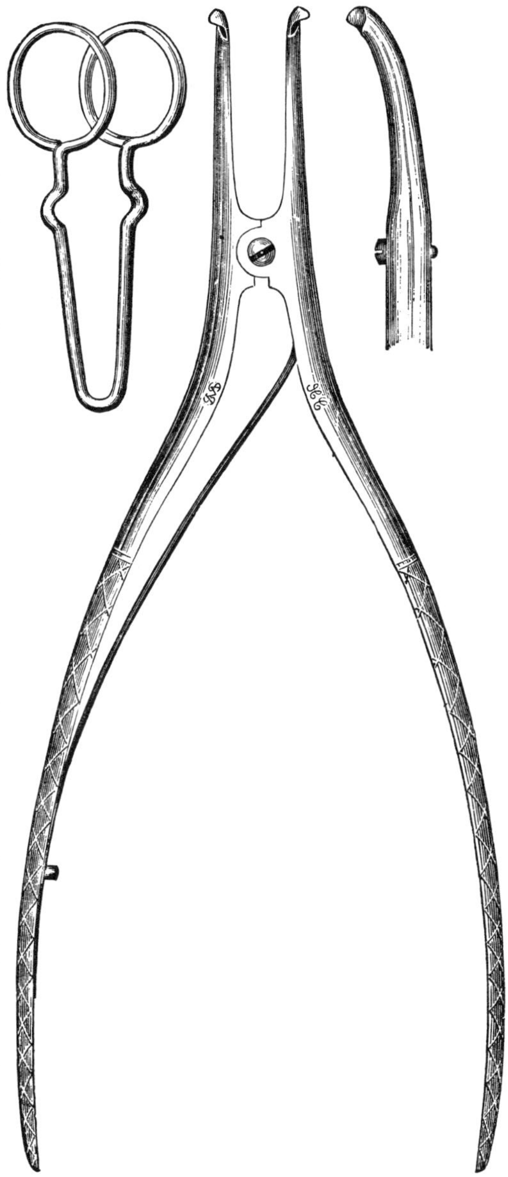

These Forceps and Spring accomplish the closure of the duct more perfectly than any other appliance we have seen. The Spring, with a pad of bibulous paper, or napkin, prevents all flow of saliva, while the lip is free to yield in operating; whereas, with a napkin crowded between the cheek and jaw, the lip is stretched tight, and very little motion frees the duct, allowing the saliva to flow.

In use, the recurved ends of the Forceps fit in the recess of the Spring, which closure of the handles will expand. Having placed the pad in position,—exactly opposite the second upper molar,—release the grasp on the handles, and the Spring will close and the Forceps be detached at once. An outer pad may be slipped under the Spring afterwards if desirable.

Forceps	per pair	$3.00
" Nickel-Plated	"	3.50
Springs, always Nickel-Plated	each	.25

A NEW FORM OF SCREW FOR SECURING GOLD FILLINGS IN DIFFICULT CASES.

PATENTED BY E. OSMOND, M.D., D.D.S., OCTOBER 7th, 1873.

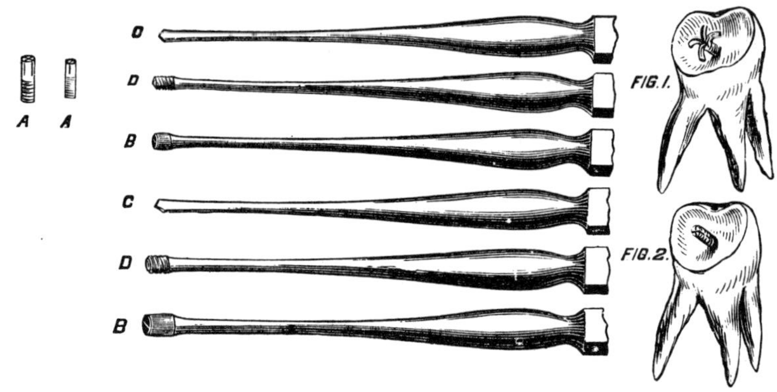

VIEW OF INSTRUMENTS AND SCREWS ENLARGED.

A A are Screws made of 20-carat gold wire, annealed, split about half-way, once or twice, so as to form two or four arms when opened. B is a Screw-Driver, surrounded by a tube for the purpose of holding the Screw and carrying it to its place in the tooth. C is a Drill, for the purpose of drilling a hole which is afterwards tapped by the Tap-Screw D.

Figures 1 and 2 are Teeth with large saucer-shaped cavities, such as we very frequently find, but other cases in which these Screws are available will readily suggest themselves to the mind of the experienced operator.

Price of set of 6 Instruments, Nickel-Plated, in Morocco Case, Velvet-lined, including one dozen large and one dozen small Screws, 20-carat gold		$15.00
Extra Screws, large	per doz.	3.00
" " small	"	2.00

Practical Directions for inserting Screws accompany each Case.

DR. CORYDON PALMER'S WEDGING PLIERS.

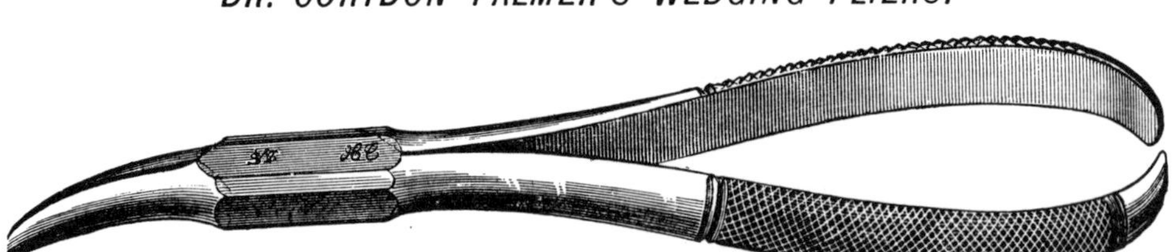

These Pliers are intended for adjusting and removing wedges.

Price . . . . each $2.50

JACK SCREWS FOR REGULATING TEETH.

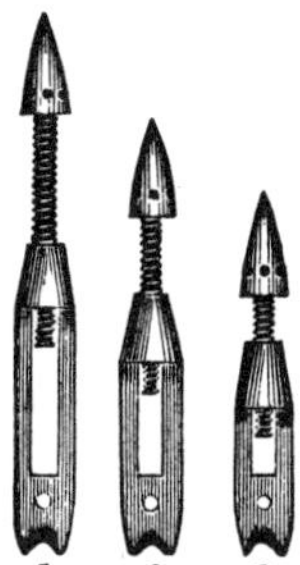

1 2 3
Old Style.

EXTENSIONS.

No. 3	will open	from	$\frac{3}{4}$	inch	to	$1\frac{1}{4}$	inches.
No. 2	"	"	$\frac{7}{8}$	"	"	$1\frac{3}{8}$	"
No. 1	"	"	1	"	"	$1\frac{1}{2}$	"

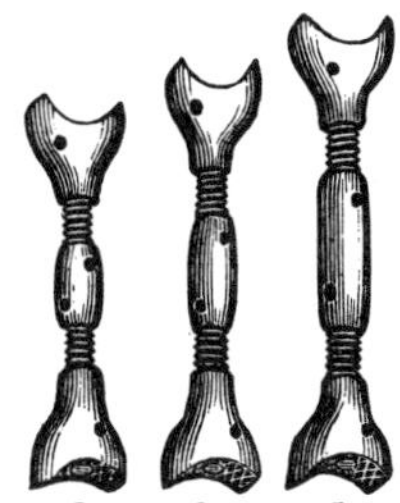

3 2 1
New Style.

We make these useful articles in the best style and with perfect Screws. We retain the Zinc plug in the old style to prevent rusting, although Nickel-Plating is expected to make them safe from that. The new style is made from patterns first supplied by Dr. A. McCollom to us. They are made with Right and Left Screws, and can be operated by the holes in the middle bar without removal. The Heads or Nuts have a hole by which they can be secured to a tooth, thus avoiding the danger of being swallowed if accidentally detached.

PRICES.

Nickel-Plated, either kind or size	each	$1.50
Bars of the new style	"	.50
One New Style Screw and two extra Bars, called a full set . . .		2.50

WEDGING WOOD SLIPS.

Dr. Palmer's Boxwood Slips, large,	6 x $\frac{3}{8}$ x $\frac{1}{8}$	per doz.	60 cents.
" " " medium,	6 x $\frac{3}{16}$ x $\frac{1}{8}$	"	24 "
" " " small,	6 x $\frac{1}{8}$ square	"	24 "

DR. BUTLER'S WEDGE SLIPS.

Made of Cotton-Wood, about 6 inches long, $\frac{3}{8}$ inch wide, $\frac{3}{16}$ inch thick.

Price . . . . per doz. 20 cents.

ORANGE-WOOD.

FOR WEDGING. SUPERIOR QUALITY.

Price . . . . per bundle 10 cents.

WEDGE CUTTERS,

To Excise the Ends of Separating Wedges, Inside and Outside of the Jaw.

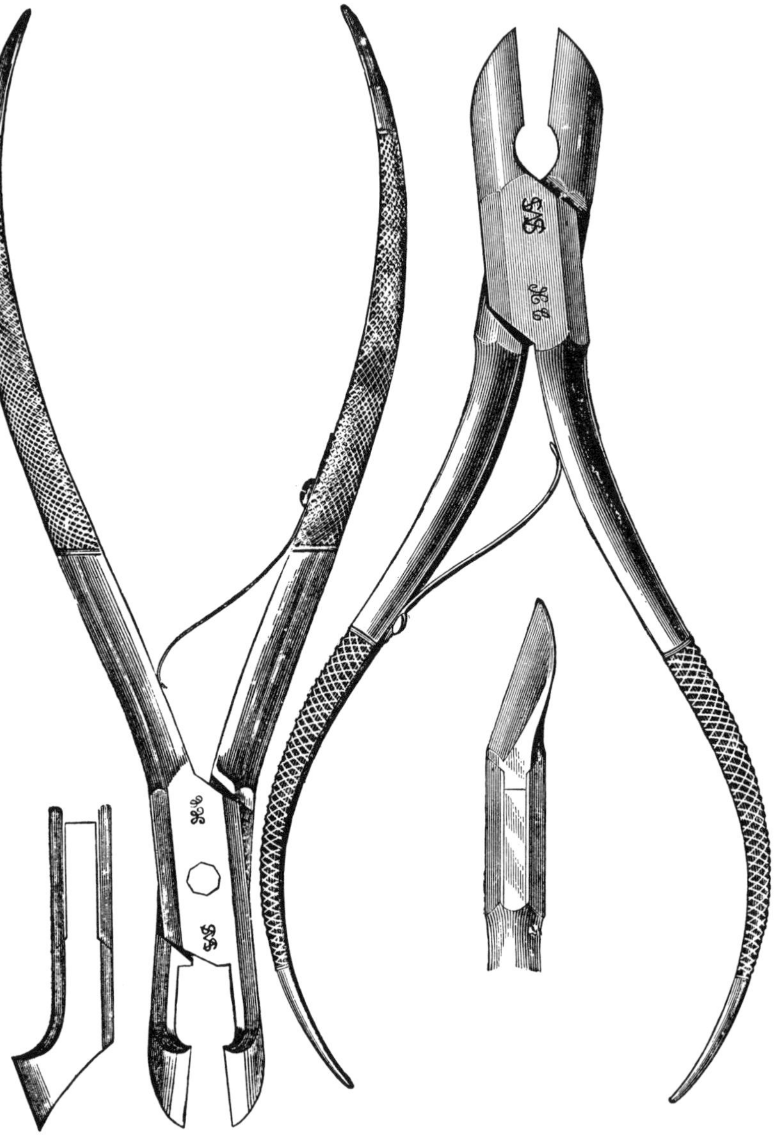

No. 1. No. 2.

Of the same style, quality, and finish as our best Forceps. Crocus-Polished.

No. 1, 6 inches long, as shown in Cut	$3.00
No. 1, 5 " "	3.00
No. 2, 5½ " " Dr. Morrison's pattern.	3.00
Dr. Corydon Palmer's Wedge Cutters	3.75

Nickel-Plated, 50 cents extra.

MATRICES AND MATRIX PLIERS.

INVENTION OF DR. LOUIS JACK.

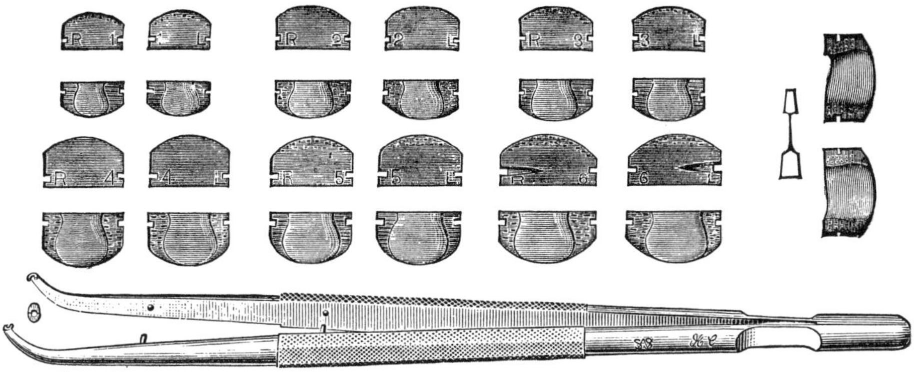

Our Cuts represent six pairs, right and left, of the Matrices, and the Pliers for placing them and the wedges in position. The small Cuts on the right, unnumbered, exhibit a Double Matrix for use in the case of two proximals.

These mechanical aids for filling proximal cavities were described by Dr. Jack in the DENTAL COSMOS for April, 1871. Since that time a great many dentists have adopted his method, and we believe many more would do so if aware of its value. The points especially notable in the use of the Matrix, are, to cut away the masticating surface of enamel to the depth of the cavity ; to prepare the edges flat and smooth ; to cut down to sound bone in the neck of the tooth, forming the base of the cavity, and shaping it so that the Matrix will fit accurately at the cervical wall. Having excavated the cavity and cut a retaining groove along the buccal and palatal walls (terminating at the very surface of the masticating walls of the enamel), select a Matrix the concaved surface of which matches the cavity. Then, after applying the rubber dam, finish and dry the cavity, place the Matrix, and secure it with wedges of boxwood, which being hard and dry require very little forcing. The filling may then be done with the ease and certainty of a crown cavity with strong walls.

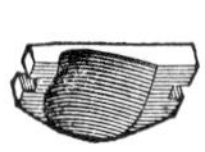

A

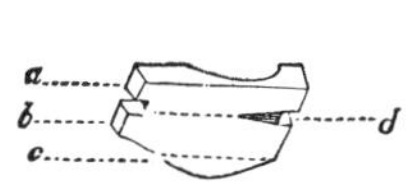

B

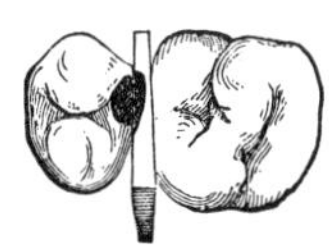

C

Figs. A and B show the concave and wedging sides of a Matrix, and C shows a Matrix placed between two teeth ready to wedge and fill. Pluggers, especially bent and slanted so as to pack the Gold extremely hard against the face of the Matrix, are included in the set of Dr. Jack's Matrix Pluggers.

PRICES.

Matrices, Single, Thick or Thin	each	$0.50
" Double	"	.75
Matrix Pliers	"	2.00
" " Nickel-Plated	"	2.50
Boxwood Slips, medium and small	per doz.	.24
" " large	"	.60
" " round, for polishing, 50 in a box	per box	.50

FOIL CARRIER AND PLUGGER COMBINED.

INVENTION OF DR. J. B. RICH.

LONG, BROAD, AND LIGHT. PERFORATED HANDLES.

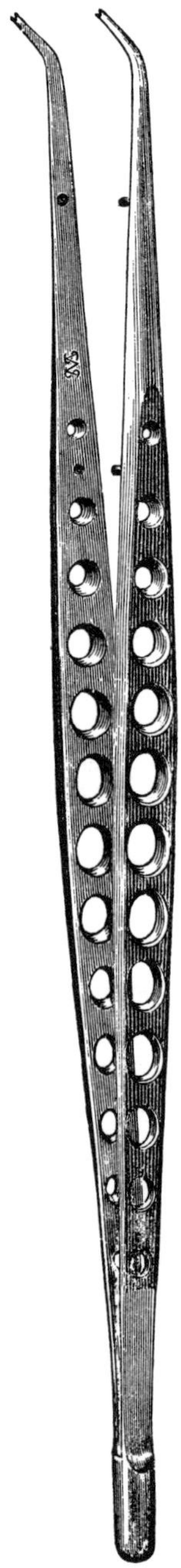

This Cut illustrates an instrument which has had great sale, eliciting the approval of many of the finest operators in this country and in Europe.

Dr. Rich, appreciating that the large Foil Carrier, by its weight, impaired the delicacy of touch so important in all of the finer dental operations, worked out the device, and gave us his original to perfect in manufacture.

These Pliers are as light in the springs and on the fingers as the very small Foil Carriers, while their efficiency and strength for the special uses of the instrument are not impaired.

The Points are of varied sizes and angles.

Our Foil Carriers of this design are made of genuine Silver Steel, and the workmanship, temper, and finish are all extra fine.

Price . . . each $2.50 Nickel-Plated . each $3.00

FOIL CARRIER AND PLUGGER COMBINED.

No. 1.

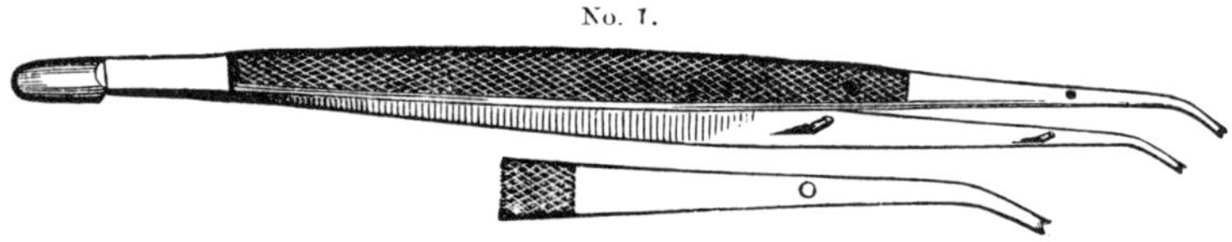

No. 2

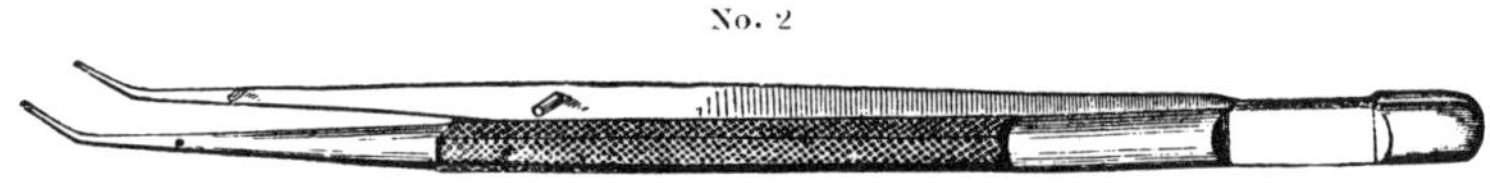

The superiority of this instrument over the ordinary Foil Tweezers consists in the additional strength, the Serrated Points, and the large, rounded end of the Handle, which permits the use of the Carrier, when desired, as a Plugger to fix the gold in the proper position.

No. 1, Flat Handle, 7 inches long $2.00
No. 2, Octagon Handle, 6 inches long 1.75
Nickel-Plated, 50 cents extra.

DR. CONNER'S HEAVY PLUGGING PLIERS

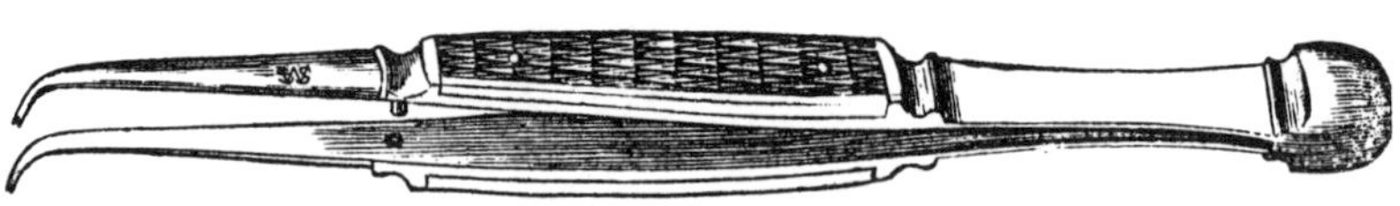

Are 5½ inches long; large, round, and heavy End, for protection to the palm of the hand in filling; mounted with Ivory; handsomely finished. The Points in the Cut are serrated, but we also make them without serrations, to be used in cylinder fillings.

Price . . . . each $2.50
Nickel-Plated, 50 cents extra.

PLUG PLIERS.

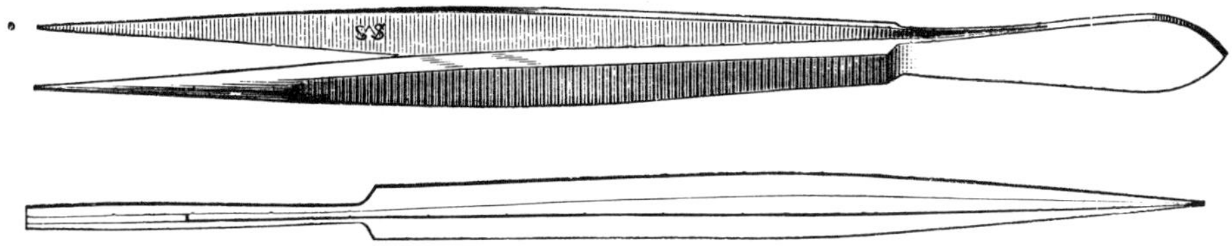

Plug Pliers for carrying Gold, 4½ inches long $0.60
" " " " 5¼ " 1.00
" " " " 6 " Brass ends 1.00
" " " " 6 " extra large, German Silver ends, fine finish 1.50
" " " " Mounted in Ivory and Shell 2.00
" " " " Mounted with Pearl . . $3.00
" " " " " " Nickel-Plated 3.50
Dr. Corydon Palmer's Foil-Carrier Pliers 2.00

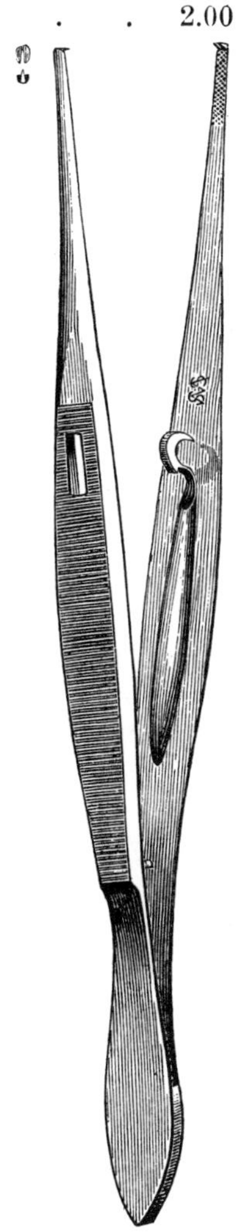

TAPE FORCEPS, OR SPRING LOCKING PLIERS.

FROM PATTERN FURNISHED BY DR E. A. BOGUE.

Our Cut represents the Surgeon's Artery Forceps, modified by Dr. Bogue to suit the requirements of Dentists. Its uses are, in his words, "The insertion and removal of tapes and rubber wedges, the removal of wooden or other wedges from between the teeth, the firm grasping of wet napkins and other slippery substances in the mouth; also the holding firmly of anything which is to be cut off with knife or scissors, and as a light weight to hang on rubber dam or napkin when it obstructs the view." The sharp points puncture the article, while the elasticity of the ends allows them to bend so that the latch-spring will close. This spring-lock, or latch-spring, holds the blades firmly together, so that, once grasped, the article is held safely until, at a touch of the thumb on the latch, the blades open and release it instantly.

The Profession owes the adaptation of this little instrument entirely to Dr. Bogue.

We are pleased to say that he has approved those of our make unqualifiedly.

Plain $2.50
Nickel-Plated 2.75

Syringes.

Gold, extra heavy, 18 Carats fine, two Pipes	$25.00
Silver, two Pipes	7.50
Coin Silver, small size, Electro Gilded, two Pipes	7.50
Silver-Plated, two Pipes	3.00
Britannia, German Silver Pipe	.63
" Silver Pipe	1.13
Vulcanized Rubber	.75
" " Silver Pipe	1.25
" " 18 Carat Gold Pipe	3.00

PEAR SHAPE NICKEL-PLATED ELASTIC BULB SYRINGE.

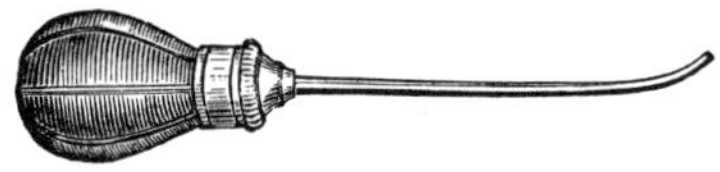

Entire length, 6 inches; diameter of Bulb, 1½ inches. In use, compress the Bulb, and insert the Point under water, when it fills itself.

Price $2.50

NICKEL-PLATED RING SYRINGE, WITH ELASTIC BULB.

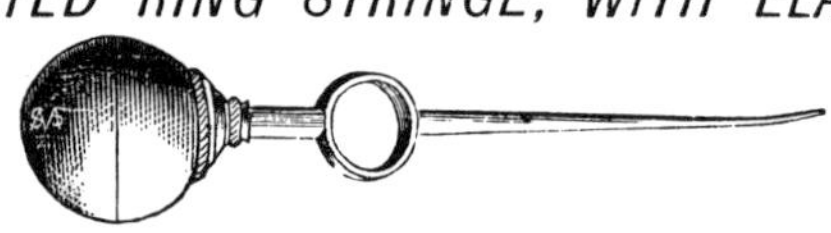

Price $3.00

DR. MOFFATT'S NICKEL-PLATED BULB TOOTH SYRINGE.

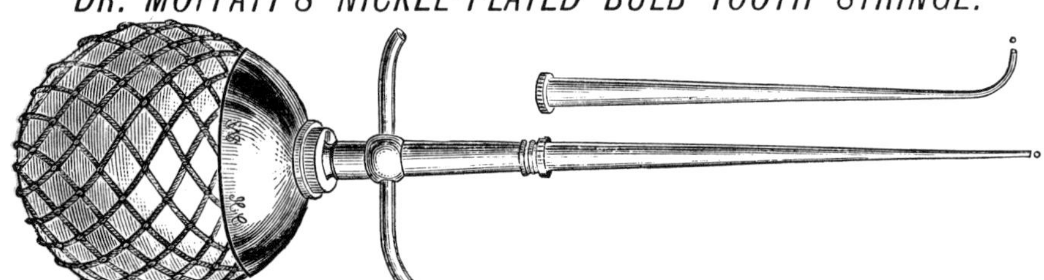

Length, 5¼ inches, Bulb covered with Silk Netting.

Price, in Case, with two Pipes as shown in Cut $3.50

RUBBER BULB CHIP SYRINGE.

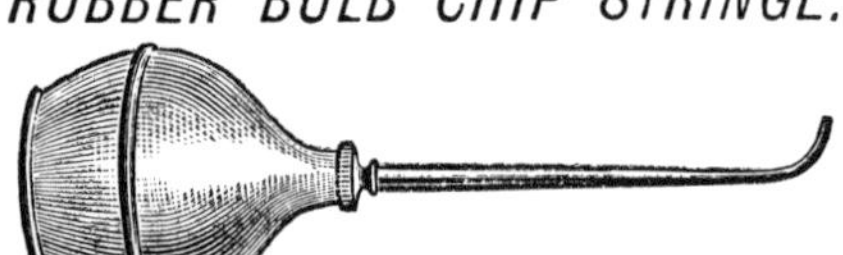

This is a Cold-Air Syringe only, for blowing the cuttings and dust from cavities. Full length of Syringe, 6 inches. Tube is Nickel-Plated.

Price $1.50

HEAVY GLASS OFFICE SYRINGE.

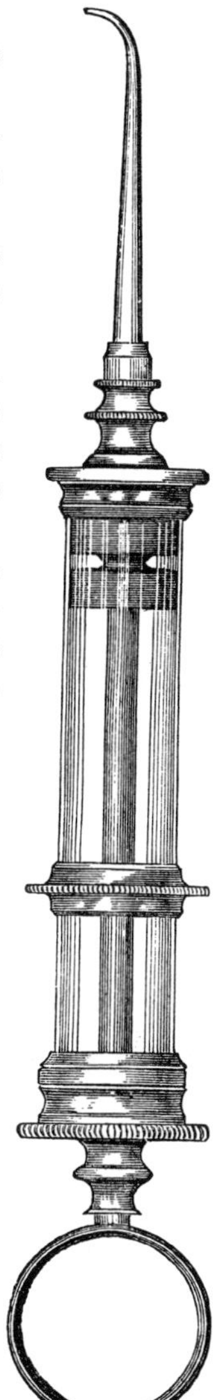

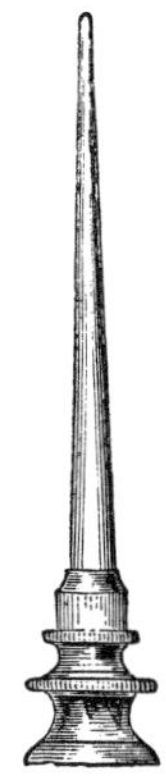

This has for a long time been accepted as the Best Dental Syringe of moderate cost.

Glass is safe and cleanly, and quite free from the unpleasantness of Hard Rubber, which also soon wears loose at the part of cylinder most used.

The thickness and strength of the Glass in this Syringe make it acceptable as avoiding the risks of the frail thin tubing heretofore used.

These are made of that kind of tubing which is used for steam gauges and other exact apparatus; being the most perfect in form and evenness inside which can be procured. It is carefully annealed, and has a bore large enough to permit a good packing.

The parts are sized and fitted to correspond, by the use of extra Hubs, with our standard Gold, Silver, and Platinum and Iridium Points, and also for the Hypodermic Injection Pipes. With the addition of these Points it may be used not only for washing out cavities, but also for injecting the various solutions used in the treatment of abscesses, and as a Hypodermic Syringe. It is extremely well made, the metallic portion being of fine German Silver, heavily Silver-Plated. This is the best cheap Syringe yet offered, and it is recommended as combining neatness, durability, and an extensive range of uses, with economy in first cost.

The No. 1 Hub or Tip fits the Hypodermic and Abscess Points; No. 2 fits the Plain Gold and Silver Points.

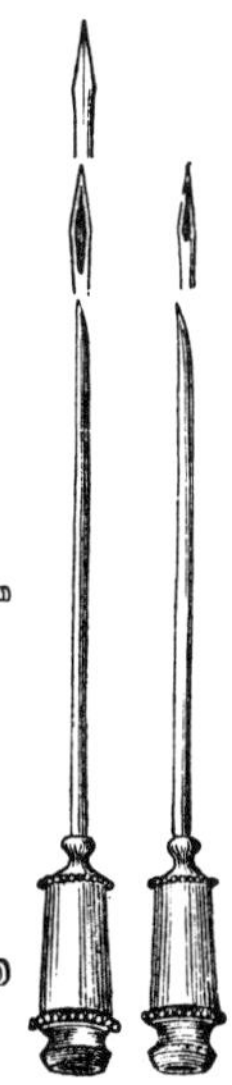

HYPODERMIC SYRINGE POINTS.

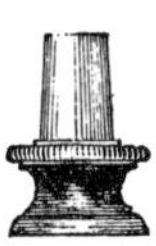

No. 2.

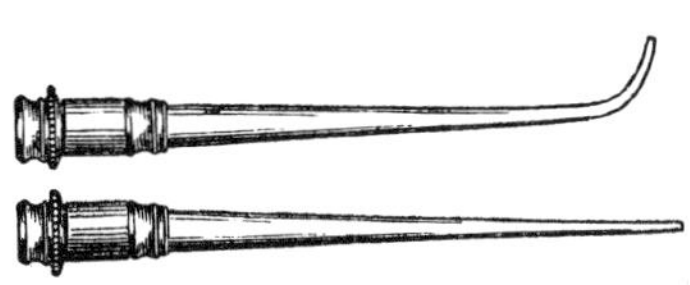

ABSCESS SYRINGE POINTS.

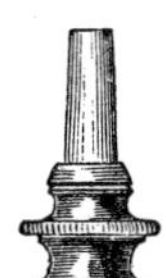

No. 1.

Price, with one Point, straight or curved . . .		$3.50
Extra Points	each	$0.50
Tips or Hubs	"	.50
Hypodermic Syringe Points	"	.75
Gold (18c.) Abscess Syringe Points, straight or curved	"	2.50
Platinum and Iridium Abscess Syringe Points, straight or curved . .	"	1.75
Plain Gold Points, such as are on Common Hard-Rubber Syringe . .	"	2.25
Plain Coin Silver Points, such as are on Common Hard-Rubber Syringe .	"	.50

HYPODERMIC SYRINGE.

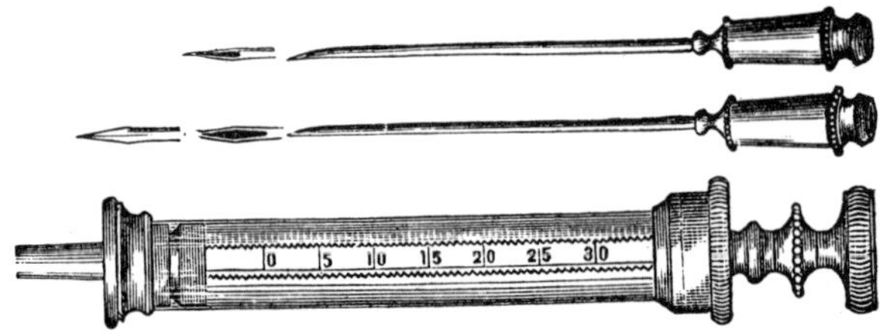

Our Cut represents the best form of instrument for hypodermic injections, with graduated Piston-Rod and Jam-Nut to set for the exact quantity to be discharged. The mountings of these are made of German Silver, and Silver-Plated. The Pipes have fine, well-formed Points. They are made of steel, tempered and finished as well as the best lancets. The Points of all our Hypodermic Syringes are of the same quality; no inferiority in shape, temper, or finish being admissible in this important part.

Price, with two Points, in Morocco Case $5.00

We also make a graduated Rod Syringe, the glass of which is cased in a metal tube, and the graduations exposed to sight as in the bulb of spirit-levels.

Price, in Morocco Case, two Points $4.50

We have a less expensive instrument of the same size as our Cut, with the graduations on the Glass instead of the Rod. Brass mountings, Silver-Plated.

Price, in Case, with two Points $3.00

HOT-AIR SYRINGE.

Patented November 2d, 1875.

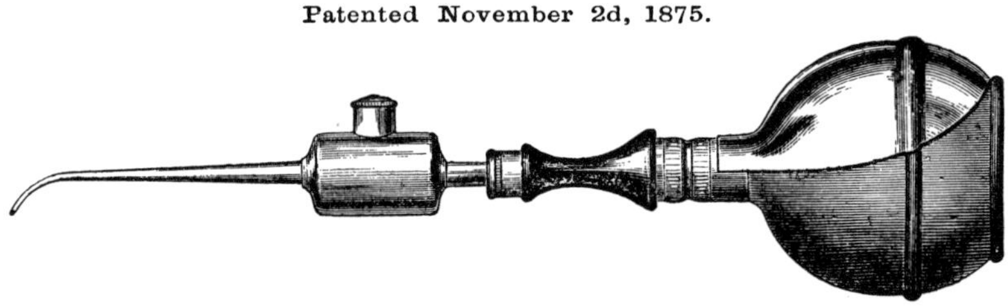

The Cut illustrates a Hot-Air Syringe for drying cavities. The Bulb is of Rubber, with a *Metal Guard*, for the purpose of getting a firm support in the palm of the hand while compressing the Bulb with the fingers. This Metal Guard is connected by a Ferrule with the Ebony Thumb- and Finger-Piece, and thus gives steadiness in working the Syringe, so that the direction of the Point can be preserved without wabbling. The section of Ebony, being a non-conductor, prevents the conveyance of heat to the injury of the Rubber Bulb. To fill the Syringe with heated air, hold the Turret of the Air-Chamber in the flame of a spirit-lamp; this Turret is provided with a Metallic Valve, which recedes as the Bulb, after being compressed, fills with air, and allows the flame to be drawn into the Chamber; the Air-Chamber is divided by partitions of Wire Gauze, which act as retainers of heat. It is a very neat and efficient instrument.

Price, with Metal Guard . . . . each $3.50

" " " and Silk Netting . . . . " 4.00

DR. MOFFATT'S WARM-AIR CAVITY DRIER.

FOR DRYING CAVITIES WITH WARM AIR, AND ALSO FOR REMOVING CUTTINGS AND BUR DUST FROM EXCAVATIONS.

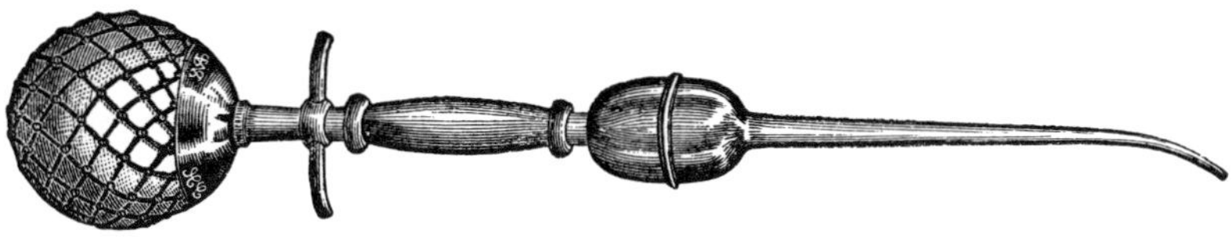

With a Rubber Air-Bulb, covered with Silk Netting; Finger Bars for holding the instrument firmly in manipulating; and a thick Metal Bulb for heating the air as it passes to and from the Rubber Bulb. The part between the Finger-Bars and the Metal Bulb being of non-conducting material, prevents the passage of heat toward the hand.

In using, exhaust the air from the Rubber Bulb before heating; then heat the Metal Bulb over a spirit-lamp for a short time, and allow it to fill with air; inject the heated air into the cavity by pressing on the Rubber Bulb. In cases of sensitive teeth, heat the air for blowing out cuttings, etc. The instrument is Nickel-Plated.

Price . . . . each $3.50

HARD RUBBER SYRINGE.

FOR INJECTING IODINE, ACID, ETC., INTO ABSCESSES.

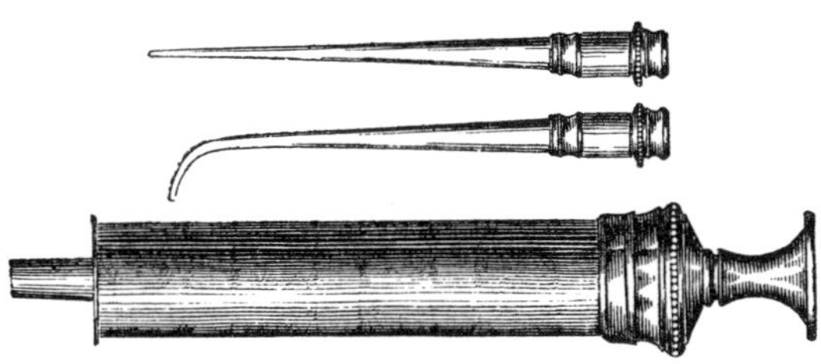

The attention of Dentists and Physicians is invited to this Syringe, as being superior in quality to any others in the market.

The Cut represents the Syringe perfectly in size and form. It will be furnished with one or more Points, of either quality as desired, at quoted prices.

The Platinum and Iridium Points are made thick and strong, are much stiffer than pure Platinum, and are said to resist the action of acids as well.

The Points fit and can be used with the Hypodermic Syringes.

Price, in a neat Morocco Case, with one Platinum, or one Platinum and Iridium Point (straight or curved)		$3.00
The same, with one Gold Point (straight or curved)		3.75
Platinum Points (straight or curved)	each	1.75
" and Iridium Points (straight or curved)	"	1.75
18 Carat Gold Points (straight or curved)	"	2.50
Hypodermic Points, Steel	"	.75

Files.

MURPHY'S FILES—PHILADELPHIA MANUFACTURE.

Separating, Nos. 00 to 8	10	cts. each ;	per doz.	$1.00
Finishing, Flat, Oval, Blunt and Pointed, Nos. 9 to 22	18	"	"	2.00
" Bevel Edge, Nos. 23 to 25	18	"	"	2.00
Finishing, for Lateral and Crown Cavities, Double-End, Nos. 45, 46, 47, 50, 51, 52, 54, 55, 56, 57, 60, 62, 66, 69, 85, 91, 92, 95, 98, 99, 101, 104, 105, 106, 108, 109	22	cts. each ;	per doz.	$2.40
Oval, Half-Round, Round, and Triangular Stump, Nos. 33 to 39, 41 to 43	18	"	"	2.00
Bicuspid (thick and thin), Nos. 27 to 30, 32, and 86	18	"	"	2.00
Molar, Single Curve, No. 78	18	"	"	2.00
" " Feather Edge, No. 87	22	"	"	2.40
" " No. 107	30	"	"	3.25
" Double Curve, No. 84	22	"	"	2.40
" " Feather Edge, No. 80	30	"	"	3.25
" " Oval Face, No. 81	30	"	"	3.25
" " Extra Thick, No. 82	30	"	"	3.25

SEPARATING.

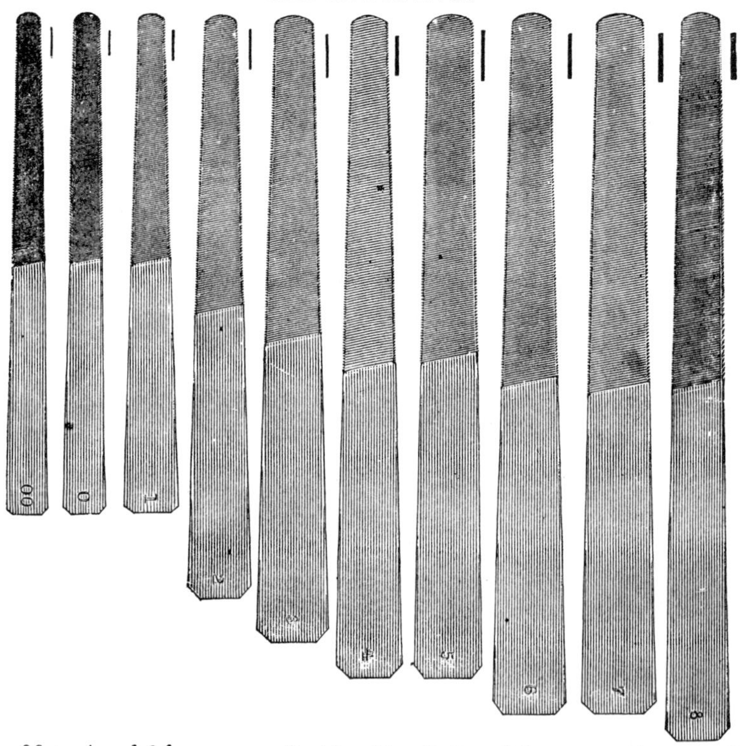

Nos. 00 to 4 and 6 have one safe side; Nos. 5, 7, and 8 are cut all over. They are also put up in packages containing one dozen assorted.

Price . . . . 10 cts. each ; per doz. $1.00

MURPHY'S FILES.

PLUG-FINISHING.

FLAT, OVAL, BLUNT, AND POINTED.

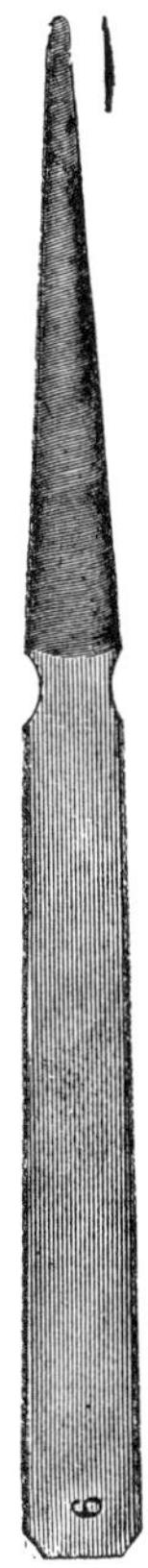

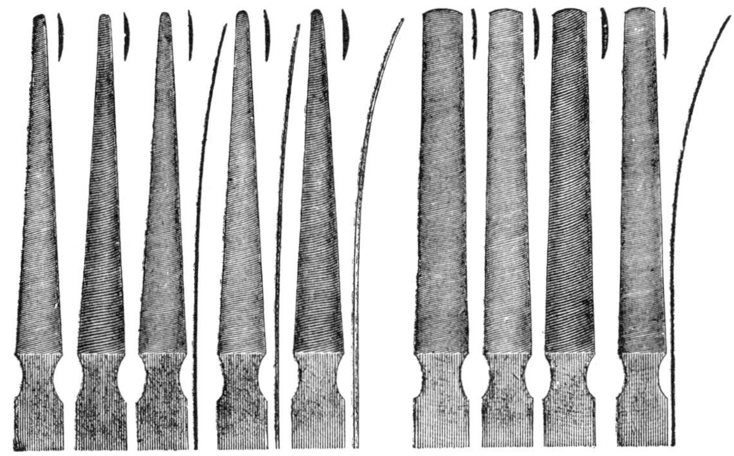

10. 11. 12. 13. 14. 15. 16. 17. 18.

BEVEL EDGE.

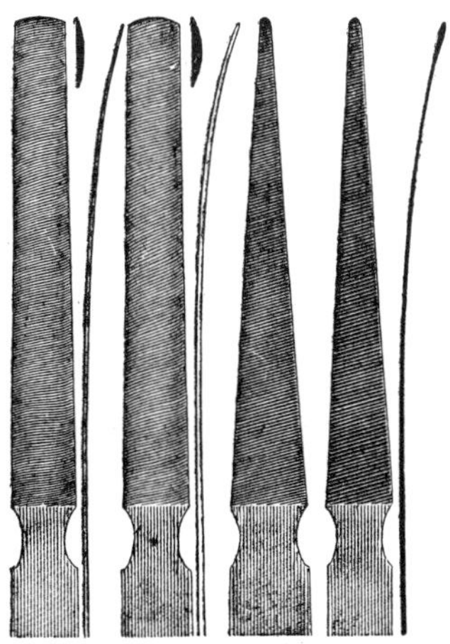

19. 20. 21. 22.

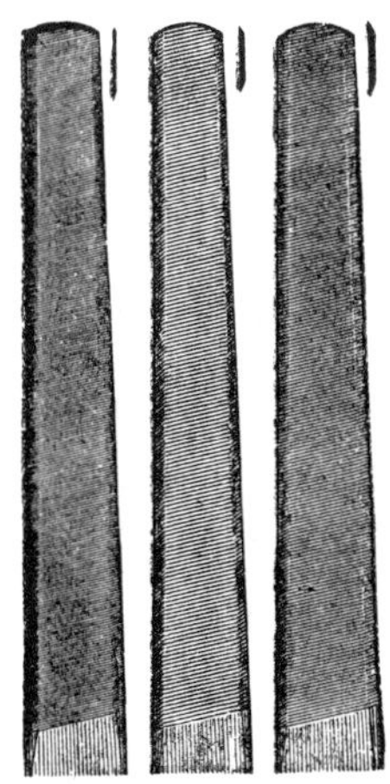

23. 24. 25.

These Files run thin, medium, and thick, and fine, medium, and coarse-cut, as shown in Cuts.

Price . . . . each 18 cents; per doz. $2.00

MURPHY'S FILES.

DOUBLE END PLUG-FINISHING, FOR LATERAL AND CROWN CAVITIES.

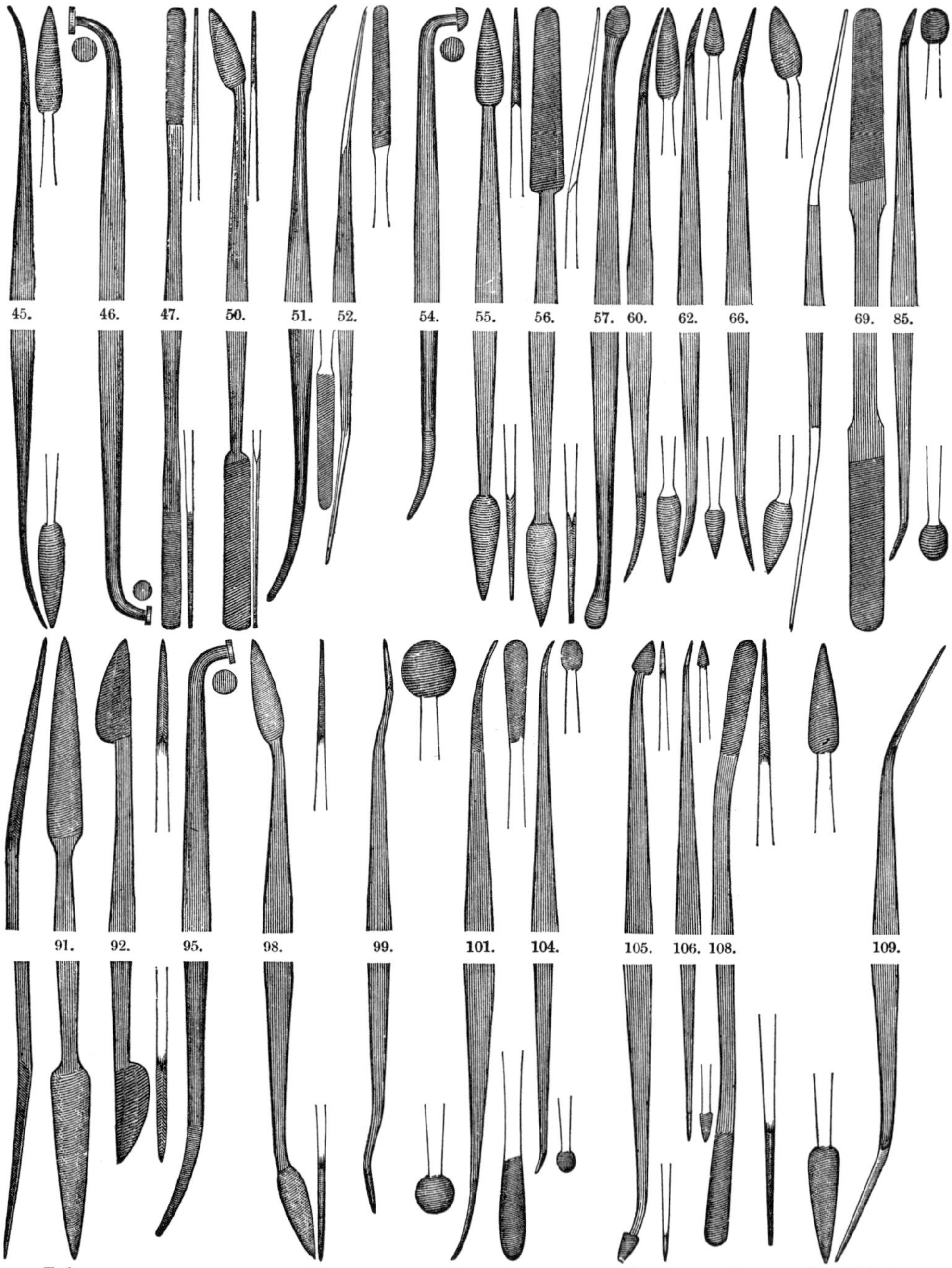

Price . . . . 22 cts. each; per doz. $2.40

MURPHY'S FILES.

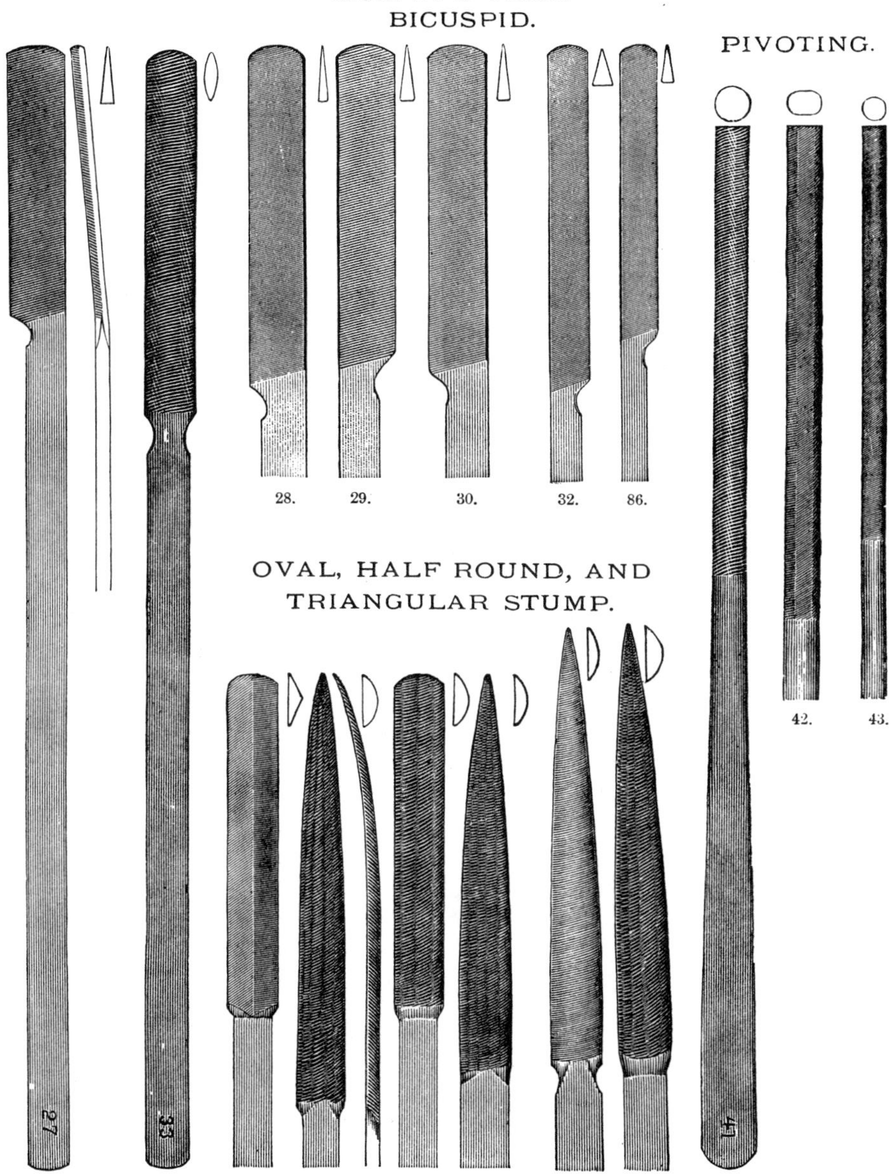

Nos. 27, 28, 29, 30. Bicuspid Files, Rights and Lefts, cut inside, outside, and all over. Nos. 28, 29, 30, are thin, medium, and thick; and fine, medium, and coarse-cut. No. 32 is an extra thick Bicuspid File, Right and Left, cut inside, outside, and all over.

Price . . . . 18 cents each; per doz. $2.00

Nos. 37, 38, 39, are cut fine, medium, and coarse, and made of three distinct sizes.

Stump and Pivoting Files . . . . 18 cents each; per doz. $2.00

MURPHY'S FILES.

SINGLE AND DOUBLE CURVE MOLAR.

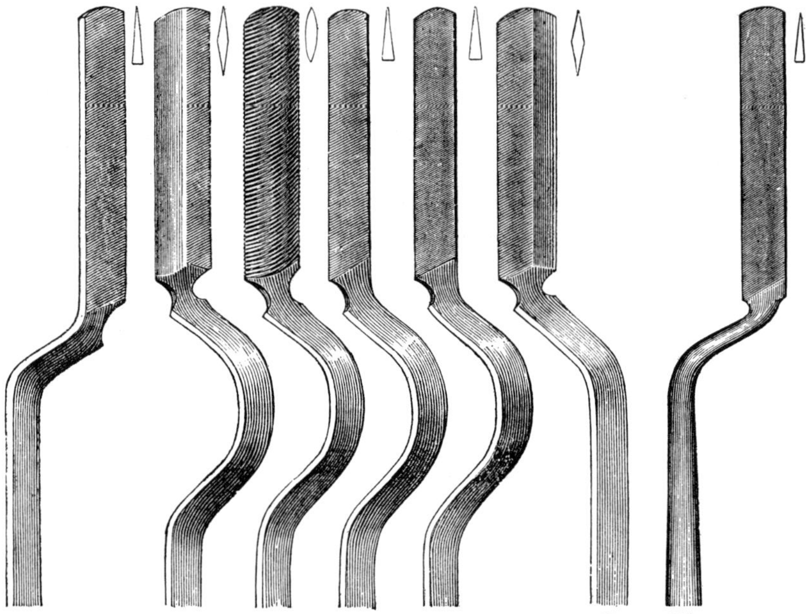

78. 80. 81. 82. 84. 87. 107.

In ordering, state whether wanted cut on one side or on both sides; whether for the right or left side of the mouth; upper or lower jaw.

PRICES.

No. 78, Single Curve	18 cts. each; or per doz.	$2.00
No. 87, "	22 " "	2.40
No. 107, "	30 " "	3.25
Nos. 80 to 82, Double Curve	30 " "	3.25
No. 84, "	22 " "	2.40

DR. TAFT'S PLUG-FINISHING FILES.

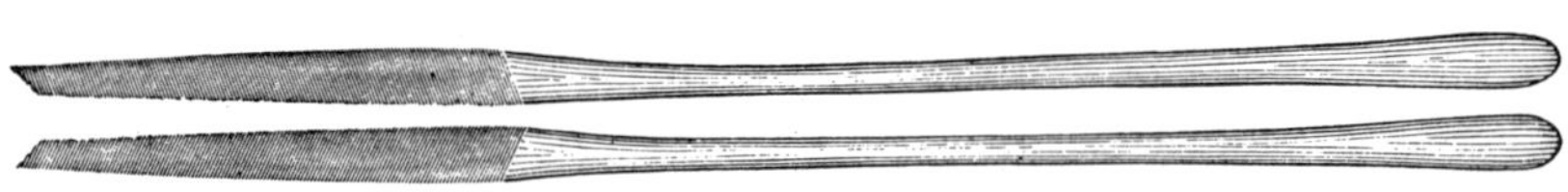

This Cut represents a small, delicate File, with Spring Temper, designed for dressing down fillings in approximal cavities.

Price, Rommetin's	per doz.	$1.75
" Murphy's	"	1.50

DOUBLE END PLUG-FINISHING FILES.

RIGHT AND LEFT.

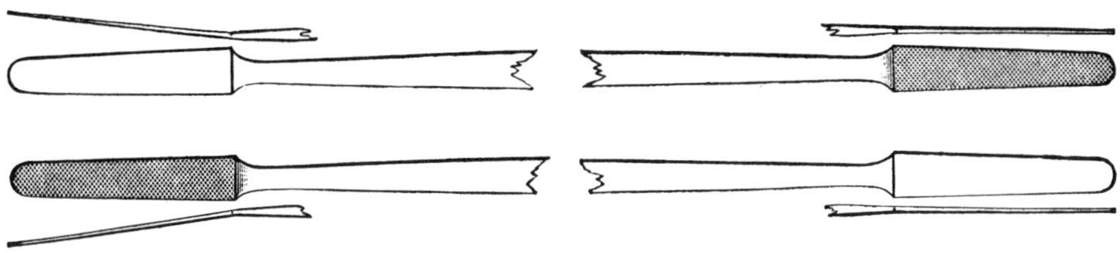

The Cut illustrates a new form of File for finishing fillings, very finely cut.

Price . . . . per doz. $3.00

FROID'S FILES.

(For Plate Files see Mechanical Dentistry.)

Separating, One Safe Side, Nos. 00 to 8	12	cts. each; per doz.	$1.25
" Cut Four Sides, Nos. 6, 7, and 8 . .	12	" "	1.25
" Curved, Cut Inside, Nos. 3 to 6 . . .	12	" "	1.25
" " Cut Outside, Nos. 3 to 6 . .	12	" "	1.25
Plug-Finishing, Pointed, Nos. 0, 1, 2, and 3. . .	14	" "	1.50
" Blunt, Nos. 0, 1, 2, and 3 . . .	14	" "	1.50
" Pointed, Curved, Nos. 0, 1, and 2 .	14	" "	1.50
" Blunt, Curved, Nos. 0, 1, and 2 . .	14	" "	1.50
Stump, Half Round, Pointed, Nos. 1 to 5 . . .	18	" "	2.00
" " Blunt, Nos. 1 to 4 . . .	18	" "	2.00
" Oval, Blunt, Nos. 0, 1, and 2	18	" "	2.00
" " Pointed, Nos. 0, 1, and 2 . . .	18	" "	2.00
Knife-Edge or Bicuspid, Pointed, Nos. 3, 4, 5, and 6 .	18	" "	2.00
" " Blunt, Nos. 1, 2, 3, and 4 .	18	" "	2.00
Bayonet, Half Round, Pointed Molar, Nos. 1, 2, and 3.	28	" "	3.15
" " Blunt " Nos. 1, 2, and 3.	28	" "	3.15
" Knife-Edge, Blunt Molar, R. and L., Nos. 1, 2, and 3	28	" "	3.15
Double Curve, Feather-Edge Molar, Nos. 1, 2, and 3 . .	34	" "	3.90

STUBS'S FILES—OUR OWN IMPORTATION.

(For Plate Files see Mechanical Dentistry.)

Separating, various cuts . . . . 22 cts. each; per doz. $2.50

Miscellaneous.

DR. FORBES'S FILE CARRIER.

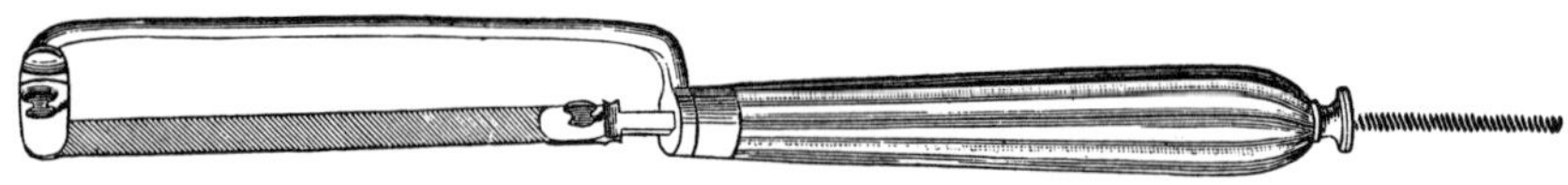

The Cut is half the size of the Instrument. The Files are 3 inches in length and from $\frac{1}{8}$ to $\frac{3}{16}$ of an inch in width, and of various thicknesses and cuts. The Shaft extends through the handle, and can be adjusted at any point by a Thumb-Screw at the end. Files of different lengths can be used and held firmly.

Ivory Handle	each	$3.50
Fluted-Bone or Ebony Handle	"	3.00
Files, Assorted	per doz.	1.00

DR. ABBOTT'S FILE CARRIER, No. 1.

TWO ANGLES, FOR UPPER AND LOWER FILLINGS.

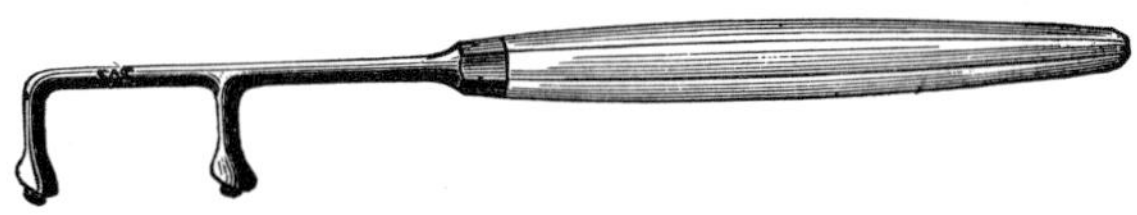

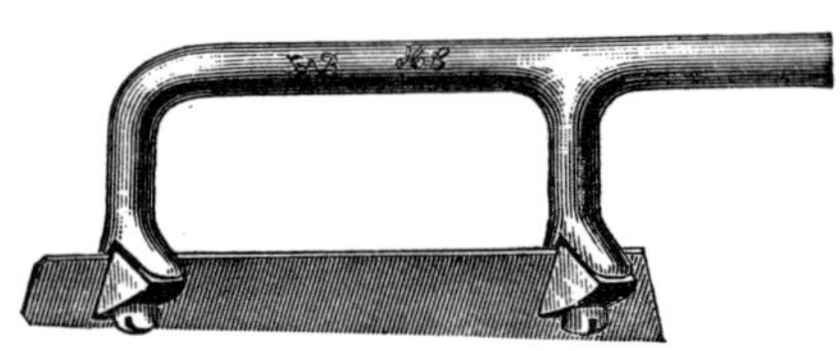

The Sectional Cut (full size) shows the Two Angles for the insertion of the File.

Ivory Handle	each	$3.00
Fluted-Bone or Ebony Handle	"	2.50

DR. ABBOTT'S FILE CARRIER, No. 2.

FOR SEPARATING.

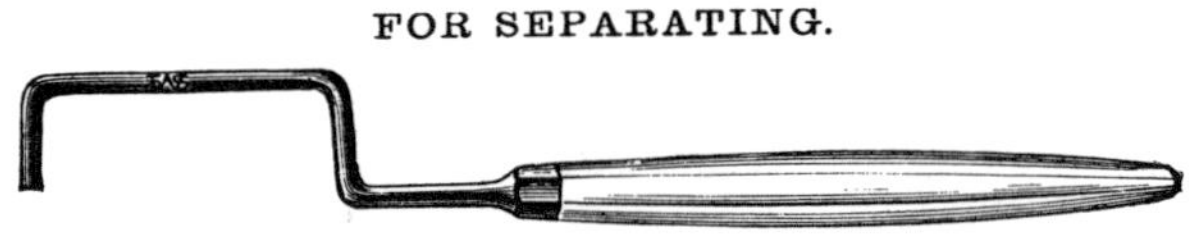

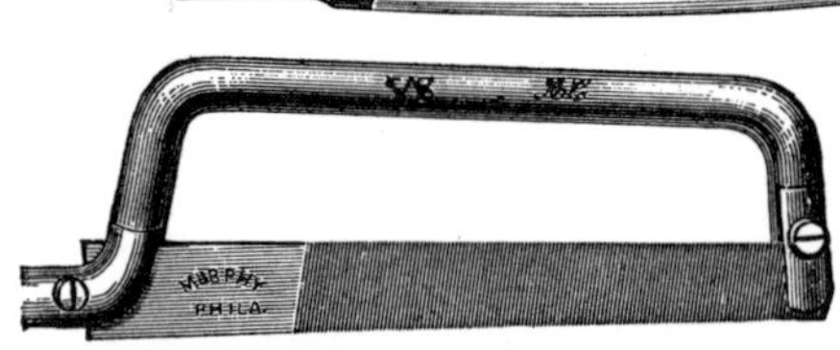

The Sectional Cut (full size) shows the manner in which the File is held in position.

Ivory Handle	each	$2.50
Fluted-Bone or Ebony Handle	"	2.00

DR. W. G. REDMAN'S REVERSIBLE FILE CARRIER.

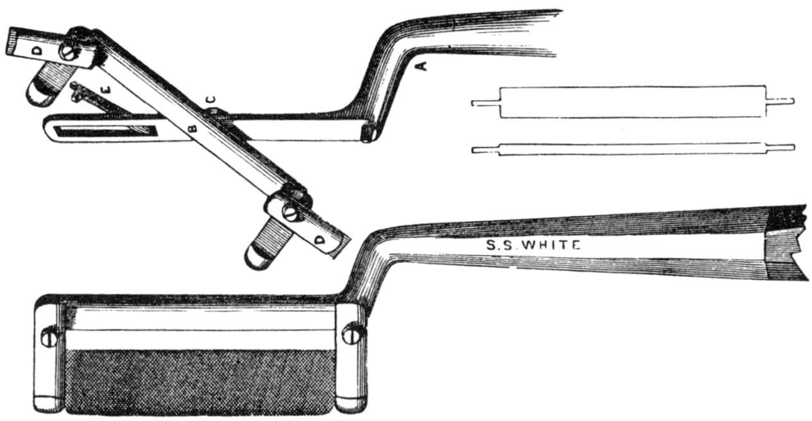

By the use of this Instrument much of the inconvenience experienced in the changing and adjusting of Files is avoided. The Shaft A having a double bend, and the Holder B being reversible, allows the easy and comfortable use of the same file in separating even the farthest molars, on either side, upper or lower. No Thumb-screws are used, nor is a Screw-driver necessary to secure the File, a single movement of the Fastenings D accomplishing this. C is the Pivot on which the Holder turns, which is securely fastened by pressing down the Lock E. Made and finished in the best manner and mounted with an Ivory Handle. The outlines on the right describe the thicknesses of Nos. 2 and 7 Files, No. 2 being the thickest. There are four intermediate thicknesses, and the set of 12 Files is arranged as follows: No. 1, Feather-edge File, cut all over, same thickness in the center as No. 2. Nos. 2, 3, 4, and 5 are Knife-edge Files, varying in thickness, one of each number cut all over, and one of each number with one safe side. No. 6 is a flat Separating File, cut all over, and No. 7 is a Bevel-edge Separating File.

Ivory Handle	each	$5.00
Ebony "	"	4.50
Files, per set of 12		2.50

FILE CARRIER FOR SEPARATING MOLARS.

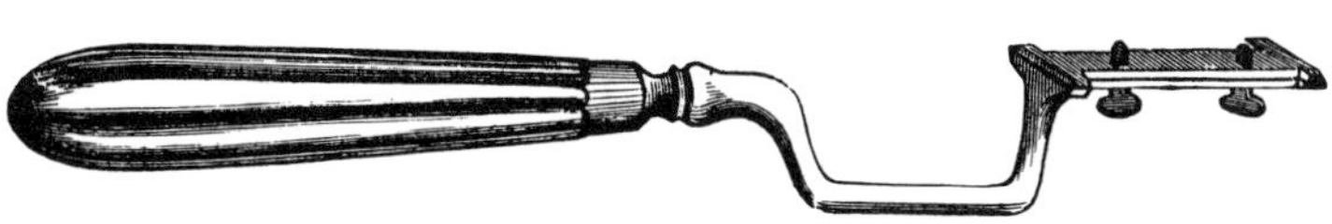

Ivory Handle	each	$3.00
Ebony or Fluted-Bone Handle	"	2.50

DR. J. C. CONNER'S FILE CARRIER.

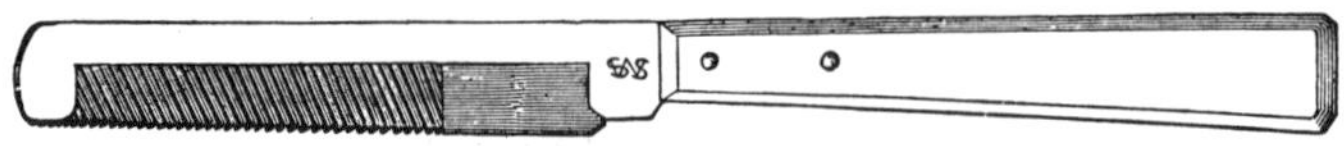

Ivory Handle . . . . each $1.00
Buffalo " . . . . " .75

BRIGHT STEEL FILE CARRIERS.

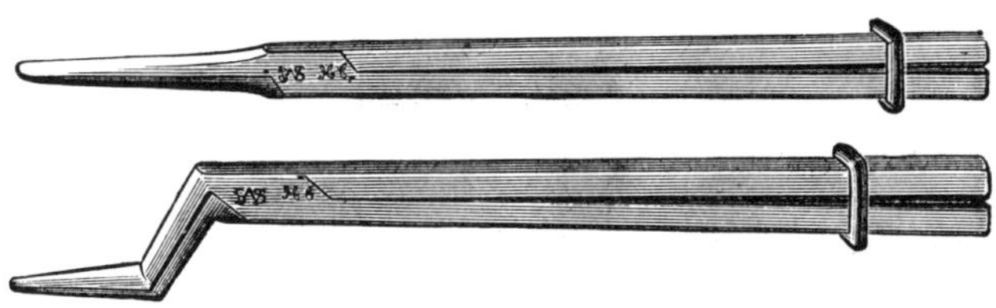

Square Joint, like Forceps, with Ring Slides. Cuts about one-half size.

Straight, Nickel-Plated . . . . each $2.50
Bayonet-Shape, Nickel-Plated . . . . " 3.50

SAW FRAMES.

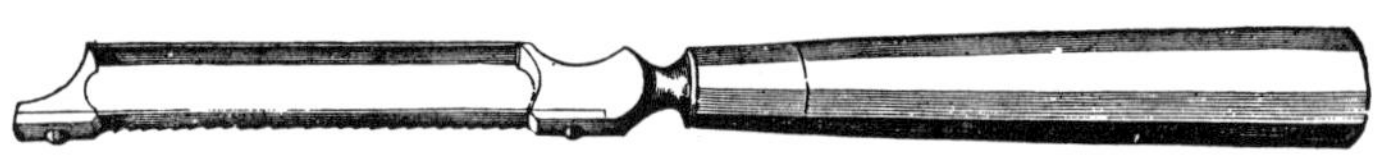

These are neat and convenient instruments for cutting off natural teeth for pivoting, or for sawing off the linings of artificial teeth to remove them from the plate.

Ivory Handle . . . . each $1.50

CREASOTE APPLIANCE.

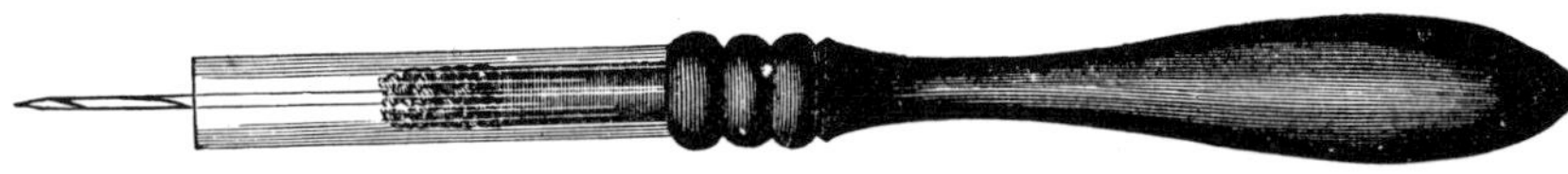

Intended to prevent fluid caustics, such as Creasote, or Solution of Nitrate of Silver, from running down and cauterizing the lips when being applied to the gums. The Cut shows the size of the Instrument. A Spiral Platinum Wire, 2 inches long, is inserted in a Handle, passing through a small piece of Sponge, over which is a Glass Tube 1¼ inches long. The Tube slides over a part of the Handle to keep it firm, and to hold the Wire in the center. When the caustic is taken up on a small piece of cotton, if any should run down it is caught in the Tube.

Price . . . . 75 cents.

PORTE-POLISHERS.

INVENTION OF DR. LOUIS JACK.

A B C

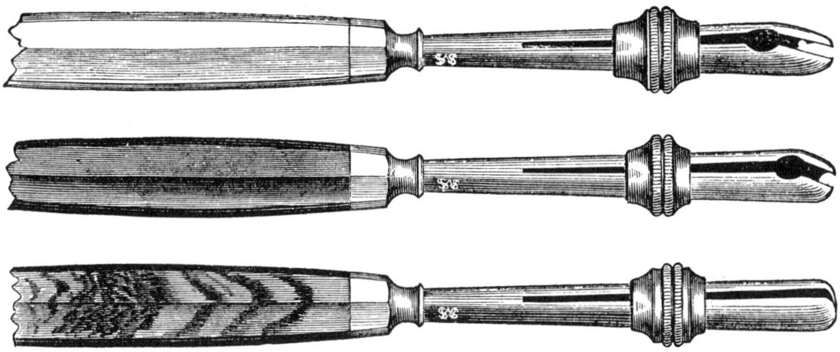

Set of 3. Split and set to spring open; closing on the wood by pushing up the Ring-Slide. One straight and two slants, each known by the Handle, which is varied, in order that the operator may thereby distinguish the one which he wishes to use.

"A," Ivory Handle, Long Slant	each	$3.00
"B," Ebony " Aslant	"	2.50
"C," Snakewood Handle, Straight	"	2.50

NEW ADJUSTABLE PORTE-POLISHER.

SUGGESTED BY DR. LOUIS JACK.

D

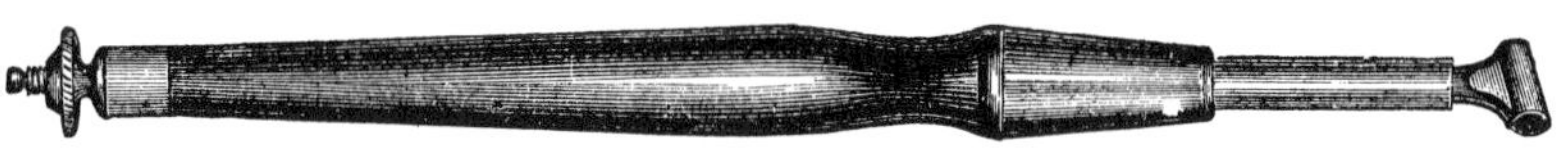

The Cut illustrates a Porte-Polisher in which the slit or opening is controlled by a neat milled Thumb-screw at the other end. There are two forms: one at angle as shown in Cut, the other straight with the Shank.

"D," Ebony Handle, Nickel-Plated	each	$1.50

PORTE-POLISHERS.

Ebony Handle, Tube End Split	each	$1.00
¼ inch File-cut, Bronzed Handle, Tube End Split	"	1.25

UNIVERSAL PORTE-POLISHERS.

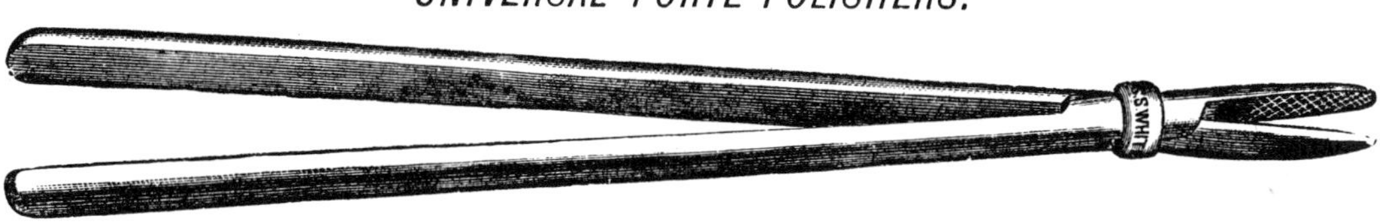

Polished Steel, Straight or Aslant	each	**$1.00**
Corundum Points, 25 in a Box	per box	**.40**

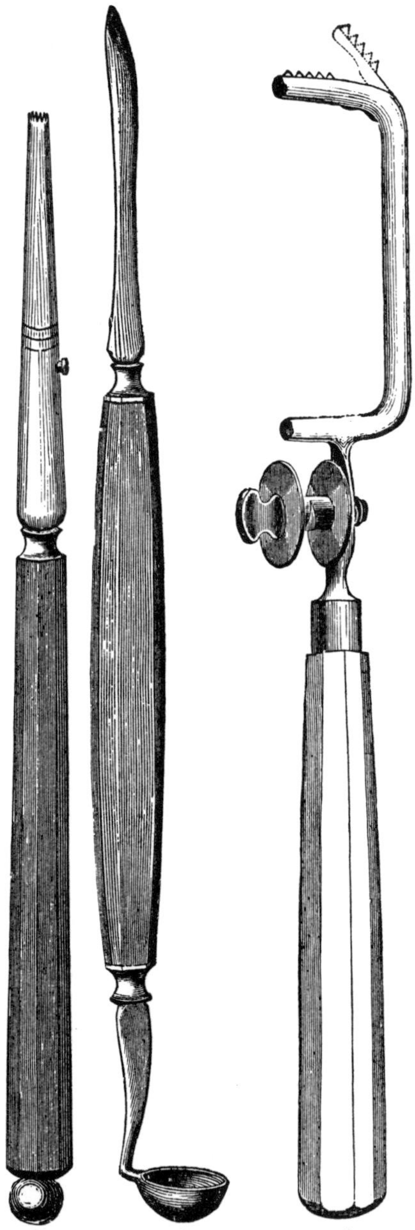

1. 2. 3.

TREPHINE FOR THE ANTRUM.

CUT No. 1.

Useful when it is desired to enter the Antrum through a tooth socket. Two sizes, the larger of which is illustrated; the smaller one is contained in the Handle—which is hollow—and may be adjusted to the same Socket by the Screw represented in the Cut.

Price $2.00

AMALGAM MANIPULATOR.

CUT No. 2.

Designed to facilitate the preparation of Amalgam for fillings, having a Cup at one end for taking up the desired amount of filings or powder, and a curved Spatula at the other end for combining the Mercury with the filings and packing it in the cavity.

Price $2.00

TAPE CARRIER.

CUT No. 3.

Made upon the principle of a File Carrier; intended to facilitate the use of Tapes, and answering the purpose admirably.

Ivory Handle $3.50

Ebony " 3.00

GOLD CYLINDER ROLLER.

INVENTION OF DR. CHARLES R. BUTLER.

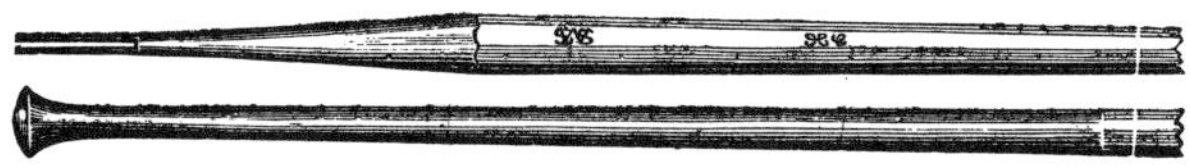

An Instrument for making Cylinders out of Gold Foil. Cut a strip of Foil or fold it up for thicker Cylinders, as wide as the length of the intended Cylinder; insert an end of it in the slit, and roll to the bulk required. The forked end is very finely finished, so that the roll may be made close without any danger of tearing the gold in its withdrawal.

Varney Style of Handle . . . . each $1.00
Plain Octagon Handle . . . . " .75

FOIL SPATULA.

A neat and convenient Instrument for the manipulation of Gold Foil. The blade is 6 inches in length by ⅝ of an inch wide, made of best quality steel, spring temper, with an ebony handle 3½ inches long.

Nickel-Plated . . . . each $1.50

PLUGGING MALLETS.

No. 1, as per Cut, showing the exact size and diameter of the Mallet; weight, 4½ ounces avoirdupois.

No. 2, as per Cut, showing the exact size and diameter of the Mallet; weight, 6½ ounces avoirdupois.

These are made of Patent Metal, and are of medium hardness, between tin and lead; Silver-Plated.

No. 3. Same size, diameter, and weight as No. 1.

No. 4. Same size, diameter, and weight as No. 2.

Made of Composition Metal, which keeps its shape pretty well, being a little harder than lead, yet giving about as dull a blow; Silver-Plated.

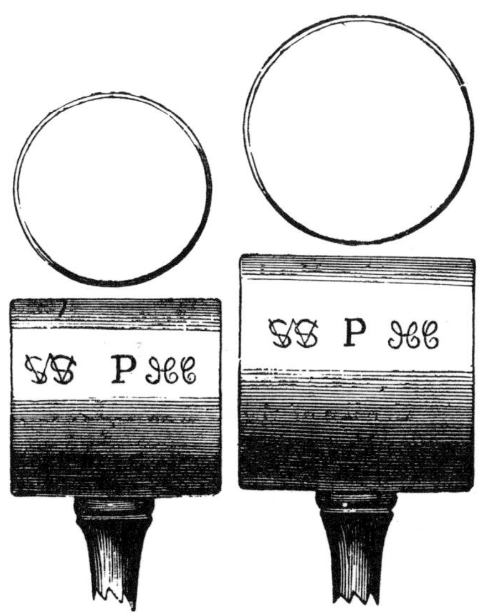

1. 2.

Price . . . . each $1.25

PLUGGING MALLETS.

Lignum Vitæ or Iron-Wood Head, with Rosewood Handle. Head 1½ inches long by 1 inch in diameter	each	$0.30
Vulcanized Rubber Head, with Ebony handle. Head 1½ inches long by 1 inch in diameter	"	.75
Vulcanized Rubber Head, with Snakewood Handle. Head 1¾ inches long by 1¼ inches in diameter	"	1.00
Dr. Colburn's Spring Attachment, one end of the Head plain, the other filled with Soft Rubber to modify the blow. Solid California Rosewood Head and Handle	"	.75
Dr. Head's Plugging Mallets	"	.75

CASE MALLETS.

INVENTION OF DR. CHAS. R. BUTLER.

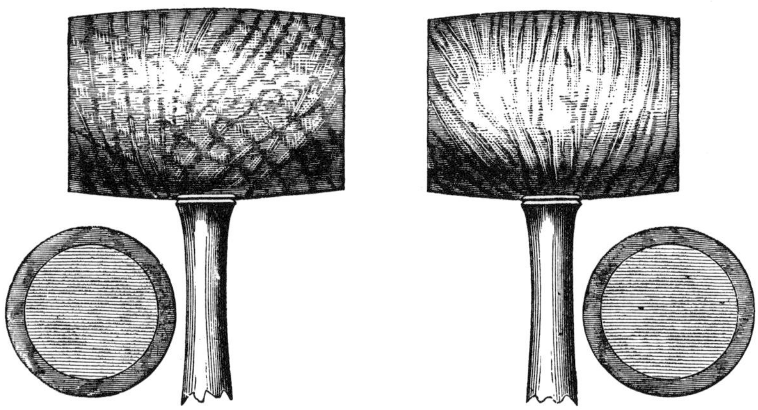

The case is made of thoroughly seasoned Laurel or Brier-Root. The filling is a Composition Metal. This, as we now make it, is approved as the best DULL BLOW Mallet yet produced.

The wood is beautifully variegated and interlaced.

There are three sizes, nearly the same diameter, differing principally in the length.

Handles of the choicest Heart Hickory, and made oval in the palm-hold, as in all our fine Mallets.

Price	each	$1.50
" C. Palmer, Special	"	2.50
" Metal Case, 6 ounce	"	2.00
" " 4 "	"	2.00
" " 3 "	"	1.50
" Pure Tin	"	1.25

STEEL MALLETS.

FROM DESIGN BY DR. A. B. ROBBINS.

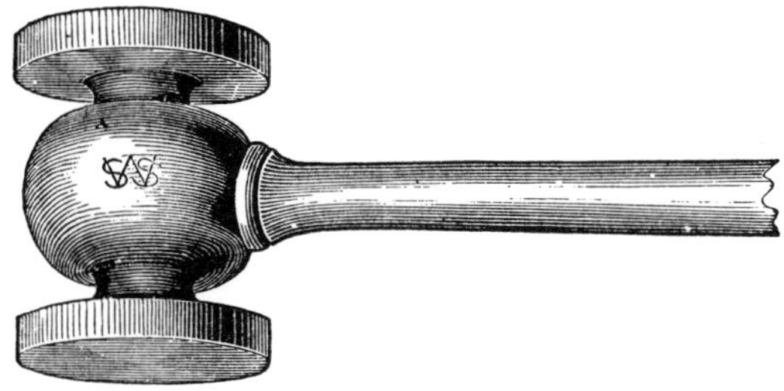

Several very eminent practitioners have approved of and adopted these Mallets, of our make, as the perfection of plugging force.

They strike a LIVE BLOW, which communicates an impetus to the Plugger; there seems to be no doubt that they pack gold faster, and with infinitely less complaint from the patient, than any other kind of Mallet.

Those which we make are of superior quality. The form gives the least weight with the greatest possible malleting face. It also cuts off all communication of vibration between the Handle and Mallet. They are made of soft steel, which, after a little use, takes on a surface-condensed face superior to any tempering, and yet does not batter the ends of the Pluggers.

Nickel-Plated, Oval Handles . . . . each $1.50

LIP PROTECTOR

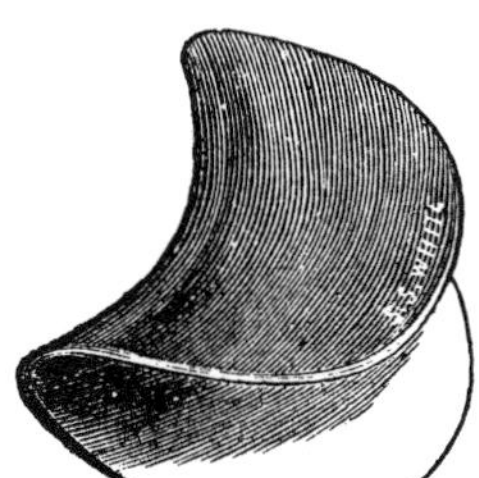

The advantage of this Instrument was suggested by the use of the ordinary Cheek Holder. It is found very useful in protecting the lips from being chafed, when using either Files, Drills, or Excavators.

Silver-Plated . . . . each 35 cents.
Gilt . . . . " 50 "

TONGUE HOLDER AND DUCT COMPRESSOR.

No. 1.

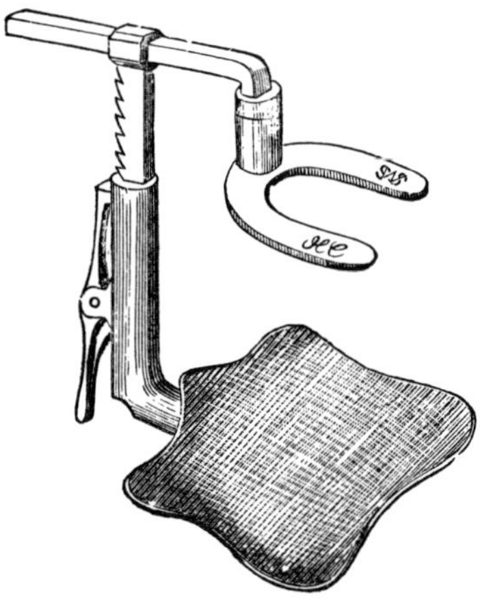

No. 2.

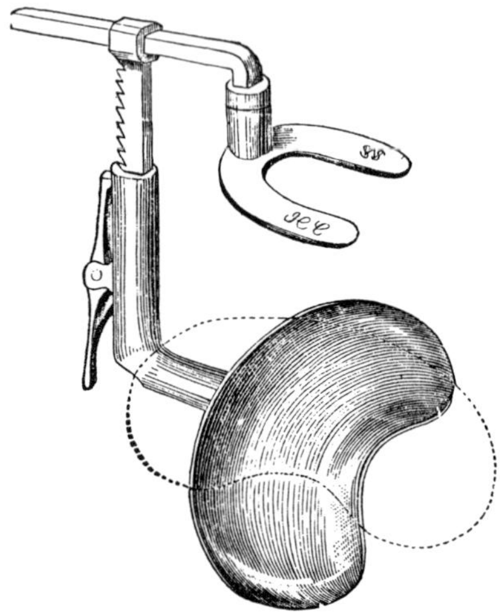

For this modification of a very useful instrument we are indebted to Dr. P. T. Smith, of Tipton, Iowa.

By its use the tongue may be clamped down in place and kept in position as long as desired. The sublingual and submaxillary ducts may be very effectually closed by placing upon them rolls or pads of bibulous or tissue paper before applying the Compress; a pad of paper or a napkin should be placed on the tongue before adjusting the instrument. The use of it is a relief to patients rather than a discomfort, holding the tongue entirely out of the way during an operation, without requiring constant effort on their part. It possesses all the advantages of the Hawes Compressor, and the additional convenience of a lateral and sliding motion of the Compressor, and a lateral motion of the Chin-Plate, by which the Post can be placed at either side out of the way of the Operator.

The Chin-Plate of No. 1 is 2 inches long by 1¾ inches wide; that of No. 2 is 2½ inches long by 1¼ inches wide.

The stationary part of the Post of each is 1⅝ inches long, and can be extended to 2¾ inches by the Ratchet and Stop.

The Compressor has a sliding motion of 1⅞ inches.

PRICES.

BRASS, SILVER-PLATED.

No. 1, Chin-Piece, Concave Shield-form, Padded with Velvet	$3.50
No. 2, shaped to fit the Chin front or sideways, Plain Burnished . . .	3.50
With both Patterns of Chin-Plate	6.00

GERMAN SILVER, SILVER-PLATED.

No. 1, Chin-Piece, Concave Shield-form, Padded with Velvet	$4.50
No. 2, shaped to fit the Chin front or sideways, Plain Burnished . . .	4.50
With both Patterns of Chin-Plate	7.00

DR. FLAGG'S TONGUE HOLDER.

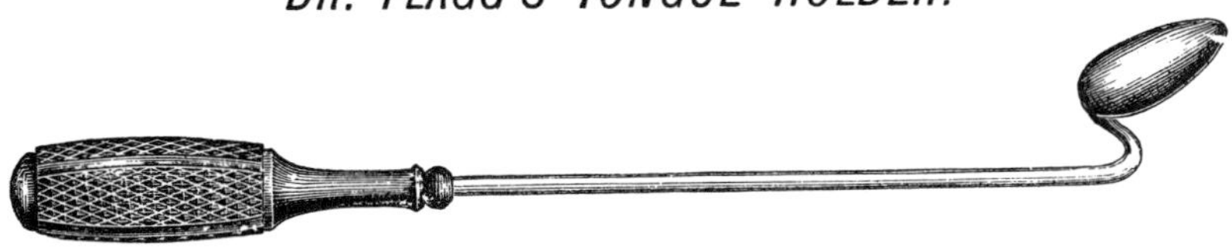

It will be found that the use of this instrument will insure additional facility to the Operator, and maintain the tongue in position with perfect comfort to the patient, producing no fatigue, no unpleasant sensations, and even removing all desire to resist constraint.

Directions for Use.—After introducing a fold of napkin, or a small piece of muslin, under the tongue, and then covering that organ by back-folding the napkin, or placing another small piece of muslin upon it, the Holder should be put in position nearest to the side where it is proposed to operate, and the patient be requested to retain it thus by means of the *right* hand if the cavity be on the *left* side, and the *left* hand if the cavity be on the *right* side, the elbow resting upon the arm of the operating chair.

Ebony Handle, Silver-Plated Wire	each	$2.00
Dr. C. Palmer's Tongue- and Cheek-Holder, Walrus	"	1.50

NAPKIN HOLDERS.

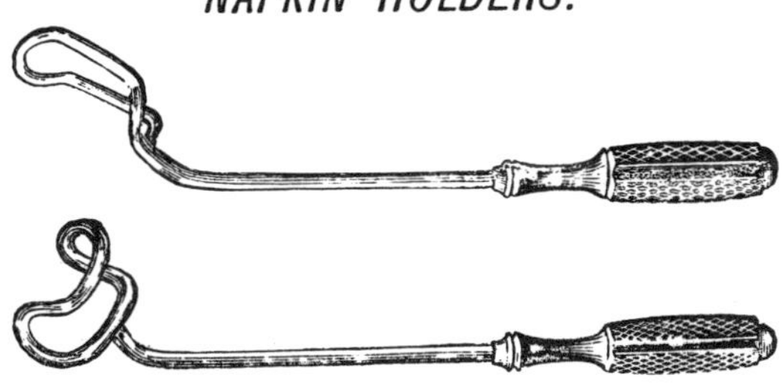

Ebony Handle, Silver-Plated Wire	each	$1.00

FOIL SHEARS AND SCISSORS.

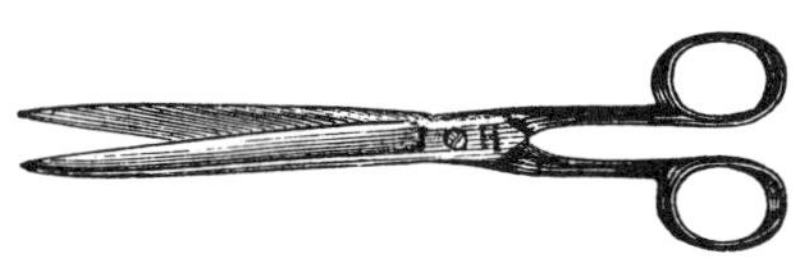

Steel, Japanned Handles, 8 inches	$1.00
Polished Steel, 8 inches	1.00
" " 9 "	2.00

(See also Pearl Handle Foil Shears.)

Steel Scissors, Small, Curved, for Trimming the Gum.	per pair	1.50
" Large, " " "	"	1.25
" Small, Straight, " "	"	1.25
" Large, " " "	"	1.00

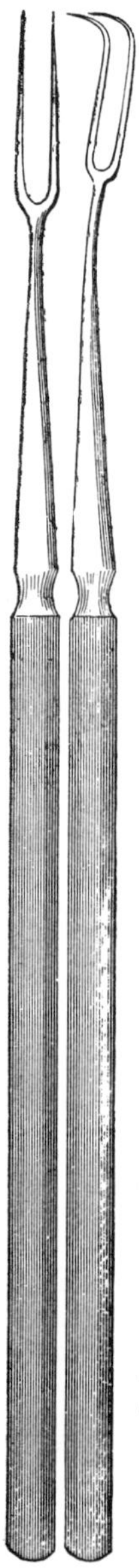

Instruments used for separating Plastic and Crystallized Gold. Cuts the exact size of the Instruments . per pair $1.00

MERCURY HOLDER.

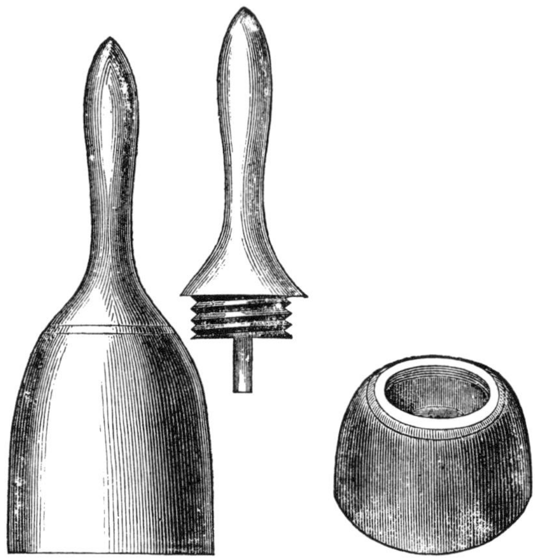

For convenience in preparing Amalgam. The Cut represents the size of the Holder, which will contain two ounces of Mercury. A small opening through the Tube allows the Mercury to escape in a very fine stream. A plug in the lower end of the Tube prevents its escape when not in use.

Holder, of Wood, nicely Polished $0.25
" Filled with Re-distilled Mercury (price fluctuates), present price 50

DOUBLE-TOP MERCURY HOLDER.

For convenient preparation of Amalgam. The Cut represents the size of the Holder, which will contain two ounces of Mercury. It has two apertures, one for filling the Holder with Mercury, and a small opening to allow it to escape in a fine stream. The screws being well cut, the joints fit accurately. The Cap prevents the escape of the Mercury.

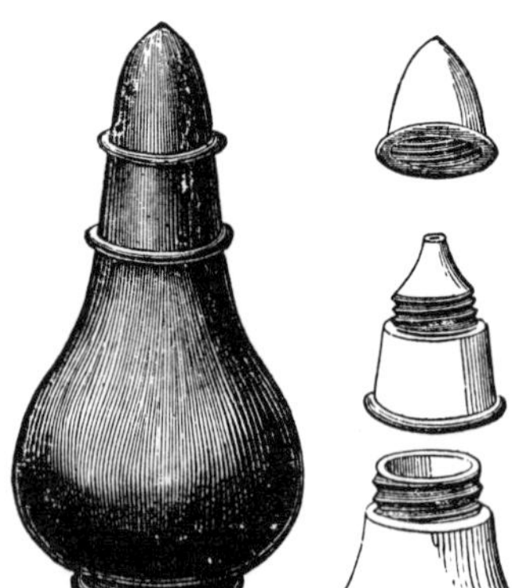

Holder of Ebony or Boxwood $0.50
" Filled with Re-distilled Mercury (price fluctuates) present price . . .75

HINGED BUR THIMBLE—IMPROVED.

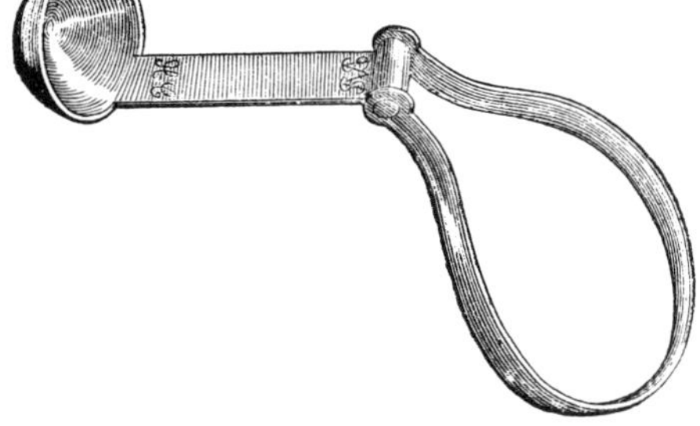

For the protection of the Hand and easy rotation of the Instrument.

German Silver, Silver-Plated . . . . each 50 cents.

DROP BOTTLES.

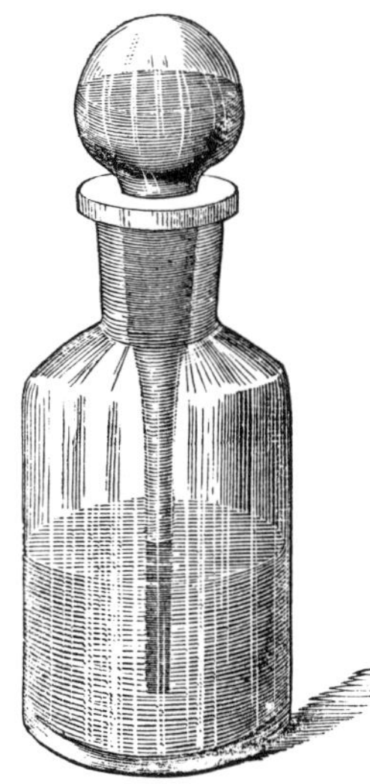

These Bottles have been prepared for using iodine, creasote, acids, etc., in the office. Warm the Bulb over the flame of a spirit-lamp, or in warm water, in order to expand the air; then immerse the point in the liquid desired, and it will slowly ascend into the Bulb as the air is condensed. This should be done in a wide-mouthed bottle or cup, as, if placed in the Bottle to which it belongs, it is apt to crack by the unequal expansion in the Neck.

When perfectly cool it may be placed in the Bottle, which should contain at least enough of the liquid to cover the point and prevent its contents from dropping. When desired for use, the warmth of the hand applied to the Bulb will force the contents out a drop at a time.

Price . . . . each 25 cents.

DENTISTS' NAPKINS.

Fine quality, all Linen, Damask Napkins, 6½ inches square . . .	per doz.	$0.60
Damask Napkins, 12½ by 11½ inches, cut and fringed . . .	"	1.25
" " 12 inches square	"	1.00

Also, for the mouth, in square and oblong pieces, stitched to prevent raveling, the following varieties, made of fine Birdseye Diaper:

Square, 3¼ inches	per doz.	$0.40
" 5½ "	"	.80
Oblong, 4 " by 7 inches.	"	.80
Also, fine Birdseye Diaper Napkins, hemmed, 10½ inches square .	"	2.00
Extra " " " " " 10½ " . .	"	2.75
" " " " " " 16½ " . .	"	3.50

DENTISTS' LAMP AND WARM-WATER CUP.

The following letter from Dr. Bogue explains the uses of this neat and efficient little apparatus:

New York, May 20th, 1875.

Dr. S. S. White:

Dear Sir,—In accordance with your request, made last summer at Detroit, I send you the model of a Lamp and Warm-Water Cup, originally devised by my former associate, Dr. J. C. Dean, of Chicago, and successively improved upon by Dr. C. F. Ives and myself.

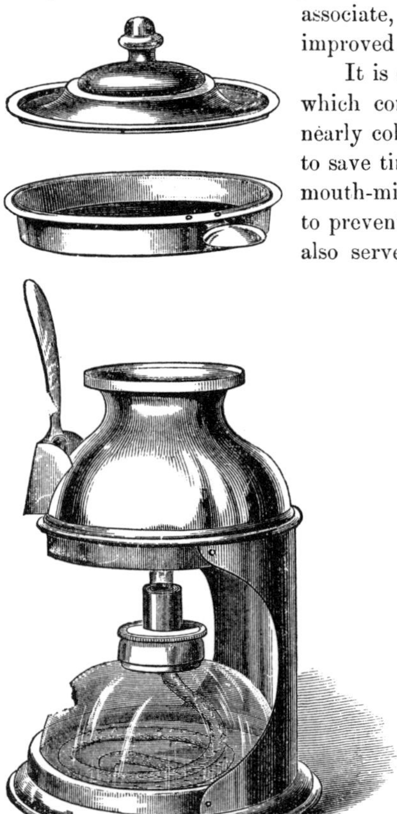

It is designed to save the great suffering to the patient which comes from the common practice of using cold or nearly cold water for syringing out cavities of decay, and to save time and annoyance to the operator, by keeping his mouth-mirror always at the temperature of the body, so as to prevent condensation of the breath upon the glass. It also serves without alteration of the flame for warming gutta-percha on a separate porcelain plate. It may be used as an Annealing Lamp when it is only designed to warm the gold; but for heating to redness I prefer to use another Lamp, so as to let the flame in this one remain always the same. By this means I am constantly supplied with warm water of the same temperature for mouth use, and my mirror is always ready; while the Lamp requires to be filled only once a week if used for this purpose alone.

The Wick should be kept level with the top of the Tube when in use.

Yours very truly,

E. A. Bogue.

The apparatus is of Brass, Nickel-Plated. The Lamp is of Glass, with Nickel-Plated Collar and Tube. Over the Tube is a Screw-Collar with a milled edge, by which, with a touch of the finger, it can be raised or lowered to control the flame as desired. The Tube is provided with a cover, to prevent evaporation of the alcohol when the Lamp is not in use.

Price . . . . each $7.50

COTTON WOOD

Recommended by those who have long used it as a superior Wood for carrying polishing powders; possessing the advantage, when wet, of retaining the powder; very useful in polishing fillings and teeth after the removal of tartar. Put up in packages of one dozen strips eight inches in length by a quarter of an inch square.

Price . . . . per doz. 20 cents.

GOLD FOIL ANNEALING LAMP.

OUR OWN DESIGN.

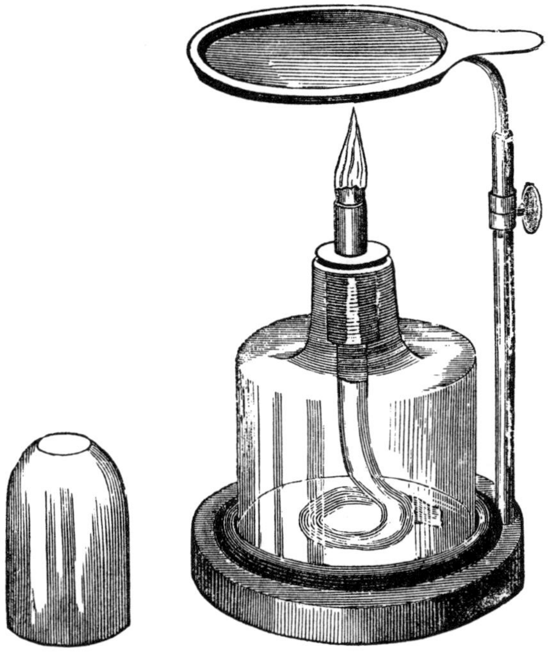

The Cut represents the Lamp half size. Base of Ebony, and Annealing Tray of German Silver.

Some of the advantages claimed for the Annealing Lamp, are: By its use all soft Gold Foils are made adhesive.

Any amount of heat sufficient to make the Foil adhesive can be produced without fear of melting the edges.

It does not make the Foil hard and unyielding, as is often the case when passed through a flame, but leaves it soft as before annealing.

It keeps the Foil warm during the operation, thereby preserving its adhesive quality in the most perfect condition.

The adhesive quality is imparted to the Foil *after it is prepared for the cavity*, obviating the annoyance often experienced, especially in warm weather, in having its adhesiveness partially destroyed by the moisture of the fingers.

Price, complete . . . . each $2.50

HOLLY STRIPS.

For polishing Gold Fillings in approximal cavities. Put up in rolls.

Price . . . . per roll $0.16
" . . . . per doz. 1.75

CUP FOR HEATING GUTTA-PERCHA FILLINGS.

DEVISED BY DR. FLAGG.

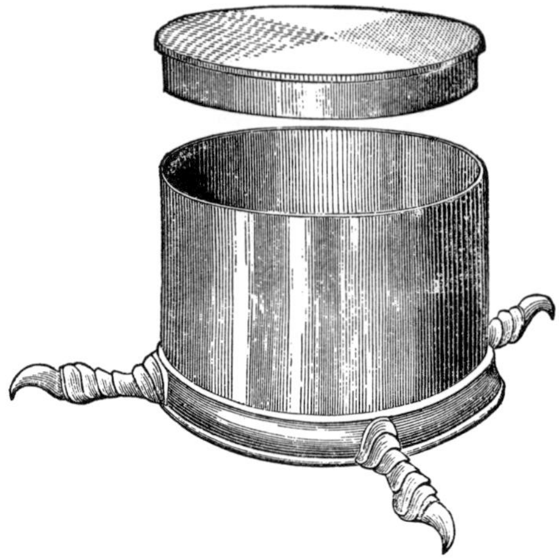

To be filled with water, and warmed over a Spirit Lamp. Cup of Brass, Silver- or Nickel-Plated. The Cut represents a size adapted to our Annealing Lamp. Another variety is made with longer arms, to fit a circle 4⅛ inches in diameter.

Price $1.00

PHYSICIANS' AND DENTISTS' DROP TUBE.

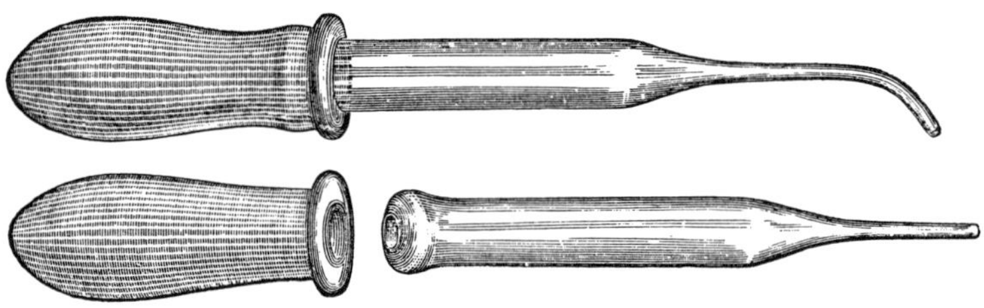

A Drop Tube adapted to the wants of the Physician in the use of preparations for the eye, etc., and for the Dentist for the convenient employment of iodine, creasote, acids, etc., especially for the liquid preparations which accompany plastic materials for filling teeth. The Tubes are of glass, with a swell at the end to prevent the Bulbs, which are of rubber, from slipping off. Can be operated at will by pressure of the Bulb between the thumb and finger.

Price . . . . each 10 cents.

POLISHING PUTTY.

Oxide of Tin, called Polishing Putty, used for polishing natural teeth after filing, chiseling, or scraping.

Price . . . . per box 20 cents.

CORUNDUM TAPE.

A superior article of Corundum Tape. This saves much time, and for many fillings is superior to Files for finishing.

Per piece of two yards . . . . 8 cents.

WATER-PROOF POLISHING TAPE.

Covered with a variety of reducing and polishing powders for finishing fillings, held in contact with the Tape, by a preparation *which is not dissolved by moisture.* There are five grades, No. 1 being the finest, and No. 5 the coarsest. Put up in pieces of two yards each.

Price . . . . per piece 10 cents.

SILEX AND BUCK-HORN TAPE.

Designed to follow the Corundum Tape. A finely polished surface can be obtained by its use.

Per piece of two yards . . . . 8 cents.

PIVOT WOOD.

50 Sticks in a box, assorted sizes . . . . per box 50 cents.

SPUNK FOR DRYING OUT CAVITIES.

A superior article for drying out cavities and absorbing saliva while filling teeth.

It is very valuable in absorbing the moisture in sensitive teeth, as the patient does not experience the pain produced by the application of paper or cotton.

Price . . . . per ounce 20 cents.

FRENCH BIBULOUS PAPER.

Direct importation from Paris.

Price	per ream	$3.00
"	per quire	.20
Bibulous Paper Pellets, for drying cavities, 900 in Box . . .	per box	.25

JAPANESE BIBULOUS PAPER.

Extra fine quality, and free from dust.

We commend this Bibulous Paper as the best article we have ever seen, and far superior to that generally offered in the market.

Price	per 100 sheets	$0.80
"	per 500 "	3.00

PREPARED COTTON FOR DENTAL PURPOSES.

A good article of Cotton, adapted especially for a reliable absorbent for drying cavities preparatory to filling teeth.

Price . . . . per package 20 cents.

SPONGOID.

A SUPERIOR ABSORBENT.

This material is prepared expressly for the use of Dentists. In its manufacture only the best materials are used, and these so thoroughly deprived of all native and other impurities as to produce an article colorless, free from grit, and chemically pure.

Put up in boxes containing one dozen sheets, 3 inches by 4 inches each.

Price . . . . per box 40 cents.

FRENCH RUBBER TUBING.

OUR OWN IMPORTATION.

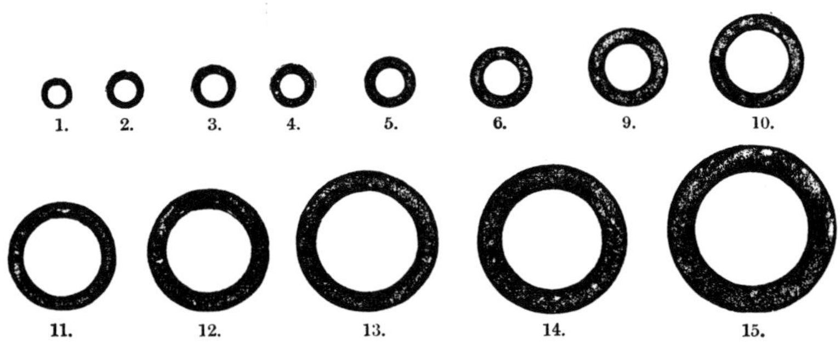

For regulating teeth and for conducting liquids or gases.

Nos. 1 to 7	per foot	20 cents.
" 9 to 11	"	25 "
" 12 to 14	"	40 "
No. 15	"	60 "

PURE RUBBER FOR SEPARATING TEETH.

Price . . . . per ounce 38 cents.

Dental Cases.

Having devoted special attention to the manufacture of Dental Cases, our arrangements are so complete as to afford unequaled facilities for supplying the demands of the Profession in variety, quality, and price.

Our assortment includes Rosewood, Walnut, Mahogany, and Leather-covered. They are mounted with Brass, or German Silver, so as to secure the best appearance with the greatest amount of strength, and are polished and finished throughout in a workmanlike manner. Special styles made and fitted to order with Drawers, Trays, or Apartments for Instruments, Vials, etc.

We give descriptions of nine of the Cases in most general use, and are prepared to furnish others still more elaborate at prices ranging from Four Hundred to One Thousand Dollars.

Our plan of affixing the price to each article in the list enables the purchaser to estimate the aggregate value of a Case and its contents, and to direct any variations from the ordinary styles that he may deem desirable.

NOTE.—When an order for a Case is received, the Instruments desired are selected specially for it, and blocks carved to fit each of them. The blocks are then fastened into the Case and covered with Velvet, so as to make a uniform lining throughout. *After this it is impossible to make changes, or add other Instruments, without spoiling the Velvet.* The selection of Instruments should therefore be carefully made when the order is given, and any article which it is desired to have in the Case should be sent at the same time, that its shape may be carved in the wood before covering.

If desired, a Tray or Drawer may be left without lining, and the Velvet furnished for covering it. The purchaser can then have it fitted to suit himself; but this plan we have not found satisfactory. As a rule, the better way is to have all the work done at the same time and place.

OPERATING CASE, No. 1.

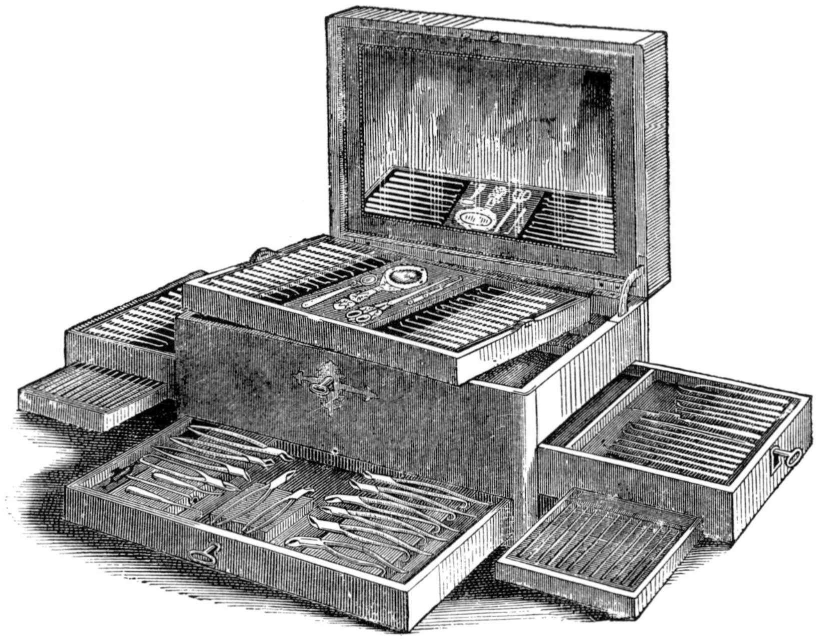

*6	$\frac{5}{8}$ inch Cameo Handle Scalers, Gold Plated Ferrules	$70.00
18	" " " " Pluggers and Burnishers, Gold Plated Ferrules	
1	Large Pearl Hand Mirror, Gold Mounted, No. 4	16.75
1	Pearl Mouth Glass, Stone set, " " 10	5.00
1	Pair Pearl Handle Foil Shears, " " 34	11.75
1	Pearl Handle Gum Lancet, " " 24	3.00
1	" Tongue Holder, Stone set, " " 21	1.50
2	Dozen large Steel Excavators, Octagon Handle, File-cut, $3.60 per doz. .	7.20
2	" $\frac{5}{8}$ inch Ivory Handle Pluggers and Scalers, German Silver Ferrules, at $24.00 per doz.	48.00
1	Improved File Carrier, Ivory Handle	3.00
1	Foil Carrier and Plugger combined	1.75
1	Revolving Head Drill Socket, Ivory	2.25
18	Socket Burs, at $2.70 per doz.	4.05
6	" Drills, at $2.30 "	1.15
2	Pairs Forceps, Upper Molar, R. and L , Octagon Joint, Ex. Quality, No. 18	6.00
1	Pair " Lower Molar, " " " 15	3.00
1	" " " Bicuspid, " " " 21	3.00
1	" " Upper " " " " 11	3.00
1	" " " Incisor, " " " 13	3.00

1	Pair Forceps, Lower Incisor,	Octagon Joint,	Ex. Quality,	No.	9	. .	$3.00
1	" Dentes Sapientiæ,	"	"	"	10	. .	3.00
1	" Excising,	"	"	"	12	. .	3.00
1	" Root, Straight,	"	"	"	1	. .	3.00
1	" " Curved,	"	"	"	3	. .	3.00
1	Pair Hullihen's Screw Forceps,	"	"			. . . .	4.00
2	Elevators, Ivory Handles, at $2.00 each						4.00
1	Improved Key, Ivory Handle						3.00
	Extra fine Rosewood Case, 20 in. by 13½ in. by 8 in., full Brass-bound Corners and Edges, with five Drawers at the sides and front, with two Trays at the top, one with Compartments for Foil, Files, Teeth, etc., and with a Mirror in the Lid to reflect the Instruments in the top Tray. Lined with extra heavy Silk Velvet						85.00
							$304.**

* The same Case, with ⅝ inch Pearl Handle Pluggers, Burnishers and Scalers, $340.00.

OPERATING CASE, No. 2.

*6	½ inch Cameo Handle Scalers, Gold Plated Ferrules						$60.00
18	" " Pluggers and Burnishers, Gold Plated Ferrules						
1	Large Pearl Hand Mirror, Gold Mounted,			No.	9		11.00
1	Pearl Mouth Mirror,	"		"	10½		4.75
1	Pair Pearl Handle Foil Shears, Gold Mounted,			No.	38		11.25
1	Pearl Handle Gum Lancet,	"		"	25		2.75
2	Dozen large Octagon Steel Excavators, File-cut Handle, at $3.60 per doz.						7.20
1	" Octagon Steel Pluggers, ¼ in. File-cut Handle						7.20
1	Improved File Carrier, Ivory Handle						3.00
1	Plugger and Foil Carrier combined						1.75
1	Revolving Head Drill Socket, Ivory						2.25
18	Socket Burs, at $2.70 per doz.						4.05
6	" Drills, at $2.30 "						1.15
1	Silver Mounted Glass Syringe						4.50
2	Pairs Forceps, Upper Molar, R. and L.,	Oct. Joint,	Ex. Quality,	No.	18	.	6.00
1	Pair " Lower Molar,	"	"	"	15	.	3.00
1	" " " Bicuspid,	"	"	"	21	.	3.00
1	" " Upper "	"	"	"	11	.	3.00
1	" " " Incisor,	"	"	"	13	.	3.00
1	" " Lower "	"	"	"	9	.	3.00
1	" " Dentes Sapientiæ,	"	"	"	10	.	3.00
1	" " Excising,	"	"	"	12	.	3.00
1	" " Root, Straight,	"	"	"	1	.	3.00
1	" " " Curved,	"	"	"	3	.	3.00
1	Pair Hullihen's Screw Forceps,	"	"			. . . .	4.00
2	Elevators, Ivory Handle, at $2.00						4.00

1	Improved Key, Ivory Handle	$3.00
	Fine Brass-bound Rosewood Case, 18½ in. by 12½ in. by 7 in., with three Trays and Drawer for Forceps. One of the Trays divided into Compartments for Foil, Files, Teeth, etc. Plate Glass Mirror in the Lid, and lined with heavy Silk Velvet. (See Cut for Case, page 209.) .	55.00
		$219.**

* The same Case, with ½ inch Pearl Handle Pluggers, Burnishers and Scalers, $240.00.

OPERATING CASE, No. 3.

*6	½ inch Cameo Handle Scalers, Gold Plated Ferrules	$60.00
18	" " Pluggers and Burnishers, Gold Plated Ferrules	
1	Pearl Hand Mirror, Gold Mounted, No. 18	7.60
1	" Mouth " " " 19½	2.50
1	" Handle Gum Lancet, Gold Mounted, No. 25	2.75
1	Pair Steel Foil Shears	2.00
2	Dozen Steel Excavators, Octagon Handle, at $2.70 per doz. . . .	5.40
1	" Small Steel Pluggers, Octagon Taper Handle, File-cut . . .	6.00
1	Improved File Carrier, Ivory Handle	3.00
1	Foil Carrier and Plugger combined	1.75
18	Socket Burs, at $2.70 per doz.	4.05
6	" Drills, at $2.30 "	1.15
1	Revolving Head Drill Socket, Ivory	2.25
2	Pairs Forceps, Upper Molar, R. and L., Oct. Joint, Ex. Quality, No. 18 .	6.00
1	Pair " Lower " " " " 15 .	3.00
1	" " " Bicuspid, " " " 21 .	3.00
1	" " Upper " " " " 11 .	3.00
1	" " " Incisor, " " " 13 .	3.00
1	" " Lower " " " " 9 .	3.00
1	" " Dentes Sapientiæ, " " " 10 .	3.00
1	" " Excising, " " " 12 .	3.00
1	" " Root, Straight " " " 1 .	3.00
1	" " " Curved, " " " 3 .	3.00
1	Pair Hullihen's Screw Forceps, " " . .	4.00
2	Elevators, Octagon Ebony Handle, at $1.50 each	3.00
1	Improved Key, "	2.50
	Fine Brass-bound Rosewood Case, 18½ in. by 12½ in. by 7 in., with three Trays, one of them stationary and divided into Compartments for Foil, Teeth, etc., and Drawer for Forceps. Lined with heavy Silk Velvet. (See Cut for Case, page 209.)	50.00
		$190.**

* The same Case, with ½ inch Pearl Handle Pluggers, Burnishers and Scalers, $211.00.

OPERATING CASE, No. 4.

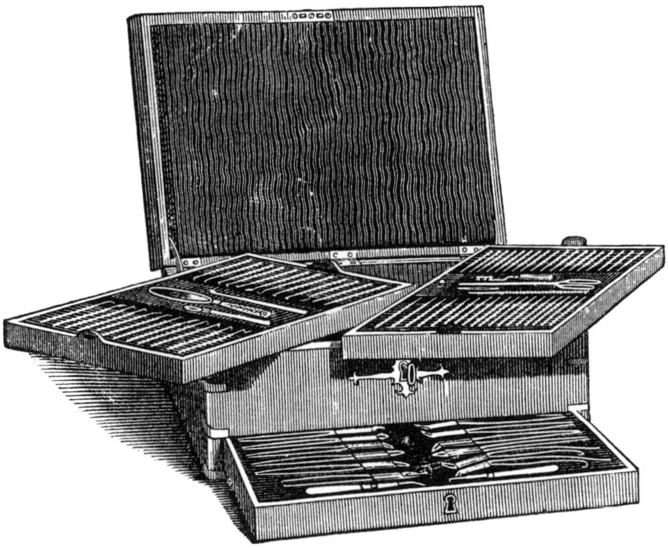

*6	⅝ inch Octagon Ivory Handle Scalers, German Silver Ferrules . .	$48.00
18	" " " " Pluggers and Burnishers, German Silver Ferrules . .	
1	Pearl Hand Mirror, No. 16	6.00
1	" Mouth Glass, " 19	2.00
1	" Gum Lancet, " 28	1.75
1	Pair Steel Foil Shears	2.00
2	Dozen Steel Excavators, Octagon Handle, File-cut, at $3.60 per doz. .	7.20
1	" small Steel Pluggers, Octagon Taper File-cut Handle . . .	6.00
1	Improved File Carrier, Ivory Handle	3.00
1	Pair Spring Plug Pliers	.60
18	Socket Burs, at $2.70 per doz.	4.05
6	" Drills, at $2.30 "	1.15
1	Revolving Head Drill Socket, Ivory	2.25
2	Pairs Forceps, Upper Molar, R. and L., Octagon Joint, Ex. Quality, No. 18	6.00
1	Pair " Lower " " " " 15	3.00
1	" " " Bicuspid, " " " 21	3.00
1	" " Upper " " " " 11	3.00
1	" " " Incisor, " " " 13	3.00
1	" " Lower " " " " 14	3.00
1	" " Dentes Sapientiæ, " " " 10	3.00
1	" " Excising, " " " 12	3.00
1	" " Root, Straight, " " " 1	3.00
1	" " " Curved, " " " 3	3.00

1	Pair Hullihen's Screw Forceps, Octagon Joint, Ex. Quality	$4.00
2	Elevators, Octagon Ebony Handle, at $1.50 each	3.00
	Fine Brass-bound Rosewood Case, 18½ in. by 12½ in. by 7 in., with three Trays, one of them stationary and divided into Compartments for Foil, Teeth, etc., and Drawer for Forceps. Lined with Silk Finish Cotton Velvet	36.00
		$160.**

* This Case, Lined with Heavy Silk Velvet, and Mirror in Lid, $180.00.

OPERATING CASE, No. 5.

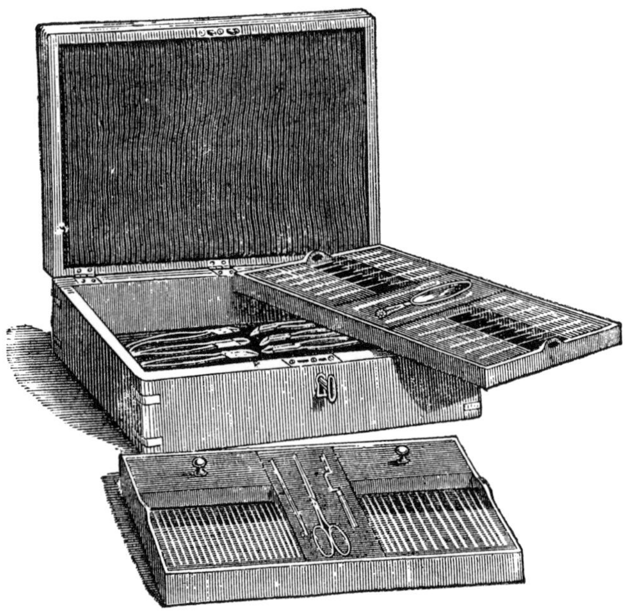

6	½ inch Ivory Handle Scalers, German Silver Ferrules	$40.00 (for these three lines)
17	" " Pluggers and Burnishers, German Silver Ferrules	
1	" " Socket for Drills, " "	
1	Pearl Hand Mirror, No. 15	4.75
1	" Mouth " " 19	2.00
1	" Lancet, " 28	1.75
1	Pair Steel Foil Shears	2.00
2	Dozen Steel Excavators, Octagon Handle, at $2.70 per doz.	5.40
1	Dozen Octagon Steel Pluggers, ¼ inch File-cut Handle	7.20
1	Improved File Carrier, Ivory Handle	3.00
1	Pair Spring Plug Pliers	.60

18 Socket Burs, at $2.70 per doz.	$4.05
6 " Drills, at $2.30 "	1.15
2 Pairs Forceps, Upper Molar, R. and L., Oval Joint, No. 18	4.00
1 Pair " Lower " " " 15	2.00
1 " " " Bicuspid and Incisor, " " 14	2.00
1 " " Upper " " " " 11	2 00
1 " " Dentes Sapientiæ, " " 10	2 00
1 " " Excising, " " 12	2.00
1 " " Root, Straight, " " 1	2.00
1 " " " Half Curved, " " 2	2.00
1 " " Alveolar, Half Curved, " " 39	2.00
2 Elevators, Octagon Ebony Handle, at $1.50 each	3.00
1 Stump Screw, " "	1.50
Brass-bound Rosewood Case, 16½ in. by 11 in. by 4½ in., with two Trays, and space for Forceps. Lined with Silk Finish Cotton Velvet	28.00
	$124.**

OPERATING CASE, No. 6.

6 ⅝ inch Bleached Bone Handle Scalers, German Silver Ferrules 17 " " Pluggers and Burnishers, Ger. Silver Ferrules 1 " " Socket for Drills, " "	$24.00
1 Pearl Hand Mirror, No. 15	4.75
1 " Mouth Glass, " 19	2.00
1 " Gum Lancet, " 28	1.75
18 Socket Burs, at $2.70 per doz.	4.05
6 " Drills, at $2.30 "	1.15
1 Dozen Steel Excavators, Octagon Handle	2.70
1 Improved File Carrier, Ivory Handle	3.00
1 Pair Spring Plug Pliers	.60
2 Pairs Forceps, Upper Molar, R. and L., Oval Joint, No. 18	4.00
1 Pair " Lower " " " 15	2.00
1 " " Upper Bicuspid and Incisor, " " 11	2.00
1 " " Lower " " " " " 14	2.00
1 " " Root, Straight, " " 1	2.00
1 " " " Half Curved, " " 2	2.00
1 " " Excising, " " 12	2.00
1 " " Dentes Sapientiæ, " " 10	2.00
2 Elevators, Octagon Ebony Handle, at $1.50 each	3.00
1 Improved Key, " "	2.50
Brass-bound Rosewood Case, 16½ in. by 11 in. by 4½ in., two Trays, and space for Forceps. Lined with Silk Finish Cotton Velvet	28.00
	$95.**

N.B.—A pair of Forceps may be substituted for the Key, if desired.

OPERATING CASE, No. 7.

6	⅝ inch Bleached Bone Handle Scalers, German Silver Ferrules	$24.00
17	" " Pluggers and Burnishers, Ger. Silver Ferrules	
1	" " Socket for Drills, " "	
1	Pearl Mouth Glass, No. 19	2.00
1	" Gum Lancet, " 28	1.75
1	Rosewood Hand Mirror, 4½ inch	.75
18	Socket Burs, at $2.70 per dozen	4.05
6	" Drills, at $2.30 "	1.15
18	Steel Excavators, Octagon Handle, at $2.70 per dozen	4.05
1	Pair Spring Plug Pliers	.60
2	Pairs Forceps, Upper Molar, R. and L., Oval Joint, No. 18	4.00
1	Pair " Lower " " " 15	2.00
1	" " " Bicuspid, " " 14	2.00
1	" " Upper Bicuspid and Incisor, " " 11	2.00
1	" " Root, Straight, " " 1	2.00
1	" " " Half Curved, " " 2	2.00
1	" " Excising, " " 12	2.00
2	Elevators, Round Ebony Handle, at 75 cents each	1.50
1	Improved Key, "	2.50
	Brass-bound Mahogany Case, 16½ in. by 11 in. by 4½ in., two Trays, and space for Forceps. Lined with Silk Finish Cotton Velvet	24.00
		$82.**

N. B.—A pair of Forceps may be substituted for a Key, if desired.

OPERATING CASE, No. 8.

11	½ inch Bone Handle Scalers, Burnishers, and Pluggers, Ger. Sil. Ferrules	$9.00
1	" " Socket for Drills " "	
12	Large Steel Pluggers, Octagon File-cut Handle, ⅜ inch	9.00
1	Pearl Mouth Glass, No. 19	2.00
1	" Gum Lancet, " 28	1.75
12	Socket Burs	2.70
6	" Drills, at $2.30 per dozen	1.15
1	Dozen Steel Excavators, Octagon Handle	2.70
2	Pairs Forceps, Upper Molar, R. and L., Oval Joint, No. 18	4.00
1	Pair " Lower " " " 15	2.00
1	" " " Bicuspid and Incisor, " " 14	2.00
1	" " Upper " " " " 11	2.00
1	" " Root, Half Curved, " " 2	2.00
1	" " Excising, " " 12	2.00
2	Elevators, Round Ebony Handle, at 75 cents each	1.50
1	Improved Key, "	2.50
	Brass-bound Mahogany Case, 16½ in. by 11 in. by 4½ in., two Trays and space for Forceps. Lined with Silk Finish Cotton Velvet	24.00
		$70.**

N. B.—A pair of Forceps may be substituted for the Key, if desired.

OPERATING CASE, No. 9.

A practical outfit for Operative Dentistry; in a compact form, selected by a first-class Operator. To be added to or curtailed, as may be desired. Designed for a Traveling or Country Dentist.

A	Brass-bound Rosewood Case, 18½ in. by 12½ in. by 7 in.	$38.00
1	Five-inch Rosewood Plate Glass Hand Mirror	.85
1	Pearl Mouth Mirror, No. 11	1.50
1	" Cheek Holder or Spatula, No. 31	.75
1	Pair Cast Steel Foil Scissors	1.00
1	Rubber Syringe, Silver Point	1.25
1	Universal Porte Polisher, and Box Corundum Points	1.40
1	Half Round Corundum File	.25
1	Arkansas Stone for sharpening	.50
18	Five-eighths Inch Ebony Handle Pluggers	18.00
12	One-quarter Inch File-cut " "	7.20
12	Three-sixteenths Inch Octagon Handle Steel Pluggers	4.00
15	Dr. Atkinson's Pluggers, assorted, suitable for Foil, Sponge, or Shred Gold, at $5.40 per dozen	6.75
1	Lignum Vitæ Mallet	.30
12	One-quarter Inch File-cut Handle Amalgam Pluggers and Burnishers	7.90
2	" " " " Burnishers	1.20
3	" " " " Chisels	1.80
3	" " " " Scalers	1 80
1	Set of 24 Nerve Extractors and Root Fillers, Drawn and Spring Temper, Arrington's	6.00
24	Plain Octagon Handle Excavators	5.40
12	" " Burs	2.70
6	" " Extra Fine-cut Burs	1.60
2	Pivot Drills, Octagon Handle	.45
2	Nerve Cavity Drills, Spear Point	.45
1	Taper Steel Handle Plug-Finishing Bur	.75
3	Molar Files, assorted	.75
3	Bicuspid Files, assorted	.50
12	Separating Files, assorted	1.00
6	Flat Oval Plug-Finishing Files, assorted	1.00
6	Double end Plug-Finishing Files, assorted	1.20
3	Stump Files, assorted	.50
1	Foil Carrier and Plugger combined	1.75
1	Pair Small Flat Nose Pliers	.40
1	Bur Thimble, Hinged	.50
1	Extension Thimble, Vulcanized Rubber	.40
1	Tongue Holder, Flagg's	2.00
1	Lip Protector	.50
1	Wedge Cutter, Polished Steel	3.00

10	Pairs Octagon Joint Forceps, S. S. White's Best Quality . . .	$30.00
3	Elevators (Hook, Punch, and Screw), Octagon Ebony Handle . . .	4.50
1	Gum Lancet	.60
1	Pair Abscess Lancets, Octagon Steel Handle	.75
6	Pieces each Cotton and Orange Wood	.12
2	" " Corundum and Silex Tape	.32
1	Box each Pumice and Silex	.20
1	Vial each Creasote, Perchloride of Iron, and Nerve Paste . . .	1.00
1	Oz. Rubber Dam for keeping Cavities dry	.50
6	Inches assorted French Rubber Tubing, for regulating	.10
1	Book Gold Foil, Globe . . . . (say)	4.25
1	" Tin "	.50
1	Oz. Townsend's Amalgam	2.00
1	Mercury Holder, filled	.50
¼	Oz. Hill's Stopping (for Temporary Fillings)	1.25
50	Assorted Pivot Teeth	4.00
1	Box Pivot Wood	.50
1	Piece Ivory for Pivot Gauge	.75
1	Box selected Asbestos (used as a non-conductor under Fillings). . .	.10
1	Quire Bibulous Paper (for drying Cavities)	.20
1	Oz Spunk (for drying Cavities)	.20
½	Dozen Linen Napkins, each, large and small	.80
1	" Common Tooth Brushes	1.25
	Chamois Skins for Instruments	1.20
		$181.00

Cases can be furnished at still lower prices than No. 8, but they do not as a rule give satisfaction. The variety of Instruments is limited, and the quality necessarily inferior, much of the outlay being in the Case and fitting.

Those who wish a set of Instruments at a small cost, would do well to make a selection from the Catalogue, and have them inclosed in a Morocco-covered Box or a neat Rolling Case.

ROLLING CASES.

Rolling Cases for Instruments, lined with Chamois,	5 Spaces . .	each	$1.50
" " " "	7 " . .	"	1.75
" " " "	9 " . .	"	2.00
" " " "	12 " . .	"	2.25
" " " "	15 " . .	"	3.00
" " " "	20 " . .	"	4.00

Any other size made to order.

Valises made of Sole Leather, with Iron Frames, for Dental Cases, from $7.00 to $12.00

PHYSICIANS' OR DENTISTS' PORTABLE EXTRACTING CASE.

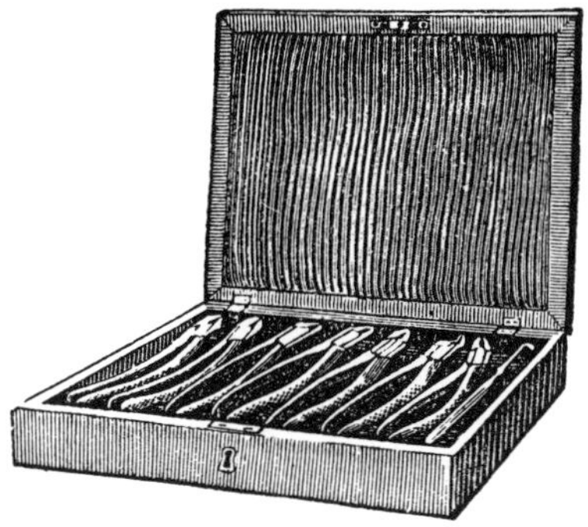

Consisting of 7 pairs of Forceps, Harris's patterns. This set is sufficient for all ordinary cases of extraction. Put up with Ebony Handle Gum Lancet in a neat, strong Mahogany Box, with lock and key. Outside measurements of Case, 11½ in. by 8½ in. by 2 in.

Octagon Joint, S. S. White's Best Quality	$26.50
" " " Nickel-Plated	30.00
" " Plain Line	23.80
Oval Joint	20.00
Knuckle Joint, English Style	18.00

U. S. ARMY AND NAVY EXTRACTING CASE.

Physicians' Portable Extracting Case, consisting of 11 pairs S. S. White's Best Octagon Joint Forceps, 2 Round Ebony Handle Elevators, and one Ebony Handle Gum Lancet, in substantial Morocco-covered Case, neat Valise form, with lock and key, such as has been adopted by the U. S. Government for Army and Navy Surgeons. Case complete as above	$41.00
The same, with Nickel-Plated Forceps	46.50
" " Plain Line Forceps	37.70

EMPTY DENTAL CASES.

LINED AND FITTED, READY FOR INSTRUMENTS.

Mahogany; 2 Trays, and space for Forceps, 16½ inches long, 11 inches wide, and 4½ inches deep, lined with French Cotton Velvet. (See Cut, page 210)	$24.00
Rosewood; same size, lined with French Cotton Velvet	28.00
Rosewood; 1 Drawer and 3 Trays, one stationary and divided into Compartments: 18½ inches long, 12½ inches wide, and 7 inches deep; lined with French Cotton Velvet. (See Cut, page 209)	36.00
Rosewood; same size and description, lined with extra heavy Silk Velvet	50.00
Rosewood; 5 Drawers and 2 Trays, one stationary and divided into Compartments: 20 inches long, 13½ inches wide, and 8 inches deep, with heavy Brass Mountings, Corners and Edges; lined with extra heavy Silk Velvet, with Mirror in Lid. (See Cut, page 206)	85.00

STUDENTS' THREE-TRAY CASE.

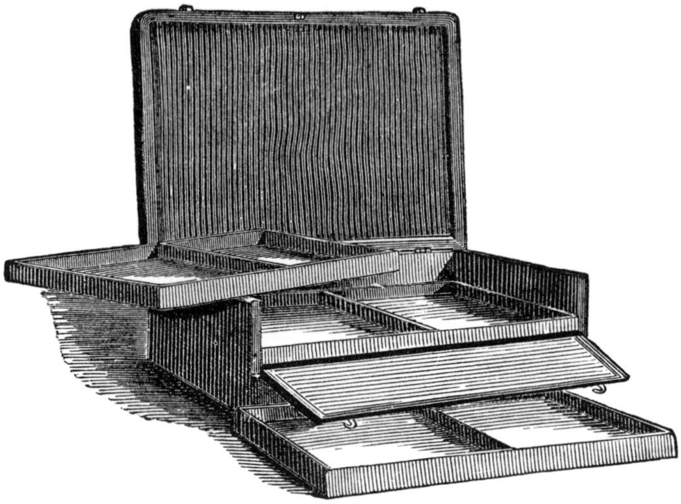

We offer Three-Tray Cases in the following varieties. They are lined with Cotton Velvet, and provided with lock and key.

Morocco Covered,	10	inches long,	6	inches wide,	4	inches deep	. . . .	$4.75
"	11	"	7	"	5	"	. . . .	6.00
"	12	"	9	"	5	"	. . . .	7.25

Same sizes, Mahogany, Varnished, at $6.00, $7.50, and $9.00.

Walnut Varnished,	10	inches long,	6	inches wide,	4	inches deep	. . . .	5.00
"	10½	"	7	"	4	"	. . . .	6.50
"	12	"	8	"	4½	"	. . . .	8.00

The above are outside measurements.

STUDENTS' PORTABLE CASE.

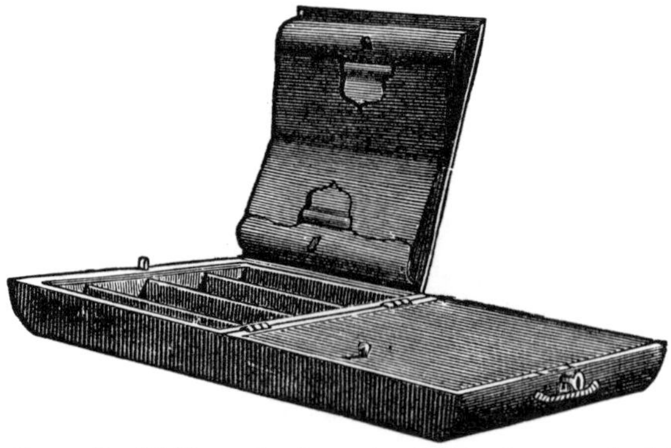

Made in the form of a Valise; the frame is of Wood, covered with Morocco. Outside measurement, when closed, 12 inches long, 9 inches wide, and 3½ inches deep. The case is divided in the center, each half having a cover to protect the Instruments. Lined with Cotton Velvet.

Price $12.00

TEETH CASES, FOR ARTIFICIAL TEETH.

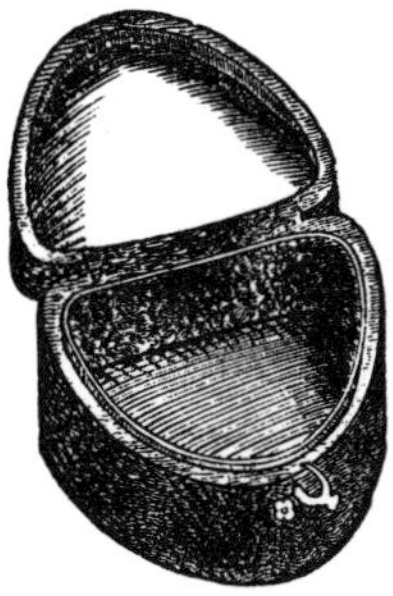

Half Oval.

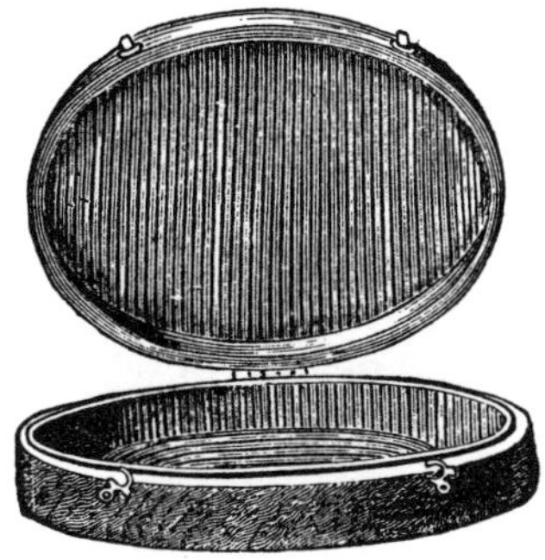

Oval.

Half Oval, Satin and Silk Velvet lined, 3¼ inches in length by 2½ inches in width by 1⅛ inches in depth, Brass Hinge	each	$0.65
Half Oval, Cotton Velvet lined, 3 inches in length by 2½ inches in width by 1½ inches in depth, Leather Hinge	each	.35
Half Oval, Cotton Velvet lined, 3½ inches in length by 2¾ inches in width by 1½ inches in depth, Leather Hinge	each	.35
Half Oval Card-Board Boxes, Paper lined, 3 inches in length by 2½ inches in width by 1⅛ inches in depth	per doz.	1.75
Oval, Satin and Silk Velvet lined, 4½ inches in length by 3¼ inches in width by 1¼ inches in depth, Brass Hinge	each	.85
Oval Card-Board Boxes, Paper lined, 3¾ inches in length by 3 inches in width by 1 inch in depth	per doz.	2.00

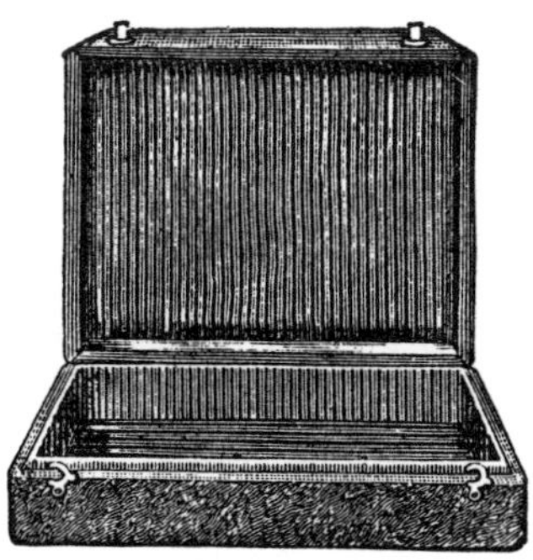

Oblong.

Oblong, Satin and Silk Velvet lined, 4½ inches in length by 3½ inches in width by 1⅜ inches in depth, Brass Hinge	each	.85
Oblong Card-Board Boxes, Paper lined, 4 inches in length by 3 inches in width by 1¼ inches in depth	per doz.	2.00
Oblong Card-Board Boxes, Paper lined, 3 inches in length by 2¼ inches in width by 1 inch in depth	per doz.	1.50

The above are outside measurements.

Pearl Goods.

PEARL HAND MIRRORS.

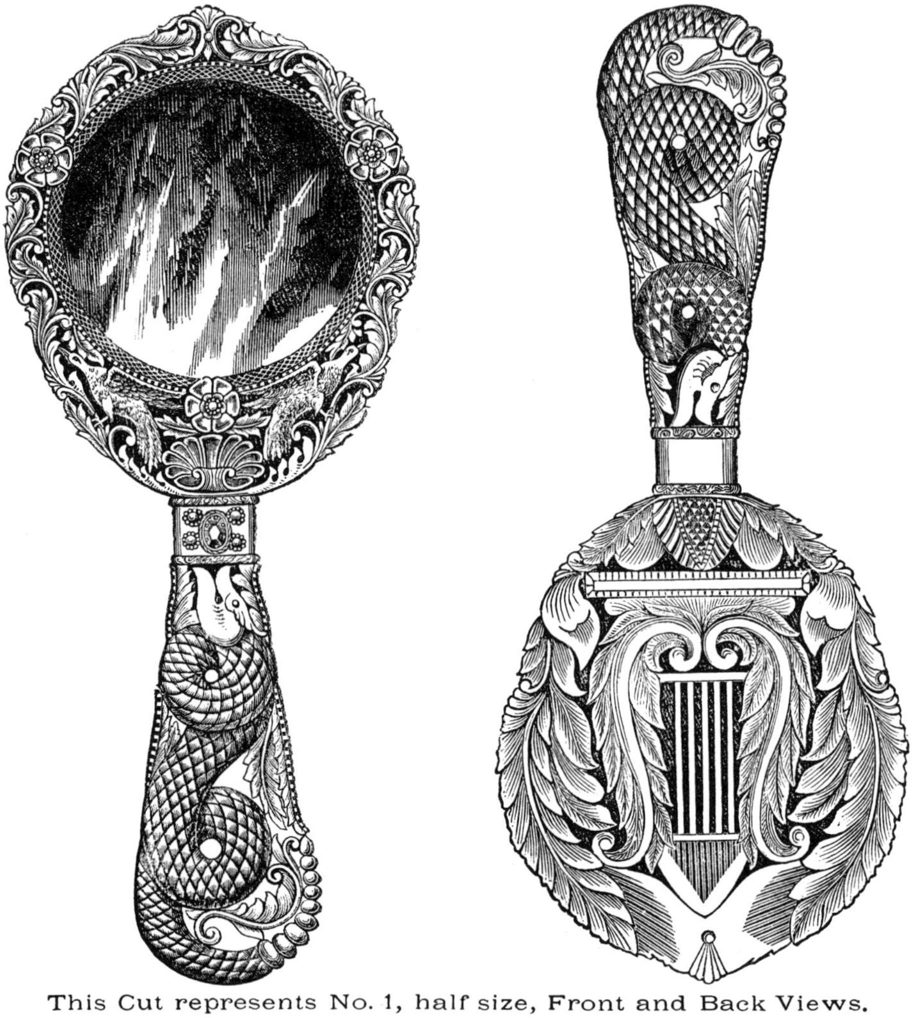

This Cut represents No. 1, half size, Front and Back Views.

Having unequaled facilities for the manufacture of articles in this line, our assortment is the most extensive in the world.

No. 1.	Gold Mounted, Saw pierced, Stone set, Carved on both sides	each	$28.00
" 2.	" " " " "	"	23.00
" 3.	" " "	"	18.25
" 4.	" " "	"	16.75
" 5.	" Setting in Ferrule	"	7.60

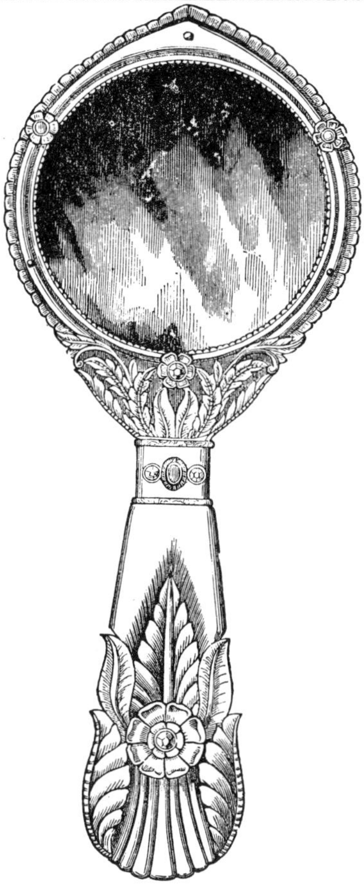

This Cut represents No. 8,
$9\frac{1}{2}$ in. long and 4 in. wide.

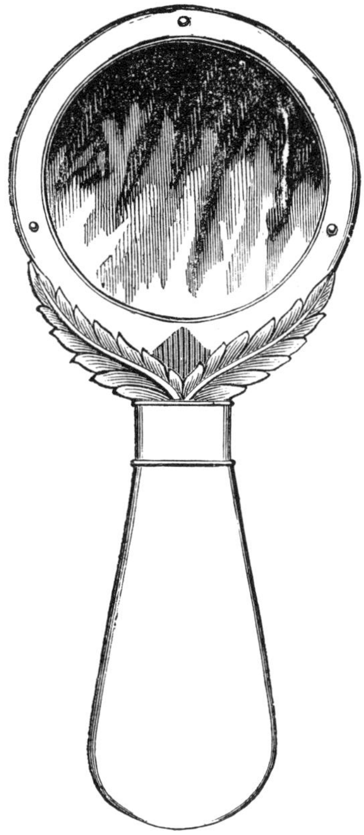

This Cut represents No. 15,
half size.

No.	$5\frac{1}{2}$.	Gold Mounted, Setting, 3 Rosettes	each $8.50
"	6.	" without Setting	" 6.75
"	7, 8.	" Saw pierced, Setting, 3 Rosettes	" 14.00
"	9.	" Setting, 3 Rosettes	" 11.00
"	$9\frac{1}{2}$.	" " "	" 11.75
"	10.	" "	" 9.50
"	11.	Silver Mounted, Plain Handle	" 6.75
"	12.	Gold Mounted, large, Setting, 3 Rosettes	" 15.25
"	13, 14.	Gold or Silver Mounted, without Setting	" 10.25
"	15.	Silver Mounted, small, Plain Handle	" 4.75
"	16.	" large, "	" 6.00
"	17.	" larger, "	" 6.75
"	18.	Gold Mounted, without Setting	" 7.60
"	19.	Silver Mounted, Plain Rim	" 6.00
"	20.	" Carved Rim	" 7.25

Extra large, beautifully Carved on both sides, and Stone set, from . $50.00 to 75.00

PEARL MOUTH MIRRORS.

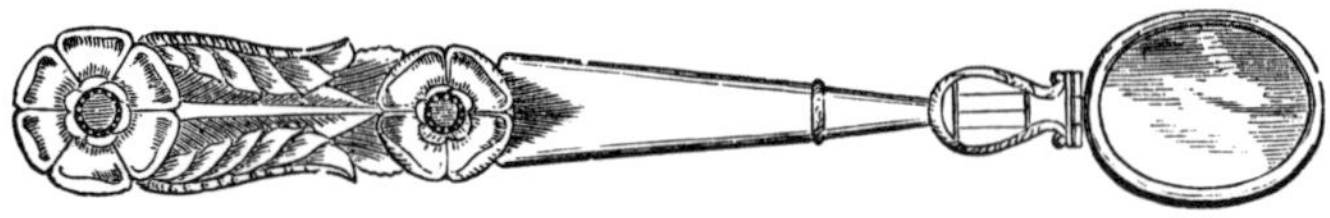

This Cut represents No. 10, half size.

No. 4.	Round Magnifying Glass, Silver Wire Shaft, Silver Mounted	each	$2.25
" 5.	Oval " " "	"	2.25
" 6.	Round, small " Silver Mounted	"	1.40
" 7.	Oval, " " "	"	1.40
" 8.	Round, Plain Glass, Pocket, Silver Mounted, with Pearl Sliding Cover for protection to glass	"	1.40
" 9.	Round, Plain Glass, Pocket, Silver Mounted, jointed to fold up	"	1.70
" 10.	Star pattern, Carved on both sides, Gold Lyre, double Glass, jointed, 2 Rosettes	"	5.00
" 10½.	Star pattern, Carved on both sides, Gold Lyre, double Glass, jointed, 1 Rosette	"	4.75

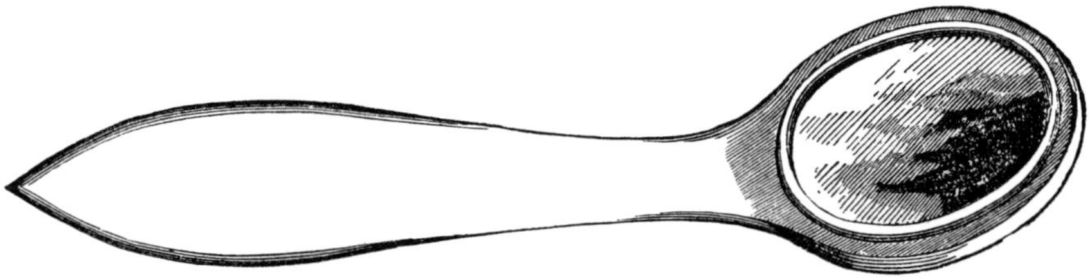

This Cut represents No. 11, full size.

No. 11.	Plain, Oval Glass, Pocket, Silver Mounted	each	$1.50
" 11½.	" " " Gold "	"	1.70

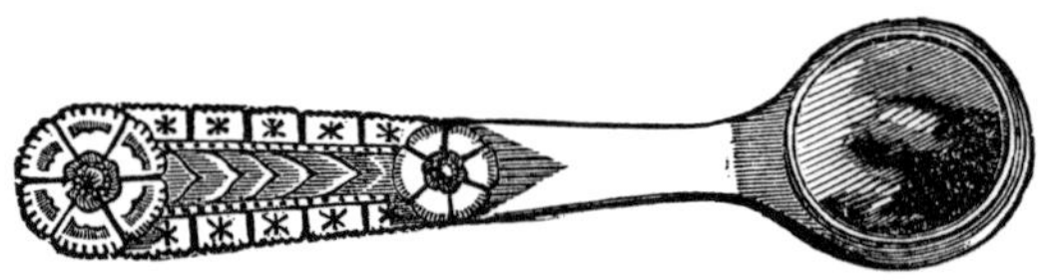

This Cut represents No. 12, half size.

No. 12.	Star pattern, Round Glass, Gold Mounted, 2 Rosettes	each	$2.25
" 12½.	" " " " 2 " Magnifying	"	2.50
" 12¾.	" Oval " " 2 " "	"	2.80
" 13.	Figured, Round Glass, Gold Mounted, 1 Rosette	"	2.00
" 13½.	" Oval " " 1 " Magnifying	"	2.50
" 13¾.	" Round " " 1 " "	"	2.25
" 14.	Dolphin, " " "	"	1.50
" 15.	" " " " Magnifying	"	2.00
" 16.	" " " Silver Mounted	"	1.50
" 17.	" Plain, Round Glass, Silver Mounted, ⅞ inch Glass	"	1.25
" 17¼.	" " " " Frame, ¾ inch Glass	"	1.25
" 17½.	" Round Magnifying Glass, Silver Frame, ¾ inch Glass	"	1.40
" 17¾.	" " " " Gold " ¾ "	"	1.60

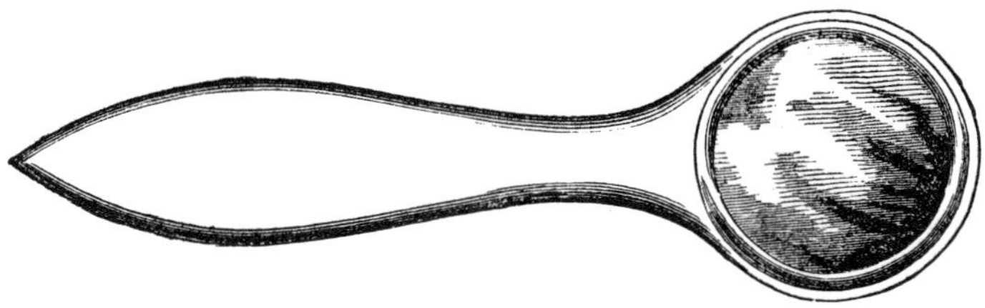

This Cut represents No. 18, full size.

No. 18.	Plain, Round Glass, Pocket, Silver Mounted	each	$1.25
" 18½.	Magnifying, Round Glass, Pocket, Silver Mounted . . .	"	2.00

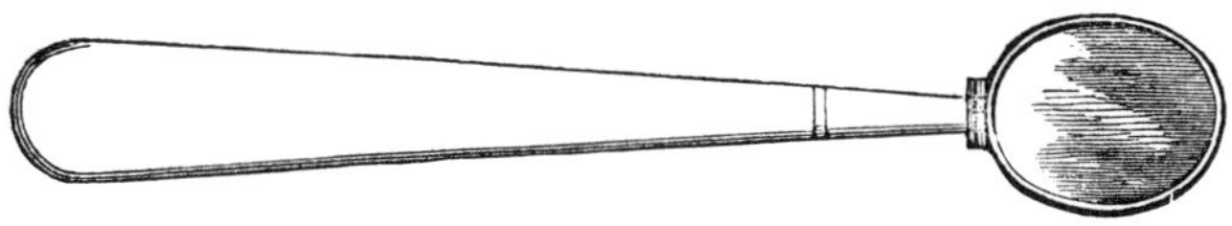

This Cut represents No. 19, half size.

No. 19.	Plain, double Glass, jointed, Silver Mounted	each	$2.00
" 19½.	Figured, " " Gold "	"	2.50
" 19¾.	Dolphin, " " " "	"	2.50
" 21.	Plain, Oval Glass, Pocket, " " Magnifying .	"	2.00
" 21½.	" " " Silver " " . .	"	1.75
" 22.	Dolphin, Oval Glass, Gold Mounted, Magnifying . . .	"	2.25
" 23.	Figured, " " "	"	2.50
" 24.	Dolphin, Gold Mounted, jointed, 1 Plain Glass, 1 Magnifying .	"	3.25
" 24½.	Figured, " " 1 " 1 " .	"	3.00
" 25.	Plain, Round Glass, Pocket, Gold Mounted, Magnifying . .	"	1.75
" 26.	Figured, Silver Mounted, jointed, 1 Plain Glass, 1 Magnifying	"	2.25
" 26½.	Plain, " " 1 " 1 " .	"	2.00
" 27.	Star pattern, Gold Lyre, " 1 " 1 " .	"	5.50
" 41.	Plain Glass, Small, jointed, Silver Mounted	"	1.25

PEARL HANDLES FOR LANCETS.

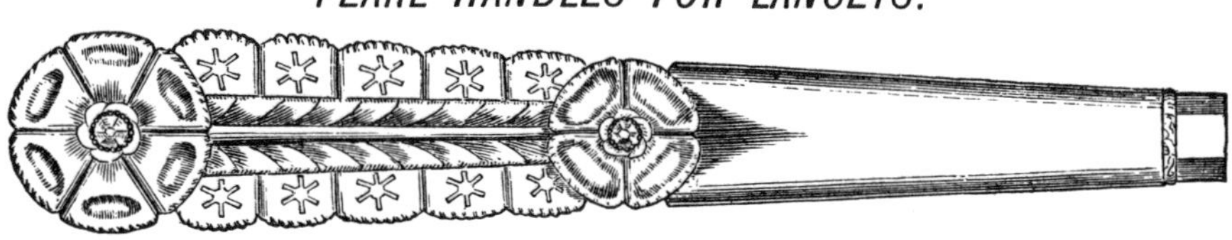

This Cut represents No. 24, full size.

No. 24.	Star pattern, Carved on both sides, Gold Ferrule, 2 Rosettes .	each	$2.00
" 25.	Shell " " " " 1 " .	"	1.75
" 26.	Dolphin " " " " 1 " .	"	1.75
" 27.	Fish " " " "	"	1.50
" 29.	Dolphin " " " "	"	1.50
" 28.	Plain Silver Ferrule	"	.75

Mounting with Lancets adds $1.00 to above prices.

PEARL HANDLES FOR SCALERS.

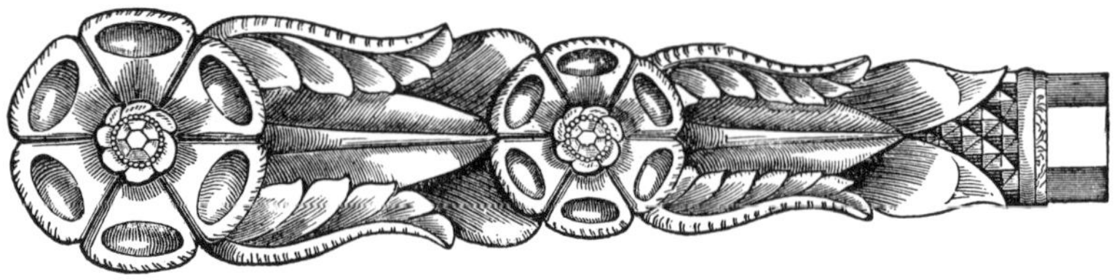

This Cut represents No. 36, full size.

No. 35. Shell pattern,	Carved on both	sides,	Gold Ferrule,	1	Rosette,	per doz.	$39.00
" 36. Fancy	"	"	"	2	"	"	45.00
" 37. Dolphin	"	"	"	1	"	"	30.00

Mounting with Scalers adds $18.00 per doz. to the above prices.

PEARL HANDLES FOR SCISSORS.

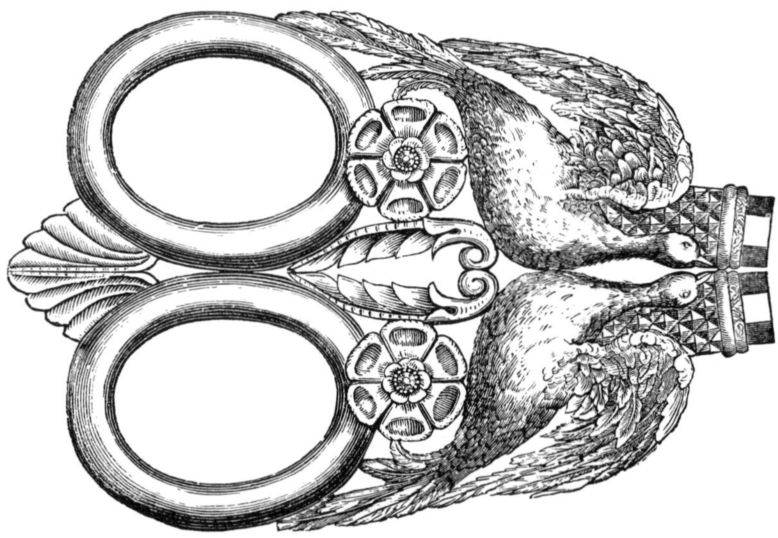

This Cut represents No. 34, full size.

No. 33. Dog pattern,	Carved on both sides,	Gold Ferrules		. . .	each	$5.50
" 34. Bird	"	"	" 2 Rosettes	.	"	6.75
" 38. Scroll	"	"	" "	. .	"	6.25
" 39. Dolphin	"	"	" "	. .	"	5.00

Mounting with Scissors adds $5.00 to above prices.

PEARL TONGUE OR CHEEK HOLDERS.

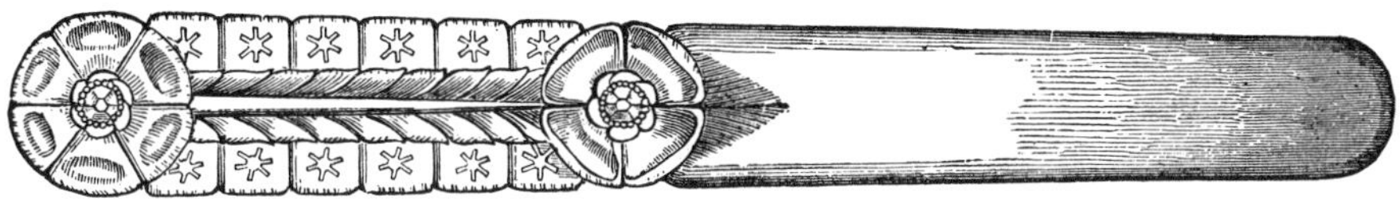

This Cut represents No. 21, three-fourths size.

No. 21. Star pattern, 2 Rosettes	each	$1.50
" 22. Fancy " 1 "	"	1.00
" 23. Dolphin " 1 "	"	1.00
" 30. Fancy "	"	.60
" 31. " "	"	.75
" 32. Dolphin "	"	.85

HANDLES FOR INSTRUMENTS.

PEARL.

Octagon, $\frac{5}{8}$ inch Plain Taper, Gold Ferrules	per doz.	$45.00
" $\frac{1}{2}$ " " "	"	33.50
" $\frac{3}{8}$ " tapering each way from the center, Gold Ferrules	"	20.00
Revolving Head Drill Socket, Gold Ferrules	each	6.00

BURGOS.

Octagon, $\frac{5}{8}$ inch Plain Taper, Gold Ferrules	per doz.	$40.00
" $\frac{1}{2}$ " " "	"	27.00

CAMEO.

A beautiful article, preferred by many to Pearl.

Octagon, $\frac{5}{8}$ inch Plain Taper, Gold Ferrules	per doz.	$23.00
" $\frac{1}{2}$ " " "	"	19.00

Any of the above with Solid Gold Ferrules, from $6 to $8 per dozen additional.

Hand Mirrors.

IMPORTED DIRECT FROM PARIS.

Rosewood, Plate Glass, $4\frac{1}{2}$ inches	each	$0.75
" " 5 "	"	.85
" " $5\frac{1}{2}$ "	"	1.50
" " 6 "	"	1.20

BEVELED-EDGE HAND MIRRORS.

IMPORTED DIRECT FROM PARIS.

We have a large stock of Heavy Glass Beveled-Edge Hand Mirrors, made of Rosewood, Satin, and Thay Wood,—four sizes, $4\frac{1}{2}$, 5, $5\frac{1}{2}$ and 6 inches, from $1.20 to $3.00 each.

NEW STYLE HAND MIRROR.

Covered with Leather. Our own Importation.

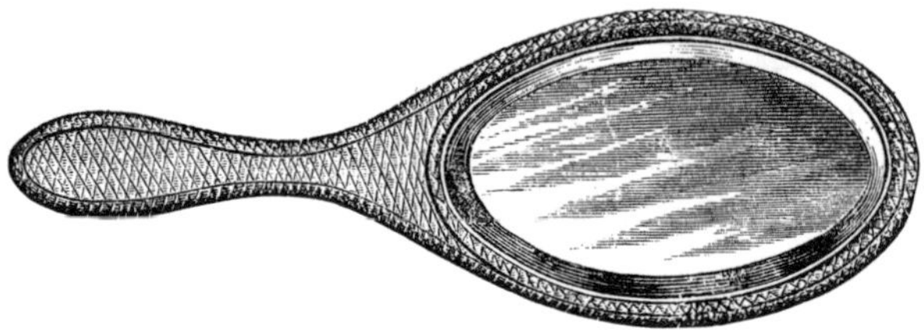

The Cut shows in miniature a new style Hand Mirror. It is covered with leather, by which the danger of warping is avoided, while there is less liability to breakage.

The Glass is thick, with Beveled edges, and perfect in every respect.

It is a very showy and durable Hand Mirror.

4½ inch	each	$1.60
5 "	"	1.75
5½ "	"	2.00
6 "	"	2.25
6½ "	"	2.50
7 "	"	3.00

Mouth Mirrors.

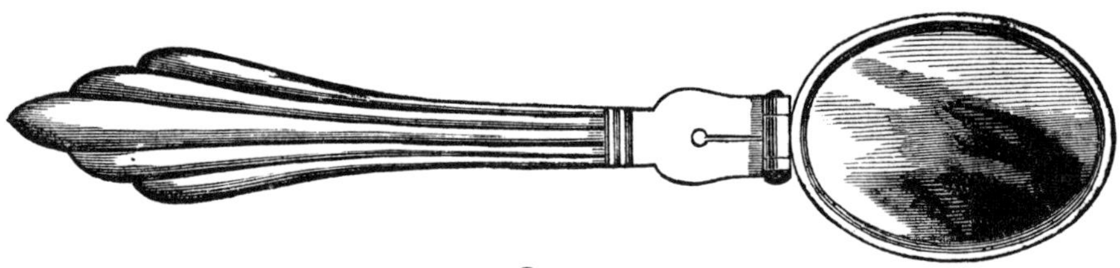

Open.

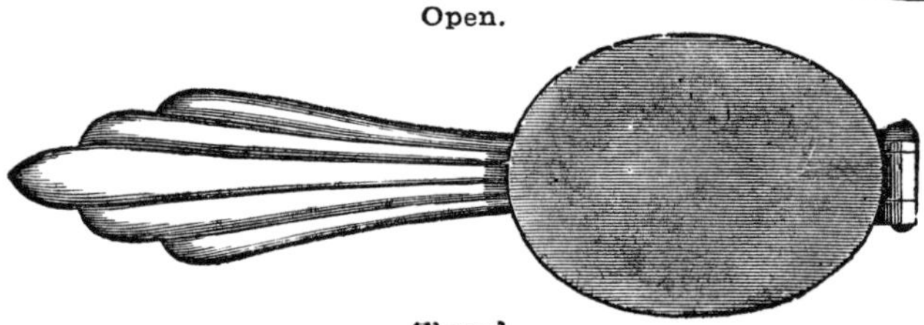

Closed.

German Silver Frame and Handle, Magnifying Glass, jointed each $2.50

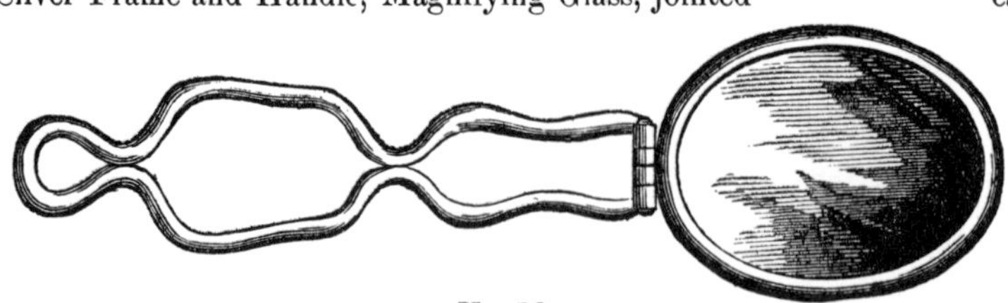

No. 20.

German Silver Wire Handle, Silver Frame, double Glass, jointed each $1.00

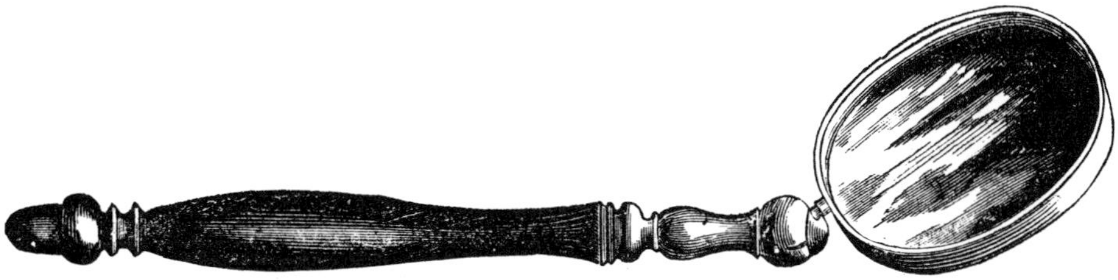

Ebony Handle, German Silver Frame, with Ball-and-Socket Joint, Magnifying Glass . . . . each $2.50

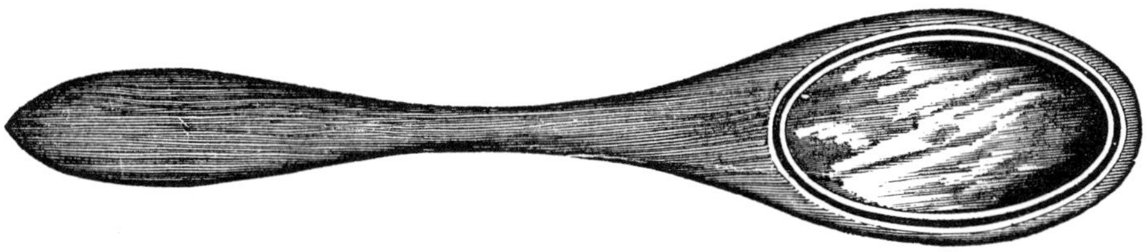

Bone, Plain Glass, Oval, Cut full size, No. 1902	each $0.60
Rosewood, “ “ “ “ “ 1903	“ .30
Bone, Magnifying Glass, Oval, Cut full size, No. 1904	“ 1.00
Rosewood, “ “ “ “ “ 1905	“ .75
Bone, Plain Glass, Round, $\frac{7}{8}$ inch diameter, 4 inches long, No. 1902 .	“ .60
Rosewood, “ “ $\frac{7}{8}$ “ “ 4 “ “ “ 1903 .	“ .30
Bone, Magnifying Glass, Round, $\frac{7}{8}$ inch diameter, 4 inches long, No. 1904	“ 1.00
Rosewood, “ “ $\frac{7}{8}$ “ “ 4 “ “ “ 1905	“ .75
Bone, Plain Glass, Oval, $1\frac{3}{4}$ inches by $\frac{7}{8}$ inch, 4 inches long, No. 1607 .	“ .65
“ “ “ $1\frac{7}{8}$ “ $\frac{15}{16}$ “ 4 “ “ 1608 .	“ .65
“ “ “ 2 “ 1 “ 4 “ “ 1609 .	“ .65

IMPERISHABLE MOUTH MIRRORS.

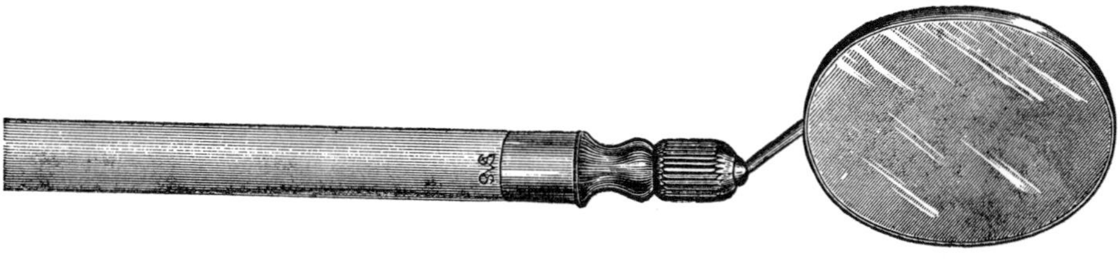

The Glass is coated with pure Silver, protected by a deposit of pure Copper, with Ball-and-Socket Joint, Nickel-Plated, Ivory Handle; five sizes of Glass.

No. 1. Oval, Magnifying Glass $1\frac{1}{4}$ by 1 inch	Price . each $3.00
“ 2. “ “ “ $1\frac{1}{4}$ by $\frac{7}{8}$ “	
“ 3. “ “ “ 1 by $\frac{3}{4}$ “	
“ 4. “ “ “ $\frac{7}{8}$ by $\frac{5}{8}$ “	
“ 5. “ “ “ $\frac{3}{4}$ by $\frac{9}{16}$ “	

ROUND MOUTH MIRRORS.

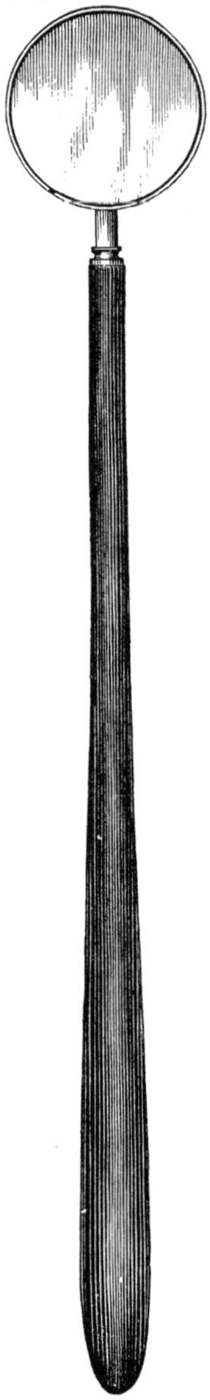

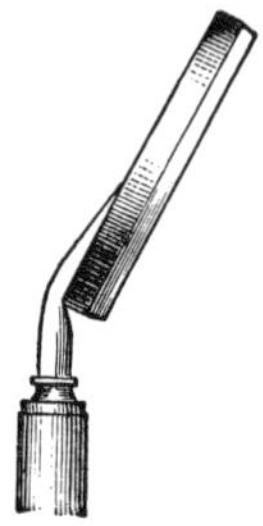

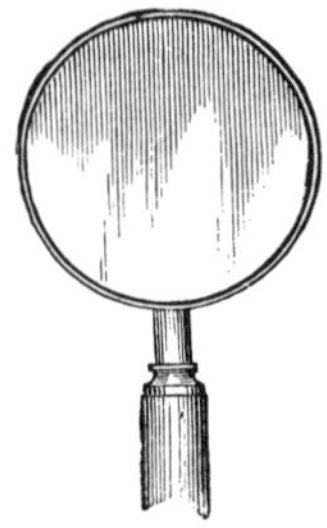

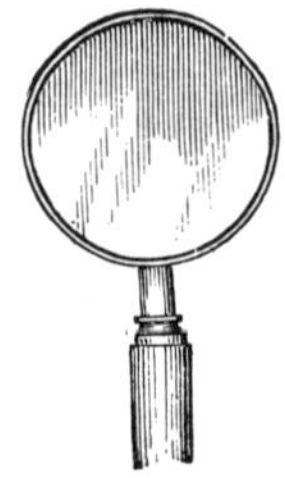

These Cuts show the sizes and form of our Round Mouth Mirrors.

The Glasses are the best quality that can be procured, of the kind called "Imperishable." Backed with an electro-deposit of Copper, they resist moisture better than any others yet produced.

The Frames are Nickel-Plated and very light. The Handles are smooth, light, and cleanly. The angle of inclination is shown in the profile cut.

In use, these Glasses, being perfectly round, occasionally get loose enough to turn in wiping; in consequence of which a few of them have had the backing worn through by rubbing. We obviate this now by concaving the Frame so that the Glass can only touch on its edge. Whenever the Glass is felt to be loose, it should be rubbed in tight, with a burnisher, on the rim.

Whenever the operator warms his Glass, either over the flame or in water, he should be careful not to heat it through. If he does so, the unequal expansion of the Glass and the Metallic Backing will cause them to part, and assume the appearance called "flaking."

Our stock comprises Plain Glasses and Magnifiers. Some of the Magnifiers are very slightly concave, making a full, clear image, which distracts the operator much less than those which greatly magnify.

Plain Glass, either size, Ebony Handle	each	$1.50
" " " Ivory "	"	2.00
Magnifying Glass, either size, Buffalo Horn Handle .	"	2.00
" " " " Ivory Handle . .	"	2.50

CHEAP MOUTH MIRROR.

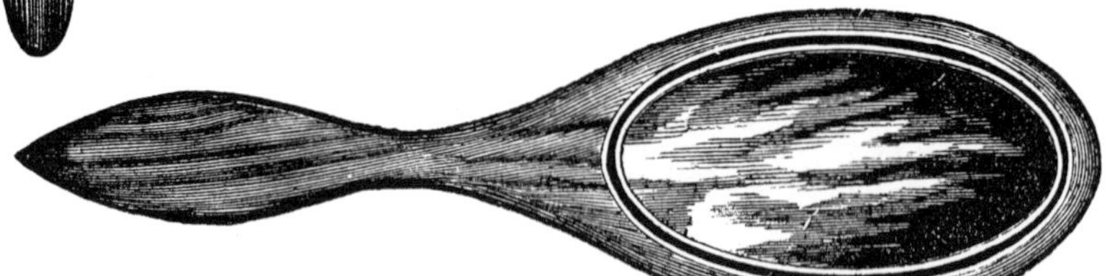

Rosewood, Plain Glass	each	$0.25

FINGER MIRRORS.

INVENTION OF DR. E. R. MULLETT.

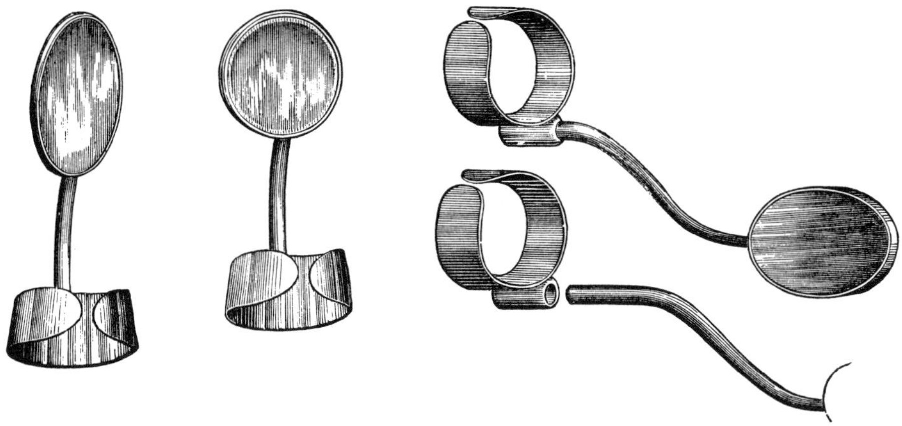

A neat and convenient mounting of Mouth Mirror, which may be retained in the hand and used with facility.

The Thimble can be opened or closed to adjust its size to the finger in a moment.

The Socket Stem is made soft and slender enough to bend easily, to adapt it for special cases in use.

All the Glasses are of the best *Imperishable* backs.

Magnifying	each	$2.00
Plain	"	1.50
Socketed Stems, extra	"	.25

MAGNIFYING EXAMINING GLASS.

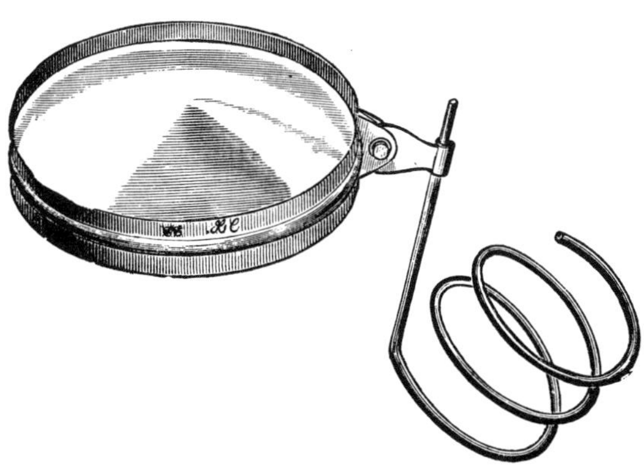

To be held on the Finger to assist the operator by magnifying the filling.

Price	each	$2.75

Nitrous Oxide Gas Apparatus.

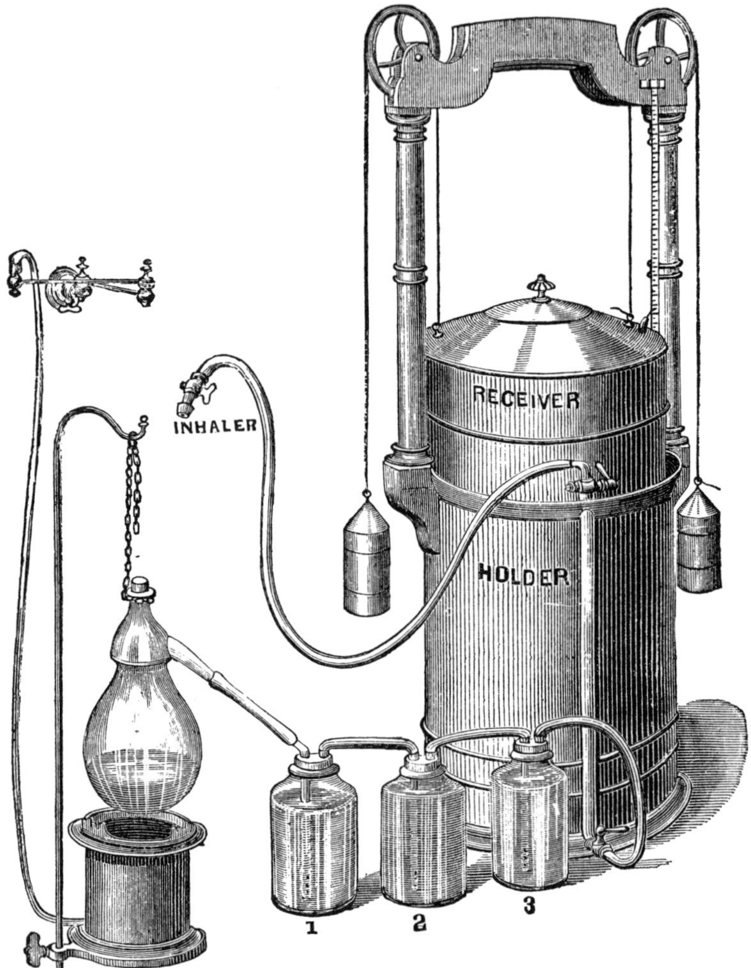

The Cut shows the Nitrous Oxide Gas Apparatus we are now furnishing. It is very complete and well adapted to the purpose for which it is designed.

The Jars and Retort are supplied with Rubber Corks, cone-shaped, which are preferred to any other arrangement we have yet tried, as they are not liable to adhere to the neck of the Retort, as glass stoppers are. They can be made perfectly air-tight by gentle pressure, and are cleanly and not liable to get out of order.

The Stand for suspending the Retort is of Iron, light, strong, and convenient. The Holder and Receiver are made of stout Zinc, Japanned. Twelve feet of $\frac{5}{8}$-inch Rubber Tubing and a Hard Rubber Valve Inhaler are furnished with the Apparatus.

The Cut shows a Gas Stove, but a Kerosene or Alcohol Lamp will be supplied instead, if desired.

Complete Apparatus, 40 gallons' capacity	$65.00
" " 50 " "	70.00
Boxing, additional	3.00

Parties desiring separate parts of the Apparatus, can have them at the following rates:

50 gallon Gas-Holder, Japanned		$50.00
1 Retort, Tubulated		1.25
1 Gas Stove		2.00
1 Retort-Holder		2.50
3 S. S. White's Wash Bottles, complete, $1.75 each		5.25
1 Hard-Rubber Valved Inhaler		4.00
4 feet ½-inch Rubber Tubing for connecting Wash Bottles	per foot	.24
12 feet ⅝-inch " for Inhaling	"	.28
12 feet ¼-inch " for Gas	"	.16

We have also a smaller Apparatus of 30 gallons' capacity.

Complete	$53.00
Boxing, additional	3.00

WASH BOTTLES AND RETORTS.

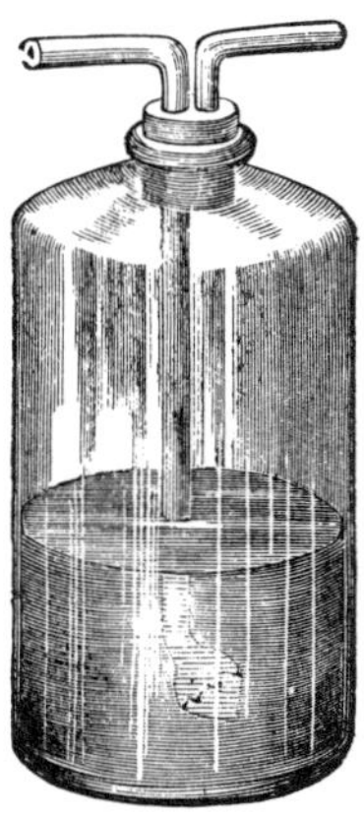

No. 1.

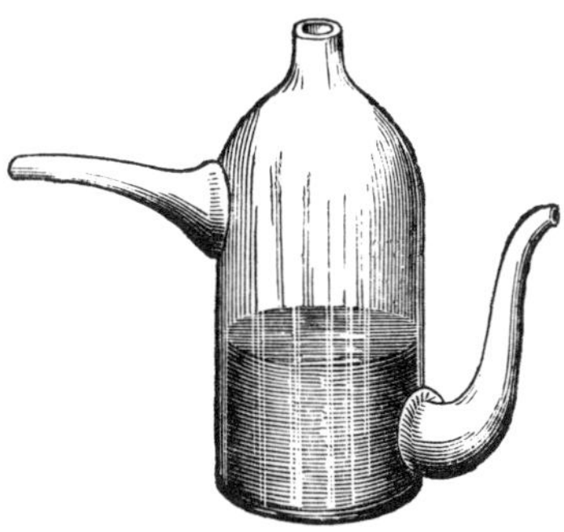

No. 2.

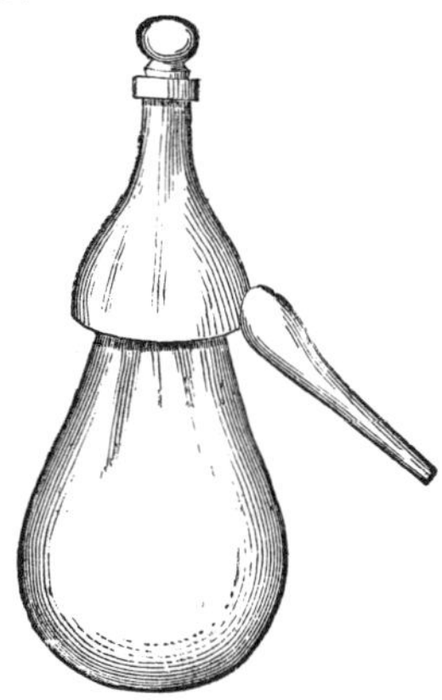

No. 3.

The Cuts represent two varieties of Wash Bottles for the manufacture of Nitrous Oxide Gas. No. 1, with perforated Rubber Cork and Glass Tubes bent at right angles; the long Tube pierced with small holes at the bottom, to compel the breaking up of the Gas, and so insure its more thorough washing. No. 2, Dr. F. R. Thomas's pattern.

No. 1	each	$1.75
No. 2	"	2.00

Cut No. 3 represents the Glass Bohemian Retort, with Rubber Stoppers, used in the manufacture of Nitrous Oxide Gas.

Price	each	$1.25
Long Neck Glass Retorts, 1 quart	"	.60
" " ½ gallon	"	1.00

NITRATE OF AMMONIA.

FUSED AND GRANULATED.

We ask the especial attention of the Profession to this article, manufactured expressly for our sales, and which we can commend for its purity.

Fluctuates. Present prices as follows:

In	5 lb. Boxes		per lb. 42 cents.
"	10 "		" 40 "
"	20 "		" 38 "
"	25 "		" 37 "
"	30 "		" 36 "
"	50 "		" 35 "
"	100 "	(Boxing, extra, 70 cents.)	" 33 "
"	5 lb. Paper Packages		" 35 "
"	1 " Bottles		" 45 "

HARD RUBBER INHALER, AND FLEXIBLE HOOD.

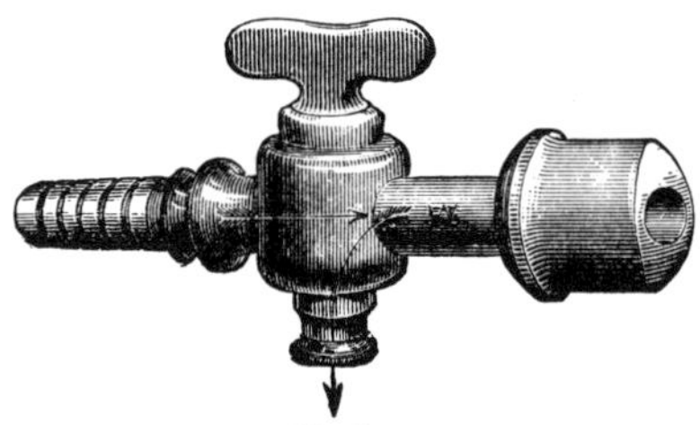

No. 1.

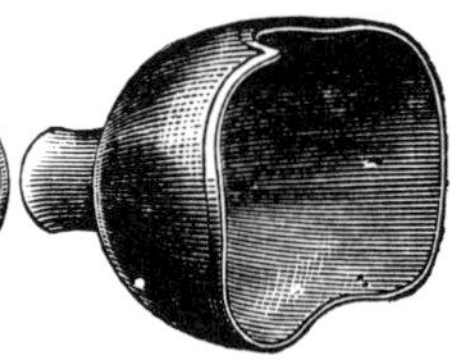

No. 2.

No. 1. Hard Rubber Inhaler, with Valve	$4.00
" " " without Valve	2.00
No. 2. Flexible Hood	1.00

NOSE COMPRESS.

INTRODUCED BY DR. S. S. NONES.

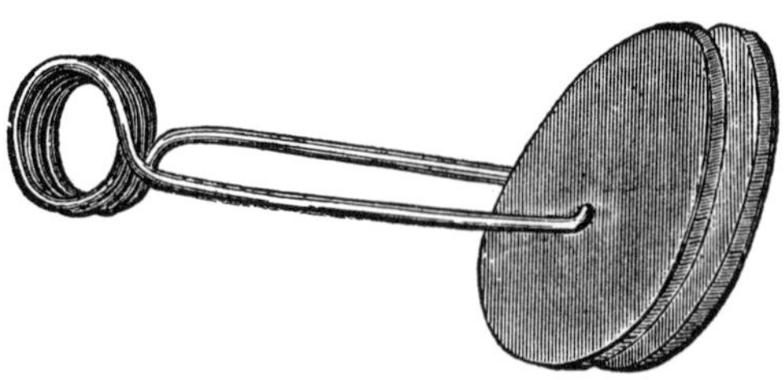

Convenient for the administering of Gas, where the Inhaler is designed to be used without a Face-piece.

Price $0.50

NITROUS OXIDE GAS INHALER.

OUR OWN DESIGN.

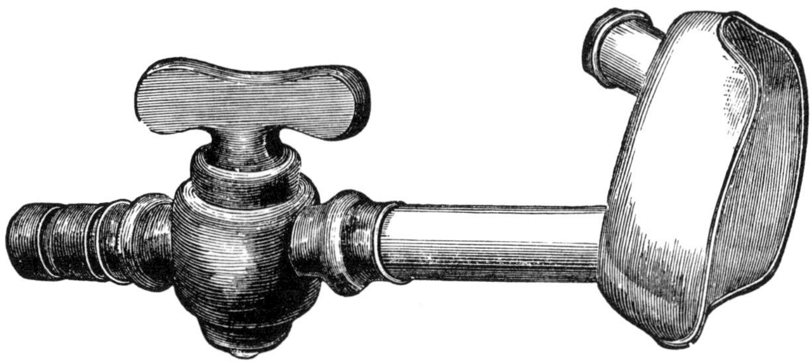

The Face-piece, which is designed to cover both mouth and nostrils, is made of Metal, Silver-Plated; the Stop-cock is of Hard Rubber. Two Valves—one for inhaling and the other for exhaling—are affixed to the bottom of the Mouth-piece, sufficiently large to allow natural respiration. Entire length of the Instrument nine inches. Inclosed in a neat Box.

Price $4.00

RUBBER CONDUCTING TUBING.

$\frac{3}{16}$ inch, inside measure	per foot	$0.12
$\frac{1}{4}$ " "	"	.16
$\frac{3}{8}$ " "	"	.20
$\frac{1}{2}$ " "	"	.24
$\frac{5}{8}$ " "	"	.28
$\frac{3}{4}$ " "	"	.34
$\frac{7}{8}$ " "	"	.38
1 " "	"	.41

RUBBER GAS BAGS, OVAL.

5 Gallons	$4.00
6 "	5.00
7 "	6.00
8 "	7.00
9 "	8.00
10 "	9.00

RUBBER GASOMETERS, SQUARE.

18 by 24 inches	$6.00
20 by 30 "	8.00
25 by 30 "	10.00
30 by 40 "	12.00

Arkansas Stone.

A SUPERIOR ARTICLE.

A large assortment of all sizes and descriptions, selected and cut expressly for our sales.

Knife-edge Slips, for finishing fillings	$0.60
Pointed Slips	.35
Square Lengths	$0.35 to .50
Small Flat Oblong Pieces, for sharpening instruments	.20 to 1.00
The same, in Walnut Boxes, very convenient	1.00
Large Flat Oblong Pieces, for sharpening instruments	1.00 to 5.00

Preparations for Office Use.

Tincture of Myrrh. 8 oz. bottles	$0.50
" Catechu. 8 oz. bottles	.50
" White Oak Bark. 8 oz. bottles	.40
" Krameria. 8 oz. bottles	.50
" Arnica. 4 oz. bottles	.30
" Calendula. 4 oz. bottles	.35
" Capsicum. 2 oz. bottles	.25
" Aconite Root. 1 oz. bottles	.15
" Iodine. 1 oz. glass-stoppered bottles	.25
" " Colorless. 1 oz. glass-stoppered bottles	.25
Wine of Opium. 2 oz. bottles	.50
Glycerin. 8 oz. bottles	.60
Chlorate of Potassa, Pulverized. 8 oz. bottles	.75
Soda Hyposulphite. 1 lb. bottles	.30
" Sulphite. ¼ lb. bottles	.25
" Bisulphite. 2 oz. bottles	.35
Saturated Solution Iodine in Creasote. ½ oz. glass-stoppered bottles	.40
" " " Glycerin. 1 " " "	.35
Iodine and Carbolic Acid. 2 oz. bottles	.25
Creasote. 1 oz. glass-stoppered bottles	.30
Pure Wood Creasote. 1 oz. glass-stoppered bottles	.50
Carbolic Acid. 1 oz. glass-stoppered bottles	.35
Carbolic Acid and Glycerin. 2 oz. bottles	.35
Dichloracetic Acid. 1 oz. bottles	3.00
Phénol Sodique 8 oz. bottles, with directions	.50
Cantharidal Collodion. 1 oz. bottles	.50
Liquid Gutta-percha. 1 oz. bottles	.40

Labarraque's Solution of Chlorinated Soda. Pint bottles, glass-stoppered	$0.40
" " " " 6 oz. bottles	.20
Monsel's Solution Persulphate of Iron. 1 oz. glass-stoppered bottles	.20
" Powder Subsulphate " 1 oz. bottles	.25
Solution of Perchloride of Iron. 1 oz. glass-stoppered bottles	.20
Sesquichloride of Iron. (Crystallized.) 1 oz. glass-stoppered bottles	.40
Styptic Colloid. 2 oz. bottles	.60
Tannin. 1 oz. bottles	.35
Elixir of Vitriol and Tannin. 2 oz. bottles	.50
Isinglass Plaster. 1 yard in box	.75
Acetate of Morphia. ⅛ oz. bottles	1.25
Nerve-Paste. (Arsenic and Creasote)	.50
Chromic Acid. ½ oz. glass-stoppered bottles	.50
Chloride of Zinc. 1 oz. glass-stoppered bottles	.30
Sulphate of Zinc. ¼ lb. bottles	.15
Nitrate of Silver, Crystals. ⅛ oz. bottles	.30
Oxalic Acid. 2 oz. bottles	.15
Permanganate of Potassa, Crystals. 1 oz. bottles	.40
Bromide of Cadmium. 1 oz. bottles	1.00
Chloroform. Pound bottles	2.00
Ether, Washed. Pint bottles	1.00
" Concentrated. Pint bottles	1.00
Hydrate of Chloral. 1 oz. bottles	.35
Tetrachloride of Carbon. 1 oz. glass-stoppered bottles	1.25
Glycerole of Thymol. 1 oz. bottles	.50
Caustic Potash. 1 lb. bottles	1.25
Copperas. 1 lb. packages	.08
Pain Obtunder. Per bottle	1.00
Chlorinated Lime. 1 lb. bottles	.40
Dental Pepsin. ½ oz. bottles	1.25
Lacto-Phosphate of Lime. ½ oz. bottles	.50
Iodoform. ¼ oz. bottles	.60
Carvacrol, "Sage's," per bottle	1.00
Salicylic Acid. ⅛ oz. bottles	.38
Mercury, Re-distilled, in ¼ lb. bottles (fluctuates), present price	.60
Best English Precipitated Chalk. Per lb.	.38
Sperm Oil. 3 oz. bottles	.20
Sandarac Varnish, for Saturating Cotton to retain preparations for destroying Nerve. 2 oz. bottles	.25

COLOGNES, ETC.

Ordinary Cologne. Pint bottles	$1.00
Bouquet Cologne. 12 oz. glass-stoppered bottles	1.50
Oriental Cologne. " " "	1.75
Bay Rum. 1¾ pint bottles	.75

TOOTH POWDERS, MOUTH WASHES, ETC.

Tooth Powder, S. S. White's,	No. 1,	4 lb.	tin cans, Rose or Wintergreen flavor	$5.00
" "	"	1 "	" " " "	1.50
" "	"	½ "	" " " "	.90
" "	"	¼ "	" " " "	.50
" "	No. 2,	4 "	" " flavor	3.50
" "	"	1 "	" " "	1.00
" "	"	½ "	" " "	.60
" "	"	¼ "	" " "	.35
" "	No. 3,	4 "	" " "	2.50
" "	"	1 "	" " "	.75
" "	"	½ "	" " "	.45
" "	"	¼ "	" " "	.25
" "	Soluble,	4 "	" " "	5.00
" "	"	1 "	" " "	1.50
" "	"	½ "	" " "	.90
" "	"	¼ "	" " "	.50

Astringent Mouth Wash, S. S.W.'s, 16 oz. bottles for office use			1.25
" " " 3 "	per doz. $3.75	per bot.	.40
Saponaceous Toilet Mouth Wash. 4 oz. bottles	" 3.75	"	.40
Tonic Mouth Wash. 2 oz. bottles	" 2.25	"	.25
Teaberry Mouth Wash. 2 oz. bottles	" 2.25	"	.25
Aromatic Mouth Wash. 4 oz. paneled-arch bottles	" 6.00	"	.75
Bouquet Mouth Wash. 6 oz. " glass-stop. bottles	" 9.00	"	1.00
Salicylic Acid Mouth Wash. 6 oz. bottles, with metal top	" 6.50	"	.75
Da Costa's Mouth Wash	" 2.50	"	.25
J. T. Rorer's Dentaria	" 2.00	"	.25
S. S. White's Tooth Paste	" 6.00	per box	.75
" " Soap	" 2.00	"	.25
Carbolic " "	" 2.00	"	.25
Lyon's Tooth Tablets	" 3.50	"	.50
Salicylic Acid Lozenges		"	.25

SOAPS FOR OFFICE USE.

Low, Son and Haydon's Manufacture, put up in boxes of 1 dozen each, containing either Elder Flower alone, or assorted, of the following varieties: Rose, Glycerin, Honey, and Elder Flower.

Price . . . . per doz. $2.00 ; per cake 20 cents.

Exquisite Office Soaps from the celebrated French Manufacturer, M. L. T. Piver. These Soaps retain their perfume until entirely consumed.

Lettuce	per doz. $6.75	each 60 cents.
Alba Rosa	" 5.25	" 45 "

The above Soaps are made expressly for our sales, and stamped with our name.

Cashmere Soap . . . . per doz. $3.00

WHITE CASTILE SOAP.

OUR OWN IMPORTATION.

We have a stock of the genuine White Marseilles Castile Soap of the celebrated manufacture of H. Arnavon, for which he received the Grand Cross of the Legion of Honor at the Paris Exposition of 1867.

PRICES.

By the Slab, weighing from 35 to 55 lbs.	per lb.	$0.25
" Bar, " " 5 to 8 lbs.	"	.30
In Cut Cakes, " " 4 to 6 oz.	"	.35
In Pressed Cakes, weighing 4 oz. each	per doz.	1.50

DENTAL FLOSS SILK.

Special manufacture of Floss Silk, made expressly and solely for our sales. We believe it to be the best article for the purpose we have ever seen.

It is made from superior stock, and warranted all Silk. 12 yards in length.

We have sold large quantities of this Silk, and have not heard a single complaint of its quality.

Price	per doz.	$1.50
"	per spool	.15

WAXED FLOSS SILK.

Manufactured expressly for dental purposes, and exclusively for our sales. It is made from superior stock, and thoroughly saturated with Wax. The spools contain 12 yards,—put up in round boxes to preserve it from dust when not in use.

Price	per doz.	$2.25
"	per spool	.20

Tooth-Brushes.

MADE EXPRESSLY FOR OUR SALES.

(SEE OPPOSITE PAGE.)

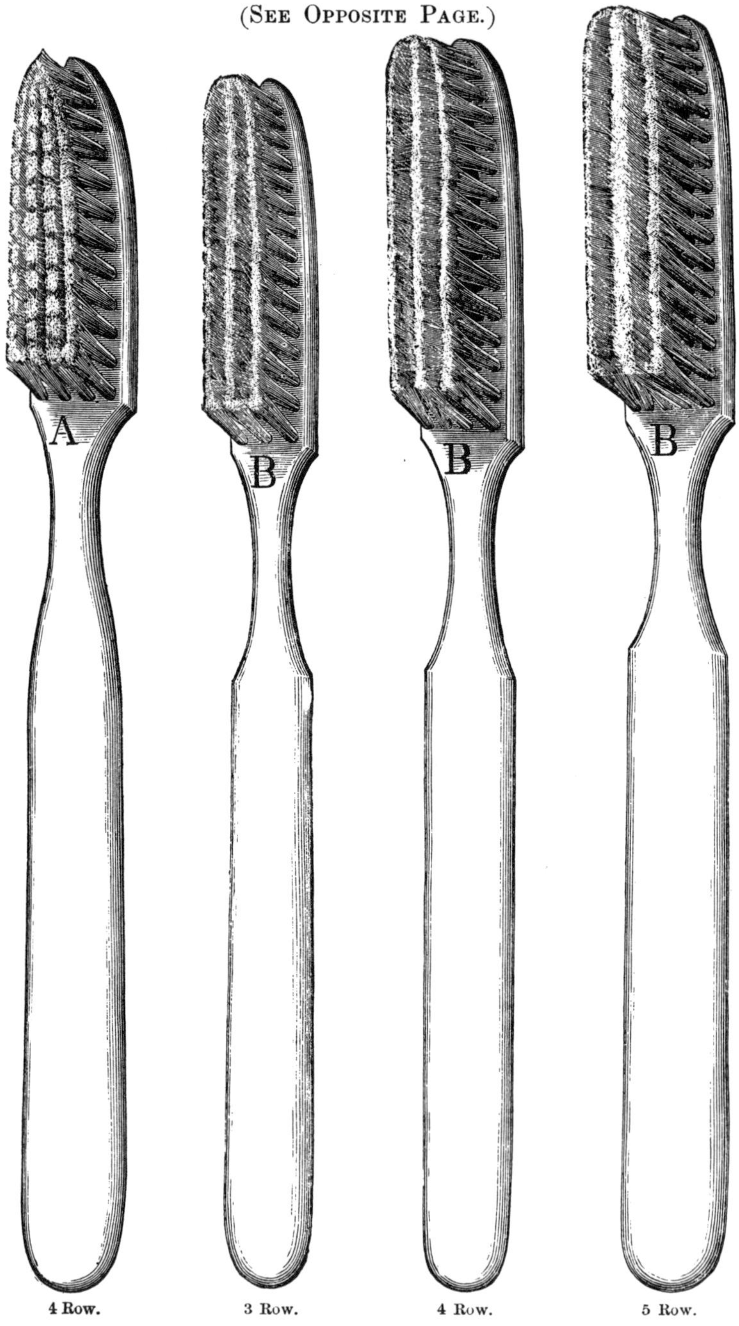

4 Row. 3 Row. 4 Row. 5 Row.

SUPERIOR FRENCH TOOTH BRUSHES.

(SEE CUTS ON OPPOSITE PAGE.)

These Brushes are made expressly for our sales, and are of the best French manufacture. Waxed Backs.

This style of brush has received the approval of many of the most intelligent practitioners. The arrangement of the bristles is such as to allow their entrance between the teeth, and into depressions and irregular spaces, thus insuring greater cleanliness than can be secured by a flat-faced brush.

A is pointed, as shown in Cut, 4 rows.

B is less pointed, and in three sizes, 3, 4, and 5 rows.

Price 3 row	per doz.	$2.30
" 4 "	"	3.00
" 5 "	"	3.80

Also, a large assortment of French Tooth Brushes ranging from 75 cents to $5.00 per dozen.

SUPERIOR ENGLISH TOOTH BRUSHES.

Manufactured expressly for our sales. We offer to the Profession a large variety of 3, 4, and 5 row Brushes of the very best quality of material and workmanship. White Cemented Backs (a new feature), in the following varieties.

By stating the number, and whether Soft, Medium, or Hard is wanted, or otherwise characterizing the Brush desired according to the following classification, parties may always be sure of obtaining the Brush ordered.

Nos. 101 to 106, inclusive, 3 rows, either Soft, Medium, or Hard	per doz.	$3.30
" 122 to 156, " 4 " " " "	"	3.30
No. 157, 4 rows, very Soft	"	3.30
Nos. 158 to 163, inclusive, 5 rows, either Soft, Medium, or Hard	"	4.00
" 168 to 172, " Palate, " " "	"	3.30
" 173 to 176, " 3 rows, running from large to small size, Dr. Coffin's Pattern, Medium grade only	"	4.30
No. 177, 4 rows, Goat Hair	"	3.30
" 178, 4 " Badger Hair	"	5.82
" 179, 4 " very Hard only	"	4.00
" 180, 4 " with sponge, either Soft, Medium or Hard	"	4.30
Nos. 181 and 182, 4 rows, Yellow Bristles, very Hard only	"	3.30
No. 183, 3 rows, Black Bristles, Soft only	"	3.30
" 184, 4 " either Soft, Medium, or Hard	"	3.30
Cemented, 4 " assorted dozens	"	1.32
" London, 4 rows, assorted dozens	"	1.55
" Improved, 4 " "	"	1.84
" Warranted, 4 " "	"	2.15
" Superfine, 4 " "	"	2.60
Best Children's, 3 " "	"	1.84

SUPERIOR AMERICAN TOOTH BRUSHES.

MANUFACTURED EXPRESSLY FOR THE DENTAL TRADE.

A large variety of 3, 4, and 5 row Brushes of the very best quality of material and workmanship. For convenience in ordering, we have had them put up in assorted dozens—each Brush differing in style. The Brushes being numbered on the Handles enables the Dentist or Dealer to select such styles as he may wish to order.

3 row Brushes	per doz.	$3.00
4 " "	"	3.00
5 " "	"	4.00

FOIL CRIMPERS.

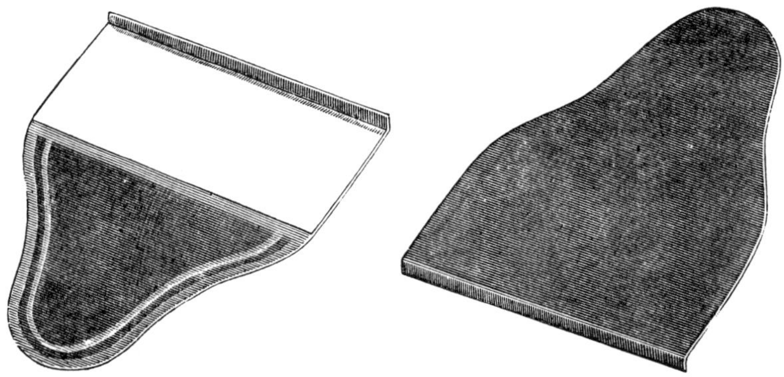

Made of thick Tin; four inches wide and five inches long; japanned on the back and face, as shown in the Cut. Two of these are used; a half sheet of Foil being laid upon one, the other is placed over it with the Flange upon the extreme edge of the Foil, and drawn to the other Flange.

Per pair $0.50

***** Articles not illustrated or classified in this Department will be found in the Mechanical or Miscellaneous Department.**

DENTAL FURNITURE.

Dental Chairs.

THE HARRIS DENTAL CHAIR.

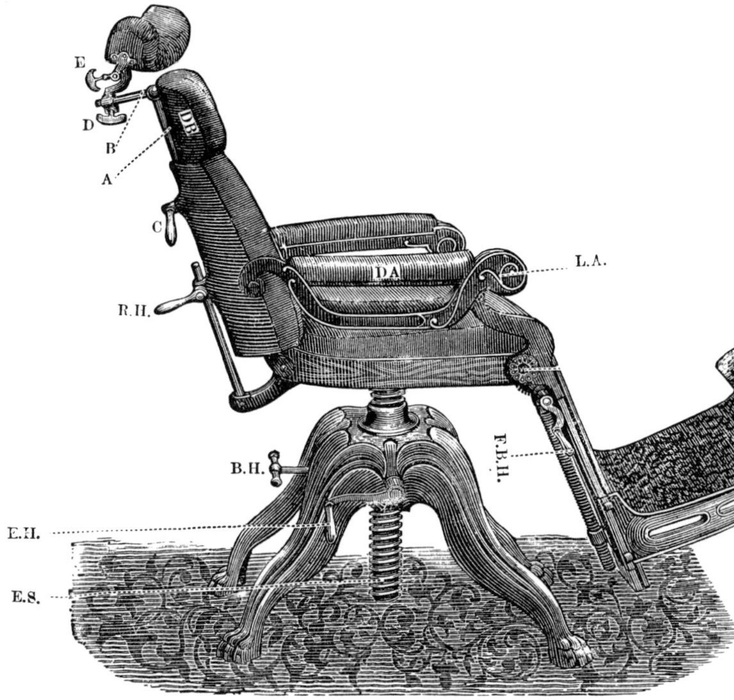

The Cut represents the Low Base Harris Chair, with recent improvements.

The Detachable Back (D.B.) permits a ready and easy adaptation of that part of the Chair to adults or children. The outline Cut shows the simple method of connecting this upper back, which does not interfere at all with the Head Rest adjustments.

The Detachable Arm (D.A.), when in place, is of equal height with the Fixed Arm on the other side, and its removal allows access to work in some cases where if permanent it would be very inconvenient to the Operator. The Low Arm (L.A.) finishes level with the Seat cushion, except at the front, where its full height is a useful rest for the patient's arm. The reclining motions of the Chair are in no way affected by this Low Arm.

The Foot-Board at its outer extremity terminates in a supplemental step Rest, 4 inches wide, which is raised 3½ inches, leaving an easy passage under it for the feet when resting on the platform.

For the information of those who have not seen the Harris Chair, we add the following Explanation of the remaining letters on the Cut. E. S. is the Elevating Screw; and E. H. the Elevating Handle, by turning which, the Chair, with the patient in it, may be readily raised or lowered 13 inches. B. H. Brake Handle, by which the Chair may be clamped so that it will not rotate when leaned against by the Operator. F.B.H. the Foot-Board Handle, whereby the Foot-Board is adjusted in height. This Handle

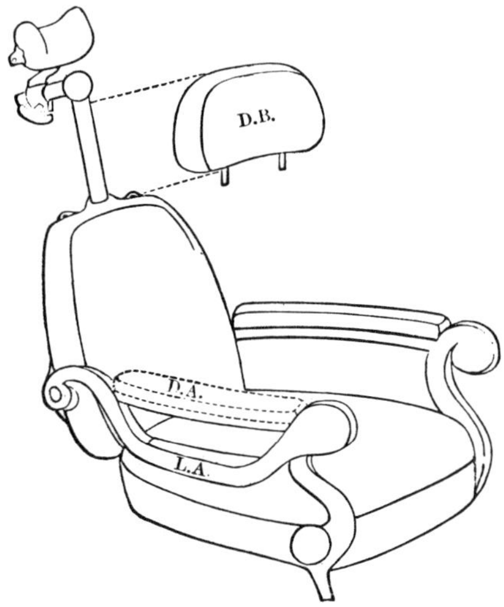

can also be used by the patient while seated, to change the height of the Foot-Rest for convenience. R.H. is the Reclining Handle. By moving this less than half a turn, the whole reclining motion of this machine is freed. It may then be moved with a very slight effort of one hand from the upright to a nearly horizontal position. When the desired incline is gained, a slight turn of R.H. locks it again immovably. In this reclining motion the patient does not assist, and is not disturbed.

The Head-Rest shown in the Cut has the following adjustments:—Up and down, fully 12 inches; backward and forward, 6 inches; the whole cushion to either side, 6 inches. Besides which the cushion has ¾ of a circle motion of inclination on its own back-rod, clamped by Screw E, and the whole Head-Rest may swing around entirely on its Stem A, being secured in its turning as well as its height by the handle C. Combinations of these motions are very varied, and will suggest themselves to the Profession.

The Medium Base Chair differs from the Low Base only in being 2 inches higher.

The High Base Chair we have ceased to manufacture.

Upholstered in Fine Green or "Red" Plush	$170.00
In Morocco, with extra quality of Carpet	176.00
In extra Fine Garnet Plush, with extra quality of Carpet	176.00
Steel Screws for Elevating and Foot-Board, extra	10.00
Tubular Cover on Elevating Screw, extra	3.00
With Double Back, extra	7.00
" " " and Low and Detachable Arm, extra	9.00
Boxing	6.00

In addition to the above, we now supply for those who wish to practice economy without any loss in usefulness, a

$150 LOW-PRICED HARRIS CHAIR. $150

There is no difference between this Chair and the others except in finish AFTER IT LEAVES THE MACHINE-SHOP. In painting and upholstering it will be inferior to our regular Harris Chair—but not at all inferior to any other chair in the market. The price will be $150, uniformly—in Plush or Leather; with Double Back, extra, $7.00; with Double Back and Low and Detachable Arm, extra, $9.00. The cost of boxing and freight being at the expense of every buyer, our Branch Houses and dealers will be obliged to sell at the above prices, with the cost of these added.

THE S. S. WHITE DENTAL CHAIR.

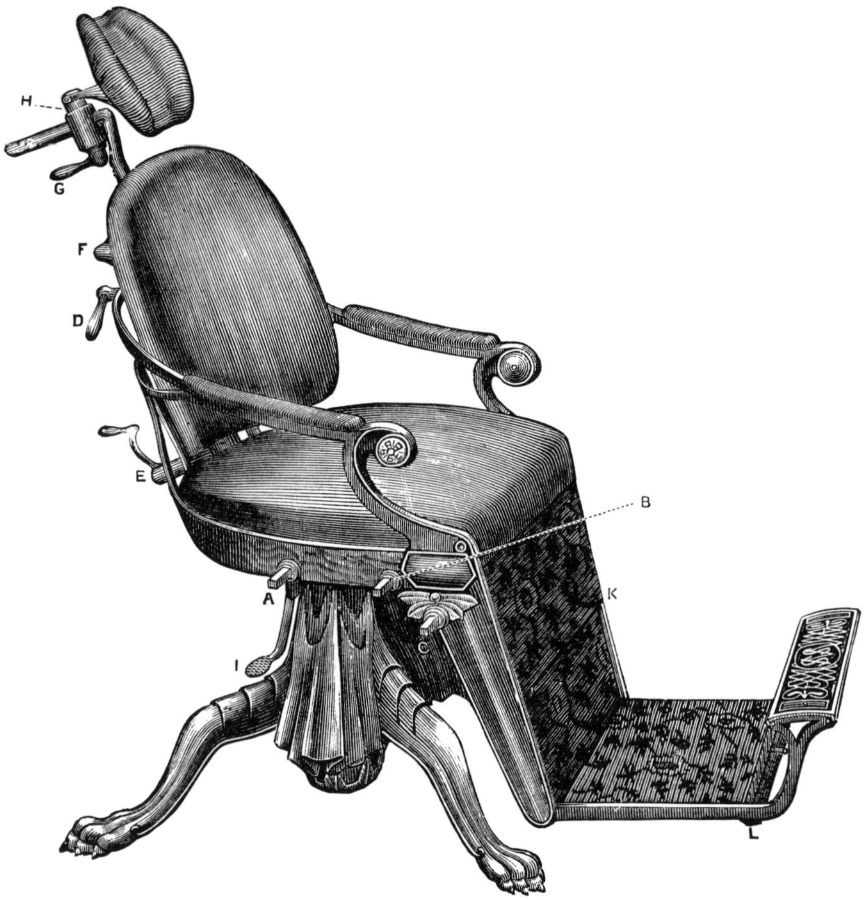

We call attention to the accompanying Illustrations of our new Chair, known by the above name. It is the result of long experience, observation, criticism, and experiment, and we have no hesitation in claiming that it combines more and greater advantages—some of them long in use, others the result of new inventions and combinations—than any other Dental Chair ever offered, and without any objectionable feature.

It requires no pawls, and each change of position is maintained without liability of slipping. It can be changed easily and rapidly from its lowest position, 21½ inches from the floor, to its highest, 32½ inches, or the reverse, having a vertical range of 11 inches. It may be thrown with equal facility into oblique positions, without disturbing the adjustment of the parts.

A special and valuable feature of this Chair is the Adjustable Back, which may be easily raised or lowered 7 inches, or varied in its angle, at pleasure, to give support where most needed to the body of the patient; these movements not interfering in any way with the adjustment of the Head-Rest or the Seat.

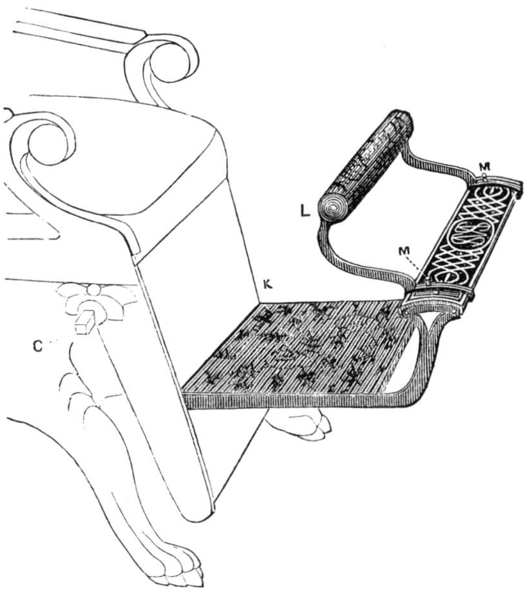

The Foot-Board is self-sustaining at any point in its range, which is 7 inches, and can be adjusted by the patient, at pleasure, when not under operation; it terminates in an additional fixed Rest, 6 inches above the platform, having an easy passage under it for the feet, and giving an opportunity to ease the limbs by a change of position. To this additional Rest is attached a supplementary Foot-Bar, pivoted so that it can be thrown up 12 inches above the platform, thus bringing it level with the Seat, and shortening the distance for children. When in use it is locked in place by the Spring-Pins MM, which need only be lifted, to swing the Bar under the Foot-Board out of the way. The whole body of the Chair revolves on its Base, and can be locked firmly at any point.

The Head-Rest is well shown by Cuts and description on page 244.

A is the Shaft by which the Chair, above the Base, may be raised 11 inches.

B, the Shaft by which the entire Chair may be thrown into an inclined position, pivoting at A.

C, the Shaft by which the Foot-Board may be raised up to the line K.

D is the Handle by which the Adjustable Back may be locked at any point.

E, a Crank attached to a revolving nut working on a screw by which the Back is set at the angle desired.

F is a Handle which locks the Head-Rest Bar, securing it in its turning as well as in its height.

G is the Locking-Handle of the Head-Rest.

H is the Pivot-Socket of the Head-Rest.

I is a Treadle connected with a Shoe, which secures the Chair from revolving.

L is the Supplementary Foot-Bar seen in the outline Cut in position for use. In the full Drawing it is as when not in use.

MM, Locking-Pins of the supplementary Foot-Bar.

Price of the S. S. White Dental Chair, in Plush or Leather $175.00
Boxing 5.00

NEW HEAD-REST.

Patented September 24th, 1867, and December 28th, 1875.

Fig. 1.

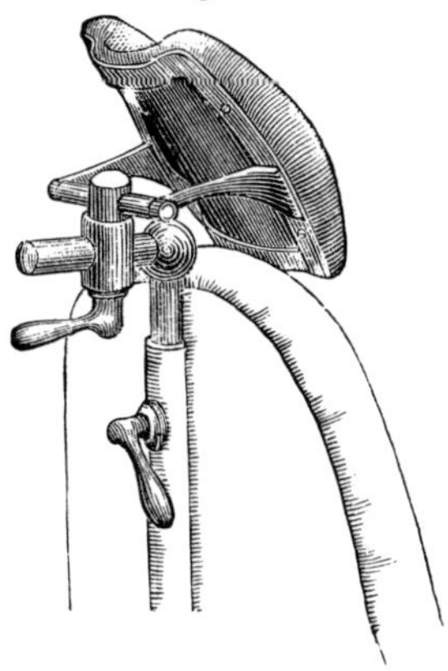

Fig. 2.

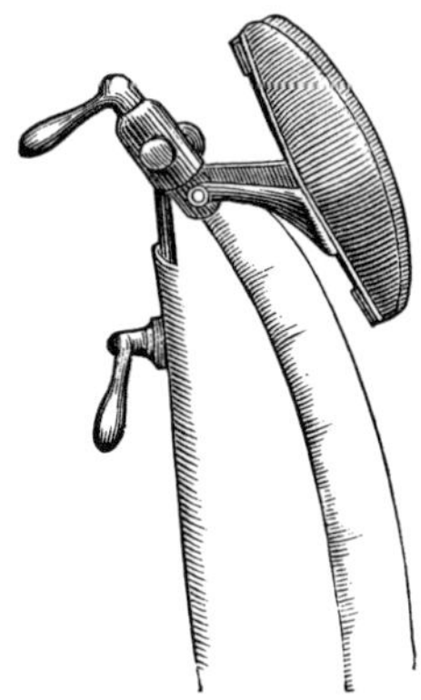

Fig. 3.

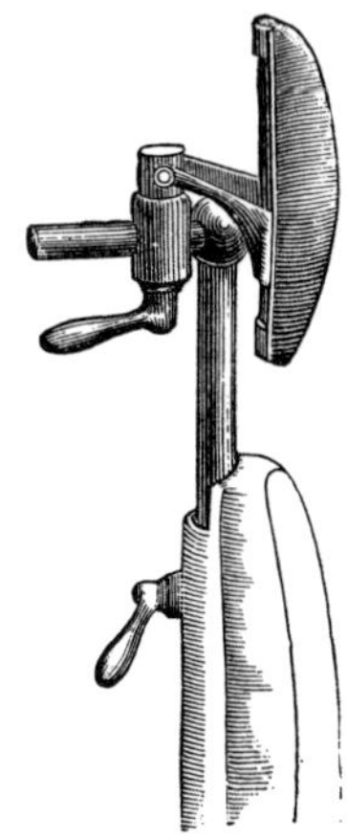

Fig. 4.

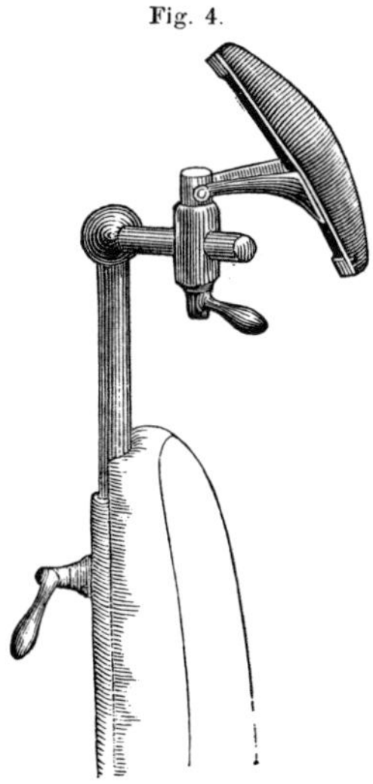

The New Head-Rest illustrated in the Cuts is believed to possess many and very decided advantages over any hitherto in the market. For lightness and strength, for facility and range of movement, for comfort to the patient and convenience to the Operator, it is without a rival. It is capable of easier and quicker adjustment, and has greater range, with fixation at any desired position, than any other Head-Rest we have ever seen; while the form of the frame and the character of the upholstering leave nothing to be desired by the patient.

Fig. 1 shows the Head-Rest at a medium position, its axis inclined to the rear.

Fig. 2 shows the Head-Rest at its lowest position, four inches below the top of the Chair, to accommodate children.

Fig. 3 shows the Head-Rest elevated, and in line with the back of the Chair,—a desirable position for operations on the lower jaw.

Fig. 4 represents the Head-Rest at the same height as in Fig. 3, but thrown forward seven inches from the line of the Chair-back,—a position well adapted for round-shouldered patients.

These illustrations, which might be greatly multiplied, will serve to show the range of movement of which the Head-Rest is capable.

It needs no modification for any of the Harris Chairs now in use, and is adaptable to any Chair which has a sliding rod in the back.

Price, adapted to the Harris Chair $12.00
" " " Morrison Chair, including the Upright Support . . 12.00

CHEAPER DENTAL CHAIRS.

(ARCHER'S.)

No. 0 is made of Walnut and upholstered in good style, with movable Head-Rest, and can be tipped backward or forward, but the Seat cannot be raised or lowered.

Covered with Figured Plush	$45.00
" " Rep or Enameled Cloth	40.00

No. 1 is made of Walnut and upholstered in good style, with all the movements complete, but with the old style of Head-Rest, same as No. 0. It is covered with Rep or Enameled Cloth.

Price $51.00

No. 2.—This Chair is a very handsome Walnut, Mahogany, or Imitation Rosewood frame, with all the movements complete, and with the patent Head-Rest. It is made with flaring Arms, Carved imitation of swan's neck and head, making the Seat wide enough for the convenience of any patient. See Cut, page 246.

PRICES.

Walnut or Imitation Rosewood, covered with best figured Green or Crimson Plush	$61.00
The same, covered with best plain Green, Crimson, or Blue Plush or Moquette	64.00
Mahogany, covered with best figured Green or Crimson Plush . . .	64.00
The same, covered with best plain Green, Crimson, or Blue Plush or Moquette	67.00

No. 3 is made of the best quality of Black Walnut or Mahogany, Carved and covered with the best quality of Plush or Moquette. It has flaring Arms, Carved in imitation of swan's neck and head. See Cut, page 247.

Price of either Walnut or Mahogany $90.00

No. 4 is made of solid Rosewood, Carved, and covered with the best quality Plush inside and outside alike, and with Silver, Gilt, or Porcelain Headed Nails. The Seat is raised by means of a Silver-Plated wheel instead of crank, and the brass work is Silver-Plated.

Price	$125.00
Mahogany or Walnut, same style and finish	110.00

Any of the above Chairs (except No. 4) upholstered with Silver, Gilt, or Porcelain Nails, $2.00 extra.

The prices above given are for Chairs only, and do not include Footstool, Spittoon, etc.

DENTAL CHAIR, No. 2.

(ARCHER'S.)

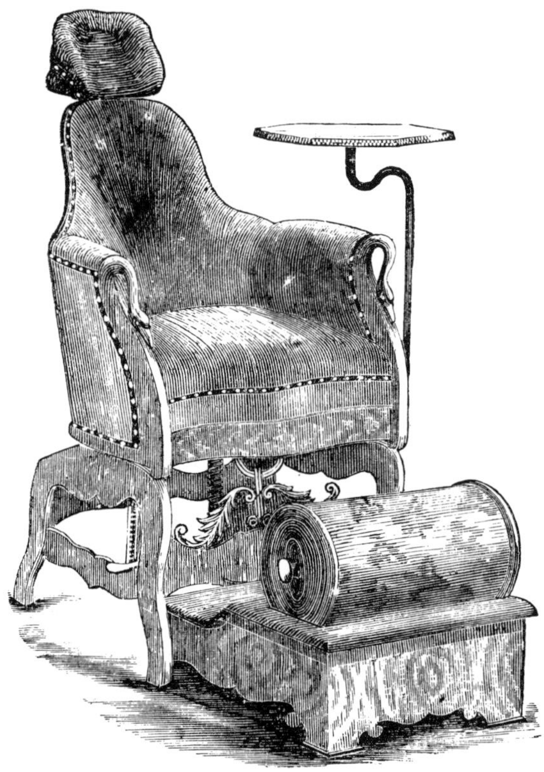

The above engraving represents a No. 2 Chair, No. 2 Footstool, and No. 1 Instrument Stand. The Chair is covered with plain Plush and trimmed with Porcelain, Gilt, or Silver-Headed Nails.

PRICES.

Chair	$66.00
Footstool	13.00
Instrument Stand	5.00

DENTAL CHAIR, No. 3.

(ARCHER'S.)

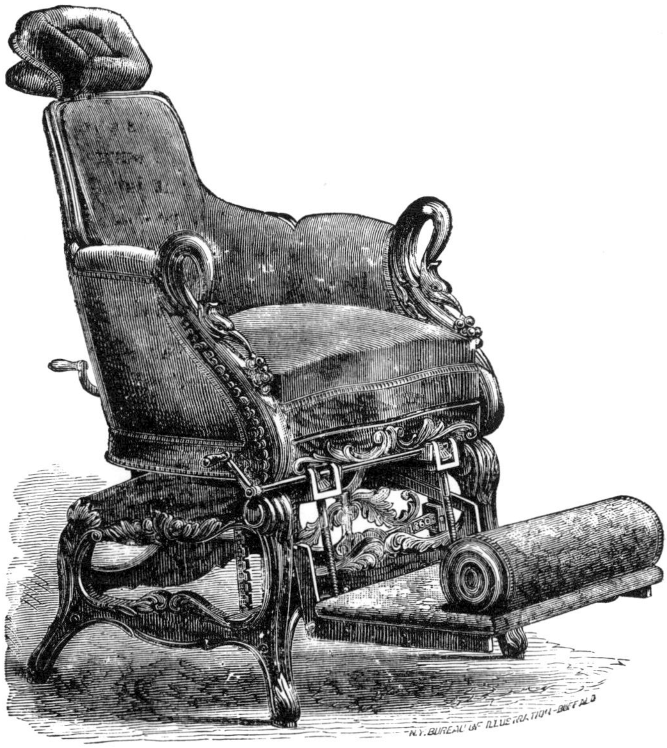

The above engraving represents a No. 3 Chair with Footstool attached. The curtain that covers the machinery has been removed in order to show the working parts of the Footstool. The Chair is Oil-finished and covered with best plain Plush. This Footstool can be attached to any of the other cheap Chairs, or the Footstool shown on page 246 will go with this Chair when preferred.

PRICES.

Chair	$90.00
Footstool	15.00

IMPROVED SELF-ATTACHING PORTABLE HEAD-REST.

INVENTION OF DR. O. C. WHITE.

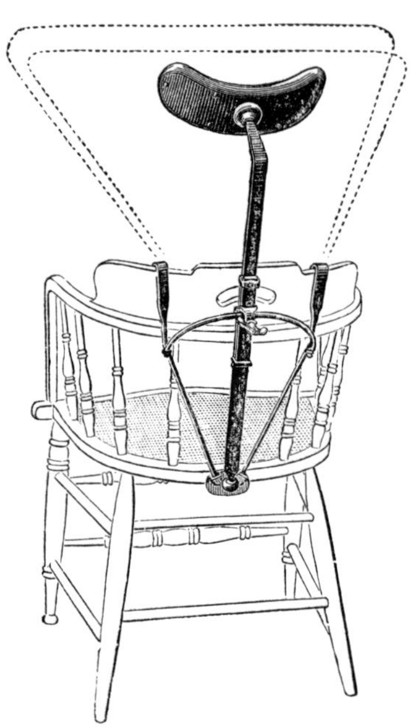

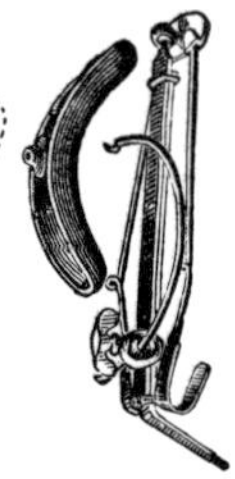

The accompanying Cuts represent Rests Nos. 6 and 7 applied to a common office-chair, with dotted lines showing its movement; and the Rest, on the same scale of size, folded up, to occupy but little space, either for transportation or to lay aside. Weight, $4\frac{3}{4}$ pounds.

It makes its own fastening to almost any style of Chair, Sofa, Lounge, or Settee.

It has full movement in all directions, and may be adjusted for a tall person or for a child, and is securely fastened by turning a *single* Thumb-Screw.

It is well adapted for Office, Travel, or the House; on Chairs for the sick it is invaluable.

No. 6, Nickel-Plated Thumb-Screw and Top-Piece, Japanned Steel Bars and Slide-Rods, upholstered in Plush . . .	$10.00
No. 7, same form, Japanned Wrought-Iron Bars and Slide-Rods, Japanned Thumb-Screw and Top-Piece, upholstered in Rep	7.50

PORTABLE HEAD-REST, No. 9.

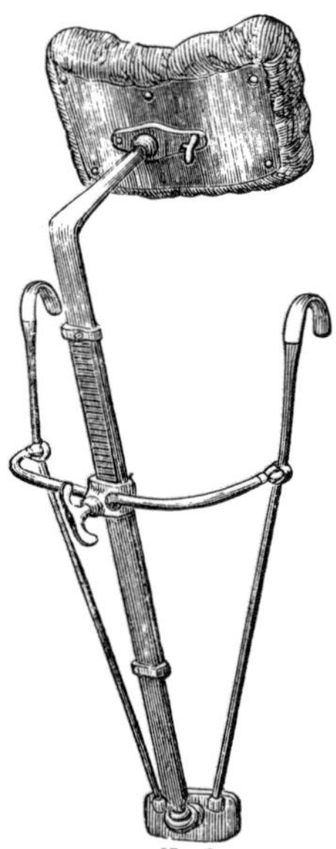

No. 9.

This Rest is much heavier than Nos. 6 and 7, and has the principal movements and advantages of a Stationary Head-Rest. It can be adapted to almost any Chair, and is thus for many purposes equivalent to an extra Operating-Chair in the office. It is especially useful for making examinations of the mouth, and in cases where frequent changes of position and light are desired. It is attached by a ball-and-socket joint.

The upholstery is of fine Plush, stuffed with curled hair, with sewed rolls to fit the head.

The Rest can be folded up so as to occupy but little space, as shown in Cut of Nos. 6 and 7. The metal portions are so arranged as to afford the greatest firmness and strength, and are made of Steel and Wrought and Malleable Iron, nicely Japanned. The Thumb-Screws and Socket-Plate are Nickel-Plated. Weight, $7\frac{1}{4}$ lbs.

Price, Complete.	Plush, Silver-Plated Mountings .	$15.00
" "	Rep, Japanned Mountings . .	12.00

Chair Appurtenances.

FOOTSTOOLS.

These Footstools (Nos. 1, 2, 3, 4), illustrated in the Cut on page 246, are strong and convenient. They can be raised and lowered to suit the rise and fall of the Chair Seat.

No. 1, Plain Walnut, covered with Ingrain Carpet	$11.00
No. 2, Mahogany, Walnut, or Imitation Rosewood, covered with Brussels Carpet	13.00
No. 3, Mahogany or Walnut, Carved, and covered with Velvet Carpet . .	20.00
No. 4, Rosewood, Carved, and covered with bėst Velvet Carpet . . .	25.00

No. 5.

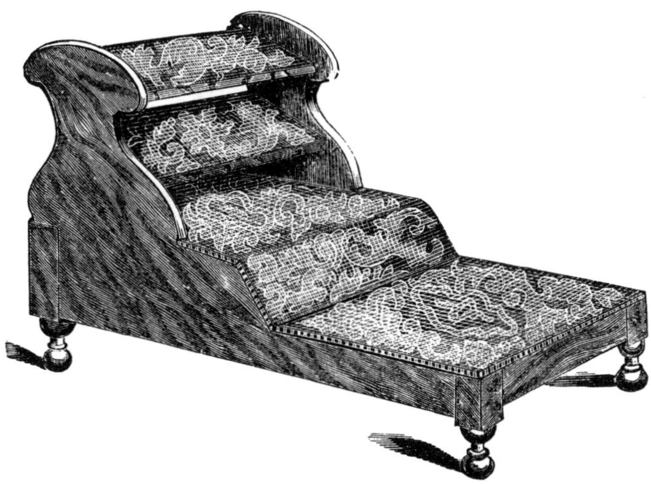

No. 5, Walnut, Oiled or Varnished, or Imitation Rosewood or Mahogany.

Dimensions.—Front, 6½ inches high; back, 20 inches high; width, 18 inches; length, 30 inches,—outside measurements.

Covered with Brussels Carpet	$12.50
Without Carpet	9.00
Brass Foot-Strips to protect the Carpet, extra	3.00

No. 6.

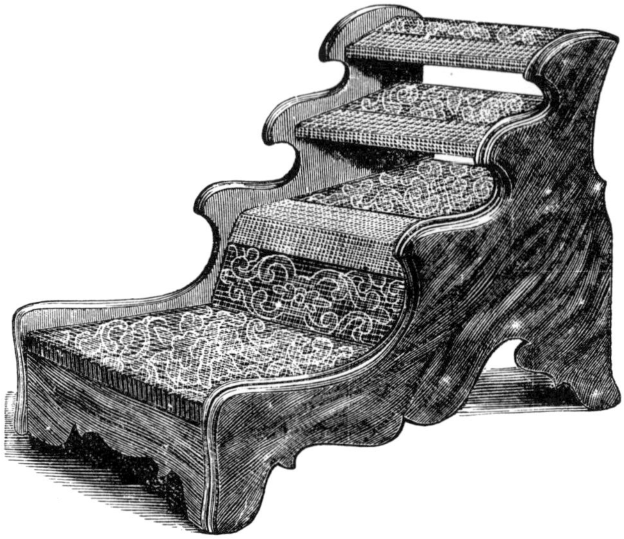

No. 6, Walnut, Oiled or Varnished, or Imitation Rosewood.

DIMENSIONS.—Front, 6½ inches high; back, 25 inches high; width, 19 inches; length, 30 inches,—outside measurements.

Covered with Brussels Carpet, with figured Brass Foot-Strips to protect the Carpet	$16.50
Carpeted, without Brass Strips	13.50
Plain, without Carpet or Brass Strips	10.00

FOOTSTOOL TO BE ATTACHED TO CHEAP CHAIRS.

This Footstool, shown on page 247, is strong and durable. It is raised or lowered by means of a crank on the side of the Chair. It can be attached to almost any wood-framed Chair.

Price $15.00

CUP FOR PLUGGERS, EXCAVATORS, ETC.

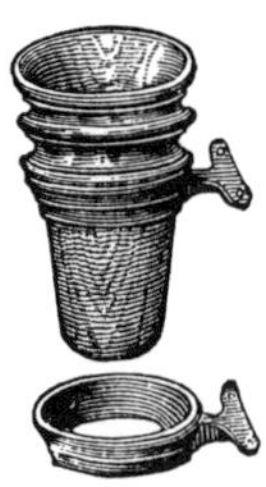

This Cup is designed to be attached to, or set into, any extension bracket or instrument table, for holding pluggers, excavators, files, etc. It is one of the most convenient attachments to a Table yet produced. It is made in the best manner. It can be set into a Table without interfering with the drawers, or can be attached by a ring shown in Cut.

Cup, Black Walnut, highly polished	each 60 cents
Ring, Japanned	" 10 "

SPITTOONS.

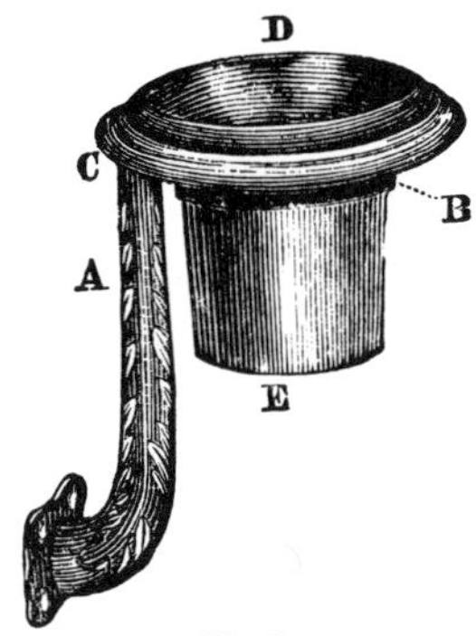

No. 1.

No. 1.—"A" is the Standard to be attached to the lower part of the Chair, which remains firm when the upper part is thrown back. "B" is the Ring attached by a strong bolt to the top of the Standard, on which it can be moved so as to throw the Spittoon toward either the front or the back of the Chair. "C' is the Marble Top, "D" the Glass Funnel, and "E" the Bowl, which, with the Funnel, can be readily removed to be cleansed. The iron work is Bronzed, and is durable.

Price $8.00

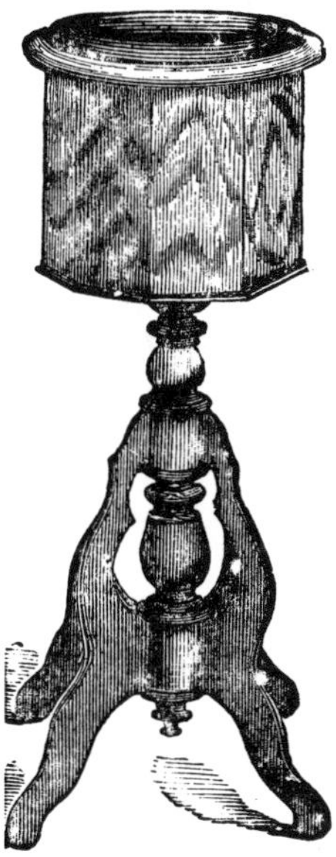
No. 2.

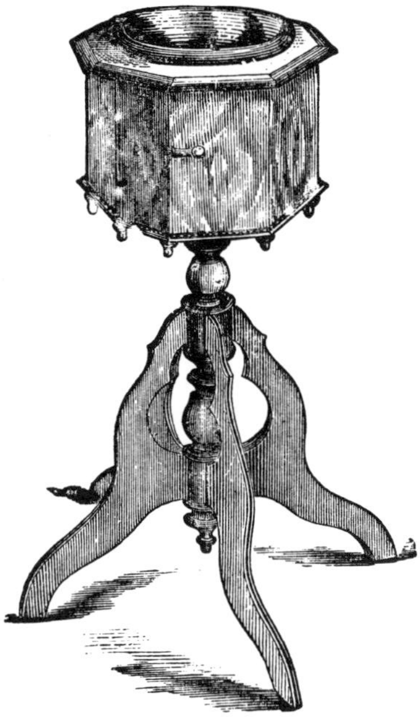
No. 3.

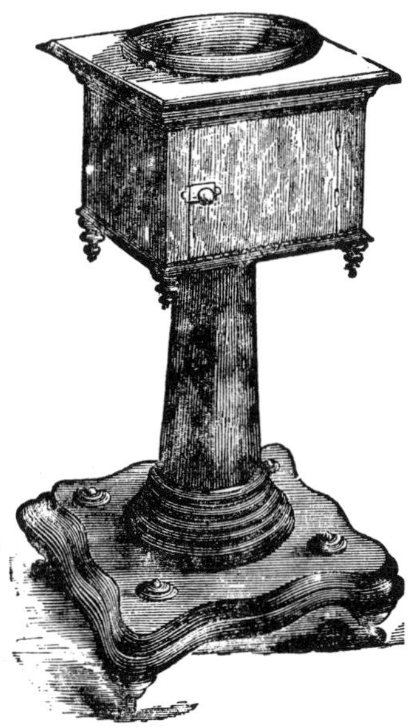
No. 4

No. 2.—Mahogany, Walnut, or Imitation Rosewood, height 32½ inches, with Marble Top and heavy claret-colored Glass Funnel and inside Bowl.

Price $11.00

Rosewood 13.00

No. 3 has an octagon Top covered with a Marble Slab 15 inches in diameter. A door in the side opens to admit an inside Bowl or Spittoon. The lower part of this Spittoon is larger and heavier than No. 2, and stands firmer on the floor. Height, 32½ inches.

Walnut. Mahogany, or Rosewood $18.00

No. 4 is covered with a Marble Slab 16 inches square, affording room to set a glass of water outside of the Glass Funnel. In one side is a door to admit an inside Bowl. The Base is on castors, and, being heavy, it stands firm on the floor. Height, 33 inches.

Walnut, Mahogany, or Rosewood $20.00

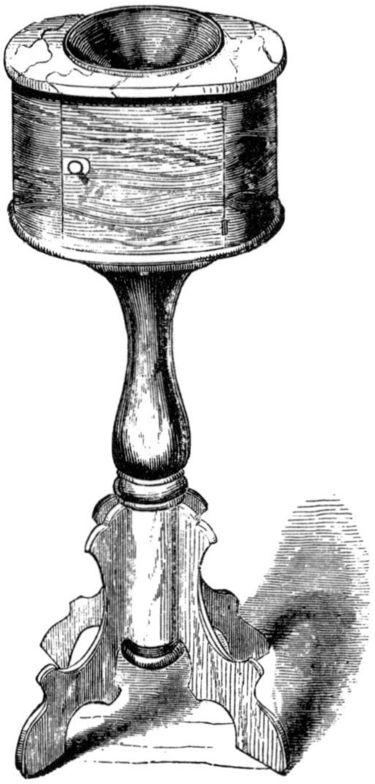

No. 5.

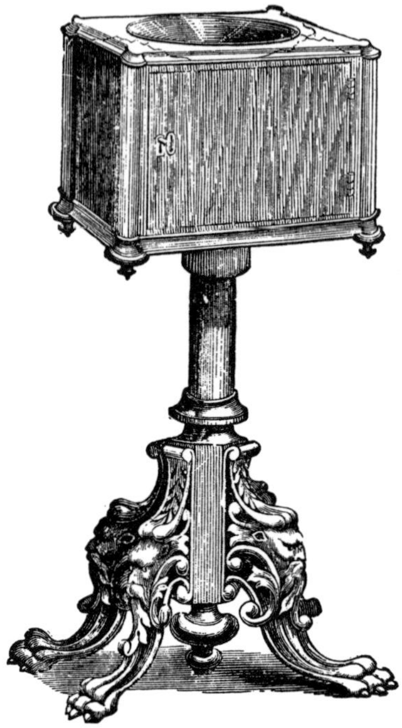

No. 6.

No. 5, Walnut, White Marble	$22.00
No. 6, Carved Oiled Walnut, White Marble	35.00
" " Tennessee Marble	36.00
Boxing, extra	1.50

Our stock in this line is extensive and varied. Only the principal styles are illustrated. The prices range from $9.00 to $36.00.

Boxing, extra $1.50

MARBLE TOPS FOR SPITTOON-STANDS.

White Italian, Square and Oval	each	$4.00
Tennessee, " "	"	8.75
Lisbon, " "	"	9.75
Mosaic, " "	"	11.50
White Italian, for Nos. 1 and 2 Spittoons	"	3.00
" " " No. 3 Spittoon	"	5.00
" " " No. 4 "	"	6.00

IMITATION MARBLE TOPS FOR SPITTOON-STANDS.

ENAMELED SLATE.

Spanish (red), Square and Oval	$4.00
Verde-Antique (green), Square and Oval	4.00
Brocatelle (yellow), " "	4.00

SPITTOON AND BRACKET FOR THE HARRIS CHAIR.

BRACKET FROM PATTERN OF DR. J. A. WOODWARD.

The Carrier for this Spittoon is adapted to the Harris Chair, to which it is attached by means of a Socket-plate, screwed to the left arm, in which the stem of the Bracket or Carrier hangs safely, has free motion, and from which it may be readily removed. It is of Steel, finely Polished and Nickel-Plated.

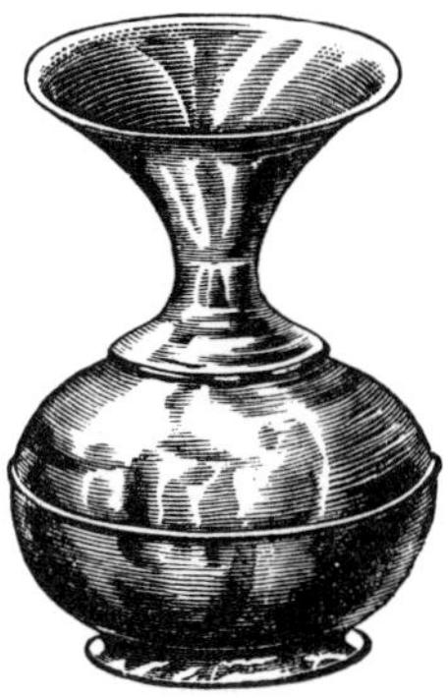

No. 2.

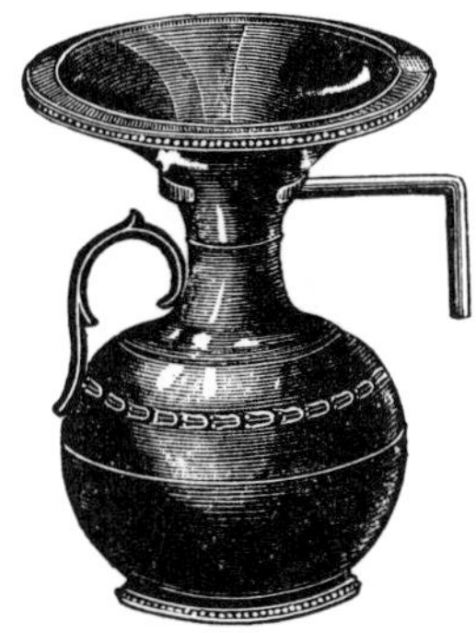

No. 3.

Cut No. 2 represents a Spittoon of Spun Brass, Nickel-Plated. Nine inches high. Funnel seven inches in diameter. The Funnel is connected with the body or base of the Spittoon by a heavy screw collar, affording facility for readily and thoroughly cleansing the same. A Gold-catcher or Cup fits into the neck, resting by a flange upon the shoulder. The saving thus effected will soon be sufficient to more than pay the cost of the Spittoon.

Cut No. 3 represents a Jet Spittoon with handle and gilt ornament. Nine and one-half inches high. Funnel seven and one-half inches in diameter.

Price of the Carrier or Bracket	$7.00
" " Spittoon No. 2, including Gold-Cup	12.00
" " Jet Spittoon, No. 3, with Handle	5.00
" " " " " without Handle	4.75

NICKEL-PLATED SPITTOON FUNNELS.

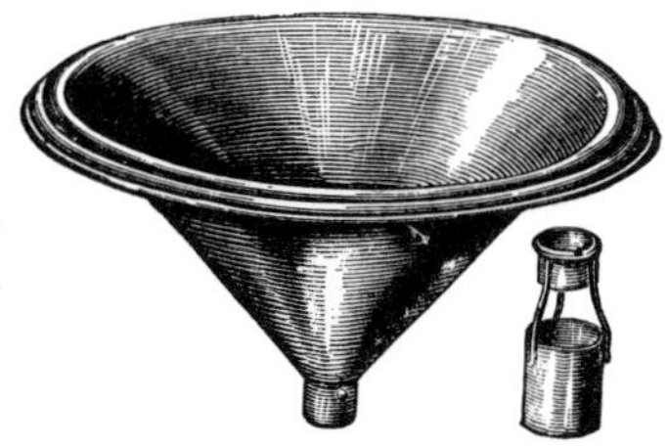

Heavy Brass, and bound with stout wire, neatly covered by the metal, and Nickel-Plated throughout; the exposed surface highly Polished. A Gold-Cup, also of Brass, Nickel-Plated, is attached, which can be instantly removed and replaced by simply turning it once around. There are three sizes, 9½, 10, and 10½ inches in diameter, 5⅝ inches deep.

Price, with Cup attached . . . . $4.25, $4.50, and $4.75

GLASS SPITTOON-FUNNELS.

Heavy Glass, Claret-colored, 7½, 9, 10, 11, and 12 inches in diameter.

Price . . . . per pound 50 cents

DR. I. W. LYON'S IMPROVED ADJUSTABLE STOOL.

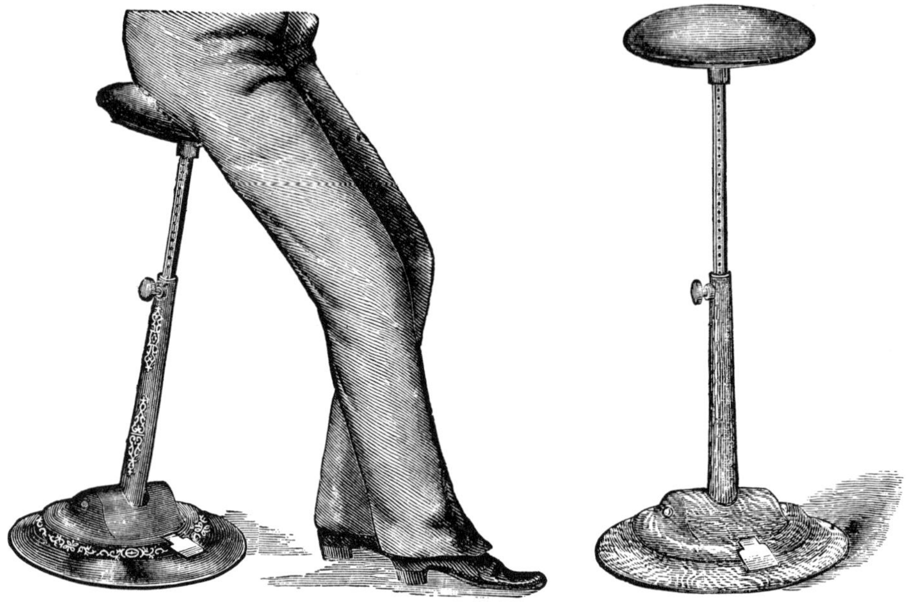

No. 1. No. 2.

A Stool designed for Dentists. The Base is Cast-iron, and the Shaft is attached to it in such a way that it may be changed from a perpendicular and held at any desired angle, by means of the Treadle. The Top revolves, and may be raised from 23 to 35 inches, and made fast at any point. It is upholstered with curled hair, and covered with Green or Crimson Plush, or Leather.

The improvement consists in a change in the shape of the Base, by which the Ratchet Lock is placed beneath, and the Treadle only (which is Nickel-Plated) projects, as shown in the Cut. The Operator can change the angle at pleasure, by placing the heel upon the Treadle, without rising from the Stool. Another improvement consists in a new form of Ratchet Lock, which holds the Stool firmly at the desired angle without danger of slipping. A still further improvement is in the means by which the Stool is held at the desired height. The Sliding-rod has a groove or slot in which holes have been drilled to receive a Plunger, which springs into place at each half-inch of the Rod, requiring only the force of the thumb and finger to withdraw it when a change of height is required.

The *inclined position* (represented in Cut No. 1) gives a peculiarly agreeable sensation of rest and comfort, coming up, as it does, *well at the back, thereby supporting the spine*, giving freedom of action to the limbs, and allowing the feet to rest upon the floor, dispensing with the necessity of a foot-rest. The Stool is now in use by many leading Dentists, who speak of it in the highest terms of praise.

No. 1.	Japanned Black, Gilt or Figured Band, Nickel-Plated Lever . . .	$18.00
" 2.	Imitation of Oak, Nickel-Plated Lever and Thumb Screw	20.00
" 3.	" of Rosewood, or Rosewood and Oak, Nickel-Plated Lever and Thumb Screw	21.00
Boxing, extra	. . . .	1.00

Dental Brackets.

THE S. S. WHITE DENTAL BRACKET, No. 1.

(Patented Nov. 2, 1875.)

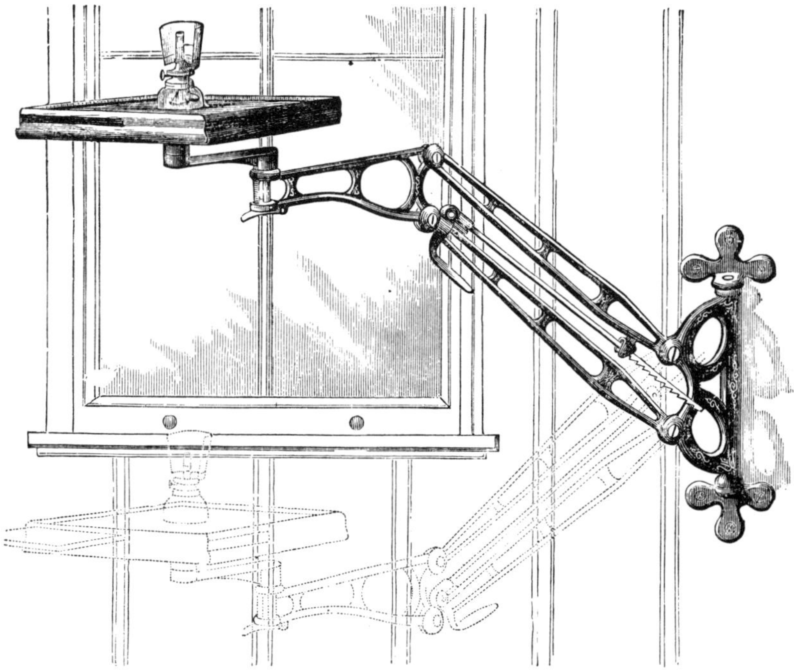

This Bracket is attached to the wall or other support by screws, swinging from its Base either to the right or left. It has a vertical range of twenty-six inches. The Cut represents the Table in its highest, the dotted lines in its lowest position.

It is raised and lowered by a Rod, having a Ratchet at the end, which holds it at any desired point within its range. The movement is as simple as lifting a door-latch, and requires the use of only one hand.

The length of the Bracket proper is thirty-eight inches, but when desired the Table may be swung beyond the Bracket, making a reach of fifty-one inches.

The Table is held solidly at either extension by a pin, which is controlled by a touch of the thumb at the end of the stationary Arm.

The Table is thirteen inches square, and contains four drawers, which are thrown out from either corner by a touch of the finger. It has a depression in the center to receive an alcohol lamp. It is covered with Velvet.

The Bracket is Japanned and neatly ornamented. The Ratchet-rod is Nickel-Plated.

Price, with Lamp	$20.00
Boxing	1.00

EXTENSION BRACKET, No. 2.

PRICE REDUCED.

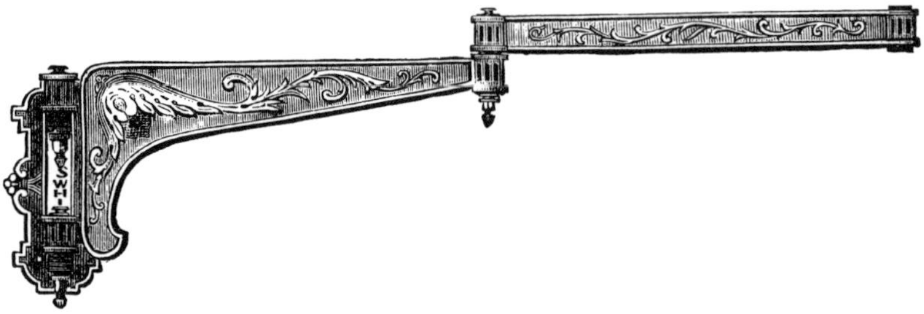

This Bracket was devised expressly for those who wish to have a fine, handsome, and tasty fixture which will bear very heavy weight. It was designed for holding a Tray which, with instruments, weighed 30 pounds, and to extend at any angle or flexure without injury under that weight. The Joints at both Main and Small Arm flexions are made with Coned Steel Pins and Friction Washers, which can be tightened as they wear, and, with proper attention, will last a lifetime.

Length, extended, to center of Tray, 31 inches.

Iron, Imitation Bronze, with Brass Trimmings (formerly $17.00), reduced to	$15.00
Brass Tray, Scalloped, Raised Rim, strengthened by Ribs underneath	4.00
The same, with Velvet Pad	5.50

EXTENSION BRACKET, No. 3.

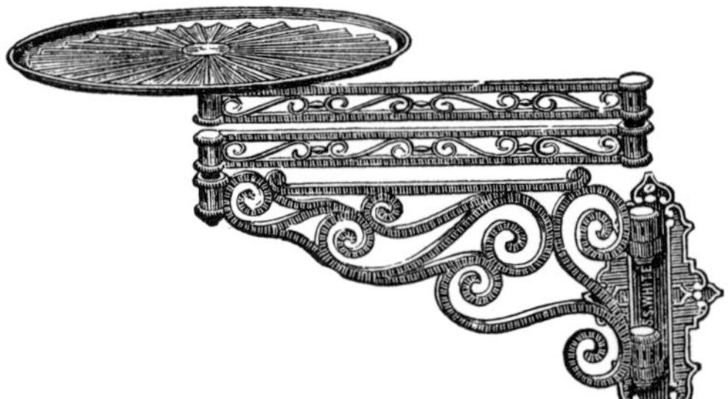

Cast-iron Extension Bracket, with three Joints or Arms, measuring 16 inches each in length. The Tray is made of Brass, 12½ inches in diameter, with a stationary Rim. The patterns of this Bracket have been carefully renewed. It is light, strong, neat, and convenient. Its great extension, with three flexions, makes it easy to place it just where desired in operating. The Joints are made with Coned Steel Pins, and Nuts to draw them down as they wear. Painted dark brown, relieved with Bronze.

Complete, Brass Tray, Japanned $12.00

ZIGZAG EXTENSION BRACKET, No. 4.

PRICES REDUCED.

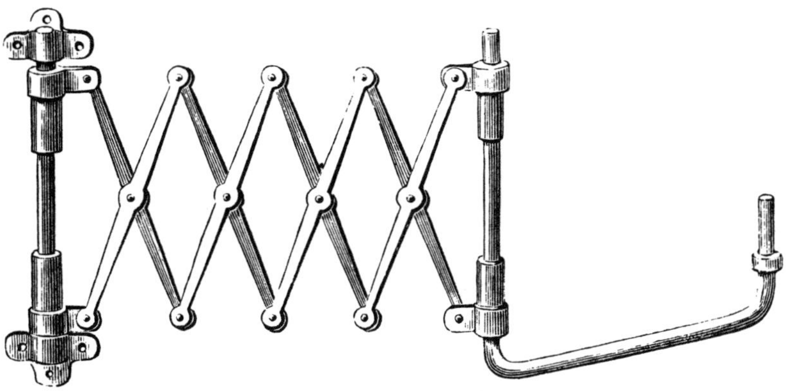

Made in several varieties of material and finish. Its full extension is 44½ inches to center of Tray. We have fitted up many of these Brackets with a small extra Tray on top of the Tray-arm. This is used for lamp, foil, gutta-percha stopping, water-cup, etc., keeping these articles apart from instruments.

Japanned, less Table	$20.00
" for two Tables	21.00
Nickel-Plated, Selected Bars, Screws in place of Rivets, less Tables (formerly $40.00), reduced to	30.00
Nickel-Plated, Selected Bars, Screws in place of Rivets, for two Tables (formerly $41.00), reduced to	31.00
Plain Round Tables for same, nicely Polished (formerly $3.00 and $4.00), reduced to	$2.00 and $3.00

Cabinets.

CABINET CASE, No. 1.

(ARCHER'S.)

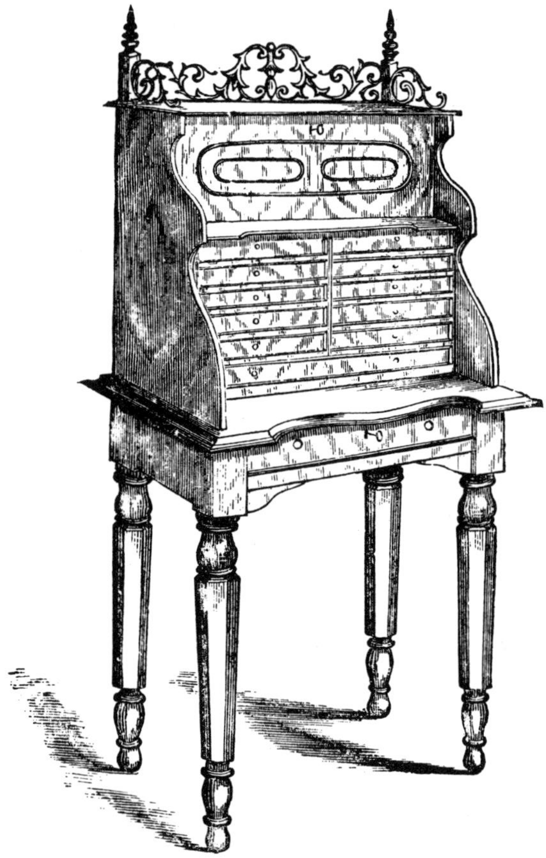

As the Engraving gives a correct idea of the style and proportions of the above Cabinet, no other description will be required than the general dimensions. The upper portion, or Case proper, is 24 inches high, 28 inches wide, and 11 inches deep. It contains one drawer the whole width of the Case, and ten smaller ones. The top part is opened by throwing down its front, which then forms a shelf or platform upon which articles in use can be laid. By a peculiar arrangement, the whole of the drawers and upper part of the Case can be locked by one key. The table contains a large drawer for instruments, the full size of the table, and a shelf which slides out above the drawer. All the drawers are lined with imitation Morocco.

Black Walnut, Varnished or Oil-Finished $40.00

CABINET CASE, No. 2.

(ARCHER'S.)

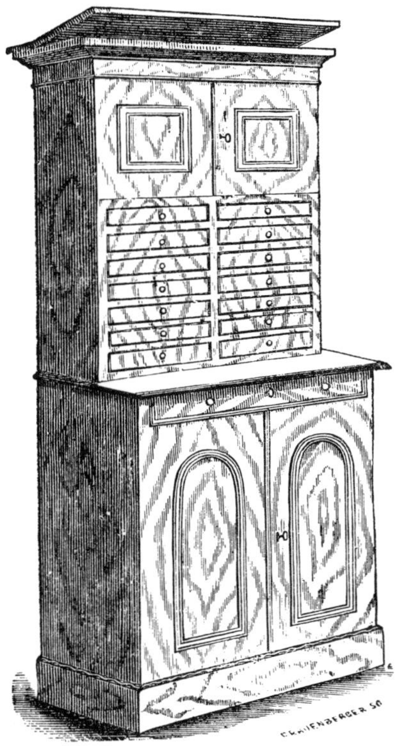

It is 5 feet 2 inches high and 2 feet 2 inches wide. The lower part, which is covered with a marble slab, contains a cupboard and a drawer for forceps, the full width of the Case and 2 inches deep. The upper part contains four drawers, 12 inches wide and 12 inches long, by 2 inches deep; also, ten drawers, 12 inches wide and 12 inches long, by $1\frac{1}{2}$ inches deep. Above the drawers are two cupboards and an apartment at the top, full width of Case and 4 inches deep. The whole of the drawers and the upper cupboards are locked with only two locks. The drawer and the cupboards in the lower part are also provided with good locks. The drawers in this Case are stained inside, as are also the apartments at the top. Lined with imitation Morocco for $5.00 extra.

Black Walnut, Varnished or Oil-Finished $50.00

CABINET CASE, No. 3.

(ARCHER'S.)

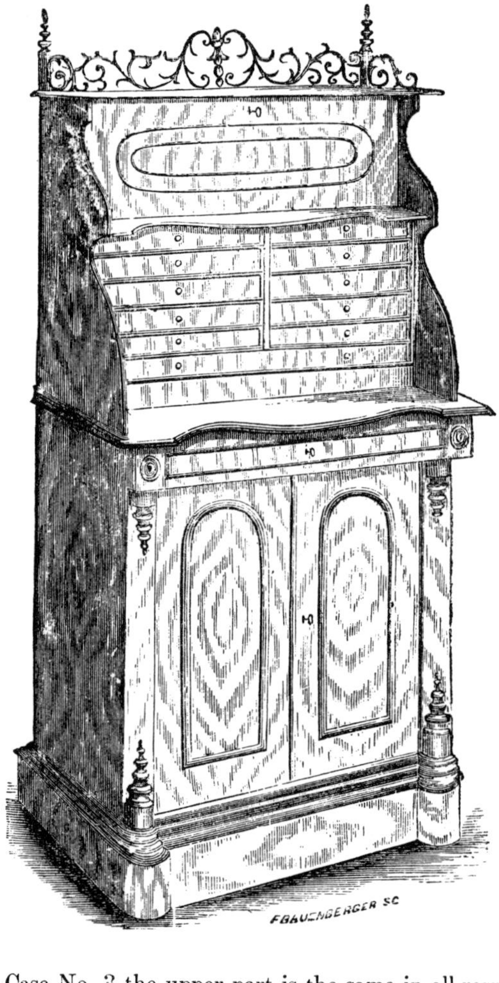

In the Cabinet Case No. 3 the upper part is the same in all respects as No. 1. The lower part contains a cupboard with an adjustable shelf. Above the cupboard is a drawer for forceps, and above the drawer a shelf slides out. The upper or lower part will be sold separately when desired.

Upper Portion	$35.00
Lower "	25.00
Complete	60.00

CABINET CASE, No. 4.

(ARCHER'S.)

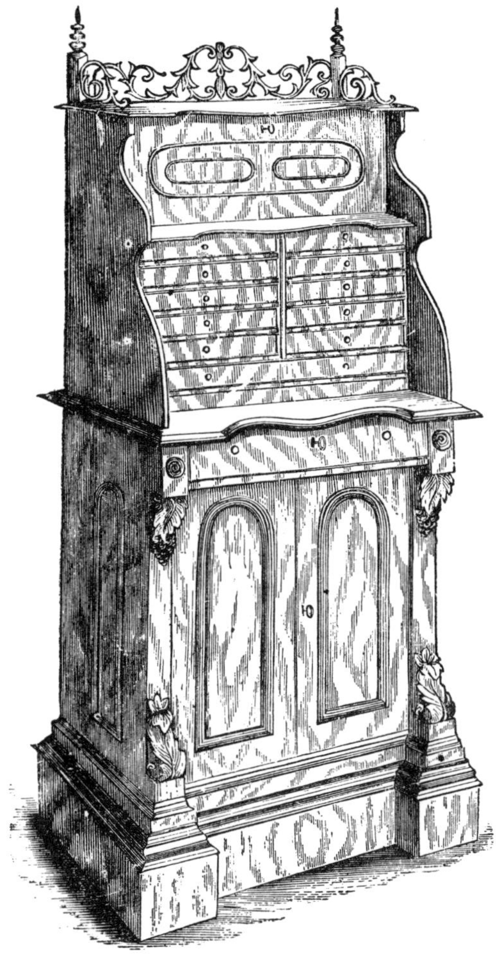

The above Engraving gives a good idea of the style and proportions of the No. 4 Cabinet Case. The upper part is the same as the No. 1 and No. 3, and the lower part is the same in all respects as the No 5. Although somewhat cheaper, many prefer it to the No. 5. The upper and lower parts will be sold separately.

Upper Portion	$35.00
Lower "	40.00
Complete	75.00

CABINET CASE, No. 5.

(ARCHER'S.)

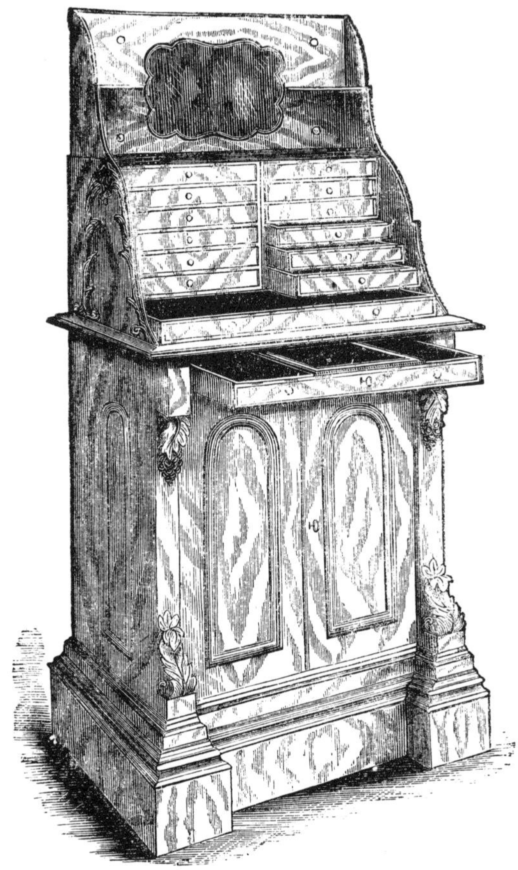

The above Engraving shows the No. 5 Cabinet Case, open. It presents a mirror at the top and a shelf above the drawers, and two small bracket shelves each side of the mirror. In the upper part there is one large drawer, 26 inches long, 10 inches wide, and 2 inches deep, and twelve other drawers, 13 inches long, 10 inches wide, and $1\frac{1}{2}$ inches deep; all lined with imitation Morocco. In the lower part is the drawer for forceps, and a shelf that slides out just above the drawer. The upper and lower portions will be sold separately.

Upper Portion	$45.00
Lower "	40.00
Complete	85.00

CABINET CASE, No. 6.

(ARCHER'S)

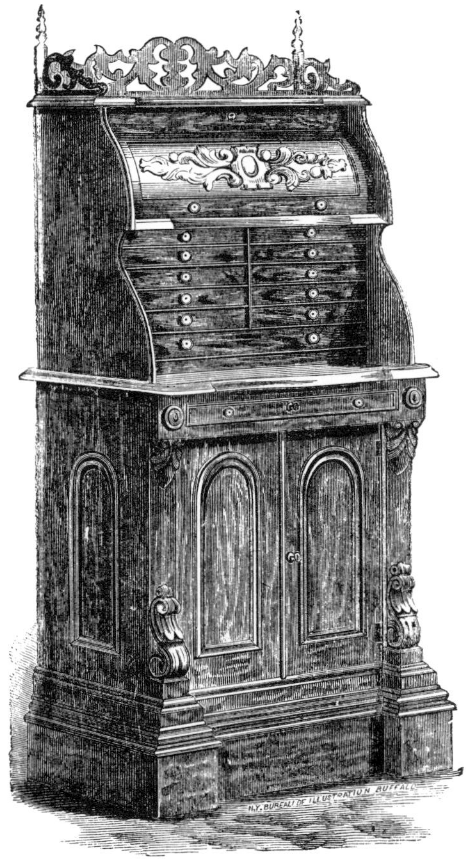

The top apartment, when opened by pushing up the circular door, is 8 inches in height, 26 inches wide, and 11 inches deep, with a mirror at the back, and marble shelf. Under the marble shelf are ten small drawers and one large one, varying in depth from one and a quarter to one and a half inches. Under the drawers is another marble shelf or top, covering the whole of the bottom part of the Cabinet. Beneath this marble and in the lower part is a slide 20 inches wide and 16 inches deep, and a drawer 22 inches wide and 16 inches deep. The cupboard, which has an adjustable shelf, is 22 inches high, 25½ inches wide, and 14 inches deep, inside measure. All the drawers and slides are lined with imitation Morocco.

Black Walnut, Oil-Finished, with Marble Shelf and Top $100.00
" " " " Walnut " " 85.00

CABINET CASE, No. 7.

(ARCHER'S.)

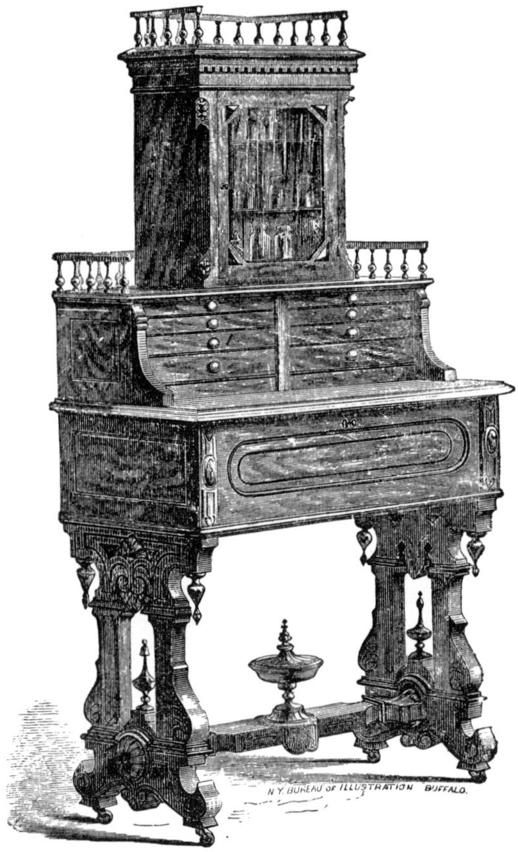

The above Cabinet Case is showy and convenient. The back is of Walnut, paneled, so that it presents a neat and finished appearance, even when standing in the center of a room. Being made entirely of Walnut, the drawers are not lined. The upper part has a glass door and mirror at the back, with two thin Walnut adjustable shelves. Next beneath are two tiers of four drawers each, from $\frac{7}{8}$ of an inch to $1\frac{1}{2}$ inches in depth, and 14 inches long by 7 inches wide, inside measure. The marble shelf is 10 inches wide and 35 inches long. Under the marble shelf are six drawers, two of them $1\frac{1}{2}$ inches deep, two 2 inches deep, and two 3 inches deep, and all of them 14 inches long by 15 inches wide. These drawers are all inclosed by a door which lets down when in use.

Grained Walnut, Oil-Finished $85.00

CABINET CASE, No. 8.

(S. S. WHITE'S.)

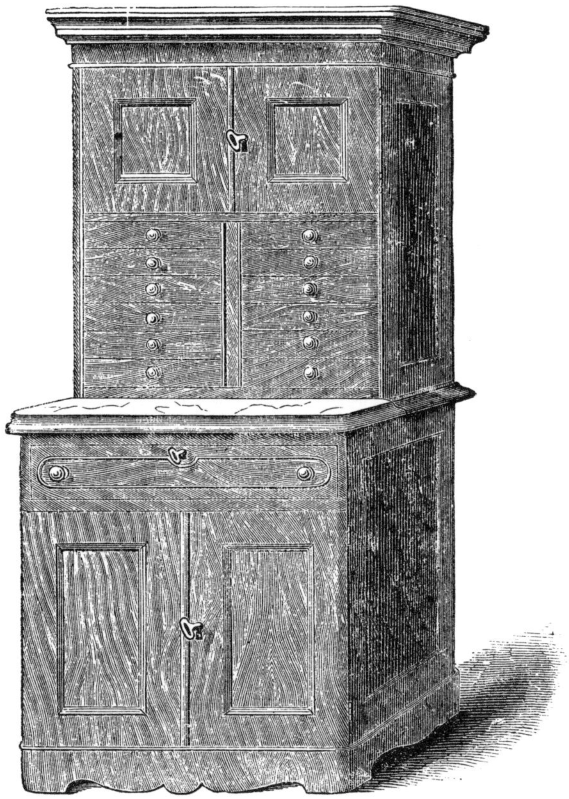

Outside measurement of entire Case as follows: height, 62 inches; width, 26 inches; depth of lower half, 17 inches; depth of upper half, 12 inches. White Marble Table-top.

Large drawer, 24 inches long, 15½ inches wide, 4½ inches deep (outside measurements); this drawer has a sliding shelf in the form of a tray, hiding forceps, etc., from view, and answering instead of a table when the drawer is pulled out. Ten of the small drawers measure 11¾ inches long, 11¼ inches wide, 1½ inches deep. The two bottom small drawers, same length and width, 3 inches deep (outside measurements). These twelve drawers are locked by a single movement of a bolt inside the top closet. Dimensions of top closet, 24 inches wide, 12½ inches high, 11¼ inches deep (inside measurements). The bottom closet, 24 inches wide, 20 inches high, 15 inches deep (inside measurements). Top of Cabinet hinged on.

Walnut, Oil-Finished	$70.00
" " Drawers lined with Silk Finish Cotton Velvet . .	85.00

CABINET CASE, No. 9.

(DR. B. F. ARRINGTON'S PATTERN.)

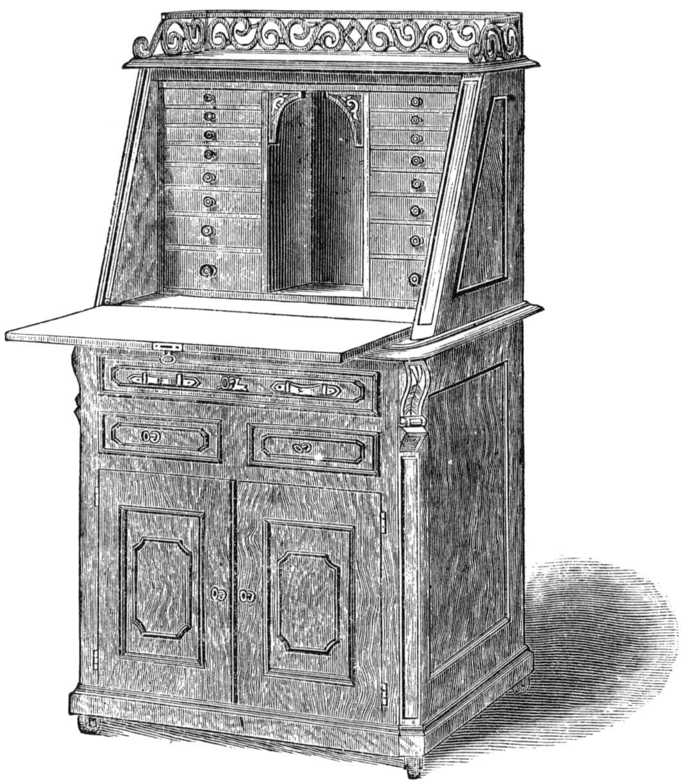

Outside measurements of entire Cabinet: width, 33¾ inches; height, 56 inches; depth, 21 inches; the upper portion being 21¾ inches high, and containing sixteen drawers, each 9 inches long and 9 inches wide, ranging in depth from ⅞ to 3¼ inches. This portion is closed by a falling lid, which, when down, can be used as a desk or support for instruments. The lower portion contains three drawers, one of which is 27½ inches long by 18 inches wide and 4¼ inches deep, the other two being 13¼ inches long by 18 inches wide and 4¼ inches deep. These three drawers each have inside movable trays. Beneath the drawers is a closet 18 inches high, 27½ inches long, 18 inches deep, containing a shelf across the center from side to side. Mounted on castors.

Walnut, Oil-Finished $80.00

MECHANICAL DENTISTRY.

GOLD AND SILVER PLATE, ETC.

Gold Plate, 18 carats fine	per dwt.	$0.90
" 20 carats fine	"	1.00
" 22 carats fine	"	1.10
" Pure (Ribbon)	"	1.12
Gold Webbing, 18 carats fine	"	1.30
Gold Plate, 18 carats fine, alloyed with Platinum, for Clasps and Backings	"	.90
Gold Wire, Round and Half Round, 18 carats fine	"	.90
Gold Spiral Springs, 18 carats fine	"	1.10
" " 10 carats fine	"	.60
Gold Solder, 18 carats fine	"	.90
" 14 carats fine	"	.75
Silver Plate, Coin	"	.08
" Pure	"	.09
Silver Wire, Round and Half Round	"	.09
Silver, Precipitated, Pure	per oz.	2.00
Silver, Granulated, Pure	"	1.80
Silver Springs	per dwt.	.15
Silver Solder	"	.08

The above are Coin prices; when sold for Currency, the current rate of Premium on Coin is added.

FRENCH AND ENGLISH PLATINUM PLATE AND WIRE.

OUR OWN IMPORTATION.

Warranted Pure. Imported to order for all uses. Price fluctuates.

Platinum, of an inferior quality, is sold at a lower price; and it is sometimes sold by Avoirdupois weight (18 dwt. 6 grs.), instead of Troy weight (20 dwt.), making the price appear lower than it really is. Remelted Platinum, if offered for sale by us, will be represented as such.

PRESENT PRICES.

Platinum Plate and Wire	per oz. Troy	$8.50
" " cut to Pattern	" "	9.00
Platinum Pins for Blocks (all sizes)	" "	9.00
Battery Platinum rolled and cut to Pattern	" "	9.50
Platinum and Iridium, cut Square	" "	9 50
" " cut to Pattern	" "	10.00

Platinum is sold at the above rates in Gold, or with the current rate of Premium on Gold Coin added.

ALUMINUM.

A superior article in Plate, cut Square	per oz. Troy	$3.00

WESTON'S NEW METAL AND IMPROVED FLASK.

This Alloy still continues to receive the approbation of the Profession as a Base for Artificial Dentures. It makes one of the cleanest styles of Base in use, because the joints are so perfectly tight that, after years of actual wear, teeth, when broken from the plate, do not show a trace of deposit between them and the Alloy backing,—a claim which cannot be made for any other metallic Base. It makes the best Base for a Lower Denture yet devised, on account of its easy and perfect adaptation, its cleanliness, and its weight. It is repaired or duplicated at a trifling cost of time and material. It is superior to any other material used as a Base, because absolutely free from liability to warp or spring. It is entirely tasteless and harmless in the mouth, containing no poisonous metal, such as antimony, lead, zinc, or copper.

The Flask consists of two rims without top or bottom, to allow for rapid escape of moisture. It is longer than the ordinary flasks, to allow room for the gate and reservoir posterior to the plate. It closes with two small bolts with nuts, and stands on feet.

Price per lb., in 1 lb., $\frac{1}{2}$ lb., or $\frac{1}{4}$ lb. packages $8.00
Flask 1.00
Solder . . . . per oz. 1.00

PATTERN METAL.

ASSORTED THICKNESSES.

This article, which is composed of Lead and Tin (the surface being Tin), is equal to pure metal for the above-named purpose.

Price . . . . per lb. 60 cents.

CHAMBER METAL.

Price . . . . per lb. 50 cents.

PLATE AND WIRE GAUGE.

BROWN & SHARPE'S STANDARD.

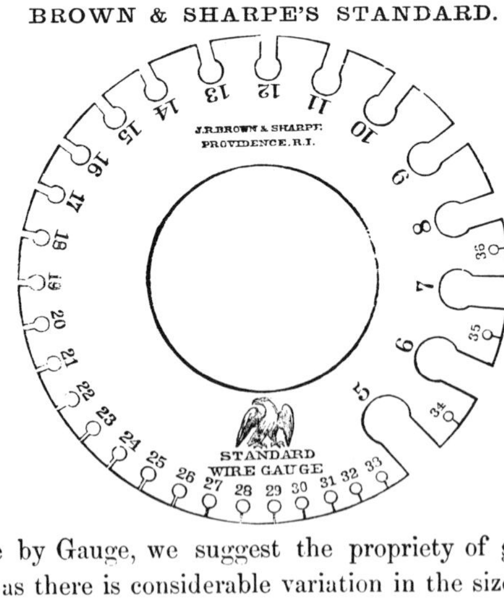

In ordering plate by Gauge, we suggest the propriety of giving the name of the maker of the Gauge, as there is considerable variation in the sizes.

Price . . . . each $4.00

FURNACES.

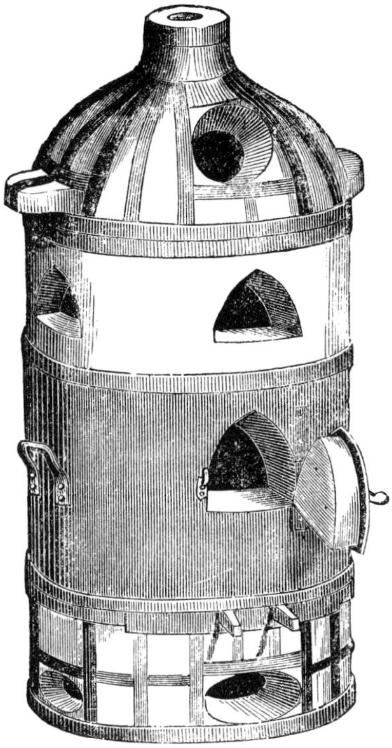

No. 1, FOR TWO MUFFLES.

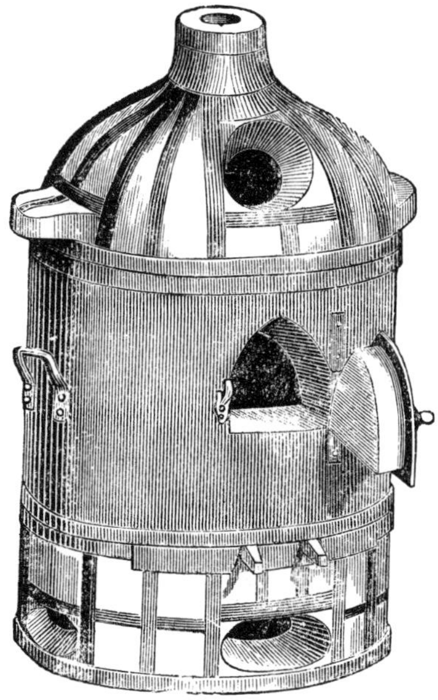

No. 1, FOR ONE MUFFLE.

These Furnaces are oval, with hinged Doors, the center sections cased with Sheet-iron, taking Muffles 12 inches long by 3¾ inches wide, inside measurements. Outside measurements of Furnaces, 43 and 34 inches high, 21 inches wide, and 16 inches deep.

No. 1, For two Muffles	$28.00
" 1, " " with 4 Muffles, 6 Slides, and half-peck Fire-clay, packed in Cask for shipping	33.75
" 1, For one Muffle	22.00
" 1, " " with 4 Muffles, 6 Slides, and half-peck Fire-clay, packed in Cask for shipping	27.50
" 2, smaller, Muffle 11 in. long by 3½ in. wide, inside measurements. Outside measurements, 33 in. high, 20 in. wide, and 14 in. deep	18.00
" 2, For one Muffle, with 4 Muffles, 6 Slides, and half-peck Fire-clay, packed in Cask for shipping	23.00
Muffles, No. 1, 12 inches long by 3¾ inches wide, inside measurements . each	.88
" " 2, 11 " 3½ " " " "	.75
" " 3, 10¼ " 3 " " " "	.60
Slides, " 1 . . . . "	.12
" " 2 . . . . "	.11
" " 3 . . . . "	.10

NOTE.—Philadelphia prices; freight and expenses added when sold at other Depots.

ROLLING MILLS.

LODGE'S.

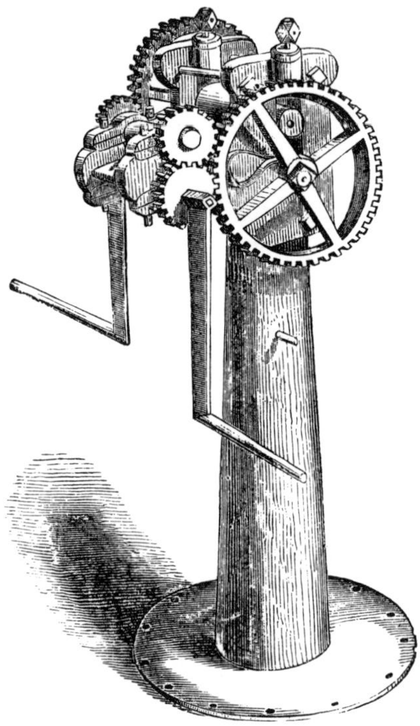

$105.00 MILL.

4 in., Double Geared, on Iron Stand.

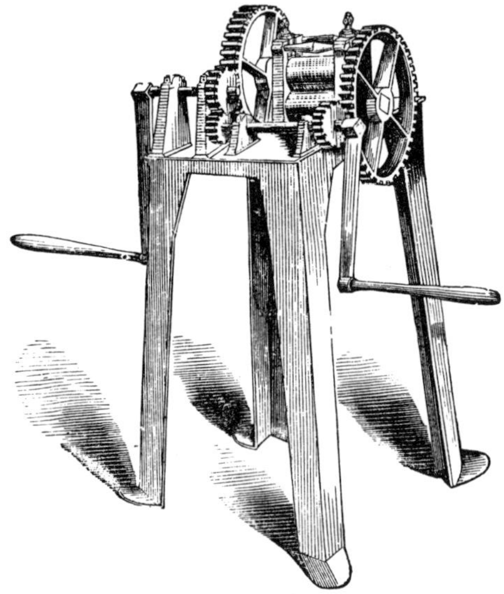

$150.00 MILL.

5 in., Extra Geared, Mounted on Iron Table.

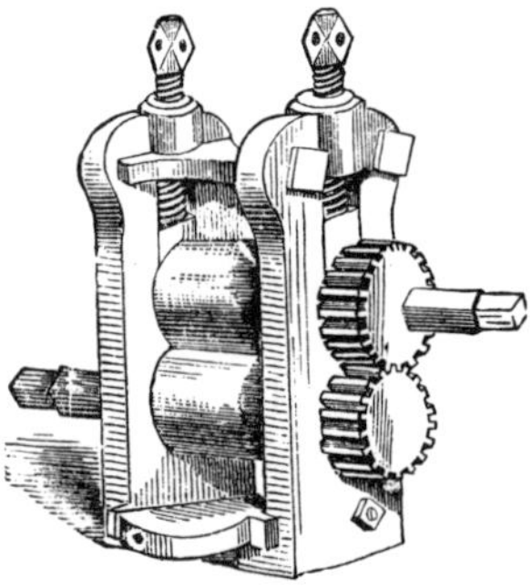

3, 3½, and 4 in. Rolls.

Sold at Manufacturer's prices. Warranted for one year.

3 inch, Plain, without Stand	$45.00
3 " Geared, "	52.50
3½ " Plain, "	52.50
3½ " Geared, "	60.00
4 " Plain, "	60.00
4 " Geared, "	67.50
Iron Stands for the above	7.50
4 inch, Double Geared, on Iron Stand, as per Cut.	105.00
5 " Extra Geared, mounted on Iron Table, as per Cut	150.00

Boxing, extra.

Any size or pattern made to order.

NOTE.—The above are Philadelphia prices; freight and expenses added when sold at other Depots.

THE S. S. WHITE DENTAL OFFICE LATHES.

No. 1.

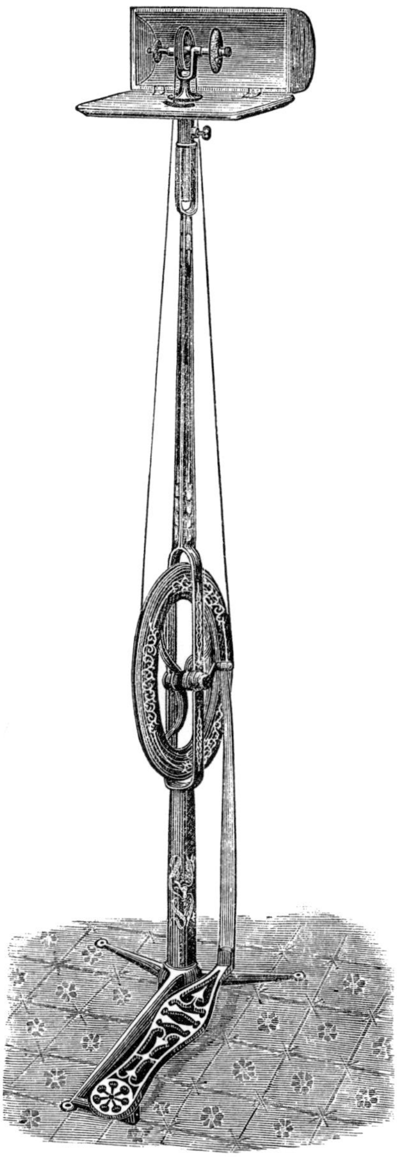

No. 2.

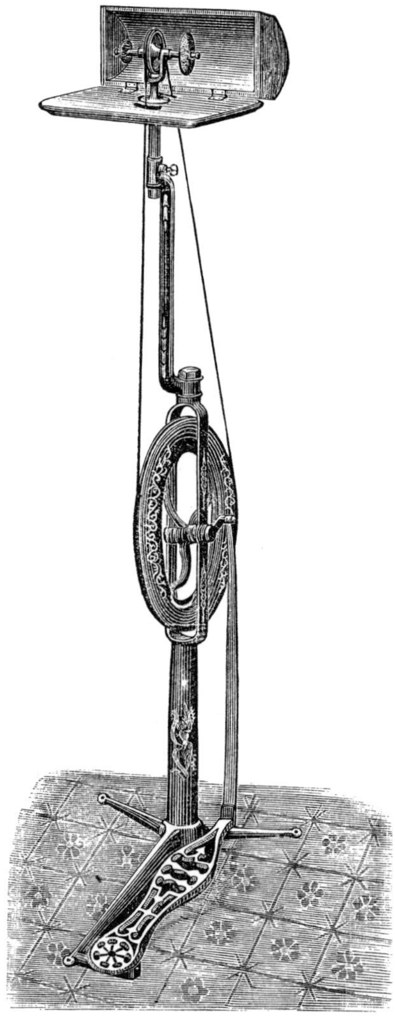

These cuts represent two very light and attractive Lathes, designed for office use. The foot-power is the novel, easily-operated, and efficient combination first used in the S. S. White Dental Engine (Patented August 4th, 1874). The table and head are so pivoted that they can be turned where the hand needs support, and bring either wheel to the operator, as desired.

No. 1 is 3 feet 8½ inches high to the center of the pulley-head, and requires the operator to stand while using it.

No. 2 is 2 feet 11 inches high to the center of the pulley-head, and, to permit the operator to sit while using it, the pulley-head has been brought forward 5 inches from the perpendicular line.

To tighten the cord, or gain additional height, the pulley-head and table of each Lathe may be raised 4 inches, and secured by a set screw.

Price of each, with a set of 6 Corundum Wheels $20.00
Boxing:—No. 1 . . . . . $1.50 No. 2 . . . . 1.00

THE S. S. WHITE LABORATORY LATHE.

No. 3.

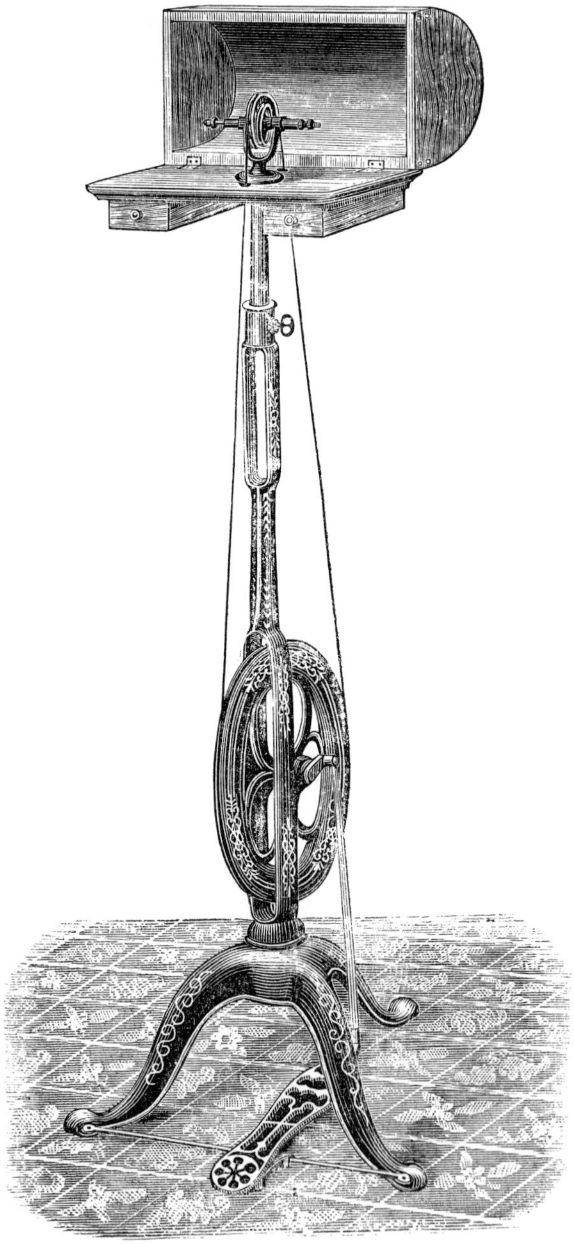

This cut represents a No. 3 Laboratory Lathe. The foot-power is the same as used in the S. S. White Dental Engine (Patented August 4th, 1874). The table and head are so pivoted that they can be turned where the hand needs support, bringing either end of the spindle to the operator, as desired.

The Lathe can be raised or lowered six inches, to tighten the cord, to adapt the cord to either groove in the pulley, or to suit the convenience of the person using it, and held in position by a set screw, as shown in the cut. The pulley-head has two grooves by which the speed may be changed as desired. Three chucks and a screw-cone, as shown in the cut on p. 276, accompany the Lathe, and are adapted to one end of the spindle. The other end of the spindle is provided with a nut-clamp, by which the burs, drills, and corundum points of the Dental Engine may be run.

Price of Lathe, with Chucks $25.00
Boxing 2.00

THE S. S. WHITE LABORATORY LATHE.

No. 4.

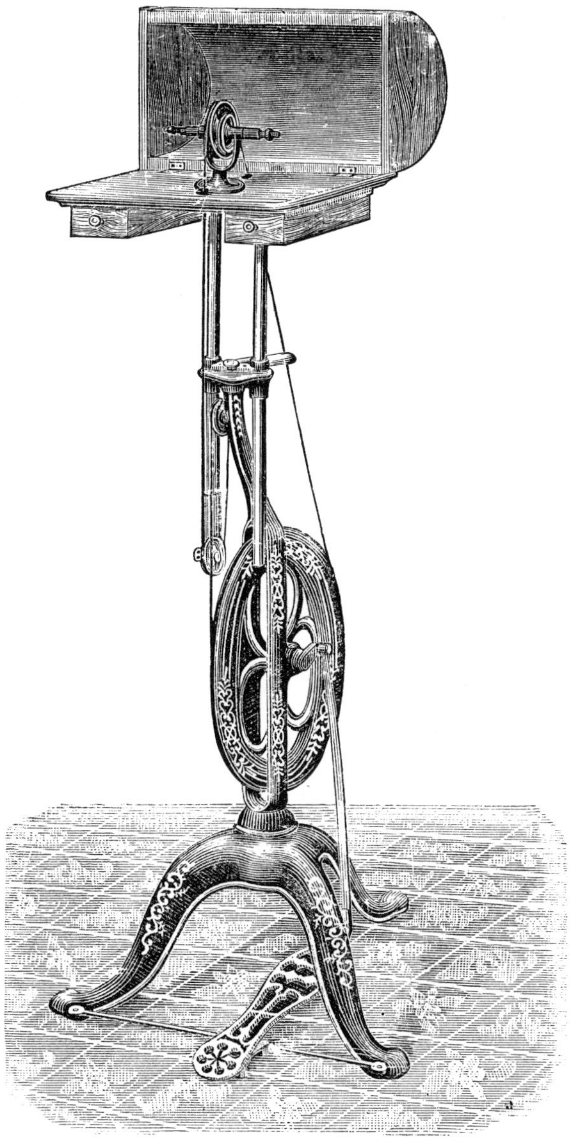

This cut represents a No. 4 Laboratory Lathe; the foot-power is the same as No. 3. THIS LATHE CAN BE RAISED OR LOWERED TWELVE INCHES, AT PLEASURE, FOR USE WHILE SITTING OR STANDING, WITHOUT CHANGING THE BELT. In other respects (except that the table and head are stationary, not pivoted) this Lathe is like No. 3, having the same arrangement of pulley, chucks, and nut-clamp.

Price of Lathe, with Chucks	$30.00
Boxing	2.00

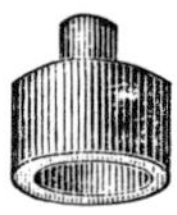
No. 1.

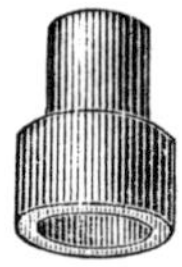
No. 2.

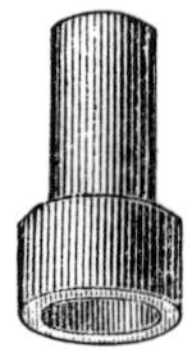
No. 3.

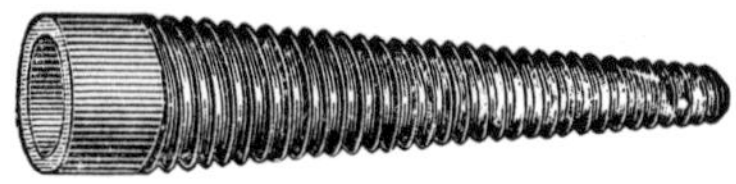
No. 4.

One each of the above Chucks accompany Lathes Nos. 3 and 4.

These Chucks are made with a plain collar on the inner end, and a screw at lower end of the hole. They run perfectly true. The Corundum Wheels are shellacked on, and can easily be removed with Chuck, and replaced by others, by reversing the Lathe.

PRICES OF CHUCKS, WHEN SOLD SEPARATELY.

Nos. 1, 2, 3	each 15 cents.
No. 4	25 "

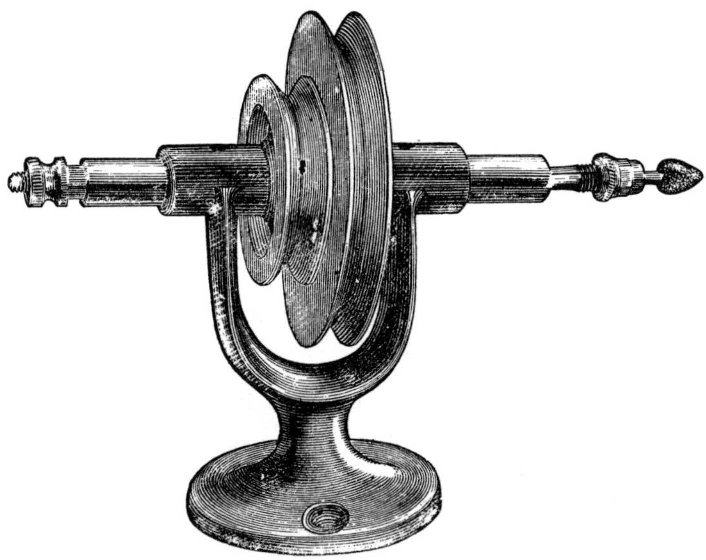

This Lathe-head is the same as used on the Nos. 3 and 4 Lathes; the pulley is provided with two grooves for the cord, securing slow or fast speed.

The spindle that holds the Chucks has a screw at one end for the Corundum Wheels, Brushes, etc.; the other is provided with a nut-clamp, and is intended to take the Burs and Drills, etc., of the Dental Engine.

Price $9.00

DR. A. LAWRENCE'S LATHE.

COMPOSED OF THE LAWRENCE DRIVING-WHEEL AND LAWRENCE LATHE-HEAD. ENTIRELY REMODELED AND IMPROVED.

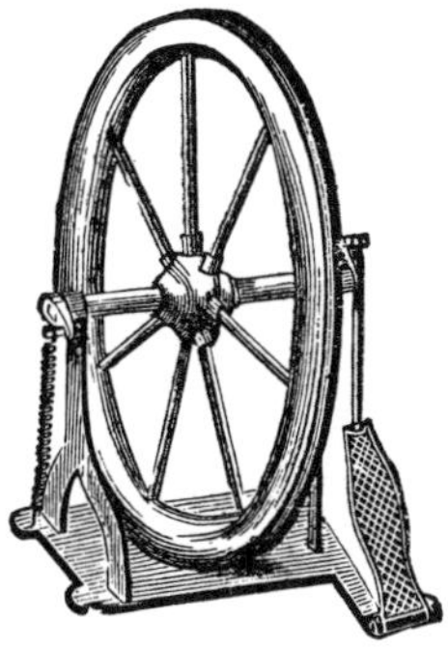

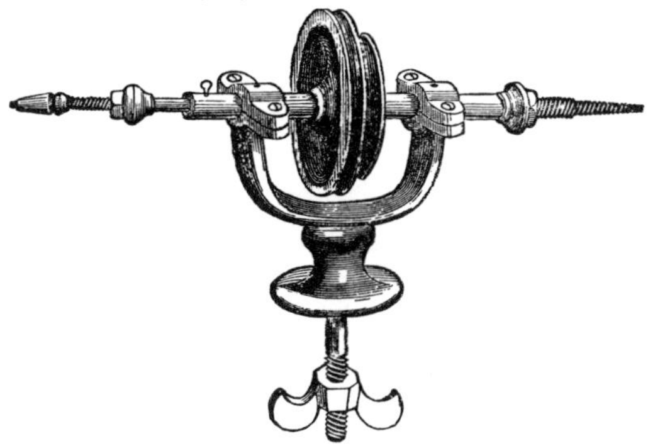

Is the best detached Lathe and Foot-Power ever offered for general use to Dentists.

The belt runs on the rim of the heavy driving-wheel, and drives the small pulley of the head at very high speed. It is simple. Being placed directly on the floor, under a table or shelf, with the Lathe-Head directly above it, and the round belt running in deep grooves, it affords the greatest use with the least trouble.

Driving-Wheel	$18.00
Head (Brass)	12.00
" (Iron)	10.00
Cord and Couplings	.75

AMATEUR LATHE.

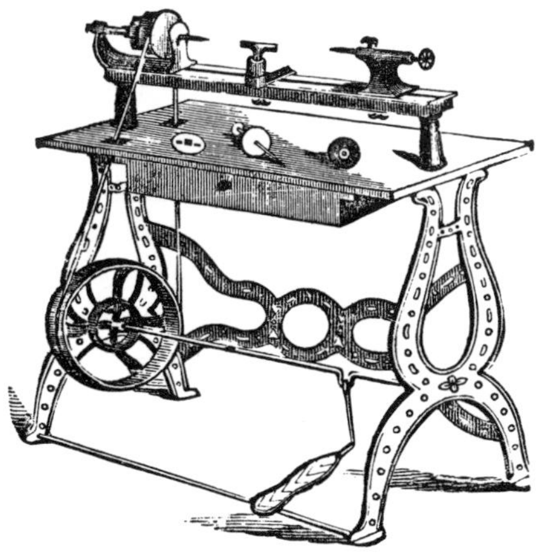

This Lathe weighs about 100 pounds. The Table is of Walnut, 16 by 20 inches, with a drawer underneath for tools. It is arranged for fast or slow speed, and is very handy for the Dentist.

Price $30.00

SS THE "BEST" LATHE-HEAD. SSW

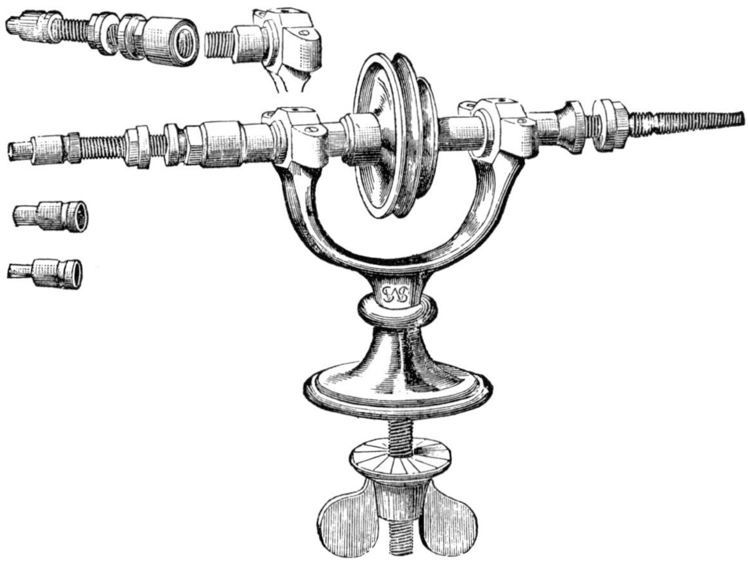

(Adapted for use with the Lawrence Driving-Wheel.)

The superiority of this Lathe-Head consists in,—

1st. The excellence of the materials used. The Frame, Bearings, and Chuck Nuts are of fine, hard, Machinist's Brass. The Mandrel and Cone-slip Mandrel are of fine Steel, and throughout the lot every piece got out is rejected for any fault as soon as discovered.

2d. The new method of setting and removing the Slip Mandrel. It is drawn into and thrown out of the socket by a sleeve nut, which always brings it up true, and removes it without any danger of bending or injury. This is of great importance when its use for carrying on its end a variety of movable chucks, which will run true at all times, is considered. Those who have been annoyed by the wabbling of other kinds will appreciate the advantage of this.

Two of these chucks are furnished with the Lathe.

3d. The workmanship and finish are greatly superior to any Dental Lathe-Head heretofore offered for sale. The screws are all originals, cut on a lathe. The fitting-up is fine and close; the work and equipment are good and complete, and, though its price is higher than any other Lathe-Heads, it has the additional value to the buyer over the cheaper articles of its kind.

Price $18.00

THE UNITED STATES LATHE.

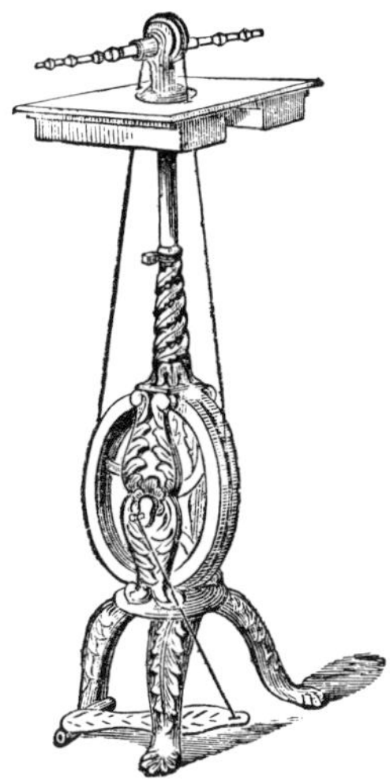

This Lathe has a Movable Column and Table, and may be elevated 8 inches, to accommodate the Operator in either a sitting or standing posture.

It can be packed in a box 16 inches square, and can be set up in a few minutes.

Lathe, Short Spindle $18.00

" with Long Spindle. (See Cut.) 18.00

TABLE LATHE-HEADS.

A.

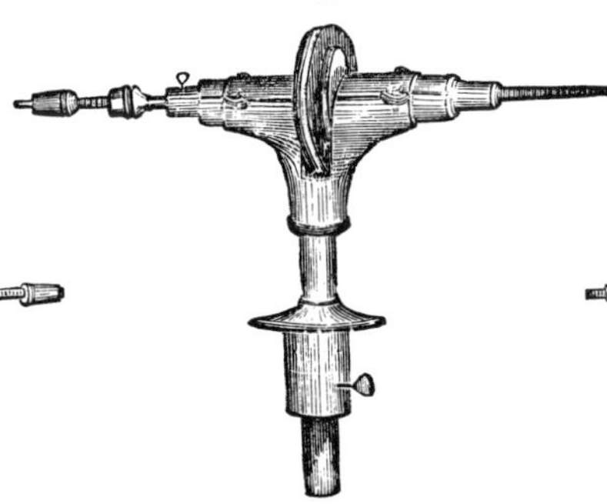

B.

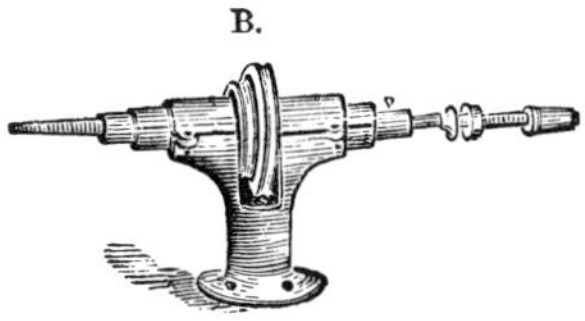

C.

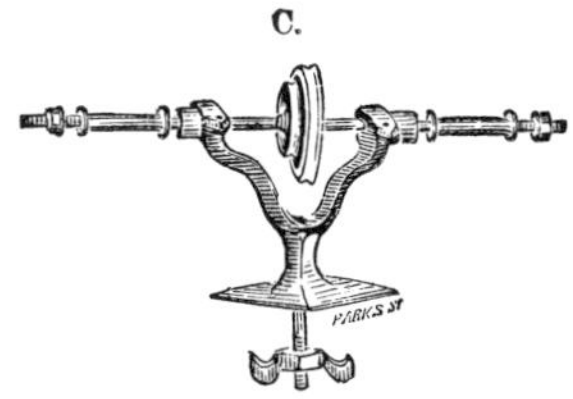

A.—Socket-Head. The Socket screws to the table and has a Set Screw in the lower part. The Head slides four inches to tighten the strap or vary the height from the table.

Price $6.00

B.—United States Lathe Head, with holes in the base to screw to any table.

Price, Short Spindle, as per Cut $5.00

" Long " 5.00

C.—Diamond Lathe Head. The Head Pulley and Spools which retain the Wheels and Brushes are of Brass. The Spindle is of unannealed hammered Steel..

Price $7.00

PORTABLE GRINDING APPARATUS.

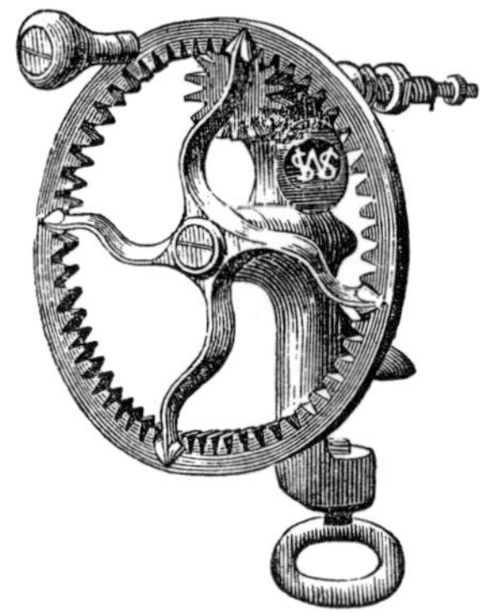

This cut represents a Portable Hand-Lathe for use in the office and for traveling dentists. Under its popular name of "The Rattlesnake" it has had an enormous sale, entirely displacing other cheap portable grinding machines. The parts are fitted up so nearly interchangeable that any one worn out or broken can be supplied at its proper price on order. This Lathe has, at the shoulder, parting nuts for holding large wheels, brushes, etc., and a bur and screw on the end of the mandrel for small corundum wheels. Extra Chucks to screw on the end are furnished to order.

The quality of the Axle Screw, Handle, Nuts, etc., and all the workmanship of this lathe, is good. It is neatly made and finished, and a thoroughly useful tool.

Price		$4.00
Extra Chucks	each	.25

NOISELESS HAND LATHE.

H. COY'S PATENT, OCTOBER 2d, 1866.

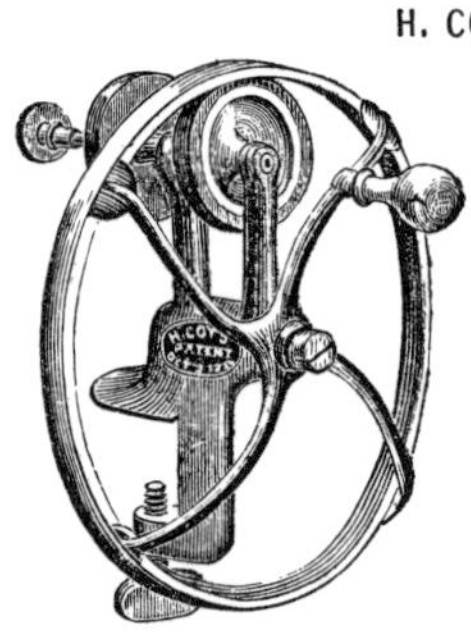

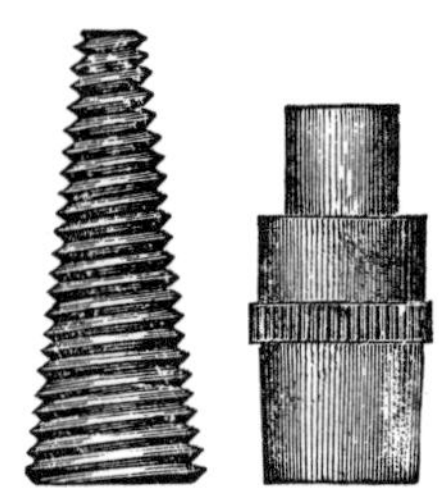

Designed especially for the office; it is entirely noiseless. Having neither cog-wheels nor belt, it is free from oil, dirt, and the trouble of adjustment. The motive-power is transmitted by contact of the inner surface of the Driving-wheel with a Soft Rubber Ring which is secured upon the small Wheel, or Pulley. In material and workmanship it is superior to any small Lathe heretofore offered, and is designed to meet all the requirements of the office, and of the traveling dentist. Driving-wheel, 6½ inches in diameter; small Wheel, 2 inches in diameter; weight, 2¾ pounds.

The Mandrel and Axle-screw of the "Extra" are of Steel, and are coned and ground in. Rim of Driving-wheel turned all over. Table-face of Clamp hollowed and float-cut, and the end of the Clamp-screw countersunk, making it very firm on the table with light pressure. The japanning and polish are also extra fine. Ivory Handle.

Our cut shows a Noiseless Lathe mounted with a 2¼-inch Corundum Wheel between the parting nuts on Mandrel, and a 1-inch Corundum Wheel on the smallest Chuck. Three Chucks go with each Lathe. The Brush-screw and large Corundum Wheel Chucks shown in side cut are full size.

Price		$7.00
" extra quality		10.00
Additional Chucks	each	.25

PARALLEL LATHE.

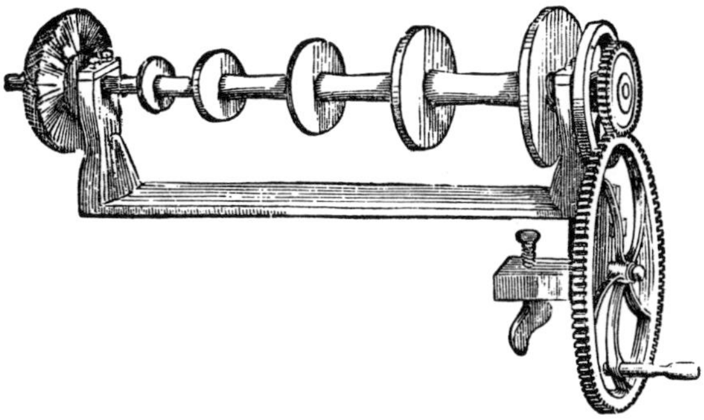

This Lathe is capable of running five Stones, a Brush, and a Drill at the same time. Outline size, 10 by 16 inches; weight, 8 pounds; Frame of Cast-Iron, with Steel Spindle and Axles. It can be easily adjusted to the table or work-bench. The Collars that retain the Grindstones are made of Wood, and their lengths are proportioned to the requirements of the hand.

Price, Corundum Wheels included $10.50
" the same without Balance Wheel 10.00

TABLE LATHES.

No. 1. No. 2. No. 3.

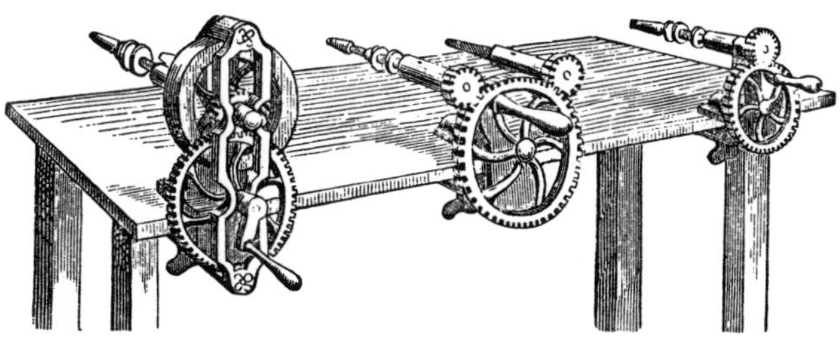

No. 1. For Hand or Foot $6.50
" 2. With two Spindles 6.00
" 3. One Spindle 4.00

N.B—No. 1 has a Treadle and Strap, to be used with the foot, not shown in Cut; also, an extra Spindle and Chuck.

PURE SPERM OIL.

The best Lubricator known for Lathes, Machinery, etc.

Three-ounce Bottles . . . . 20 cents.

DRIP CUP AND SPONGE FOR LATHES.

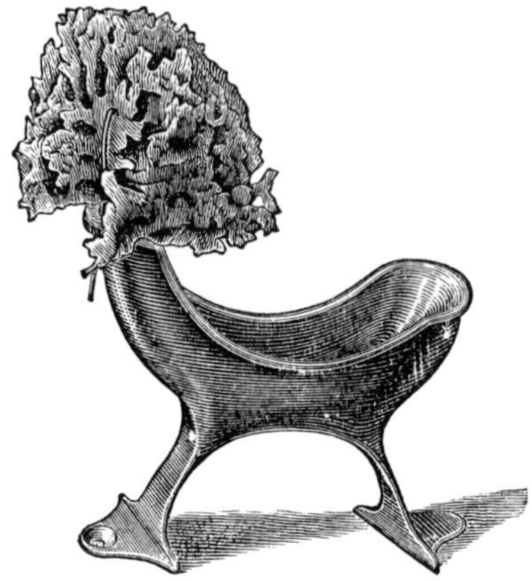

The Cut illustrates a useful little device for keeping the Corundum Wheel wet, while in motion, and catching the drip. It is of Iron, and lacquered to prevent rusting.

Price, with Sponge . . . . 50 cents.

HOT BLAST BLOW-PIPE.

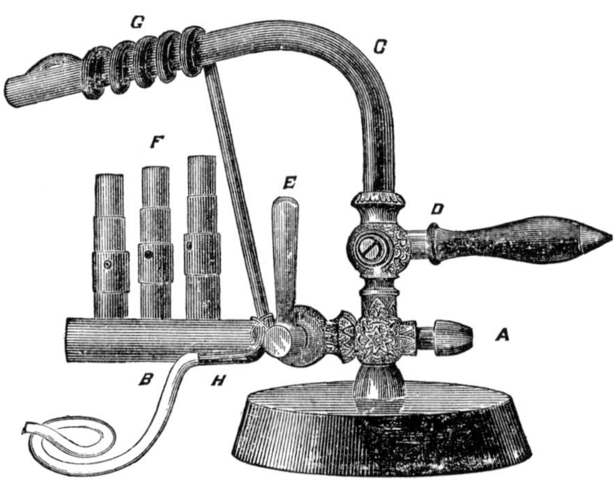

As compact and easily used as the ordinary Blow-pipe, while the heat is sufficiently intense to produce most of the effects which have hitherto been unattainable, except with costly and troublesome apparatus.

The Tubes, Coil, and connection are made of Brass, and the Base of Iron.

The Gas Tubing is attached at A, allowing the Gas to pass into both the upper and lower tubes, B C, and the supply can be regulated by the stop-cocks, D E. The Burners, F, heat up the Wire Coil, G, through which the breath passes, and it is thus thrown upon the surfaces to be acted upon in a heated condition. The Mouth Tubing is attached at H.

Price $6.50

THE BURGESS PATENT BLOW-PIPE.

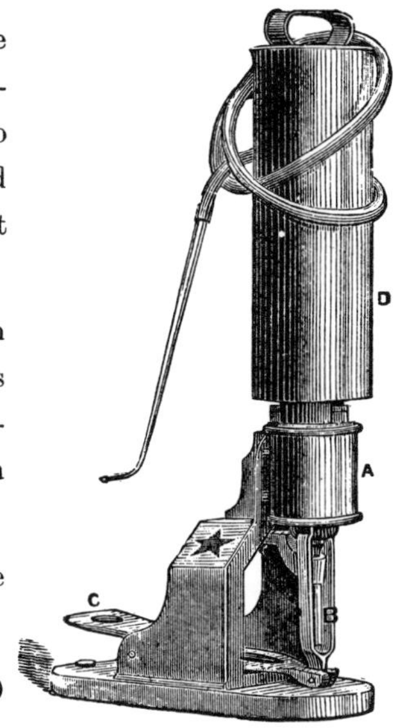

A very convenient and efficient Blow-pipe for use in the Laboratory. It is a simple, durable, and complete instrument for Dental purposes. Those who have occasion to employ the Blow-pipe frequently will economize time and breath by its use. Its efficiency is spoken of in the highest terms by those who are using it.

A is the Cylinder of the Pump, which is 2½ inches in diameter, allowing a 3-inch stroke. B, Piston-rod. C is Heel and Toe Treadle for driving the Pump. D, the Receiver, 12 inches high by 3 inches in diameter, into which the air is forced.

The whole height of the machine is 24 inches; the base is 12 inches by 5.

Price $16.00

MACOMBER'S GAS BLOW-PIPE.

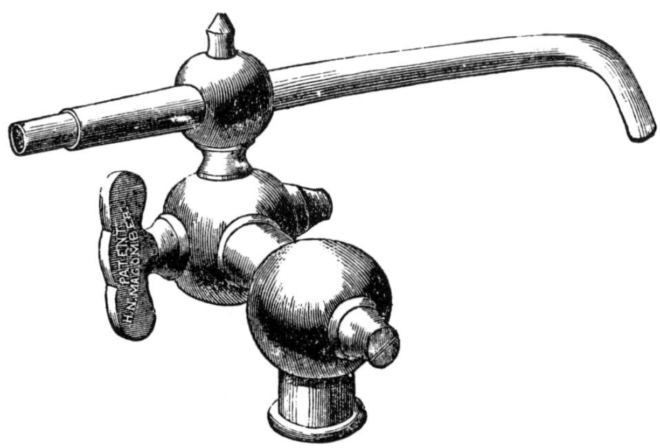

An appliance designed to be attached to a Gas-pipe, for using Gas instead of Oil or Alcohol. The Tube is double, or rather one Tube inclosed in another, the atmospheric air being driven through the inside Tube, adding force and giving a cylindrical form to the flame.

Price $3.50

SELF-ACTING BLOW-PIPE.

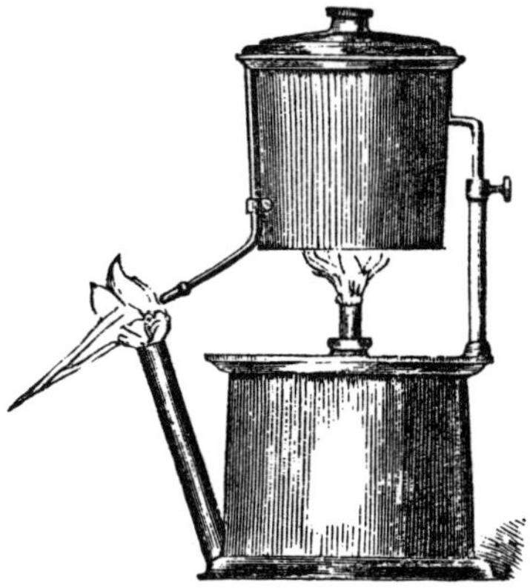

The Lamp is made of Tin, japanned, and the Boiler of Brass, each holding half a pint of Alcohol. It has a Set-Screw on the Upright, allowing the Boiler to be moved up or down; also two Nozzles to be attached to the Pipe, whereby the flame can be regulated. It is perfectly safe, as, in addition to being substantially made, it has a Safety-valve in the top of the Boiler. For cheapness and utility it has no equal.

Price $5.50

N.B.—One of the Nozzles will be found screwed on the top of the Safety-valve.

MOUTH BLOW-PIPES. (BRASS.)

9 inch Plain	each	$0.15
10 " "	"	.18
11 " "	"	.20
12 " "	"	.23
13 " "	"	.28
11 " Extra Heavy, Mouth-end Tinned	"	.50
13 " " " "	"	.55
15 " " " "	"	.60
15 " with Chamber and Screw-Joint	"	.75
13 " " Bulb	"	.75

IMPROVED SOLDERING PAN OR FURNACE. (RUSSIA IRON.)

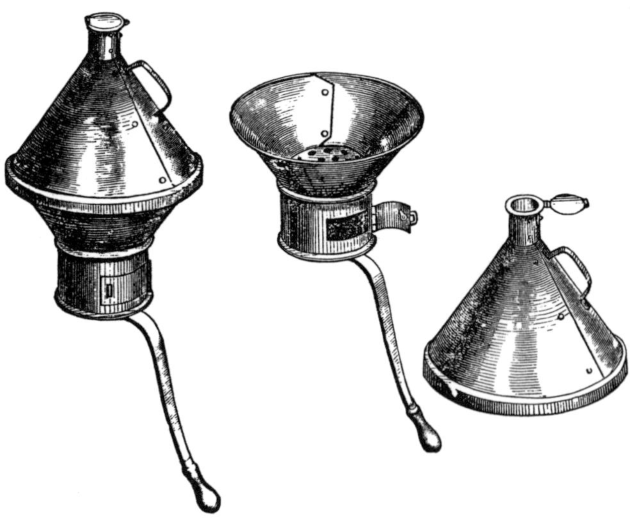

Dimensions: height, 5 inches; diameter, 6½ inches. A Cover with movable Lid, to put on while heating up the case before soldering; also to be placed on after soldering, with the Lid and Door closed to prevent rapid cooling; Handle attached by a pivot to allow the Furnace to revolve.

Complete . . $1.75

SOLDERING LAMP, No. 1.

FRANKLIN'S SAFETY.

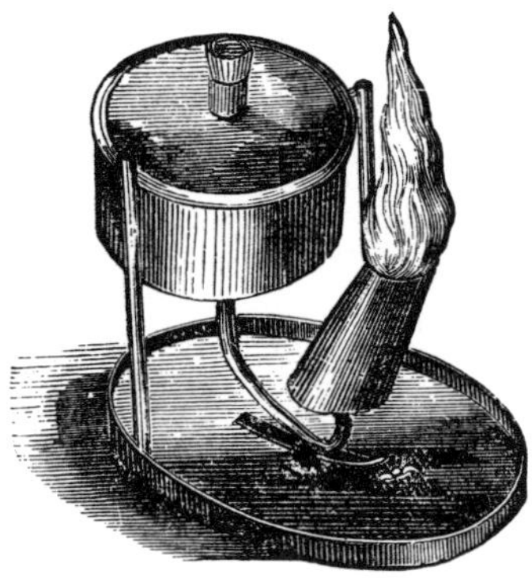

A perfectly safe Lamp, the reservoir of Alcohol being some distance from the Wick.

Price $1.00

SOLDERING LAMP, No. 2.

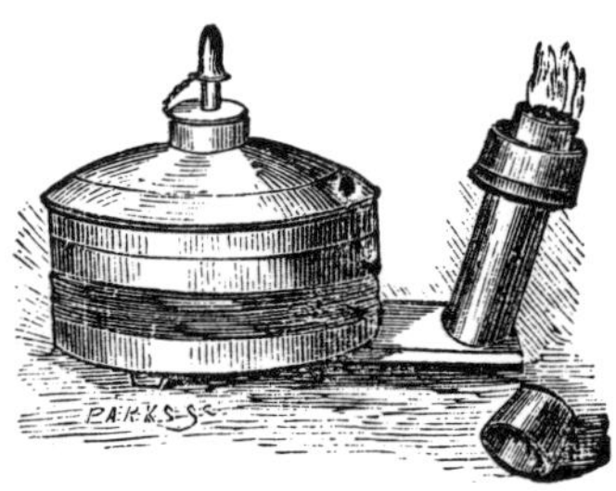

This non-explosive Soldering Lamp is very popular, and gives great satisfaction.

Price, adapted to the use of Alcohol . . . . each 90 cents.
The same Lamp, adapted to the use of Oil . . . . . . " 90 "

ALCOHOL LAMP.

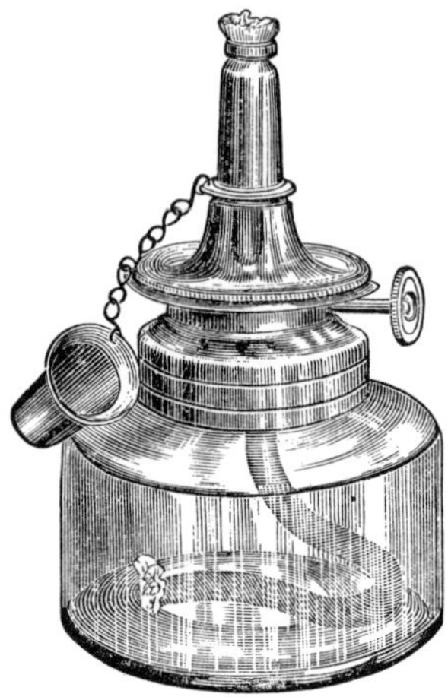

A new style of Alcohol Lamp for office use: size, 2½ inches in diameter. It is of Glass, the mountings Nickel-Plated. The Wick is raised and lowered by means of a Thumb-Screw at the side. The Wick-Tube is made conical at the end, corresponding to a similar shape of the Cap or Cover, so that when not in use the Lamp can be made air-tight.

Price	$1.00
With Shield to protect flame, extra	.30

GLASS ALCOHOL LAMPS.

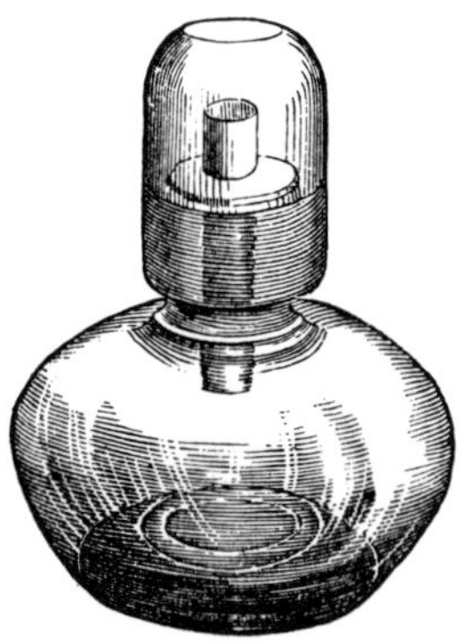

Oval.

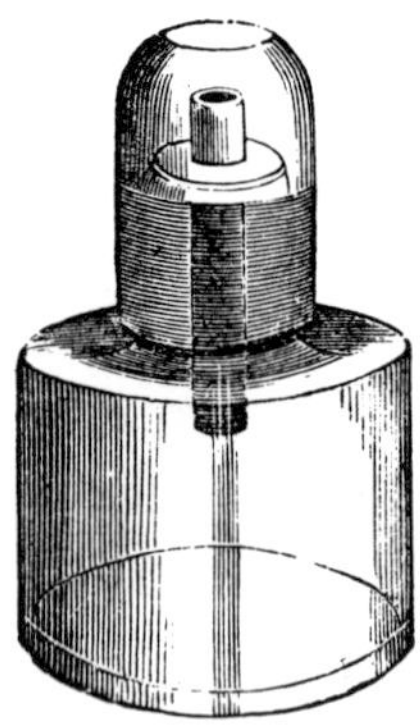

Square.

Oval,	4 inches high,	3 inches wide	. . . .	each	75 cents.
Square,	4 "	" 2½ "	. . . .	"	75 "
"	3 "	" 2 "	. . . .	"	50 "

GAS STOVE.

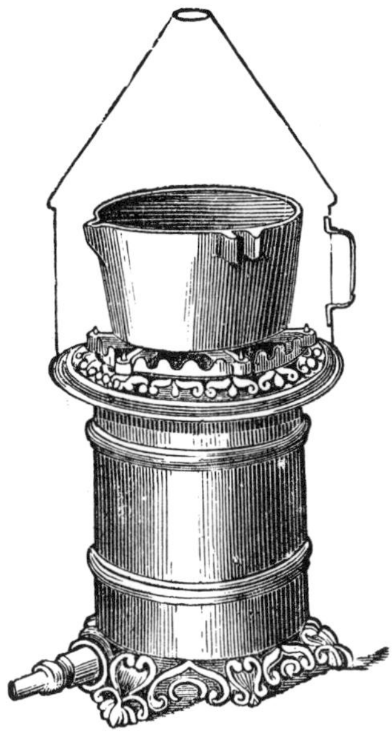

For heating up Vulcanizers, melting Zinc or Lead, and for general Laboratory purposes	$2.00
With Sheet-Iron Cover (as shown in Cut)	3.00
Ladle, Heavy Cast-Iron, with detached Handle	.80

KEROSENE STOVES.

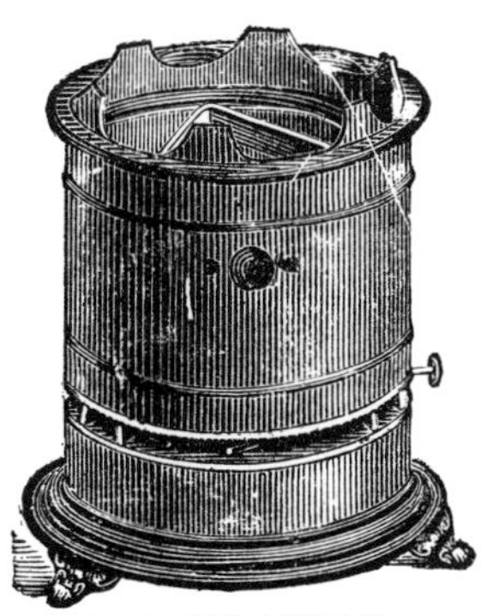

No 1 (ONE BURNER).

Union Kerosene Stove, No. 1 (one Burner)	$2.25
" " " 2 (two Burners)	3.00
" " " 3 (three Burners)	4.00
" " " 4 (four Burners)	5.00

PLATE SHEARS.

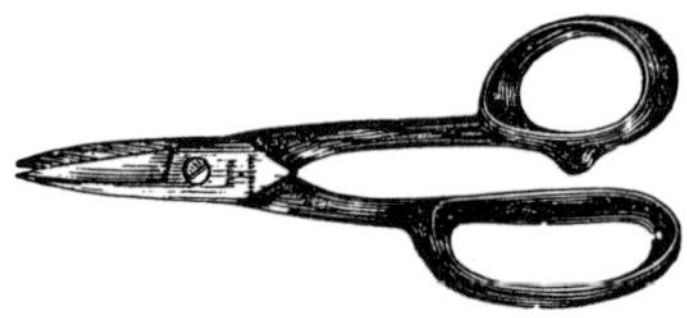

With Scissors form of Handles, Screw Fastening					$1.00
"	"	"	Nut	"	1.25
"	"	"	Curved		2.50
Stubs's Plate Shears,		5 inch,	Straight		.75
"	"	6	"	"	1.00
"	"	7	"	"	1.25
"	"	5	"	Curved	.90
"	"	6	"	"	1.25
"	"	7	"	"	1.50

NIPPERS.

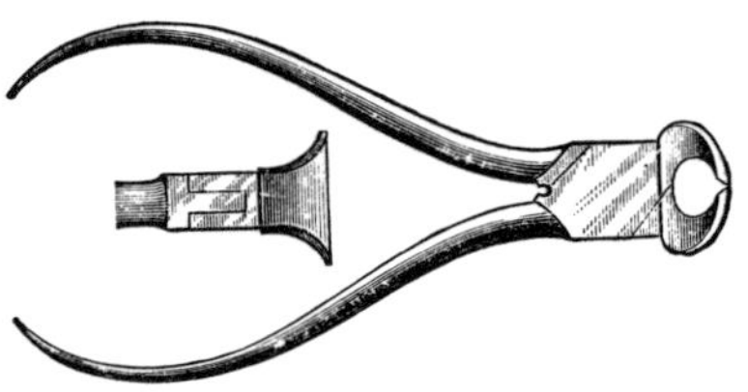

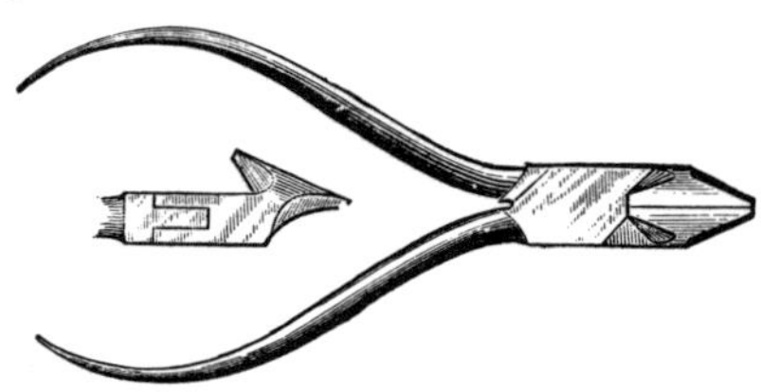

Stubs's Side Nippers,		4 to 4½	inches	each $1.25
"	Front "	4 to 4½	"	" 1.25
German Side	"	4 to 4½	"	" .50
"	Front "	4 to 4½	"	" .50

PLIERS.

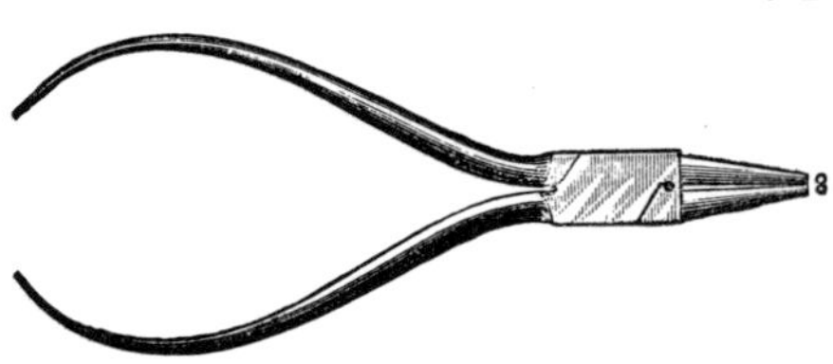

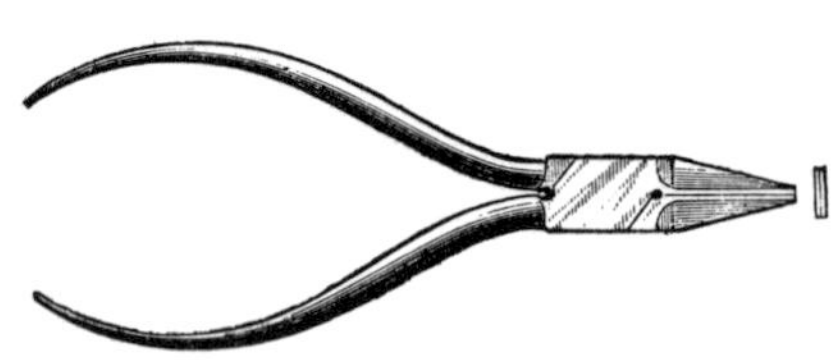

Stubs's Flat Nose Pliers,				4 to 4½	inches	each $0.65
"	"	"	"	5	"	" .75
"	"	"	"	6	"	" 1.00
"	Round Nose	"		4 to 4½	"	" .65

MECHANICAL FORCEPS.

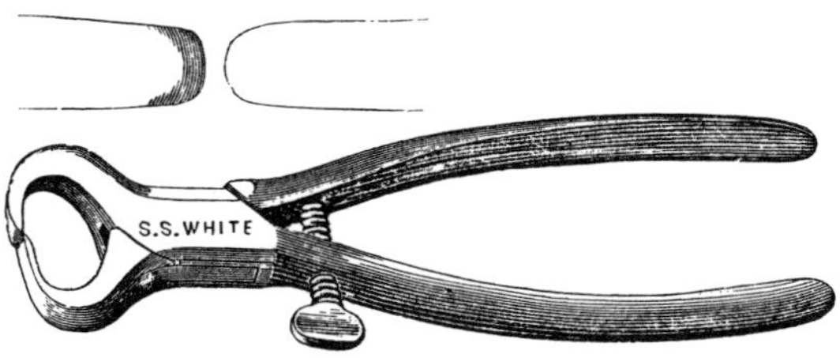

Nipper for cutting out chambers, and cutting off backings from Plates. Cutting-edge regulated by a Set-Screw $2.75

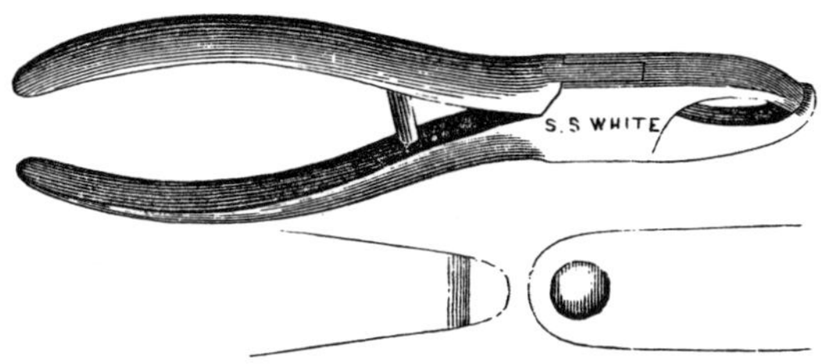

Nipper, for cutting out Plate $2.75
" " " " Stubs's 2.90

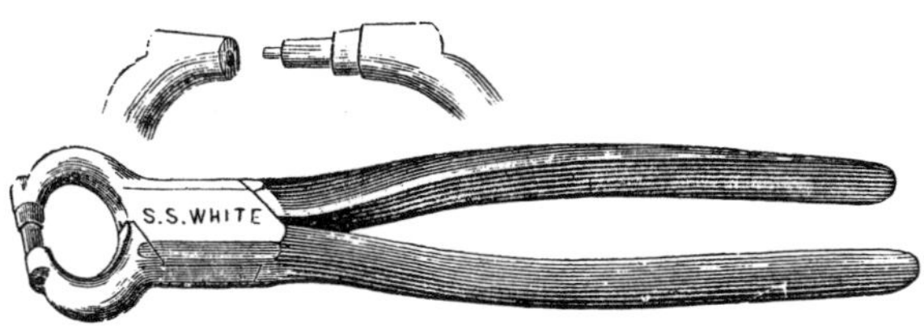

Punch, for Rivet Holes $2.75
" " " Plain Line 2.25

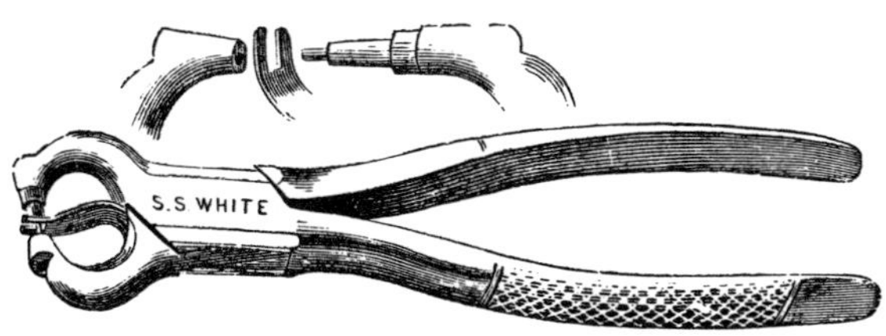

Improved Punch, for Rivet Holes, Plain Handle $3.50
" " " " Checkered Handle, as per Cut 3.75

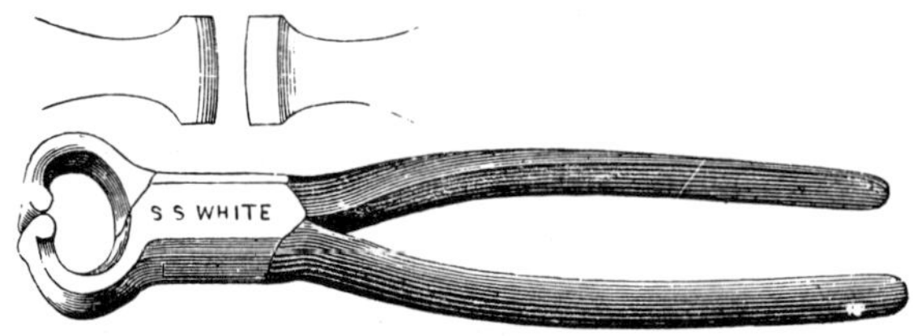

Plate Bender, for Upper Plate $2.75

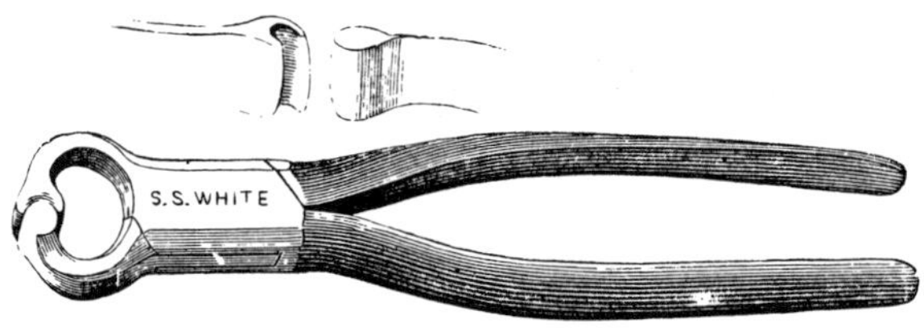

Plate Bender, for Lower Plate $2.75

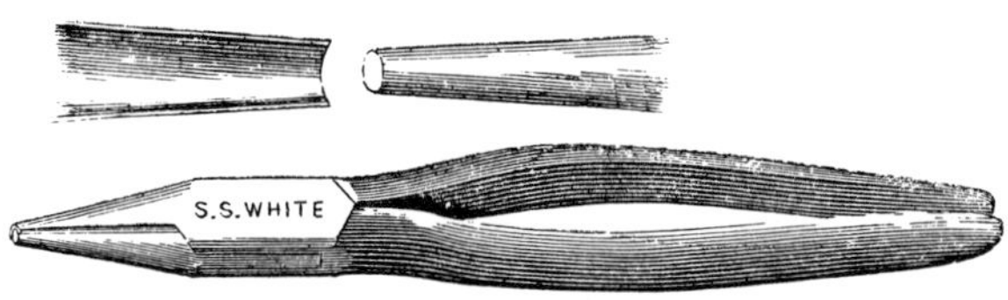

Clasp Bender $2.50

CRUCIBLE TONGS.

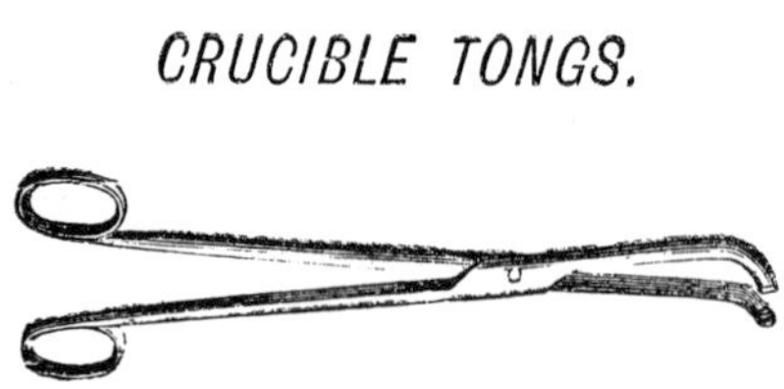

Polished, with Scissors form of Handles, from 9 to 12 inches in length (see Cut). $1.75
Iron, Spring Handle, from 16 to 20 inches long 50
Steel, with Joints, from 18 to 24 inches long 1.25

HAMMERS FOR RIVETING.

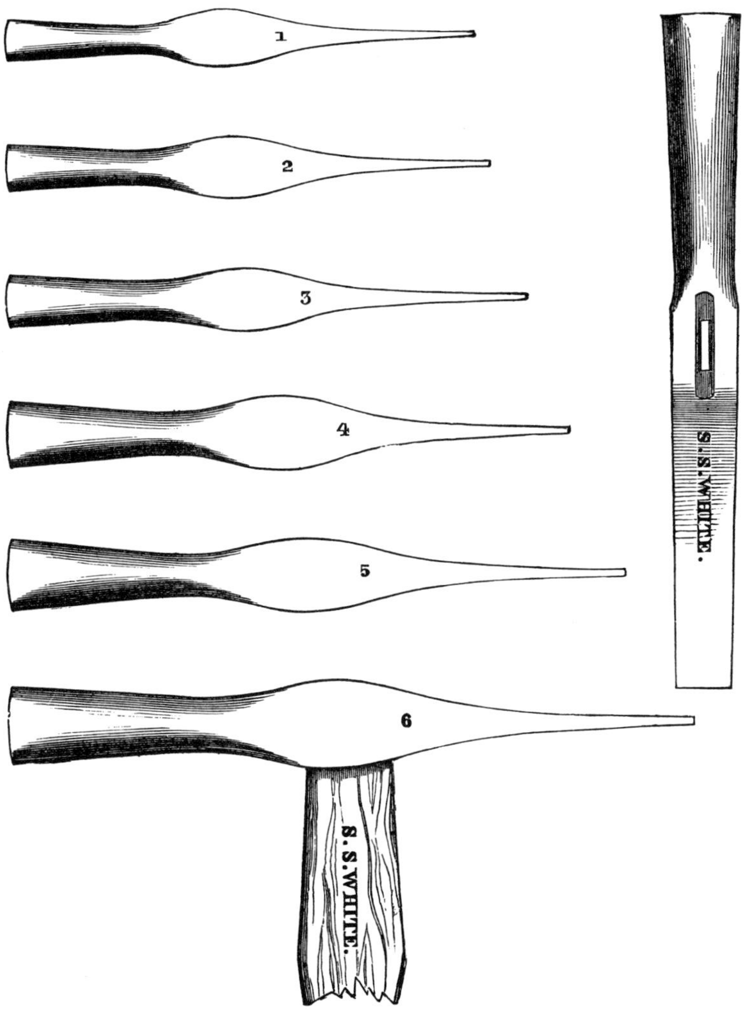

Price, with Handles . . . . each 70 cents.
" without Handles . . . . " 50 "

SOLDER BURS.

FOR TRIMMING OFF SUPERFLUOUS SOLDER.

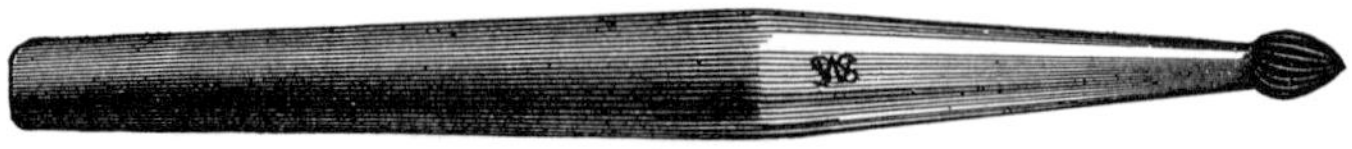

No. 1. (Full Size.)

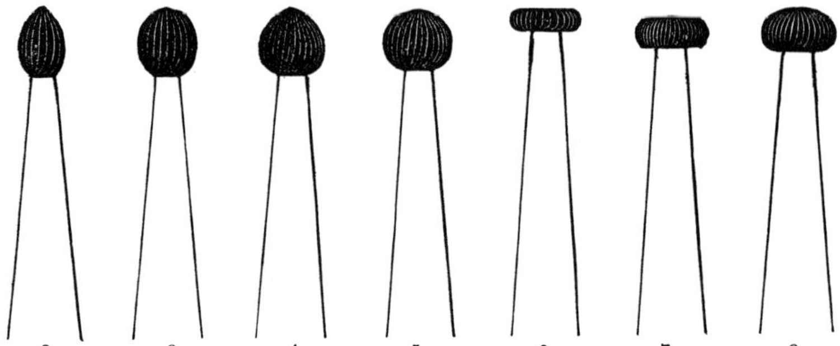

2. 3. 4. 5. 6. 7. 8.

Price . . . . each 75 cents.

FROID'S PLATE FILES.

DIRECT IMPORTATION.

Flat, Half-Soft, resembling Stubs's Bastard,	3 inch	. 14 cts. each;	per doz.	$1.60
" " " "	3½ "	. 14 "	"	1.60
" " " "	4 "	. 16 "	"	1.90
" " " "	4½ "	. 20 "	"	2.20
" " " "	5 "	. 22 "	"	2.44
" " " "	6 "	. 28 "	"	3.15
" Soft, " Stubs's Smooth,	3 "	. 18 "	"	2.00
" " " "	3½ "	. 18 "	"	2.00
" " " "	4 "	. 20 "	"	2.35
" " " "	4½ "	. 24 "	"	2.66
" " " "	5 "	. 25 "	"	3.00
" " " "	6 "	. 34 "	"	3.85
Half-Round, Half-Soft or Bastard,	4½ inch . . .	. 18 "	"	2.10
" " "	5 " . . .	. 20 "	"	2.20
" " "	6 " . . .	. 25 "	"	3.00
" Soft or Smooth,	4½ " . . .	. 22 "	"	2.45
" " "	5 " . . .	. 24 "	"	2.66
" " "	6 " . . .	. 28 "	"	3.32
Round, Half-Soft or Bastard,	4 inch	. 15 "	"	1.75
" " "	5 "	. 20 "	"	2.20
" " "	6 "	. 25 "	"	3.00
Triangle, " "	4 "	. 13 "	"	1.50
" " "	5 "	. 14 "	"	1.66
" " "	6 "	. 20 "	"	2.32
" Soft or Smooth,	2 to 3 "	. 15 "	"	1.80

STUBS'S PLATE FILES.

DIRECT IMPORTATION.

Half-Round, Bastard, 4 inch	. . . .	each	$0.32
" " 4½ "	. . . .	"	.35
" " 5 "	. . . .	"	.38
" " 5½ "	. . . .	"	.44
" " 6 "	. . . .	"	.50
" Smooth, 4 "	. . . .	"	.35
" " 5 "	. . . .	"	.44
" " 6 "	. . . .	"	.56
" Bastard, 3 to 3½ inch	. . . .	"	.25
" Smooth, 3 to 3½ "	. . . .	"	.30
Round, Bastard, 4 inch	. . . .	"	.22
" " 5 "	. . . .	"	.28
" " 6 "	. . . .	"	.35
Flat, " 4 "	. . . .	"	.22
" " 5 "	. . . .	"	.28
" " 6 "	. . . .	"	.40
Half-Round, Bastard, Steel Handles, 4 inch	. . . .	"	.38
" " " 5 "	. . . .	"	.44
" " " 6 "	. . . .	"	.56

MURPHY'S DOUBLE-END SOLDER FILES.

Six forms . . . . each 20 cents.

WAX PREPARATIONS.

WHITE AND YELLOW WAX FOR IMPRESSIONS.

Warranted pure ; put up in thin Cakes, convenient for use and adapted for the purposes for which they are intended, in half-pound Boxes.

White . . . . per box 60 cents.
Yellow . . . . " 38 "

WAX COMPOUND.

This Compound is tough, firm, and takes a very sharp impression.

Put up in half-pound Boxes . . . . per box 60 cents.

GUTTA-PERCHA AND WAX.

This Combination is pronounced a very superior article for taking impressions of the mouth. It is plastic, tough, and easily softened, either by dry heat or in warm water.

Put up in half-pound Boxes . . . . per box 50 cents.

WAX AND PARAFFIN.

White and Pink, for taking impressions. These Preparations are highly recommended by many Operators who have long used them. Soften with a dry heat, taking care to avoid overheating. Previous to taking the impression, the parts should be wiped dry with a napkin. Put up in half-pound Boxes.

Price . . . . per box 50 cents.

WAX FOR BASE PLATES.

Wax in thin square sheets, for Base Plates in Vulcanite work.

Half-pound Boxes . . . . per box 50 cents.

Gutta-Percha and Wax, in sheets as above, for same purpose.

Half-pound Boxes . . . . per box 50 cents.

MOULDING SAND FOR DENTAL USE.

A superior article. Put up in Barrels and packed securely for shipping.

Per Barrel $3.00
Per Quart 06

MODELING COMPOSITION FOR TAKING IMPRESSIONS OF THE MOUTH AND OTHER ART PURPOSES.

This Preparation is recommended by many Practitioners as superior to Wax or any of its compounds for taking sharp and accurate impressions.

Four varieties are offered, as follows :

No. 1. Soft. This variety is desirable for use in cold weather and in tender mouths, as after recent extraction of teeth. It softens sufficiently at a very low temperature, and is consequently longer in hardening, requiring two minutes to set before withdrawal from the mouth. Put up in Red Boxes.

No. 2. Medium. This variety is adapted to ordinary uses ; requires a higher temperature to soften it than No. 1, and sets more quickly,—one and a half minutes will suffice. Put up in White Boxes.

No. 3. Hard. This variety is adapted to use in warm weather and for edentulous cases. It requires a higher temperature to soften than No. 2, and sets in about one minute. Put up in Blue Boxes.

No. 4. Extra Soft. This variety answers very well for "taking bites," but is especially recommended to be used in restoring either of the other grades which may be considered to have lost their properties by age or use. Equal parts, more or less, may be mixed with either No. 1, 2, or 3. The best way to mix them is under hot water with a stout iron spoon. Put up in Green Boxes.

A dry heat answers the best for softening either variety.

Put up in half-pound Boxes . . . . per pound $2.00

BAILEY'S FLASKS FOR MAKING METAL DIES.

Fig. 1.

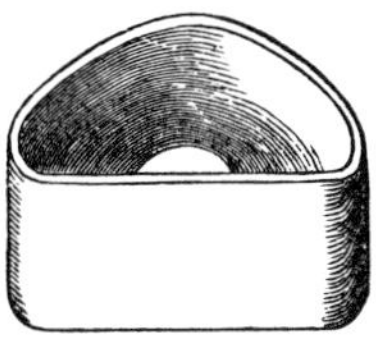

Fig. 2.

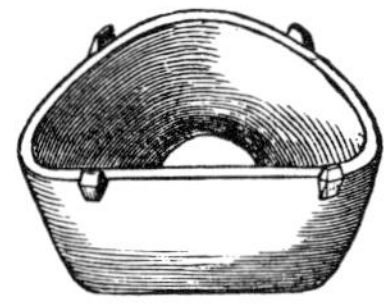

Fig. 3.

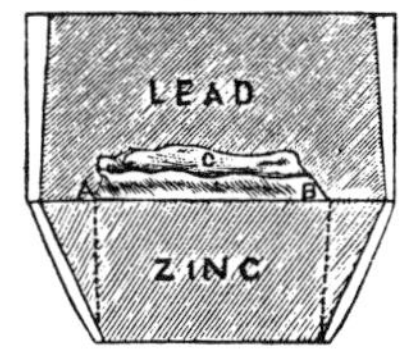

DIRECTIONS FOR USE.—Place a shallow Plaster Cast, A, B, C, on a level surface; turn over it the lower half of the Flask (Fig. 1), with joint side down; pack the sand in it, and level off the top; turn up the Flask, remove the superfluous sand, tap the cast lightly, when it can be easily lifted out; pour in the Zinc; when the impression is filled, place over it the upper half of the Flask (Fig. 2), and fill up immediately; knock out the sand, invert the whole Flask, and pour the Lead upon the Zinc; when cooled, part and remove the Flasks, and with a few sharp blows at the joint the Dies will separate.

Per Pair	$0.50
" Set	1.00

MOULDING FLASKS.

(HAWES'S.)

Fig. 1.

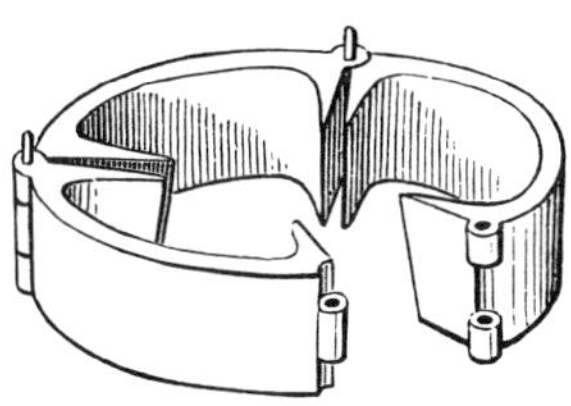

Fig. 2.

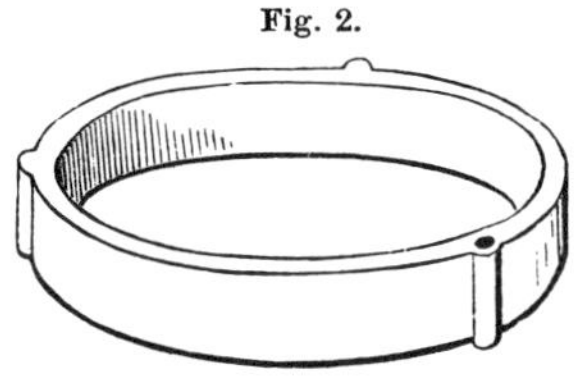

Fig. 3.

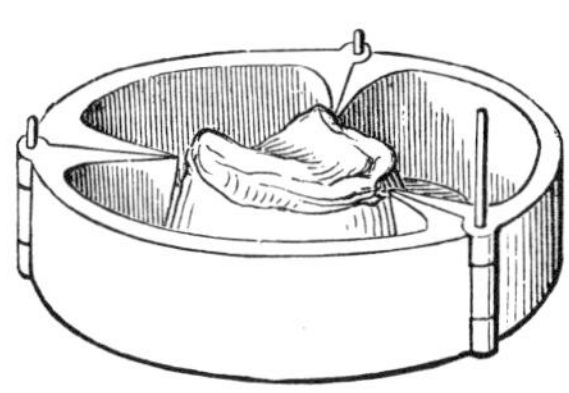

Fig. 1 represents the lower section of the Flask, slightly opened, to show the Joints. Fig. 2 is the upper section. When ready for use, the lower section is closed and confined by a Pin, and the Plaster Model placed in it, as represented in Fig. 3.

Price	$3.00

COATINGS FOR PLASTER CASTS.

Collodion, in 2 oz. bottles, with Brush	$0.40
" 6 oz. "	.80
Sandarac Varnish, in 2 oz. bottles	.25
Transparent " 2 oz. "	.25
White " 2 oz. "	.25
Extra Shellac Varnish, in 2 oz. bottles	.25
Liquid Silex, in 2 oz. bottles	.20
" " 2 oz. " with Brush	.25

DOUBLE-END SPATULA FOR SAND MOULDING.

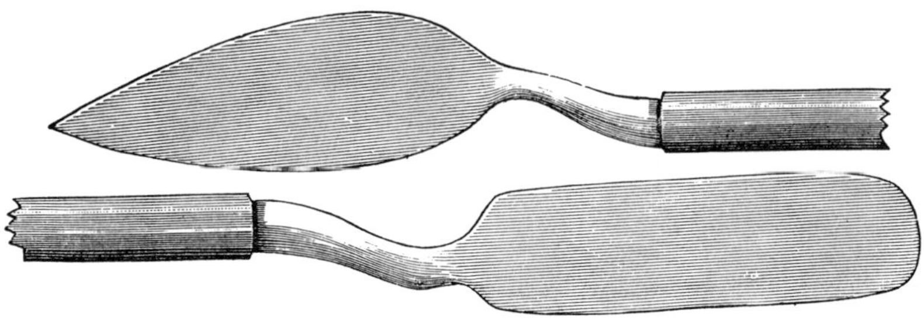

The Cut shows the size and form of the Instrument; represented in two parts on account of its length.

Price $1.00

DENTAL PLASTER.

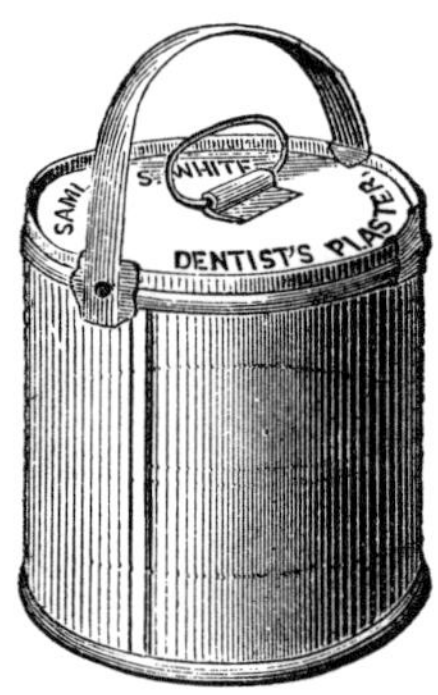

Plaster in painted Air-tight Sheet-iron Cans, containing from six quarts to three pecks, at the following prices:

Six-quart Cans	$0.75
Twelve-quart Cans	1.25
Half-bushel Cans	1.60
Three-peck Cans	2.25
ALSO,	
Quarter Barrel	1.75
Half Barrel	2.75
One Barrel	4.00

The above are the prices at the Philadelphia Depot. Boxing Cans, extra. Porterage additional on Barrels, half Barrels, and quarter Barrels, when shipped separately.

Freight and Expenses will be added when sold at other Depots.

Impression Trays.

These Trays are made of Britannia Metal, of the best quality, and of uniform thickness. They are light enough to allow of alteration by pliers or mallet, or for many cases, with the fingers, so as to adapt them to any peculiar formation of the maxillary. They are superior in form and finish to any heretofore offered to the Profession, while the price has not been advanced.

UPPER IMPRESSION TRAYS.

Fig. 1.

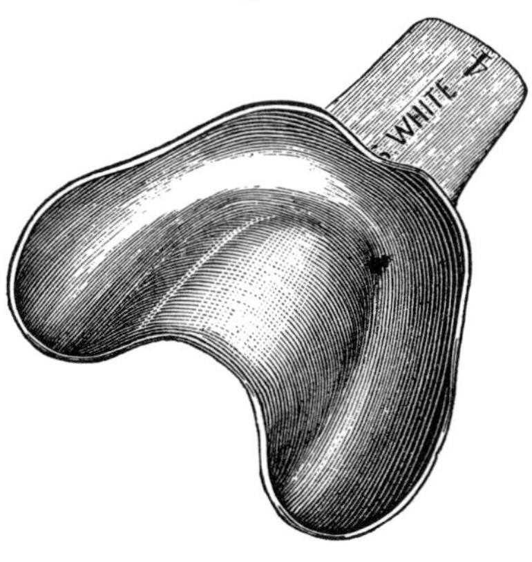

Fig. 1 illustrates the shape of a Set of 8, Nos. 1 to 8, for Full Upper Dentures. Especial attention is invited to the modifications in form—to the dip at the sides, to accommodate the prominences of the malar processes; and in front to avoid the labial frænum; and to the length (1½ inches) and position of the handle, which, being below the line of the base, gives more room for the lip.

The exact size of each Tray of the set is outlined, with its number attached, by which it may be ordered. The side views show, by the dotted line, the height of the palate portion of the Tray.

Price . . . . each 50 cents.

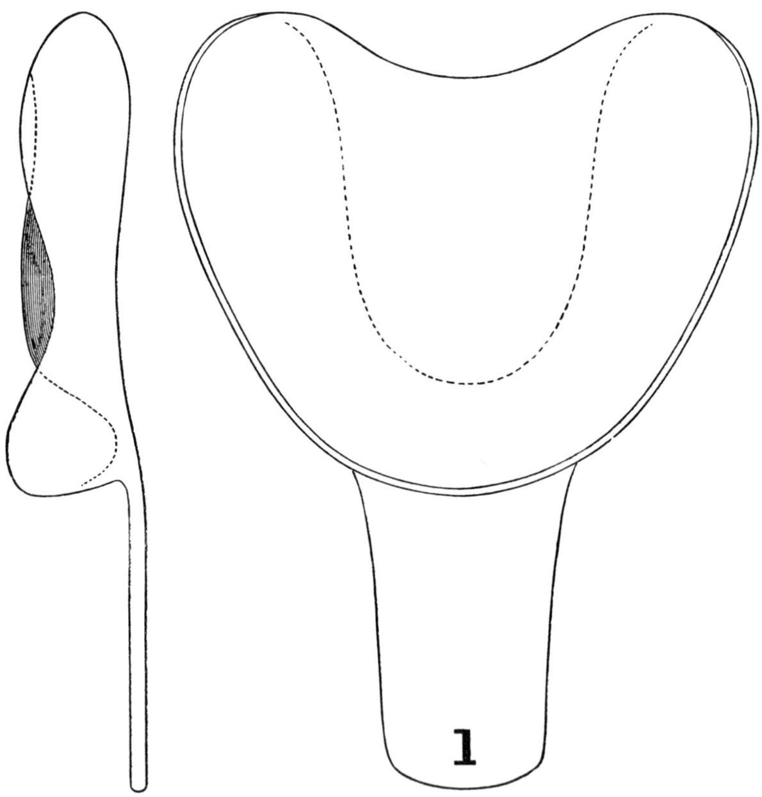

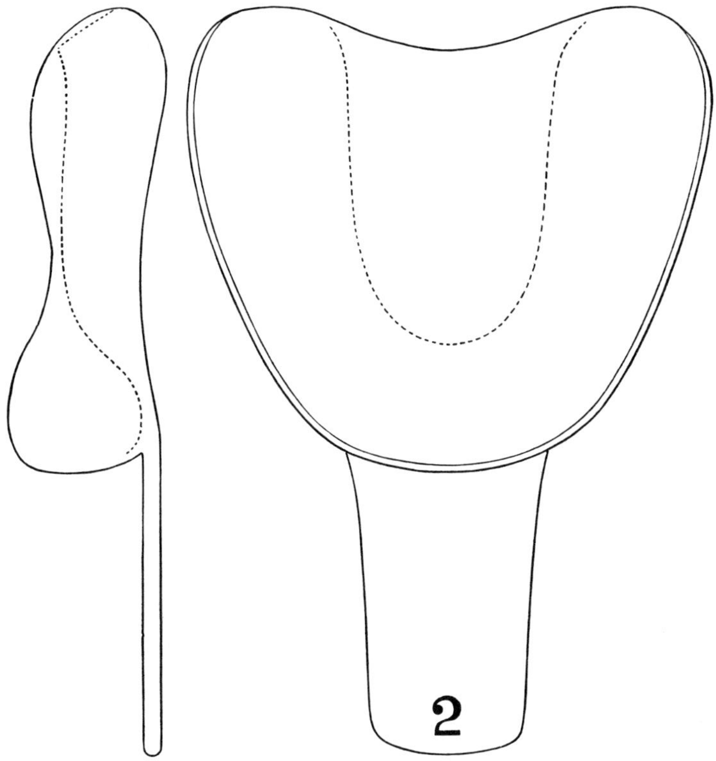

2

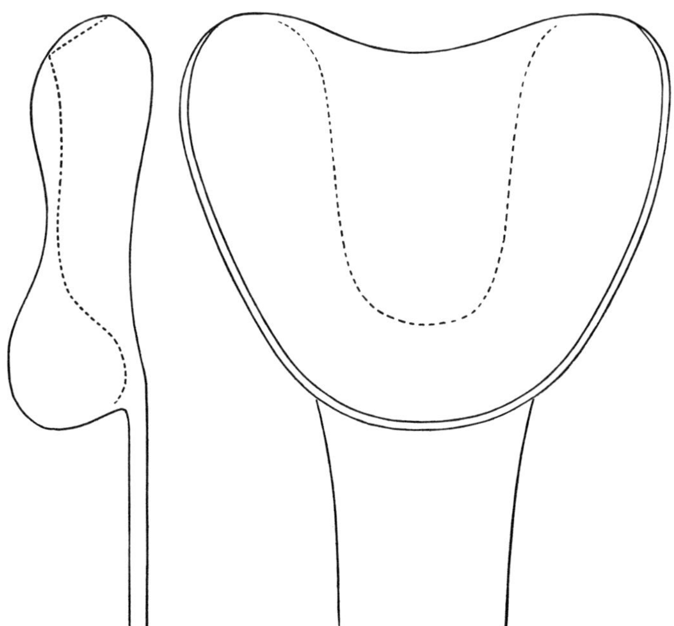

3

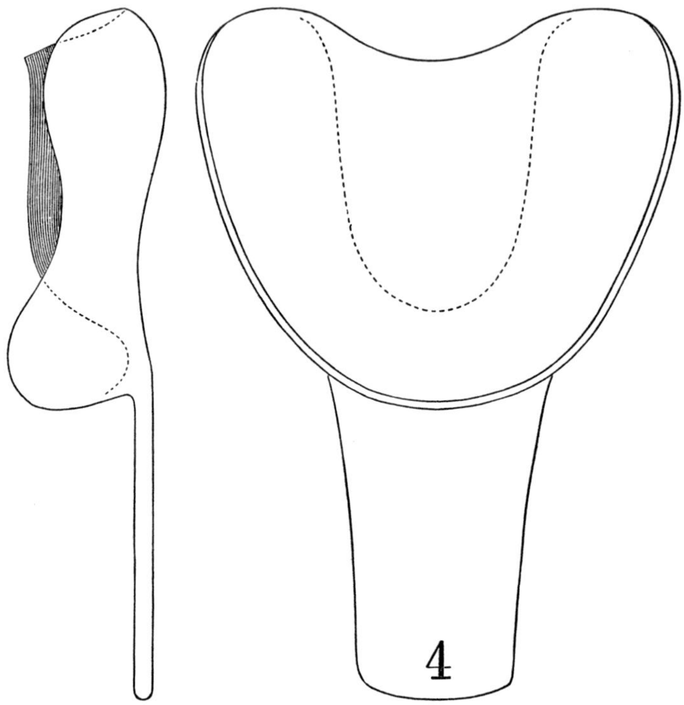

4

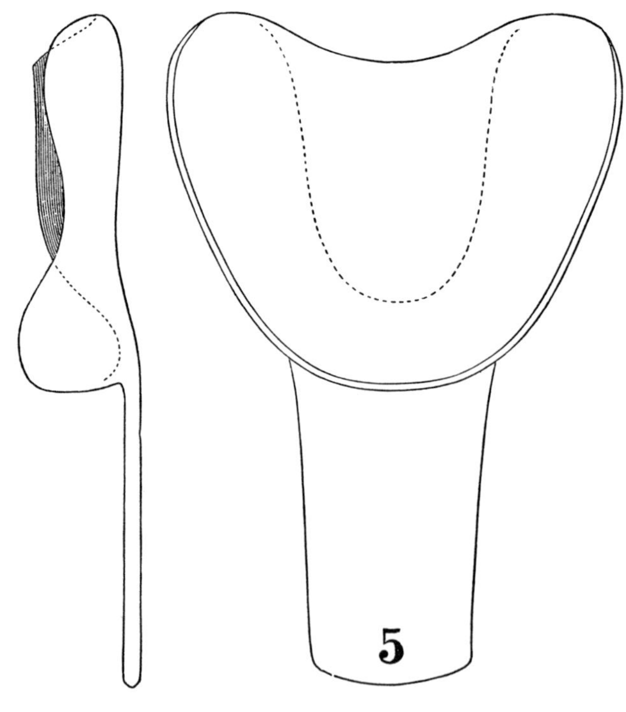

5

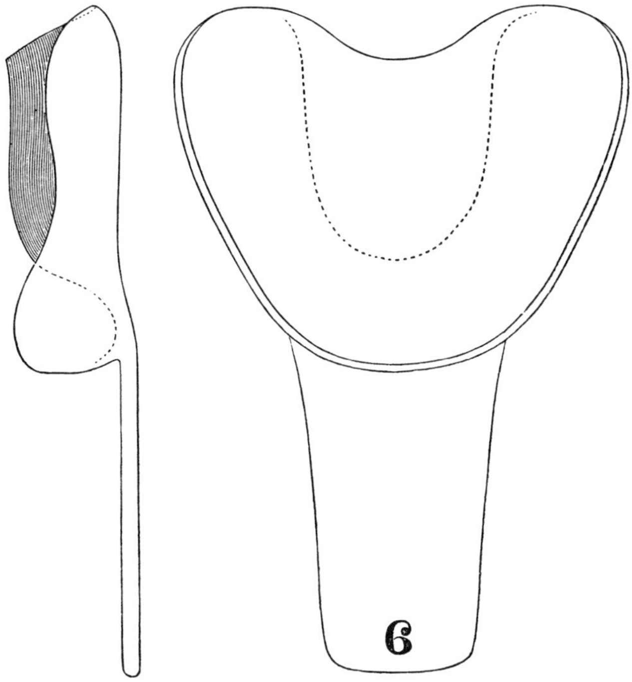

6

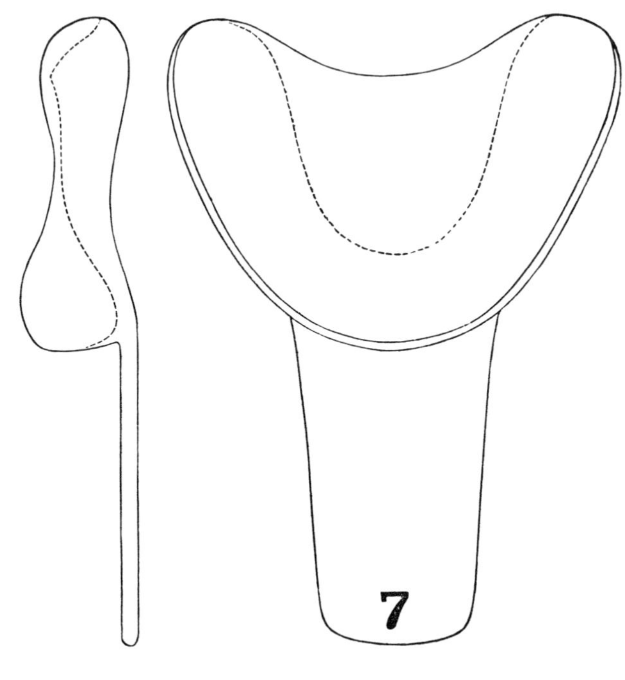

7

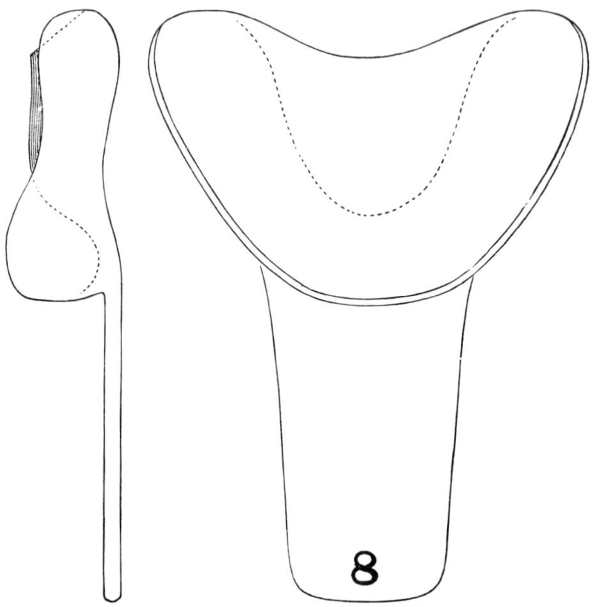

Fig. 2 illustrates the shape of a Set of 5, Nos. 12 to 16, for Partial Upper Dentures, with flat bottom and square sides; the handle, $1\frac{1}{2}$ inches in length, set below the line of the base.

The exact size of each Tray of the set is outlined, with its number attached, by which it may be ordered. The side views show, by the dotted line, the height of the palate portion of the Tray.

Price . . . . each 50 cents.

Fig. 2.

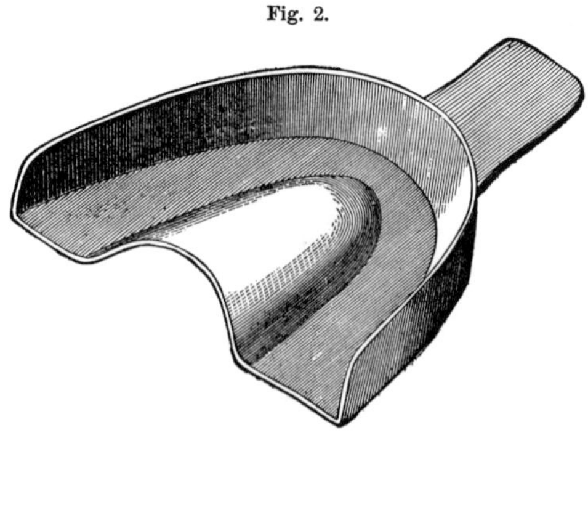

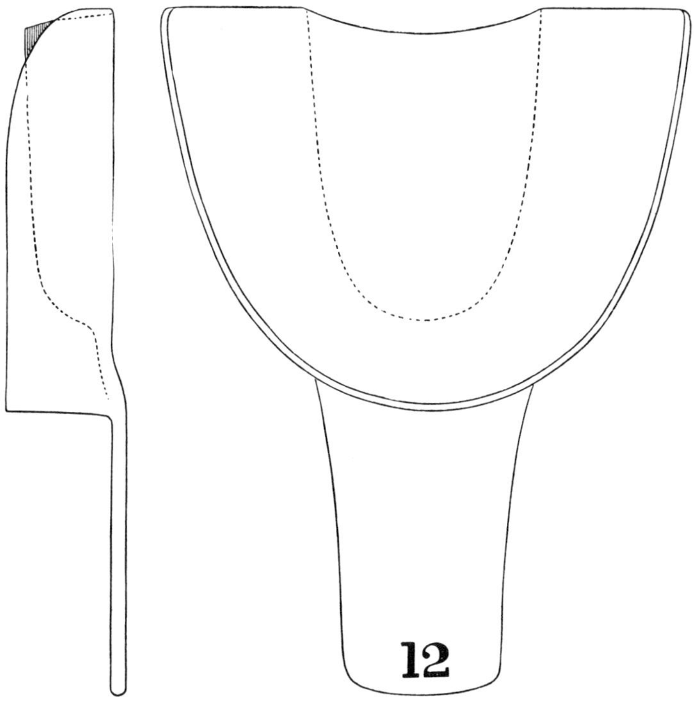

12

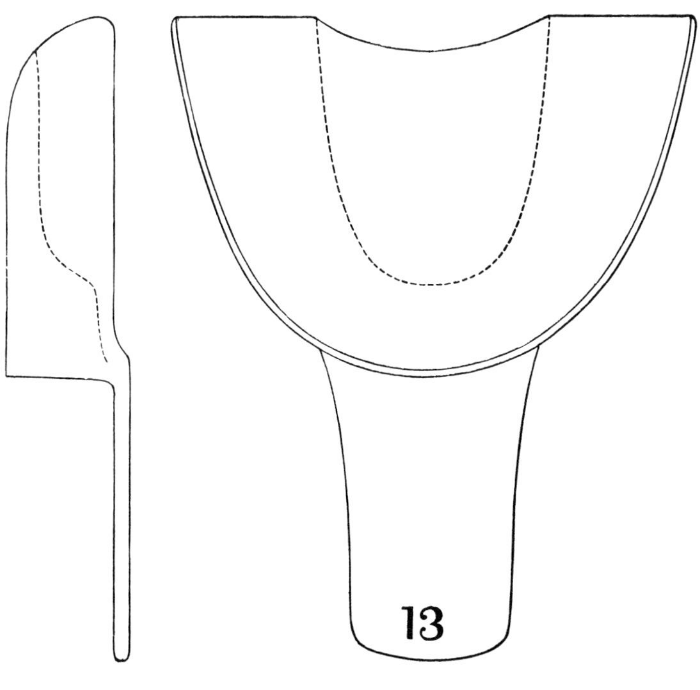

13

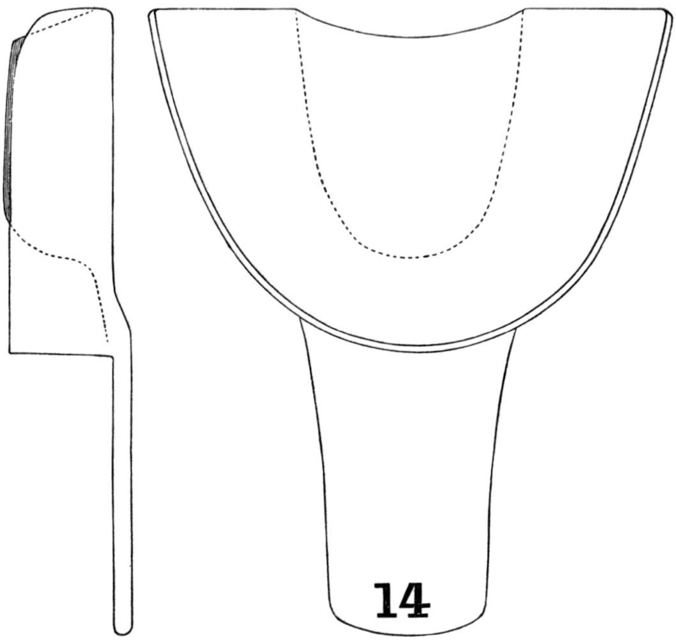
14

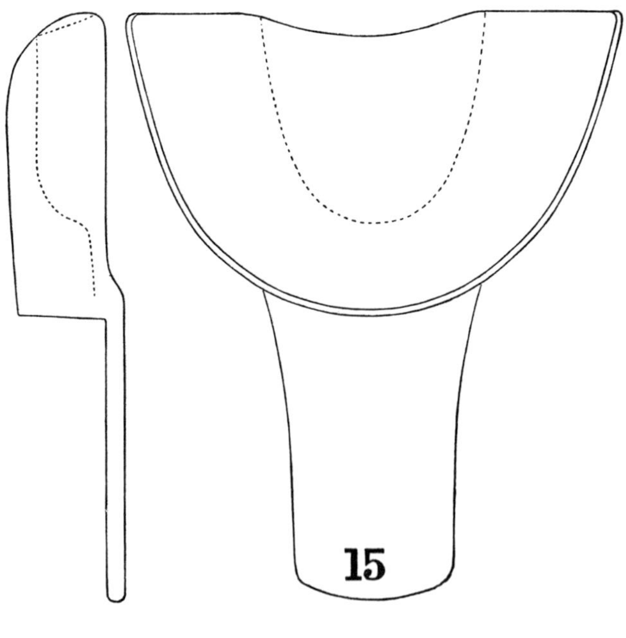
15

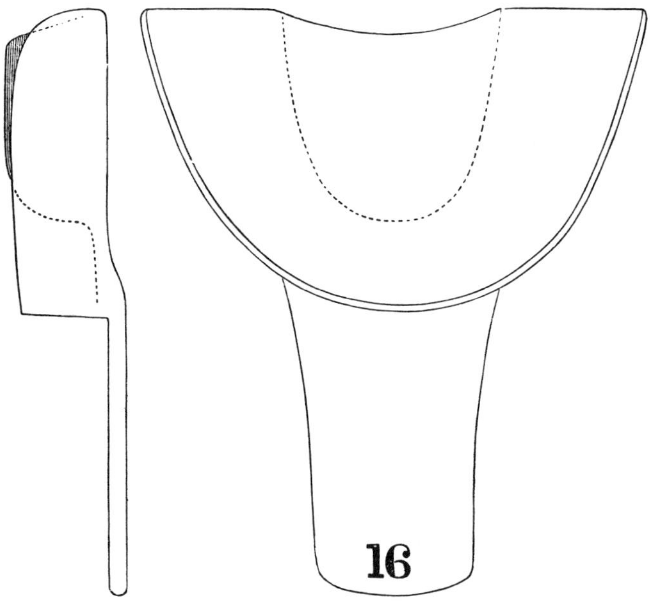

LOWER IMPRESSION TRAYS.

Fig. 3 illustrates the shape of a Set of 7, Nos. 1 to 7, for Full Lower Dentures.

Fig. 3.

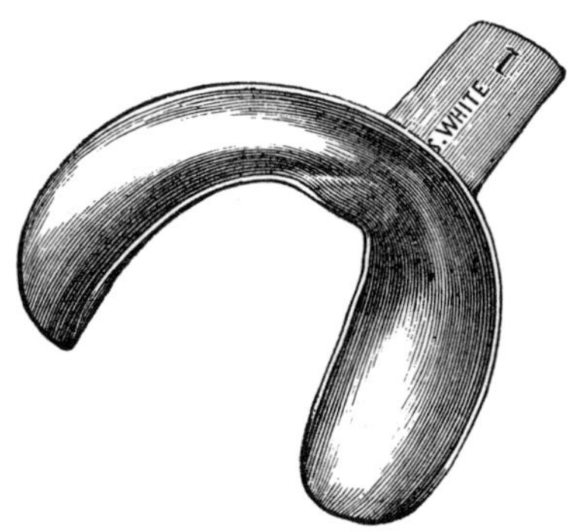

These are formed on models taken from impressions of the mouth. The handle is $1\frac{3}{4}$ inches in length, and so curved as to raise it $\frac{3}{8}$ of an inch above the base, giving room for the lip, and allowing the Tray to set well down on the maxillary. These have a special shape on the inner line designed to avoid the lingual frænum.

Nos. 5 and 6 are specially designed for cases where great absorption has taken place, and the muscles of the mouth are on a level with the maxillary ridge.

The exact size of each Tray of the set is outlined, with its number attached, by which it may be ordered. The side views show, by the dotted line, the relative dip of the outer and inner edges of the Tray.

Price . . . . each 50 cents.

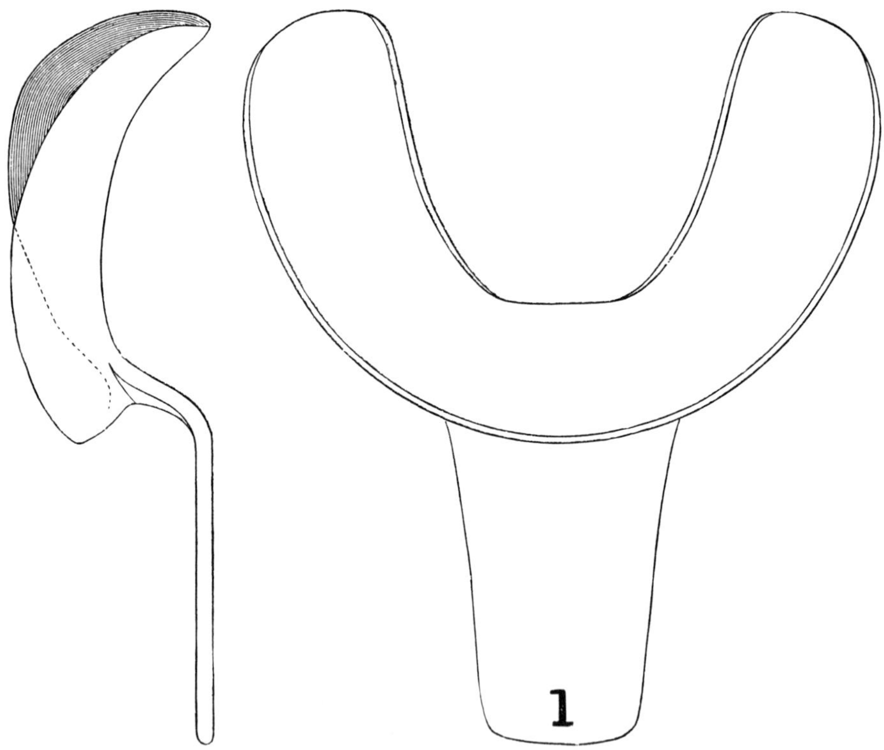

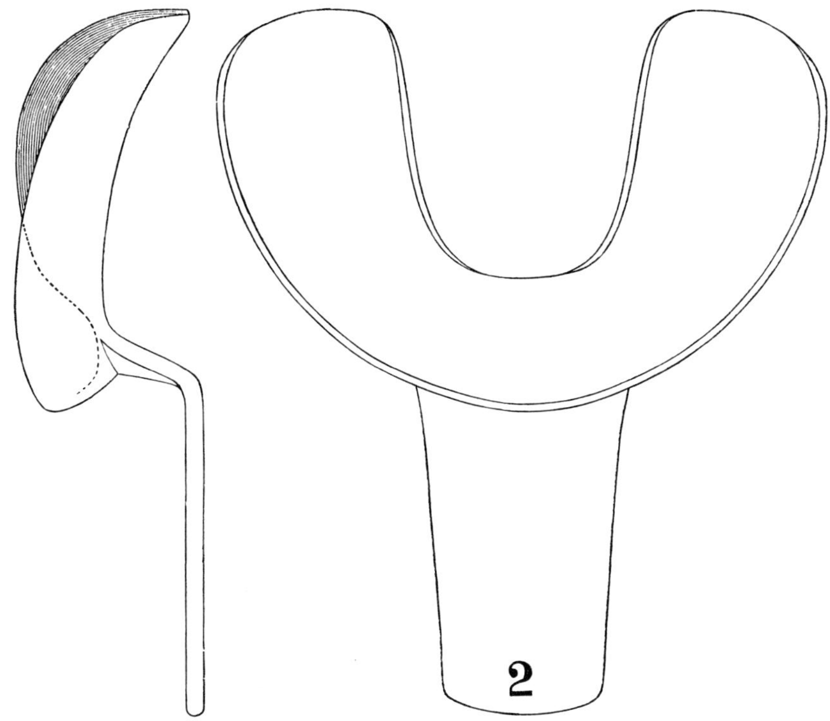

2

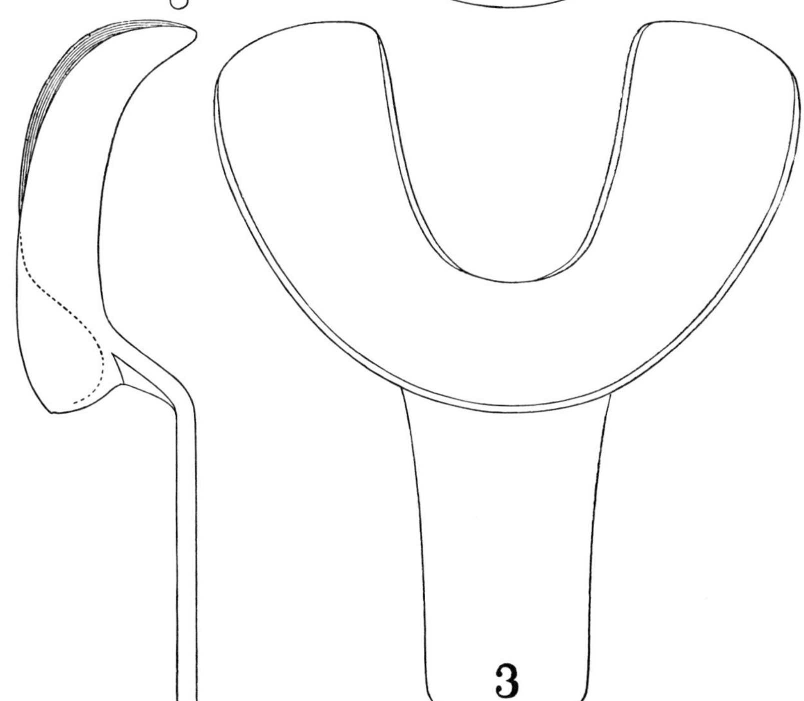

3

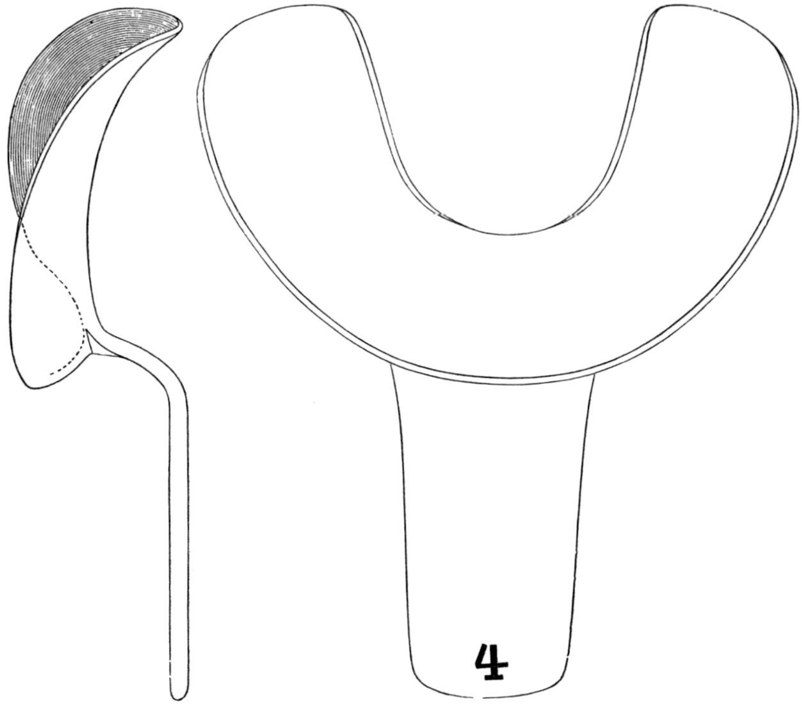

4

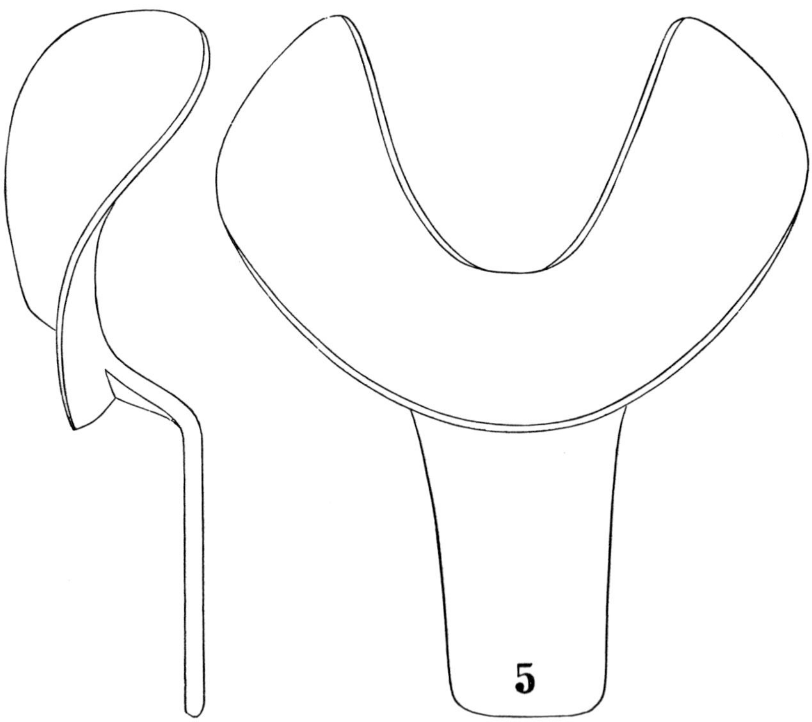

5

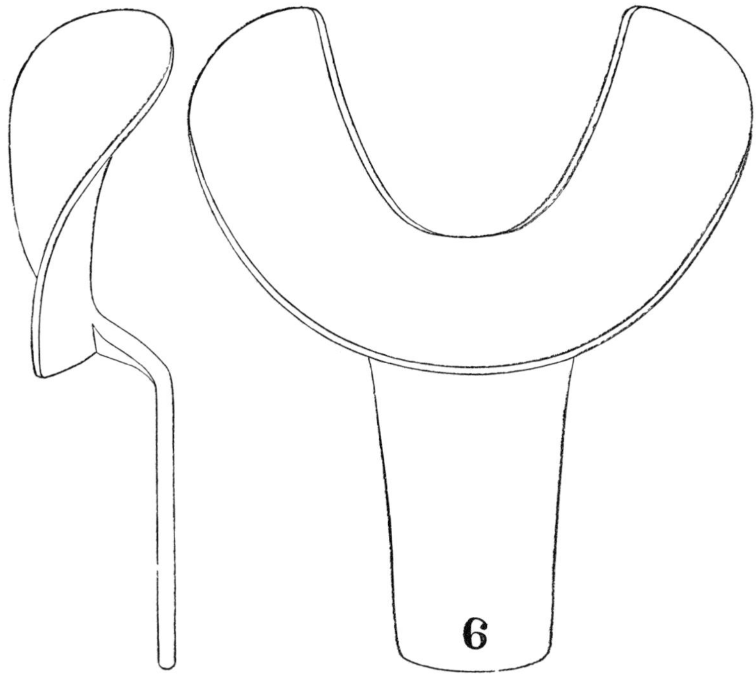

6

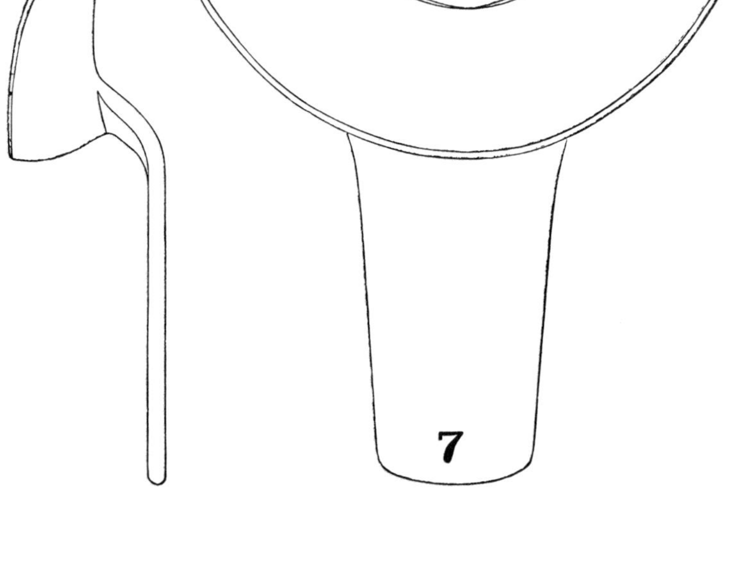

7

Fig. 4 illustrates the shape of a Set of 4, Nos. 10 to 13, for Partial Lower Dentures, having a *cavity* open to allow the front teeth to pass through, and the Tray to pass down to the maxillary ridge. The handle is 1½ inches in length, and attached to the base of the Tray at its highest point.

The exact size of each Tray of the set is outlined, with its number attached, by which it may be ordered. The side views show, by the dotted lines, the relative dip of the outer and inner edges of the Tray.

Price . . . . each 50 cents.

Fig. 4.

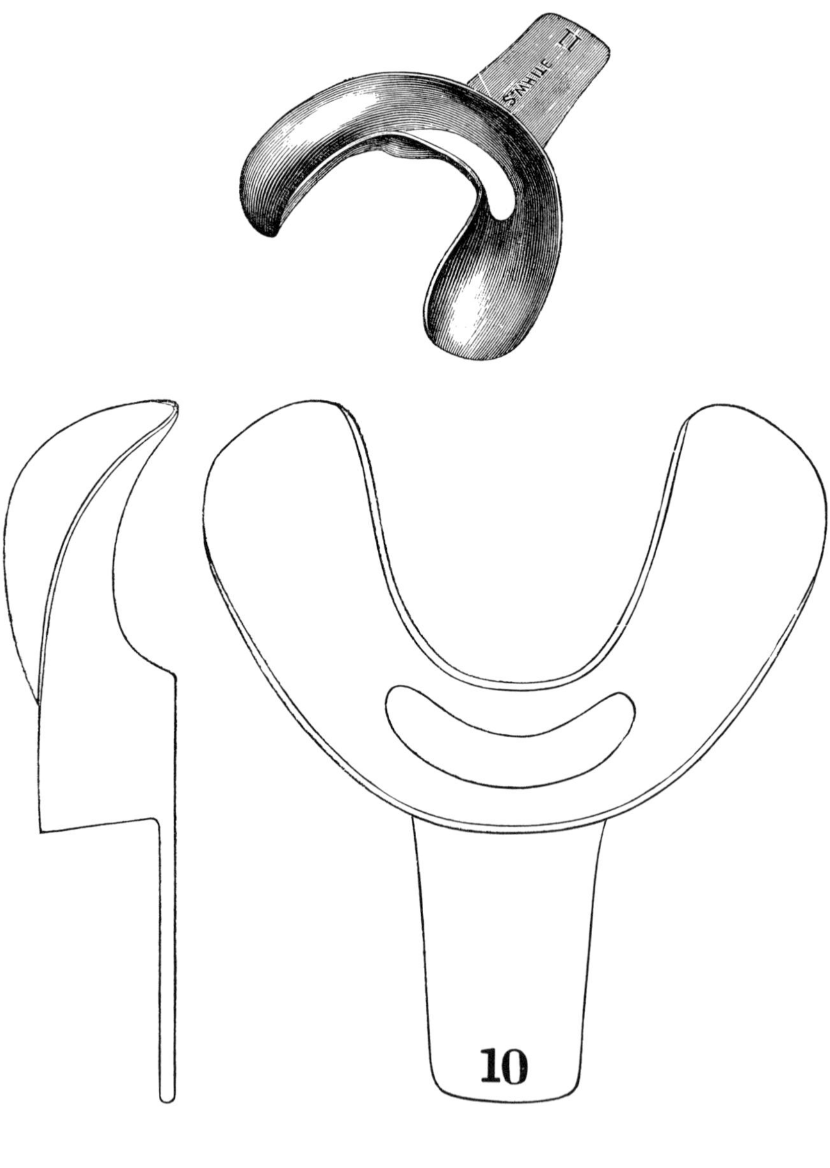

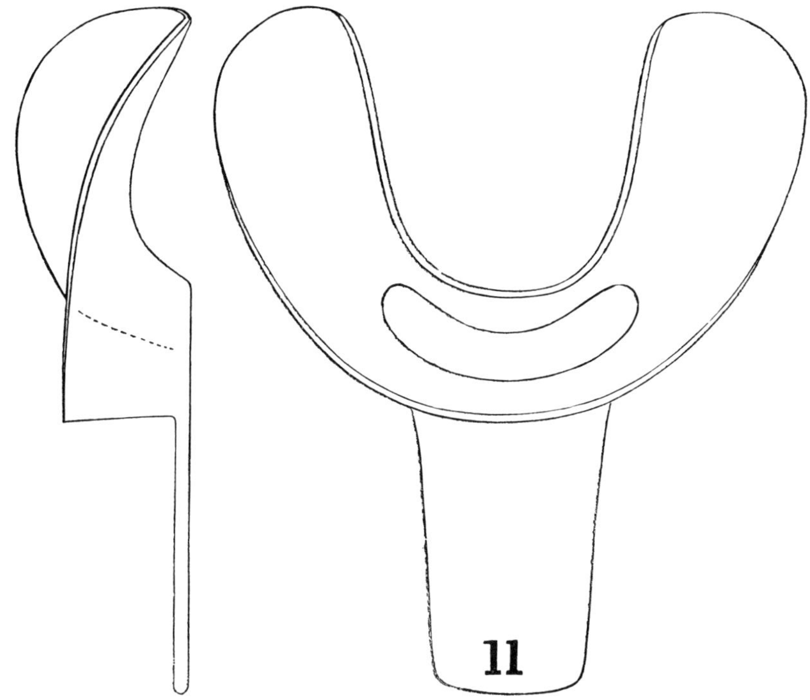

11

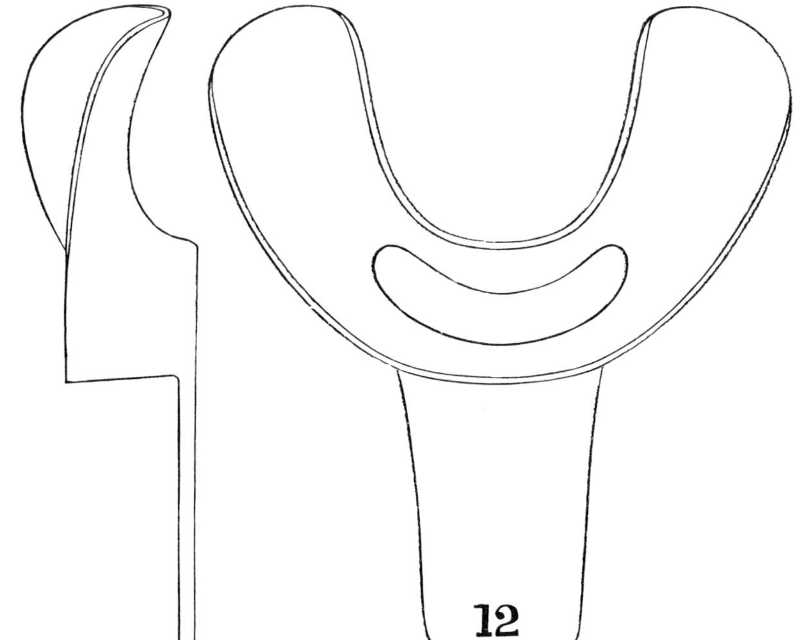

12

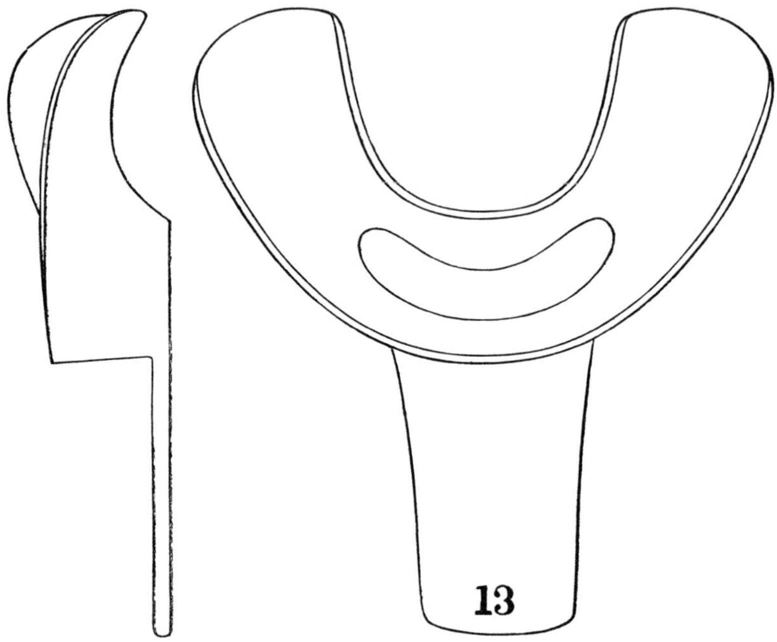

Fig. 5 illustrates the shape of a Set of 3, Nos. 14 to 16, with flat bottoms and square sides, designed especially for taking impressions of Lower Teeth, by which to obtain the antagonizing model for Upper Dentures.

The exact size of each Tray of the set is outlined, with the number attached, by which it may be ordered. The side views show the position of the handle, and the height of the body of the Tray.

Price . . . . each 50 cents.

Fig. 5.

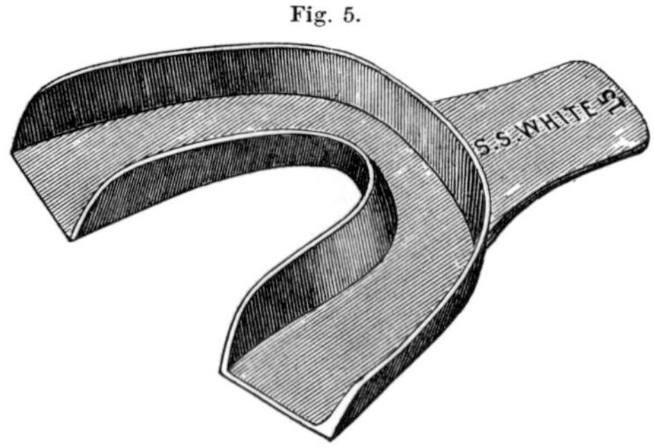

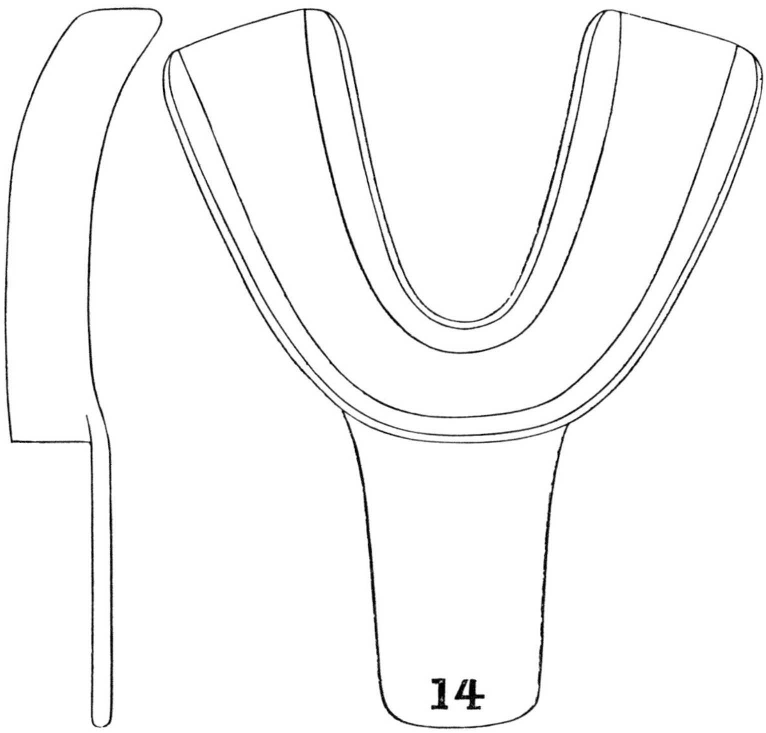

14

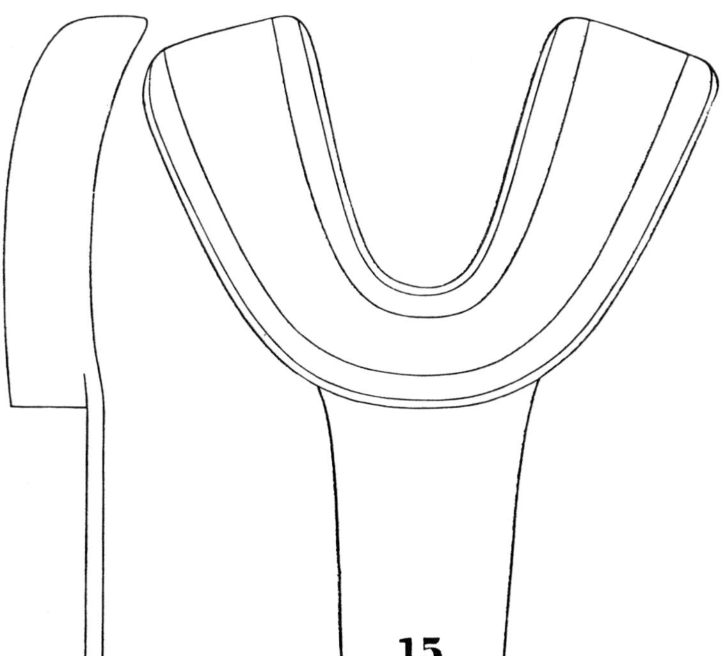

15

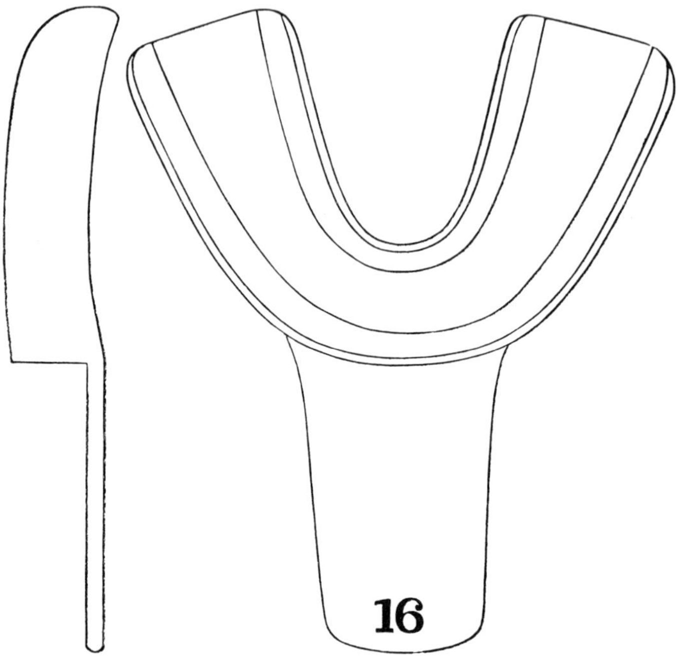

Fig. 6 illustrates Dr. B. W. Franklin's Impression Tray, of which there are three sizes, for taking impressions in plaster for Lower Dentures.

Price . . . . each 75 cents.

Fig. 6.

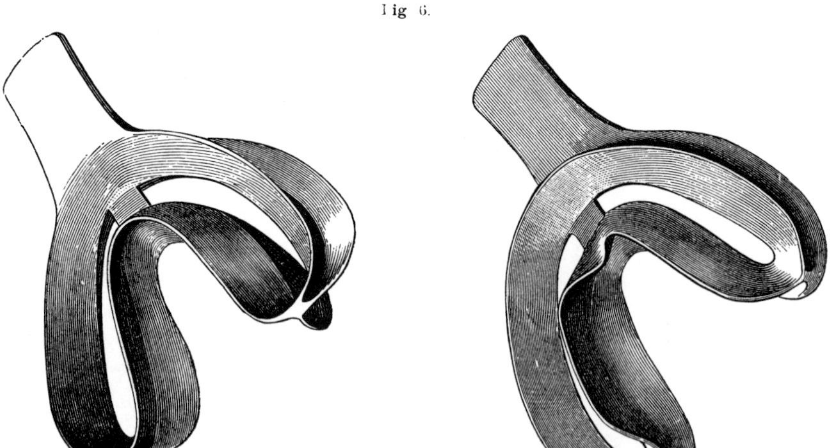

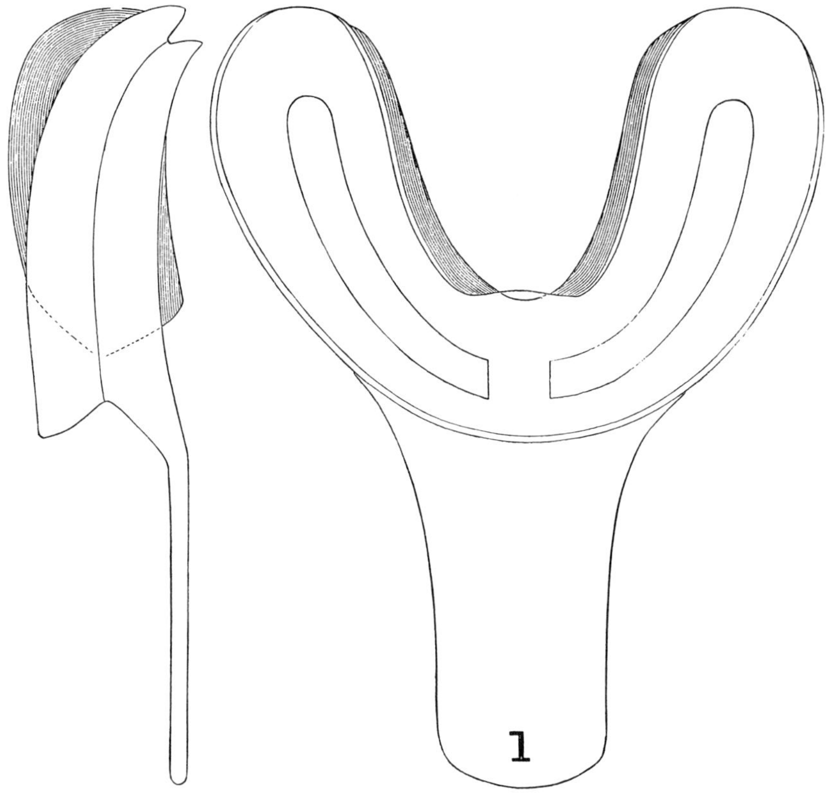

1

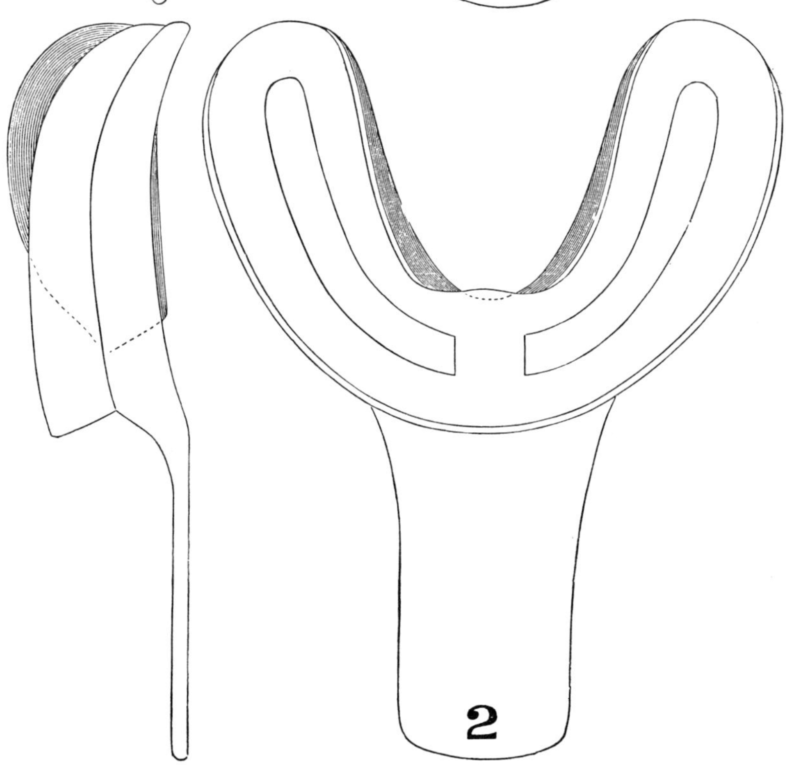

2

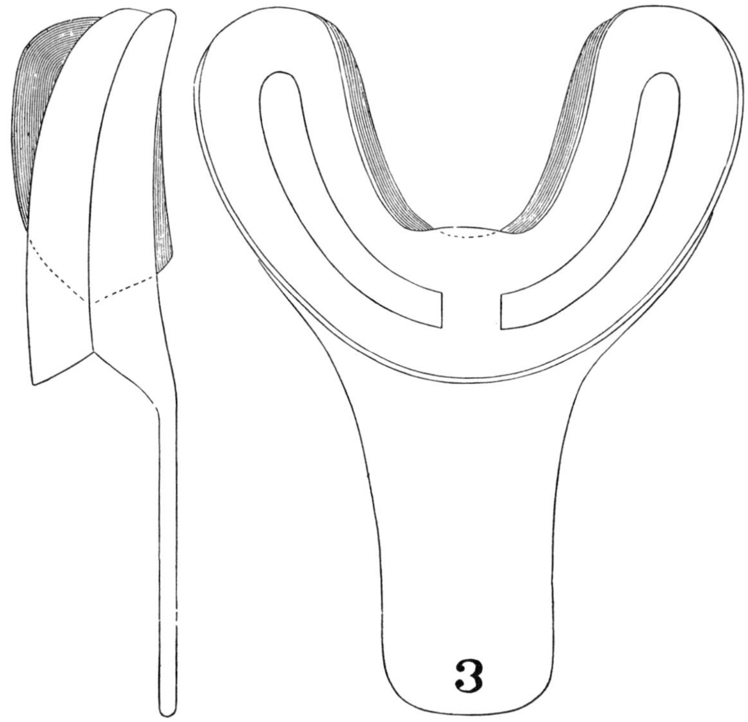

Fig. 7 illustrates Dr. Thomas Wardle's Movable Palate-Plate Tray.

Price of Tray, with two Palate-Plates Complete		$1.25
" " without Palate-Plate		.75
" Palate-Pieces	each	.25

Fig. 7.

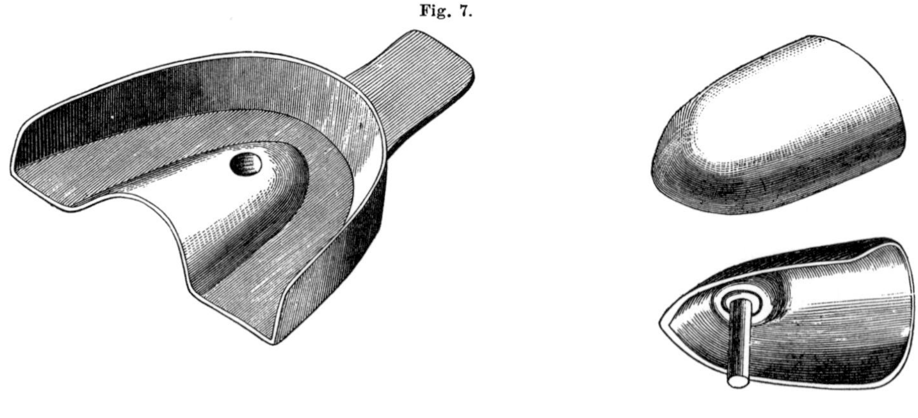

FULL SIZE SKELETON VIEW OF THE MOVABLE PALATE-PLATE TRAY.

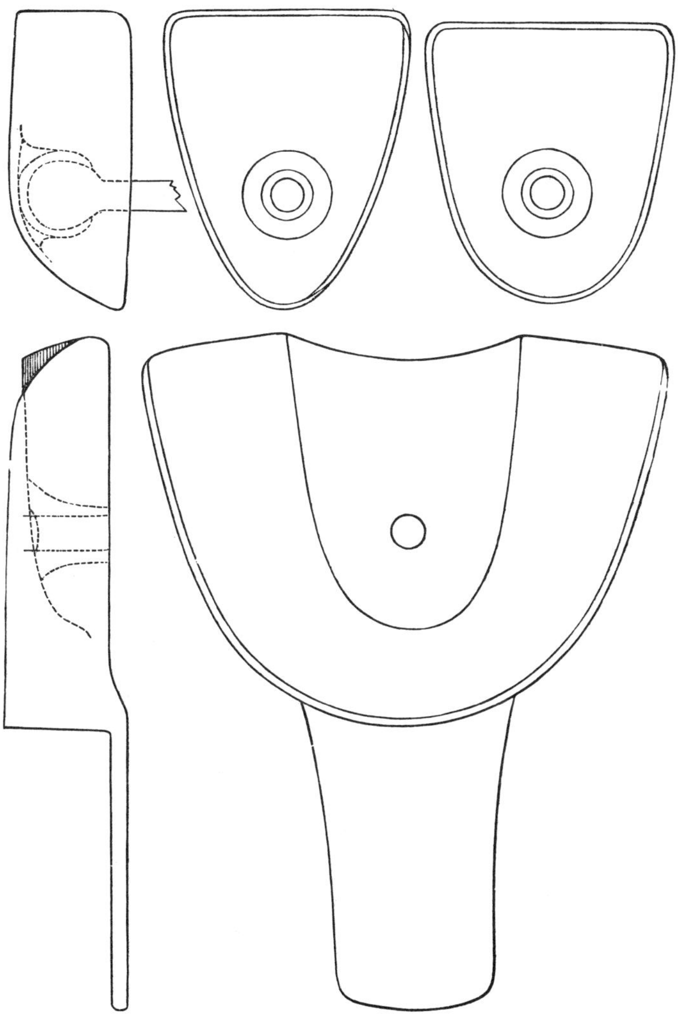

PORCELAIN IMPRESSION CUPS.

Patterns, similar to our regular Metal Cup, and which are far superior to any others heretofore offered.

These Cups commend themselves because of their neat and cleanly appearance.

The Set comprises twelve numbers, 9 Upper (Nos. 2, 3, 4, 5, 6, 7, 12, 13, and 14) and 3 Lower (Nos. 2, 4, and 6).

Price . . . . each 50 cents.

ARTICULATOR, No. 1.

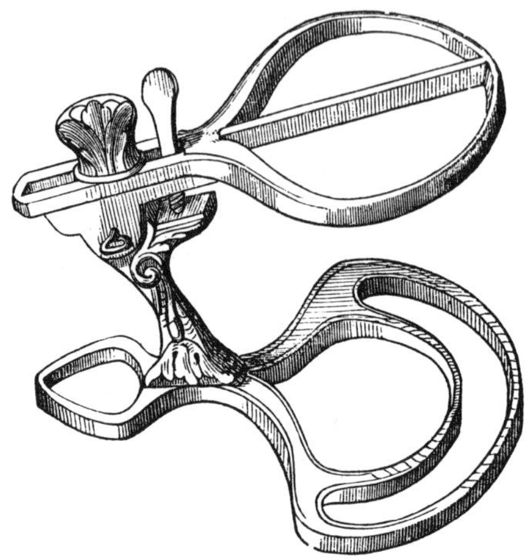

Made of Brass, having a Screw and Hinge, whereby it can be adjusted to any desired angle; also a Set-Screw, allowing the Top Plate to slide either backward or forward. It has met with general favor from those who have used it.

Price $1.00

ARTICULATOR, No. 2.

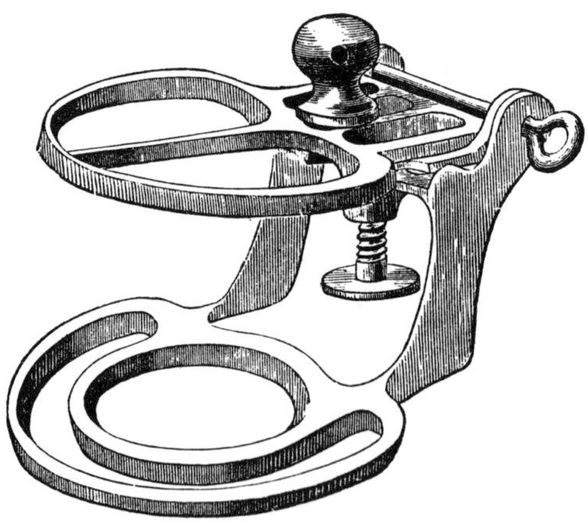

This is a more substantial article and of better finish than No. 1. It has the same movements, with the advantage that the Top Plate can be thrown all the way back, and that the Set-Screw for raising the Top Plate is more conveniently arranged.

Price $2.50

ARTICULATOR, No. 3.

Patented May 19th, 1868.

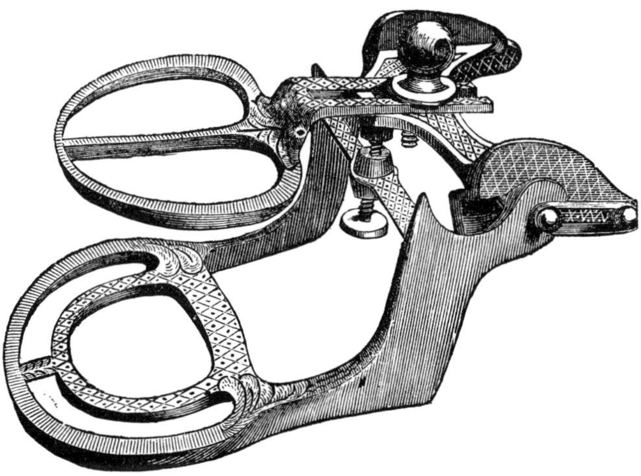

This Articulator has all the movements necessary for obtaining a correct Articulation for Artificial Dentures. The Lower Plate is modeled from the natural jaw, and moves on cone-shaped Pivots in V-shaped Grooves (without Hinges), being retained in position by elastic rubber Bands or Rings. A backward, forward, and lateral motion is provided for, corresponding with the movements of the natural jaw, by which the arrangement of the Denture can be practically tested without disturbing the Articulation. The Upper Plate has a backward and forward movement of two inches, and may be retained at any point by the Set-Screw. The Upper Plate has a double bend, so that when reversed from the position shown in the Cut an increase of one inch in the space is obtained between the Plates, allowing for both Upper and Lower Dentures. The Instrument is substantially made and nicely finished.

Price $3.00

BRUSH WHEELS.

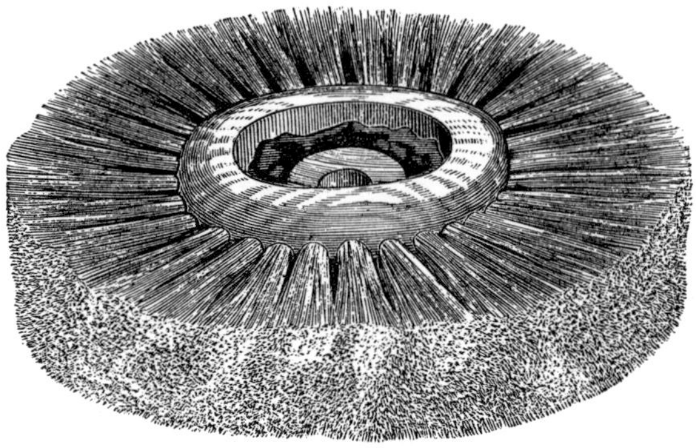

STRAIGHT BRISTLES.

Cut represents No. 26.

No.	3.	1 Row,	Stiff Bristles,	1¾	inches	diameter	. . . . . .	$0.10
"	4.	1 "	"	" 1⅞	"	"	. . . . . .	.14
"	101.	1 "	Soft	" 2¼	"	"	. . . . . .	.18
"	102.	1 "	Medium	" 2¼	"	"	. . . . . .	.18
"	103.	1 "	Stiff	" 2¼	"	"	. . . . . .	.18
"	104.	1 "	Soft	" 2½	"	"	. . . . . .	.18
"	105.	1 "	Medium	" 2½	"	"	. . . . . .	.18
"	106.	1 "	Stiff	" 2½	"	"	. . . . . .	.18
"	107.	1 "	Soft	" 2¾	"	"	. . . . . .	.18
"	108.	1 "	Medium	" 2¾	"	"	. . . . . .	.18
"	1.	2 Rows,	Stiff	" 1½	"	"	. . . . . .	.15
"	2.	2 "	"	" 1½	"	"	. . . . . .	.15
"	10.	2 "	Soft	" 1¾	"	"	. . . . . .	.18
"	6.	2 "	Medium	" 1¾	"	"	. . . . . .	.18
"	8.	2 "	"	" 1¾	"	"	. . . . . .	.18
"	5.	2 "	Stiff	" 1¾	"	"	. . . . . .	.18
"	7.	2 "	"	" 1¾	"	"	. . . . . .	.18
"	9.	2 "	"	" 1¾	"	"	. . . . . .	.18
"	11.	2 "	Soft	" 1⅞	"	"	. . . . . .	.20
"	14.	2 "	"	" 1⅞	"	"	. . . . . .	.20
"	13.	2 "	Medium	" 1⅞	"	"	. . . . . .	.20
"	12.	2 "	Stiff	" 1⅞	"	"	. . . . . .	.20
"	110.	2 "	Medium	" 2	"	"	. . . . . .	.22
"	112.	2 "	Stiff	" 2	"	"	. . . . . .	.22
"	19.	2 "	Soft	" 2½	"	"	. . . . . .	.25
"	22.	2 "	"	" 2½	"	"	. . . . . .	.25
"	21.	2 "	Medium	" 2½	"	"	. . . . . .	.25
"	20.	2 "	Stiff	" 2½	"	"	. . . . . .	.25
"	168.	2 "	Medium	" 3	"	"	. . . . . .	.45
"	169.	2 "	Stiff	" 3	"	"	. . . . . .	.45

No.	57.	2 Rows,	Soft Bristles,	3¼	inches	diameter	$0.40
"	60.	2 "	Soft "	3¼	"	"	.40
"	59.	2 "	Medium "	3¼	"	"	.40
"	58.	2 "	Stiff "	3¼	"	"	.40
"	56.	2 "	Soft "	3½	"	"	.45
"	55.	2 "	Stiff "	3½	"	"	.45
"	171.	2 "	Medium "	3¾	"	"	.56
"	172.	2 "	" "	3¾	"	"	.56
"	173.	2 "	Stiff "	3¾	"	"	.56
"	18.	3 "	Soft "	2	"	"	.28
"	17.	3 "	Stiff "	2	"	"	.28
"	26.	3 "	Soft "	2¾	"	"	.34
"	25.	3 "	Stiff "	2¾	"	"	.34
"	50.	3 "	Soft "	3	"	"	.37
"	31.	3 "	" "	3½	"	"	.50
"	34.	3 "	" "	3½	"	"	.50
"	174.	3 "	Medium "	3½	"	"	.60
"	175.	3 "	Stiff "	3½	"	"	.60
"	39.	3 "	Soft "	3¾	"	"	.70
"	42.	3 "	" "	3¾	"	"	.70
"	30.	4 "	" "	3	"	"	.44
"	29.	4 "	Stiff "	3	"	"	.44
"	38.	4 "	Soft "	3½	"	"	.62
"	37.	4 "	Stiff "	3½	"	"	.62
"	46.	4 "	Soft "	3¾	"	"	.72
"	45.	4 "	Stiff "	3¾	"	"	.72
"	64.	6 "	Soft "	3	"	"	.65
"	63.	6 "	Stiff "	3	"	"	.65

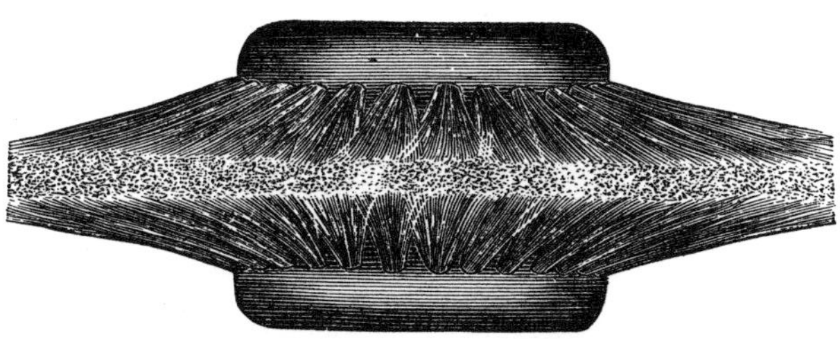

CONVERGING BRISTLES.

Cut represents No. 27.

No.	114.	2 Rows,	Medium Bristles,	2¼	inches	diameter	$0.22
"	115.	2 "	Stiff "	2¼	"	"	.22
"	118.	2 "	" "	2¾	"	"	.28
"	54.	2 "	Medium "	3½	"	"	.45
"	53.	2 "	Stiff "	3½	"	"	.45
"	16.	3 "	Medium "	2	"	"	.28
"	15.	3 "	Stiff "	2	"	"	.28

No.	154.	3 Rows,	Medium	Bristles,	2½	inches	diameter	$0.30
"	24.	3 "	"	"	2¾	"	"	.34
"	23.	3 "	Stiff	"	2¾	"	"	.34
"	47.	3 "	Soft	"	3	"	"	.37
"	49.	3 "	Medium	"	3	"	"	.37
"	48.	3 "	Stiff	"	3	"	"	.37
"	159.	3 "	"	"	3	"	"	.37
"	33.	3 "	Medium	"	3½	"	"	.50
"	32.	3 "	Stiff	"	3½	"	"	.50
"	177.	3 "	"	"	3½	"	"	.50
"	41.	3 "	Medium	"	3¾	"	"	.70
"	40.	3 "	Stiff	"	3¾	"	"	.70
"	179.	3 "	Soft	"	4	"	"	.70
"	180.	3 "	Medium	"	4	"	"	.70
"	181.	3 "	Stiff	"	4	"	"	.70
"	28.	4 "	Medium	"	3	"	"	.44
"	27.	4 "	Stiff	"	3	"	"	.44
"	36.	4 "	Medium	"	3½	"	"	.62
"	35.	4 "	Stiff	"	3½	"	"	.62
"	182.	4 "	Soft	"	3¾	"	"	.72
"	44.	4 "	Medium	"	3¾	"	"	.72
"	183.	4 "	"	"	3¾	"	"	.72
"	43.	4 "	Stiff	"	3¾	"	"	.72
"	185.	4 "	"	"	3¾	"	"	.72
"	186.	4 "	Soft	"	4¼	"	"	.90
"	187.	4 "	Medium	"	4¼	"	"	.90
"	62.	6 "	"	"	3	"	"	.65
"	61.	6 "	Stiff	"	3	"	"	·65
"	164.	6 "	Medium	"	3½	"	"	.75

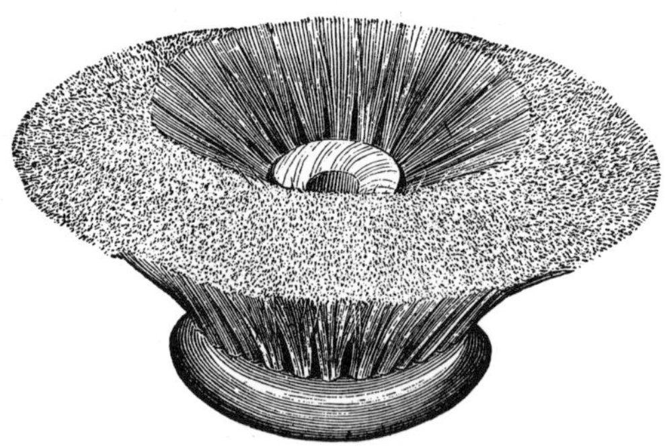

CUP SHAPE.

Cut represents No. 76.

No.	67.	1 Row,	Medium	Bristles,	2	inches	diameter	$0.14
"	68.	1 "	Stiff	"	2	"	"	.15
"	122.	1 "	Soft	"	2½	"	"	.20

No. 123.	1 Row,	Medium	Bristles,	2½	inches diameter	$0.20
" 124.	1 "	Stiff	"	2½	" "	.20
" 126.	1 "	Medium	"	3	" "	.28
" 127.	1 "	Stiff	"	3	" "	.28
" 132.	2 Rows,	Medium	"	2½	" "	.22
" 141.	2 "	"	"	2¾	" "	.32
" 135.	2 "	"	"	3	" "	.30
" 76.	3 "	Soft	"	2½	" "	.30
" 78.	3 "	Medium	"	2½	" "	.30
" 77.	3 "	Stiff	"	2½	" "	.30
" 145.	3 "	"	"	2¾	" "	.45
" 69.	3 "	Soft	"	3	" "	.34
" 71.	3 "	Medium	"	3	" "	.34
" 137.	3 "	"	"	3	" "	.34
" 70.	3 "	Stiff	"	3	" "	.34

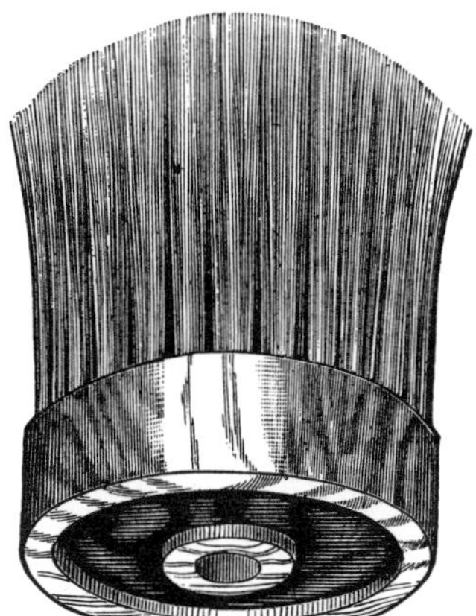

HUB SHAPE.

Cut represents No. 73.

No. 147.	Medium	Bristles,	1¼	inches diameter	$0.32
" 146.	Stiff	"	1¼	" "	.32
" 74.	Soft	"	1½	" "	.32
" 72.	Medium	"	1½	" "	.32
" 73.	Stiff	"	1½	" "	.32
" 148.	Medium	"	2	" "	.38
" 149.	Stiff	"	2	" "	.38

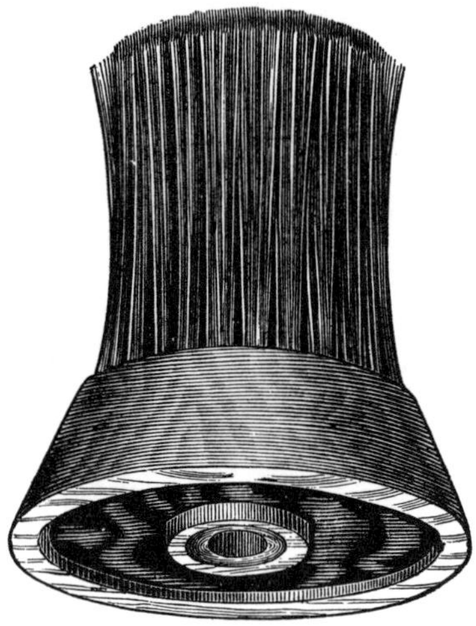

HUB-SHAPE, BROAD BASE, CONVERGING BRISTLES.

Cut represents No. 87.

No. 85.	Stiff Bristles, $\frac{3}{4}$ inch diameter through bristles	$0.18
" 86.	" " 1 " " " "	.22
" 87.	" " $1\frac{1}{8}$ inches " " "	.30

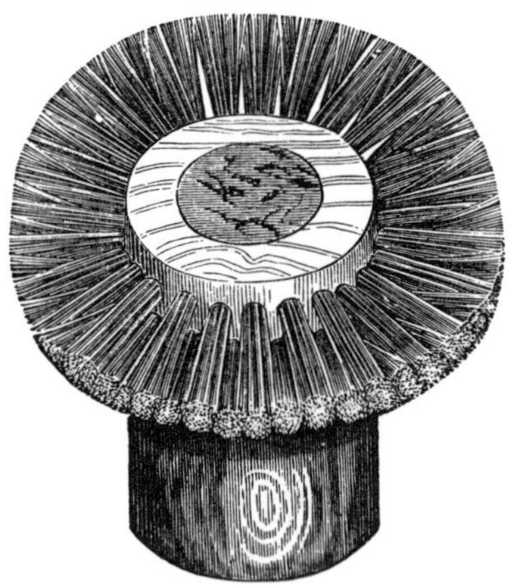

STRAIGHT BRISTLES, LONG WOODEN SHANKS.

Cut represents No. 66.

No. 52.	2 Rows, Stiff Bristles, $1\frac{3}{4}$ inches diameter	$0.18
" 66.	2 " " " $1\frac{7}{8}$ " "	.24

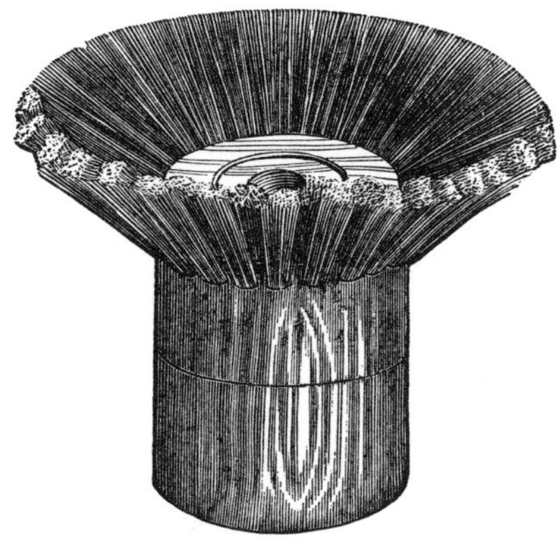

CUP-SHAPE BRISTLES LONG WOODEN SHANKS.

Cut represents No. 65.

No. 51.	2	Rows,	Stiff Bristles,	1¾	inches	diameter	$0.18
" 65.	2	"	" "	1⅞	"	"	.24
" 150.	2	"	Soft "	2¼	"	"	24

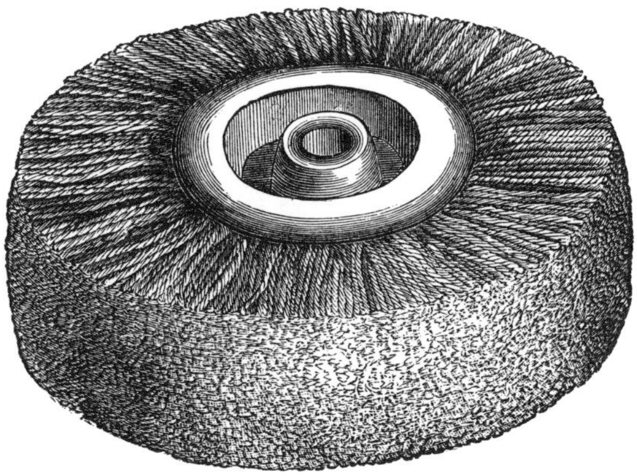

COTTON WHEELS.

Cut represents No. 83.

No. 79.	1	Row,	1¾	inches	diameter		$0.12
" 1.	1	"	2¼	"	"		.12
" 80.	2	Rows,	1¾	"	"		.20
" 81.	2	"	2	"	"		.20
" 82.	2	"	2¾	"	"		.24
" 20.	2	"	3½	"	"		.38
" 83.	3	"	2¾	"	"		.34
" 85.	3	"	2¾	"	"	stitched	.43
" 22.	3	"	3	"	"		.46
" 24.	3	"	3½	"	"		.56
" 84.	4	"	3	"	"		.40
" 25.	4	"	3½	"	"		.74
" 16.	6	"	3	"	"		.62

FELT, RUBBER, AND WALRUS-LEATHER WHEELS AND CONES.

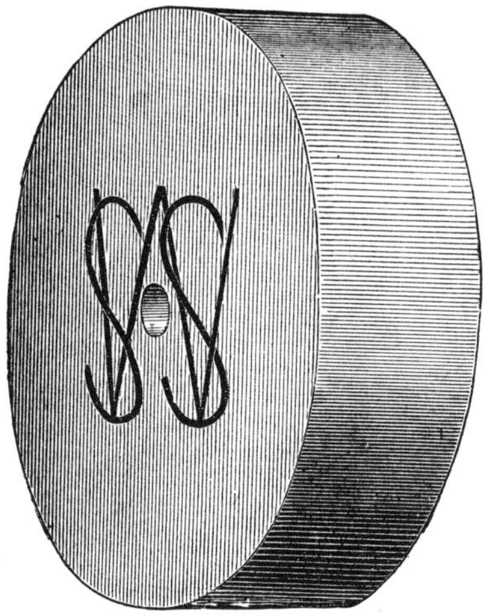

Cut represents No. 4 Felt Wheel.

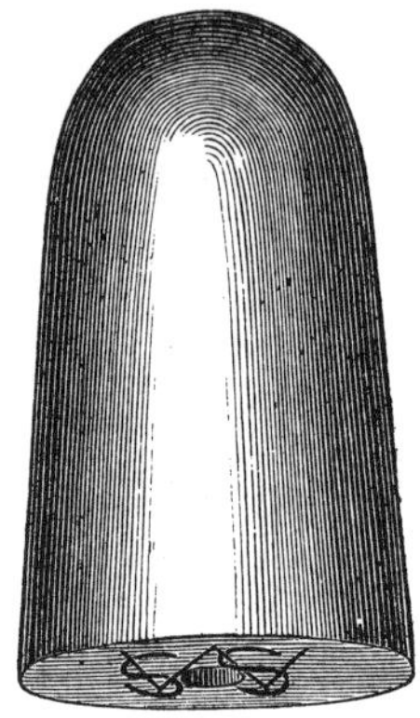

Large Felt Cone.

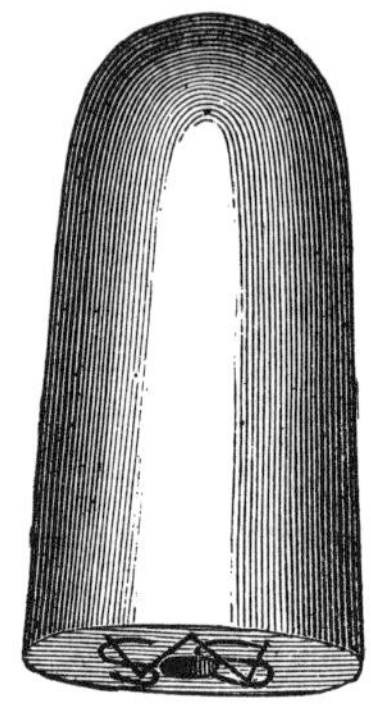

Small Felt Cone.

No. 1. Felt Wheel, 1⅛ inches diameter	each	$0.20
" 2. " " 1⅝ " "	"	.20
" 3. " " 2¼ " "	"	.40
" 4. " " 2½ " "	"	.40
Small " Cone, ¾ inch " 1½ inches long	"	.20
Large " " 1 " " 1¾ " "	"	.40
No. 1. Rubber Wheel, 1⅛ inches diameter	"	.15
" 2. " " 1⅝ " "	"	.15
" 3. " " 2¼ " "	"	.30
" 4. " " 2½ " "	"	.30
Rubber Cone, 1 inch " 1¾ inches long	"	.20
No. 1. Walrus-Leather Wheels, 2 inches diameter	"	.25
" 2. " " " 2½ " "	"	.40
Walrus-Leather Cones, ¾ inch diameter, 1½ inches long	"	.40
" " " 1 " " 1¾ " "	"	.50

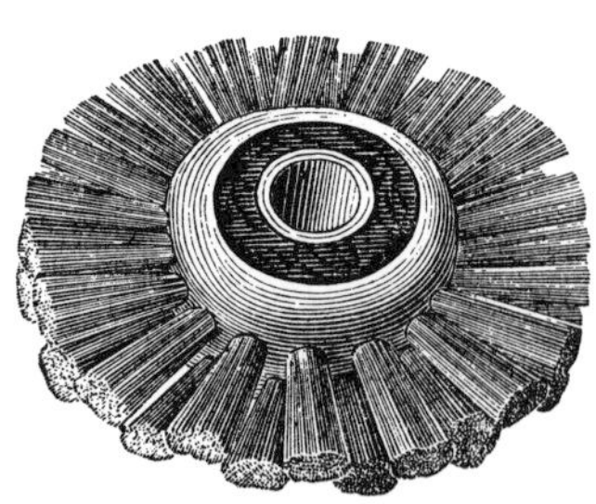

LARGE WIRE WHEEL.

SUGGESTED BY DR. J. M. WHITNEY.

For cleaning Engine Tools (Burs) and Files, and dressing down Celluloid and Rubber Plates. The Cut is full size, 1⅝ inches in diameter, two Rows and of fine Steel Wire.

Price . . . . each $0.75

POLISHING POWDERS.

We have prepared several additional Powders for polishing and finishing purposes, and the variety now offered will probably meet all preferences. These Powders are intended for use with felt and leather buffs, wood points, brush-wheels, and cotton wheels, and will be found particularly useful with the soft rubber points.

PRICES.

Hindostan Stone Powder	per box	12 cents.
Arkansas " "	"	25 "
Pumice " " (per lb. 15 cents)	"	10 "
Emery " " 25 "	"	10 "
Buck-Horn " (small box)	"	12 "
" " " (large box)	"	38 "
Corundum Flour	"	25 "
" " Extra Fine	"	25 "
Rouge	"	20 "
Rotten-Stone	"	10 "
Tripoli	"	10 "
Crocus	"	10 "
Prepared Chalk	per 1 lb. package	15 "

SOFT RUBBER POINTS.

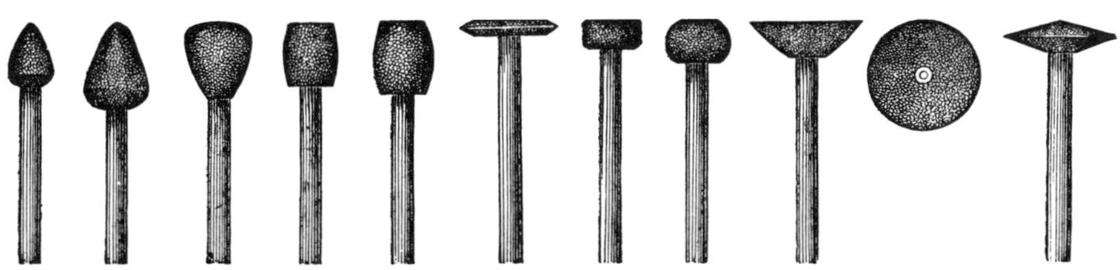

1. 2. 3. 4. 5. 8. 9. 10. 11. 12.

These Points can be used on Lathes Nos. 3 and 4, when mounted on plain Screw Engine Mandrels, for polishing around the necks of teeth in Rubber and Celluloid sets, when plain teeth are used.

Points, not mounted	per doz.	$0.75
" mounted on Mandrels	"	1.50

CORUNDUM WHEELS.

(See Cut on Opposite Page.)

					Thickness.		
			$\frac{1}{4}$ inch.	$\frac{3}{8}$ inch.	$\frac{1}{2}$ inch.	$\frac{5}{8}$ inch.	$\frac{3}{4}$ inch.	1 inch.
No. 00.	$\frac{3}{4}$ inch diameter		$0.07					
" 0.	$\frac{7}{8}$ "	"	.09					
" 1.	1 "	"	.12	$0.15	$0.18	$0.20	$0.25	$0.35
" 2.	$1\frac{3}{8}$ inches	"	.16	.18	.20	.25	.30	.40
" 3.	$1\frac{5}{8}$ "	"	.20	.25	.30	.35	.40	.50
" 4.	$1\frac{3}{4}$ "	"	.25	.30	.35	.40	.45	.60
" 5.	$2\frac{1}{8}$ "	"	.30	.35	.45	.50	.60	.80
" 6.	$2\frac{1}{2}$ "	"	.40	.50	.60	.70	.80	1.00
" 7.	$3\frac{1}{8}$ "	"	.60	.75	.90	1.00	1.20	1.50
" 8.	4 "	"	1.00	1.25	1.50	1.75	2.00	2.50
" 9.	5 "	"	1.50	1.80	2.10	2.50	3.00	4.00
" 10.	6 "	"	2.25	2.75	3.25	3.75	4.25	5.25
" 11.	7 "	"	3.25	4.00	4.75	5.50	6 25	7.00

ARTICULATING CORUNDUM WHEELS.

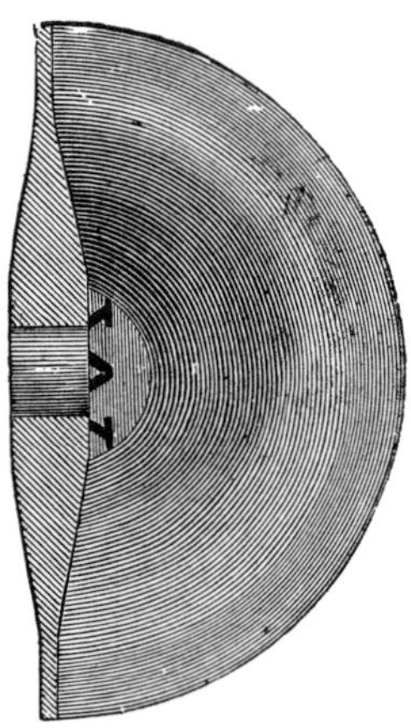

(Diameter, $2\frac{3}{16}$ inches; thickness of cutting edge, $\frac{1}{16}$ inch.)

These Wheels are intended for re-shaping the cutting edges of artificial incisor and canine teeth after they have been ground off in adapting them to the antagonizing teeth.

Price . . . . each 35 cents.

CORUNDUM WHEELS.

(SEE OPPOSITE PAGE.)

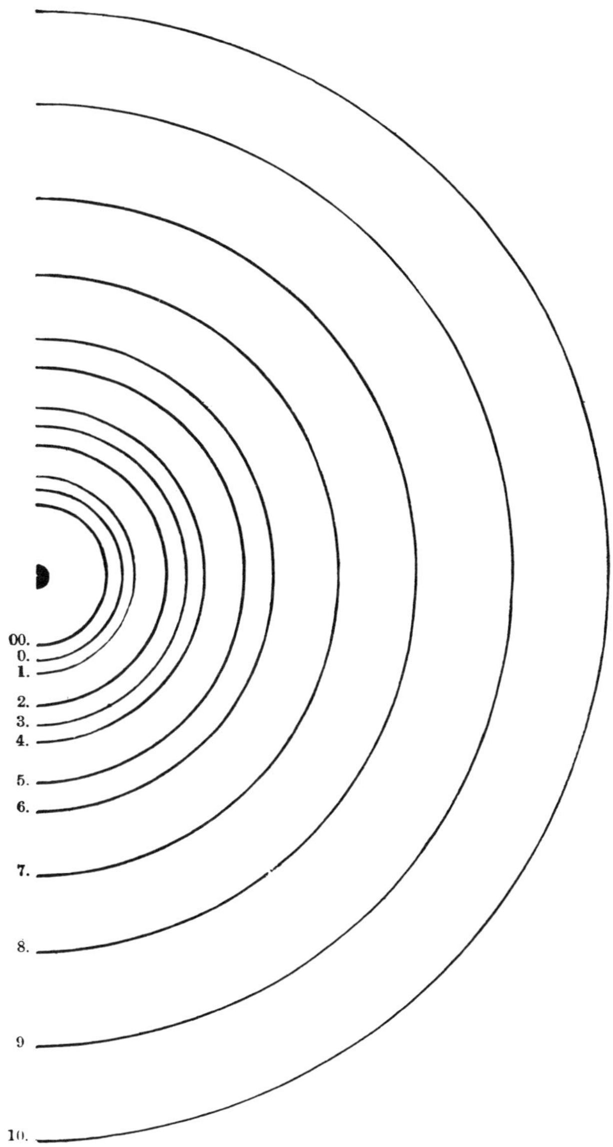

CORUNDUM FILES, ETC.

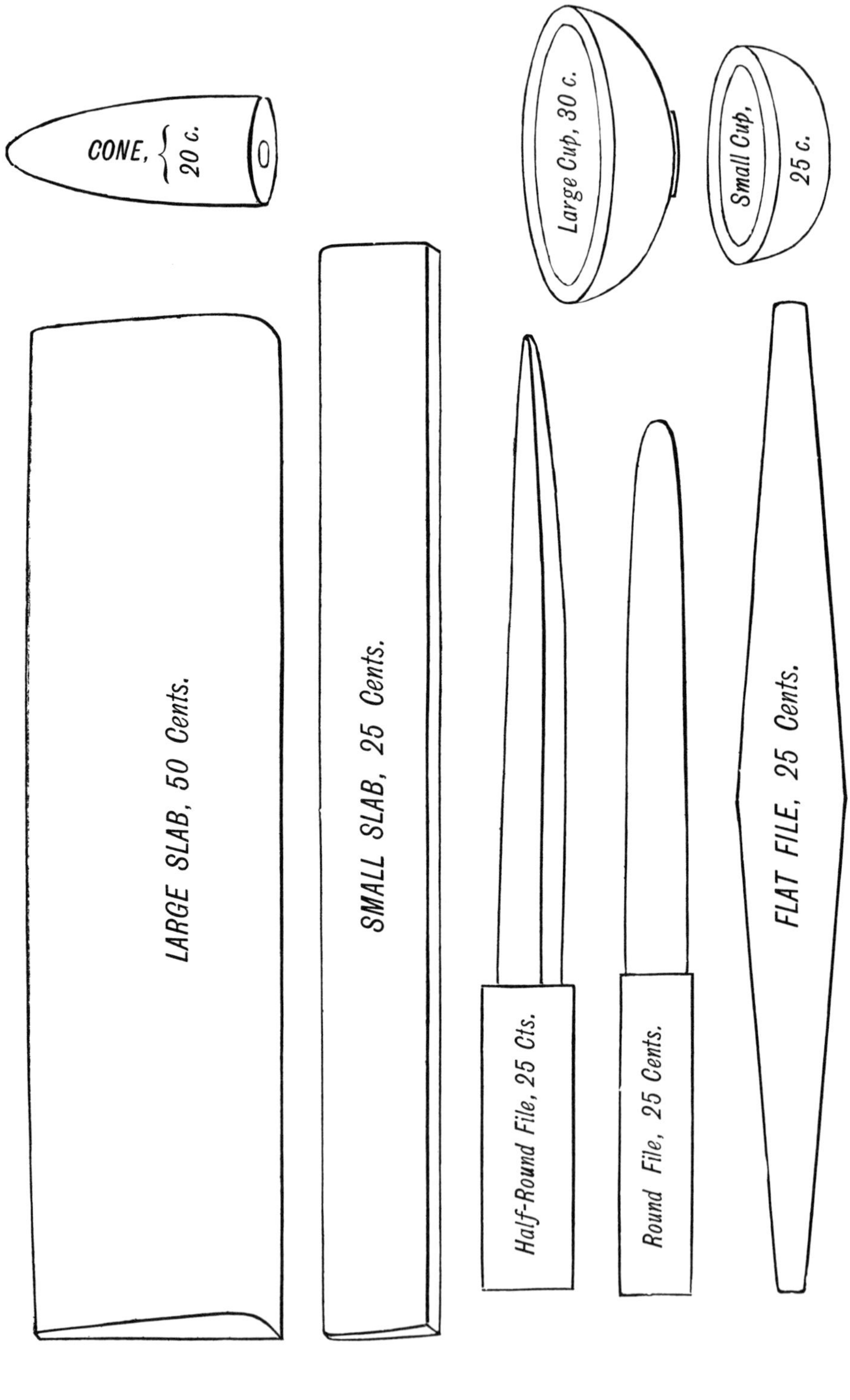

Miscellaneous.

Asbestos	per lb.	$0.37
Acid Pans, Copper, for heating Acids for Pickling	each	.75
" Bottles, with Cover	"	1.00
" " without Cover	"	.60
Anvils	"	1.25
" in Lead Bases	"	1.75
Binding Wire	per spool	.25
Brushes, Hand, for Plate	each .35 to	.55
Burnishers, Blood-stone, for Plate	" 1.00 to	2.50
" Steel, for Plate	each	.50
Body, Allen's, for Continuous Gum Work	per oz.	1.50
Block Body, S. S. White's	per lb.	2.00
Bunsen's Burners, Gas, Single Jet	each	1.50
" " " Spread Flame	"	2.00
Chamois-Skins	.40 to	1.25
Couplings for Lathe Cords, Steel	each	.25
Casting Rings, Sets of 4	per set	.75
Cotton Cones, for Polishing	each .45 to	.55
Crucibles, Nests of 3	each	.06
" Nests of 4	"	.08
Clamps for holding Plate while Swaging	"	.75
Cork Wheels and Cones, for Polishing	"	.05
Draw Plates, 30 Holes, Stubs's	"	1.60
" " 24 " Large, Stubs's	"	2.75
Enamel for Point and Base	per oz.	.38
" Gum, Allen's, for Continuous Gum Work	"	2.50
" " for Blocks	"	2.00
Emery Cloth	per sheet	.07
" Paper	"	.02
English Rose Red, Best	per oz.	1.50
Handles of Wood for Files, Scrapers, etc.	each .06 to	.10
Ingot Moulds, Iron, Broad Base, to slide with Handles	each $2.50 and	3.00
" " " " without Handle		3.00
Kaolin, Prepared	per lb.	.12
Ladles of Cast-Iron, No. 5, with Wrought-Iron Handles	each	.50
" " " " 6, " " "	"	.60
" " " " 7, " " "	"	.75
" " " 2 Ladles and 1 Handle, detached	per set	.90
" " " without Handles, extra large	each	.50
Leather Cord for Lathes	per foot	.07
Lead. (Price fluctuates.)		
Magnets for removing Steel from Filings, 2½ inches	each	.12
" " " " 3 "	"	.20

Magnets for removing Steel from Filings, 5 inches	each	$0.50
Mallets, Horn, for Plate	"	.38
" Wood, "	"	.20
Mortars and Pestles, Wedgewood	each .50 to	5.00
Oil Cans, Zinc, Spring Bottom	each .15 and	.25
Platinum, Sponge	per dwt.	.75
" Scraps put into Plate or Wire	per oz.	.80
Plaster Knives	each	.25
Plate Scrapers	"	.25
" " Triangular	"	.50
Pin Holders	"	.35
Plaster	per quart	.08
Spelter (Zinc). (Fluctuates.)		
Saw Frames, mechanical	each	1.00
Spatulas, English, 4 inch	"	.25
" " 5 "	"	.30
" " 6 "	"	.40
Scotch Stones	each .10 to	.15
Solder Tweezers	each	.10
" Tongs, 7, 9, and 12 inches	each .45, .50, and	.55
Silex, Coarse, for Slides	per lb.	.25
" Fine	"	.50
" Extra Fine	"	1.00
" Double Fine	"	2.00
Saws, attached to Shaft for Lathe	each .25 and	.35
" Small Circular, for cutting Teeth off Plate	" .38 "	.50
" for Frames, French	per doz.	.20
" " " wide	"	.25
Spar, Prepared, Common	per. lb.	.12
" " for Enamel	"	.75
" " for Body	"	.50
Tablets, Soft Rubber, $\frac{3}{16}$ in. thick, 8 in. long, and 5 in. wide, used under work to protect it	each	1.25
Tablets, same as above, 3 inches square	"	.50
Tin in Bars. (Fluctuates.)		
Tooth-Holders, for holding Teeth while grinding	each	.10
Vises for Bench, 4 in., Plain	"	3.12
" " 4½ in., "	"	3.25
" " 5 in., "	"	3.38
" Hand, Wood Handle, 3, 3½, and 4 in.	"	1.00
" Pin, Hollow	"	.80
" " with Screw	"	.80
" " with Slide	"	.80
Zinc or Spelter. (Fluctuates.)		

Other Articles, not illustrated or classified in this Department, will be found in the Celluloid and Vulcanite Department.

CELLULOID AND VULCANITE.

Celluloid.

We have assigned to Dr. S. S. White the exclusive right to sell the Celluloid Base under all our American patents, for Dental uses. All orders from the trade or Profession should be directed accordingly.

I. SMITH HYATT,

Newark, N. J., January, 1874. Secretary Celluloid Manufacturing Company.

The Celluloid Company make the following claim:

"We have added new shapes and styles to our variety of Plates, and are producing each number of uniform size. We know also that we are steadily improving the Celluloid Plates in respect to color, texture, strength, and reliability, and are confident that the hopes of the Profession as well as our own regarding this Base will be fully realized."

PRICES.

Full Plates, Upper or Lower	each	$0.60
Partial Plates	"	.30
Plumper Plates	"	1.00

ALCOHOL LAMP FOR HEINDSMANN'S HEATER.

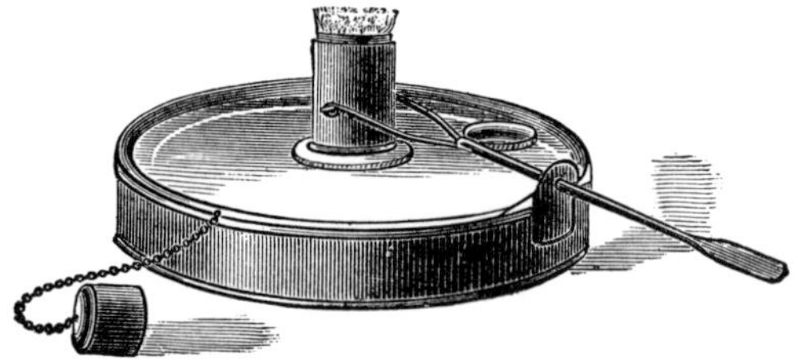

The Cut shows the Lamp furnished with Heindsmann's Heater.

Price, separate $1.00

HEINDSMANN'S HEATER.

Patented July 6th, 1875.

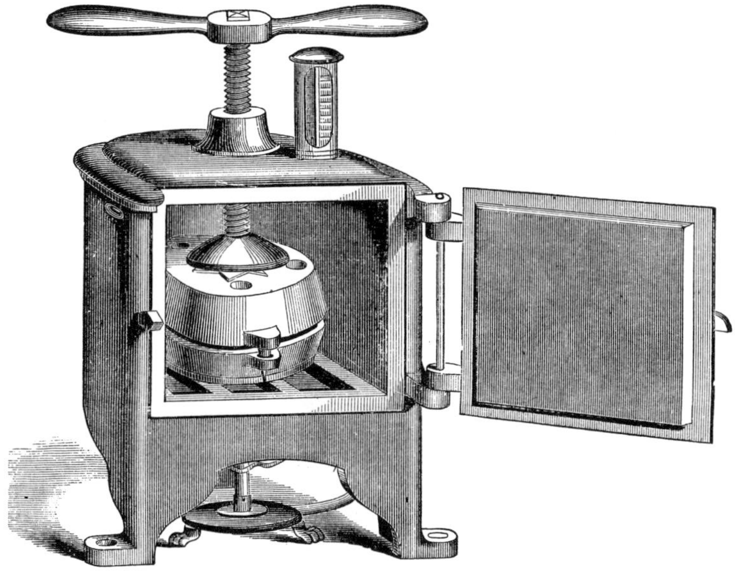

The Cut illustrates an invention for packing, while heating, Celluloid Plates. It is essentially a miniature stove-oven having an inner and outer chamber, the latter affording a continuous circulation of heated air. The bottom is ribbed, the spaces between the ribs being filled with plaster to prevent too rapid heating of the bottom of the flask. This plaster-bed may be moistened with water before heating. The door is hinged like that of an ordinary stove, opening and shutting easily, and giving access to the inner chamber, in which the Flask containing the teeth and plate is set. A clamp-screw, three-fourths of an inch in diameter, is set through the top of the Heater, and has attached to the inner end a revolving washer. The handle is fitted to the shaft of the clamp-screw, so that it may be lifted off when desired, to prevent its becoming heated.

The Flask is the patent Star Reversible. The Oven may be heated by either gas or alcohol. A thermometer, to indicate when the proper heat (believed to be 280°) is attained, is set through the top into the Oven.

After the Flask has been closed it may be removed from the Oven and placed in a vise or a flask-clamp, and allowed to cool gradually and thoroughly, the Oven meanwhile being ready for another case.

The principle involved in the process of working Celluloid by this method is the production, from the evaporation of the water in the plaster, of a moist heat, which gradually becomes more and more dry as the heat is increased or continued. It has the advantage over other methods, of driving off any excess of camphor remaining in the compound, besides admitting of the patching or repair of plates better than by the use of oil or glycerin, or by the ordinary steam apparatus.

Price, with Flask and Lamp or Gas-Burner $12.00

CELLULOID STEAM APPARATUS.

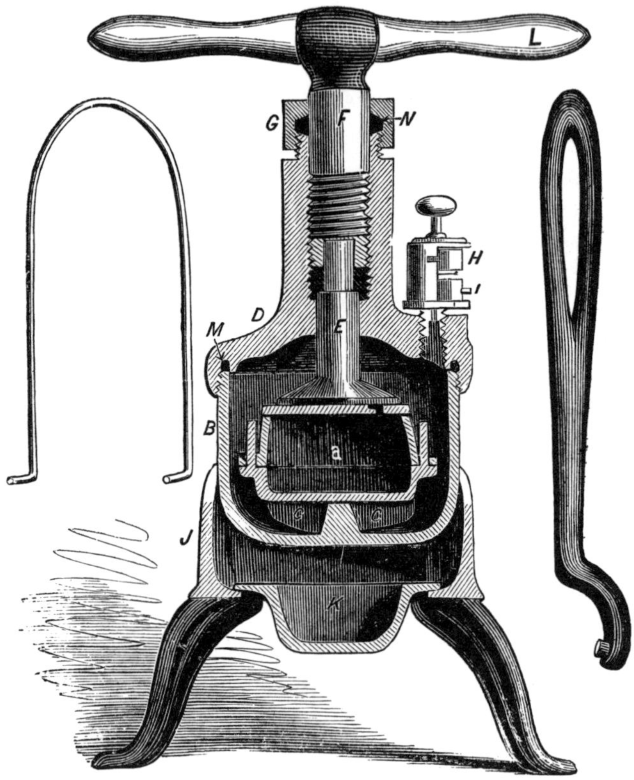

The Celluloid Company say of their Steam Apparatus:

"We have recently perfected, and now offer to the Profession, a NEW APPARATUS for moulding Celluloid Plates, in which steam instead of oil is used for the heating medium. It is cleaner, safer, and better in all respects. Samples are on exhibition at Dr. White's depots in Philadelphia, New York, Boston, and Chicago."

The Cut illustrates the Steam Apparatus, by a view through a central vertical plane. A represents the flask; B, the boiler; C, the radial ribs to support the flask; D, the cover to the boiler; E, the plunger in contact with the flask; F, the screw for forcing the plunger upon and closing the flask; G, gland for packing the screw F, to prevent the escape of steam; H, the upper section, and I, the lower section, of the safety-valve; J, the heater; K, cup to contain alcohol for generating steam, which may be removed if it is desired to use gas; L, handle; M, rubber steam-packing ring; N, hemp or other steam packing.

With each Apparatus are instructions fully explaining the method of manipulating the Base.

Apparatus complete $15.00

Dental Rubbers.

BOW SPRING RUBBER.

THE STRONGEST, MOST ELASTIC, AND MOST EASILY PACKED.

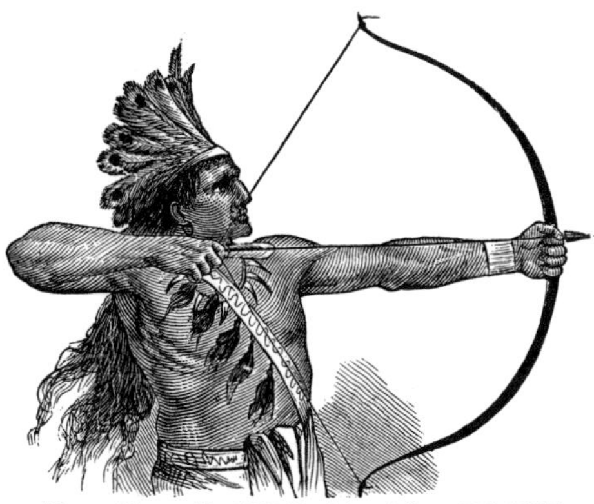

(TRADE-MARK, No. 1847, Registered June 23d, 1874.)

Those who are still willing to use Rubber as a Base for Artificial Dentures are naturally desirous of producing the best results of which the material is capable ; but satisfaction in the working and wearing of it depends not alone on the skill and care of the manipulator, but, to a very great extent, on the quality of the material.

If the Rubber is of inferior quality, or overloaded with earthy matter, it will be brittle and will not take a high polish ; while if pure, and the materials incorporated with it have been properly selected, prepared, and combined, and are not in excess, then, with care and skill, the result will be a compact, tough, strong, elastic, whalebone-like compound.

The objects in combining earths with the Caoutchouc are for purposes of economy, as they are less expensive than the gum ; and to tone down by their whiteness the vermilion used in coloring, so as to produce a light or flesh tint.

All the skill expended in this direction has, however, failed to produce a resemblance to the natural gum, and the excessive quantity of vermilion employed is asserted to have been the cause of sore mouths and constitutional disturbances in those wearing plates so composed, while the excess of earthy matter made necessary to overcome the intense redness of the vermilion has resulted in making the plates brittle.

To avoid these objectionable features, many have contented themselves with a *Black* Rubber, because free of vermilion and stronger, though unsightly in appearance.

To meet the increasing demand for an article free from these liabilities, we have caused careful experiments to be conducted by intelligent and experienced parties, with a view to the production of a rubber combining all the qualities desirable in a Dental gum, and practically free from deleterious substances. The result we offer to the profession under the name of

BOW SPRING RUBBER.

It is made of the best Para gum, carefully selected from large quantities of the crude article, is thoroughly freed from foreign substances, and is manufactured by improved processes.

It contains more gum to the pound than ordinary rubbers,—having less specific gravity,—and is cheaper to the user, not only because it takes more sheets of it to make a pound, but because it is, when properly vulcanized, much stronger, and can therefore be made into thinner plates. It is capable, by reason of its fine texture, of receiving and retaining a high polish, and possesses an elasticity or springiness which will allow it to be bent without fracture.

It is softer and packs more easily than any other rubber, requires less force to close the flask, and is therefore less liable to displace or break the block.

The relative qualities may be tested—the texture with a fine file; the strength and elasticity by bending it until it breaks, and noting the fibrous character of the fracture.

We believe it to be the BEST GUM in the market.

It is desirable that the Rubber should not be exposed to too great a heat after packing and before the flask is put together, as, when thus treated, it is liable to become spongy.

Close the flask, place the bolts in position, bring the two halves of the flask gently together, and heat up either in hot water or in the oven of a stove until steam begins to be given off; then screw it together.

Vulcanize one hour at 320° F.

It would be well not to open the flask until it is entirely cold.

It is put up in *tin boxes* to prevent the Rubber from drying.

Manufactured *exclusively* for us.

Price . . . . per lb. $3.50

CAUTION.—The purity of the Bow Spring Rubber requires that it should be more carefully vulcanized than any other. Ordinary rubbers contain much more foreign substances, clays or coloring matters, which separate the particles of gum and allow the sulphureted hydrogen gas to escape, thus effecting a more speedy vulcanization. The Bow Spring Rubber, however, should not be packed like these, with dry heat,—that is, the flask containing the Rubber should never be exposed in an open fire, as is often done with other rubbers Our experiments with the Bow Spring indicate that the best results are attained by allowing the heat 15 minutes to reach 260°, then raising it gradually to 320° and keeping it at that point for 50 minutes. Other experiments in England, with a vulcanizer of different construction from those used in America, give 300° at 45 minutes. If the plate is unusually thick, a *longer* time at a *lower* heat is to be preferred.

The point to be borne in mind is, that the heat should be allowed to penetrate the whole plate and effect a perfect vulcanization *from within outward*, instead of the imperfect results of the contrary way. By exercising the care here suggested the Bow Spring Rubber will produce the strongest and most elastic Rubber Denture known.

OTHER DENTAL RUBBERS.

S. S. White's No. 1 Improved Dental Gum	**per lb.**	**$2.75**
S. S. White's Black Rubber	**"**	**3.00**
Doherty's Rubbers, Nos. 1 and 2	**"**	**2.75**
Star Rubber	**"**	**3.75**
Whalebone Rubber	**"**	**3.50**
English Pink Dental Rubber (Deep), No. 1x	**"**	**8.00**
" " " " (Pale), No. 1	**"**	**8.00**
" White " "	**"**	**6.50**
" Black " "	**"**	**3.50**

The above are supplied in one-pound and half-pound packets, with directions for vulcanizing.

SUPERIOR GUTTA-PERCHA FOR BASE.

Price . . . . per lb. $3.00

RUBBER GAUGE.

For ascertaining the quantity of Rubber required for any given Case. The vessel being about half filled with water, set the lower Pointer to the level of the water; throw in every particle of the Model Plate, set the upper Pointer to the rise of the water; empty the vessel, and again fill with water to the lower Pointer; add a sufficient quantity of Rubber to cause the water to rise to the upper Pointer, and there will be just enough to fill the mould. Allowance can then be made for surplus.

Price $1.25

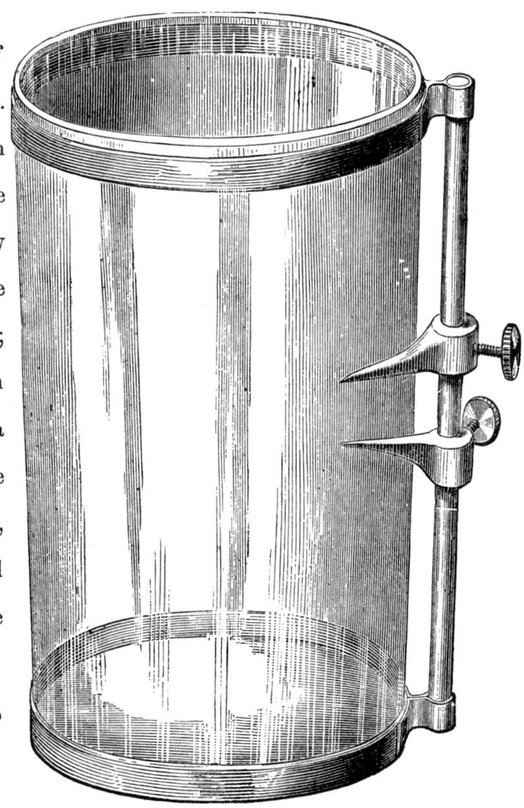

WHITNEY'S VULCANIZING MACHINE.

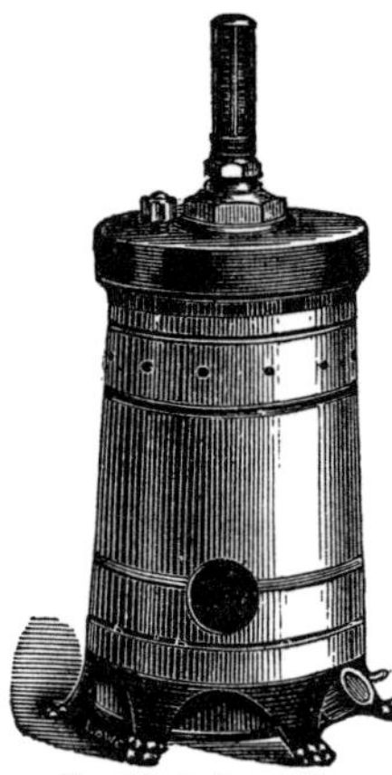
For Alcohol and Gas.

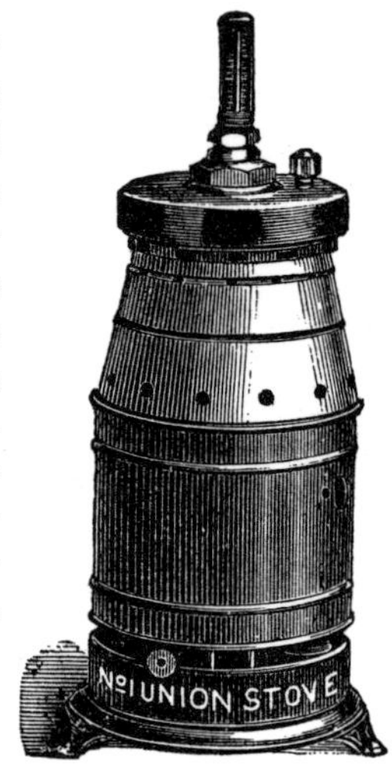

For Kerosene.

The Heater is composed entirely of Copper and Brass; is of two pieces only, a Copper Pot, and Brass Head screwed on to the Pot, dispensing with all bolts and nuts. They are uniformly 3⅞ in. diameter inside, for two cases 5 inches, and for three cases 7 inches deep. The whole complete for use weighs only from 4 to 5¼ pounds, according to the size, whether for two or three cases. Hayes's Patent Mercury Bath is adapted to this Vulcanizer, by which the liability of the thermometer to accident is very much decreased.

Special directions for using accompany each machine.

The heat is applied by either Gas, Alcohol, or Kerosene. Apparatus for burning either is furnished as required. The Kerosene Stove is also excellent for Laboratory use in heating flasks, for packing, etc. This Stove is adapted to all Vulcanizers, and will always be sent out with the Whitney Vulcanizer, unless other heating apparatus is specially ordered.

PRICES.

No. 1, Vulcanizer, Gas or Alcohol	$15.00
" 2, " " "	16.00
" 3, " " "	17.00
Union Kerosene Stove, extra	1.25

WHITNEY'S VULCANIZING FLASKS.

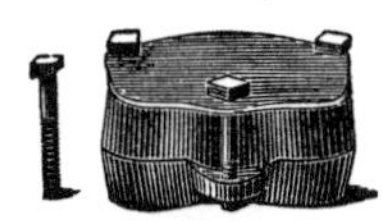
Old Style.

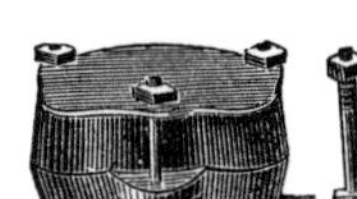
New Style.

We offer the following styles of this well-known Flask:

The "Old Style," with the bolts screwing into the lower section of the Flask.

The "New Style," with bolts and nuts.

The "Large Flask," which measures 3¾ inches across the widest part.

The "Deep Flask," which is of the ordinary size, but half an inch deeper; for partial cases, repairing, etc.

PRICES.

Flasks, Malleable Iron, Old and New Styles	$1.00
" Large Size	1.00
" " Deep	1.00
Bolts for Flasks, Old Style, per set of 3	.18
" " New Style (with Nuts), per set of 3	.25

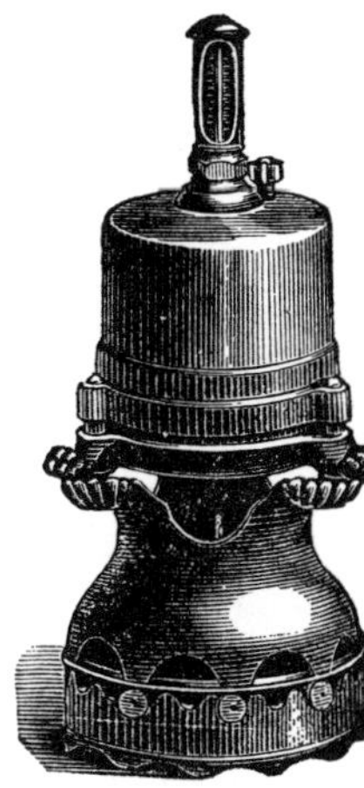

HAYES'S IRON-CLAD OVENS.

FOR ONE OR TWO CASES.

Patented March 5th, 1861, and April 3d, 1866.

These Ovens are small and compact. They are lined with Copper of the usual thickness, which is surrounded by a shell of Malleable Iron ⅛ inch thick, and strong enough of itself to withstand many times the strain required in Vulcanizing. They may therefore be safely used till the Copper is entirely destroyed by corrosion, which may then be renewed at small expense.

PRICES.

No. 1, Complete	$15.00
" 2, "	16.00

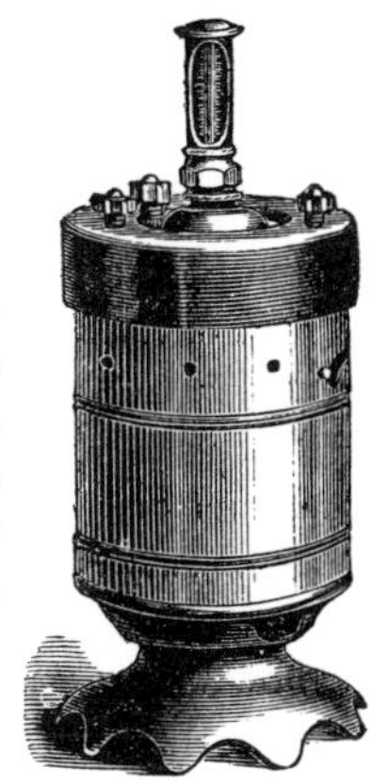

HAYES'S IRON-CLAD BOILERS.

FOR TWO OR THREE CASES.

Patented July 8th, 1862, and April 3d, 1866.

These Boilers are made with and without the Iron-Clad Shell. The cover is secured by three set-screws, which play in a movable screw collar, and produce direct pressure upon the packing joint. The Thermometer bulb is immersed in a mercury bath outside the steam chamber. These Vulcanizers are heated by Gas, Alcohol, or Kerosene. The Union Kerosene Stove will be supplied with the Hayes Boiler, if other heating apparatus is not specified.

PRICES.

No. 2, Copper	$16.00
" 3, "	17.00
" 2, Iron Clad	17.00
" 3, "	18.00
Union Kerosene Stove, extra	1.25

HAYES'S IMPROVED FLASK AND CLAMP.

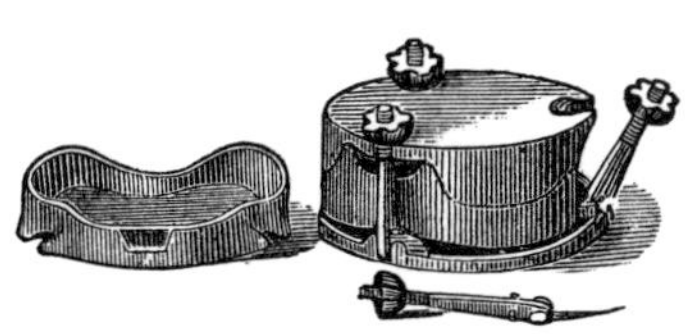

This Flask is now furnished from new patterns, and will receive a model about ¼ inch larger than the old style.

The lug-joint of the Clamp is so constructed that all the strain comes upon the casting. The pin only serves to keep the lug in place when not in use. The several pieces are attached to each other; therefore not liable to get lost or mislaid.

PRICES

Flask for Vulcanizing Oven or Boiler	50 cents.
Clamp for Flask	50 "

PRICES FOR REPAIRING VULCANIZERS.

No. 1. Boiler, Cover and Thermometer, Hayes or Whitney, Copper		$12.00
" 2. " " " " " "		13.00
" 3. " " " " " "		14.00
" 2. " " " (Iron Clad), Hayes		14.00
" 3. " " " " "		15.00
Pot to Hayes's No. 2 Copper Boiler		7.00
" " " 3 " "		8.00
" " " 2 Iron Clad		8.00
" " " 3 " "		9.00
Screw Collar to Hayes's Vulcanizer		3.00
Set Screws for Hayes's Screw Collar (per set)		.25
Cap to Hayes's Vulcanizer		3.00
Hayes's Thermometer Case, without Thermometer		1.00
Ring with Bolts to Hayes's Oven, O. S.		2.00
Packing Ring to " "		1.00
Iron-Clad Covering to Hayes's Oven		5.00
Copper Lining to " "		4.00
Bottom to " "		5.00
No. 1 Pot for Whitney Vulcanizer		6.00
" 2 " " "		7.00
" 3 " " "		8.00
Thermometer Case and Tube, complete, Hayes or Whitney		2.00
Outside Thermometer Case, Whitney		.50
Inside " " "		.50
Whitney Cap, less Thermometer Case		6.00
Altering to Mercury Bath		2.00
New Ring to Copper Vulcanizer		2.00
" Bottom " "		2.00
Safety Valve Metal, per package		.50
Automatic Lamp (Hayes), Gas or Alcohol		1.50
" " " " " Large		2.00
Round Wrench, for Pot of Whitney Vulcanizer		.50
Straight " Double End, for Whitney Vulcanizer		.25
Flask " Hayes and Whitney combined		.10
Gas Burner or Laboratory Lamp		1.00
Flask and Clamp (Hayes)		1.00
Flask and Bolt (Whitney)		1.00
Bolts for Whitney's Old Style Flask (Set of 3)		.18
Bolts and Nuts for Whitney's New Style Flask (Set of 3)		.25
Bolts for Hayes's Flask Clamps (Set of 3)		.25
Packing for Hayes's Vulcanizer	per strip	.10
" Whitney's "	"	.05
Kerosene Burner, Union Stove No. 1		2.25
Jackets for Hayes's or Whitney's Vulcanizers		.40

STAR REVERSIBLE FLASK.

Patented by E. T. Starr, August 14th, 1866.

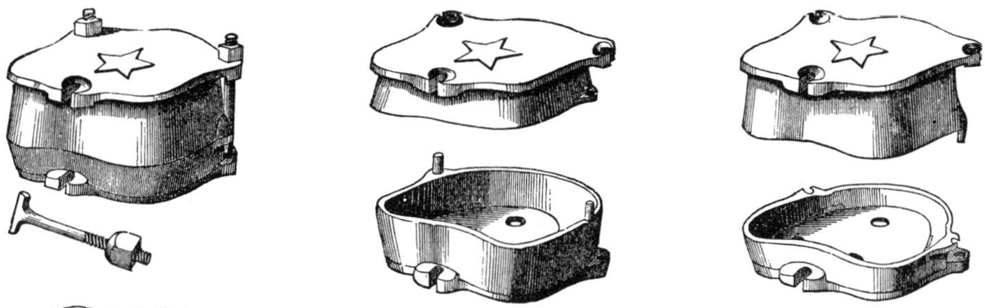

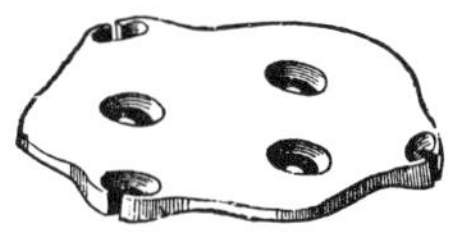

The Rings of this Flask are of different widths, either of them fitting the Top or Bottom accurately, as may be required. By using the wide Ring next to the Bottom, an admirable Flask is obtained, for deep cases and partial sets, or where the artificial gum rests on the natural. The narrow Ring is used next the Bottom Plate, for whole dentures, where the parting is at the rim of the Plate. The Bottom has three counter-sunk holes, through which the Plaster runs, which, when set, holds the accompanying Ring securely to it. The fastenings of the Flask are T-shaped at one end, and fit the slots in the Bottom Plate; and, being free at both ends, are more easily adjusted than ordinary bolts. The Flask being in four pieces (two Rings and two Plates), the Plaster is removed without the usual trouble. The Cuts are faithful representations of the Flask in different positions.

Brass	$2.00
Malleable Iron	1.50
Bolt and Nut	.12

WRENCH AND BED-PLATE.

INVENTION OF DR. THOMAS MURRAY.

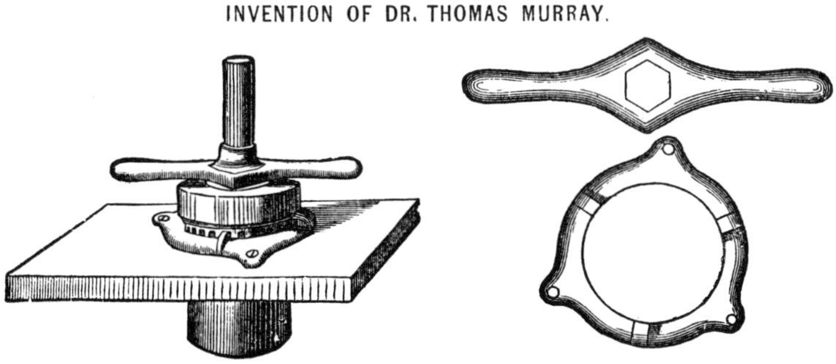

Adapted to Whitney's Vulcanizers. A hole is cut in a table, work-bench, or box, the size of the Bed-plate, which is secured over it by three screws. It is a very efficient arrangement.

Very Heavy, as per Cut	per set $1.00
Malleable Iron	" .55

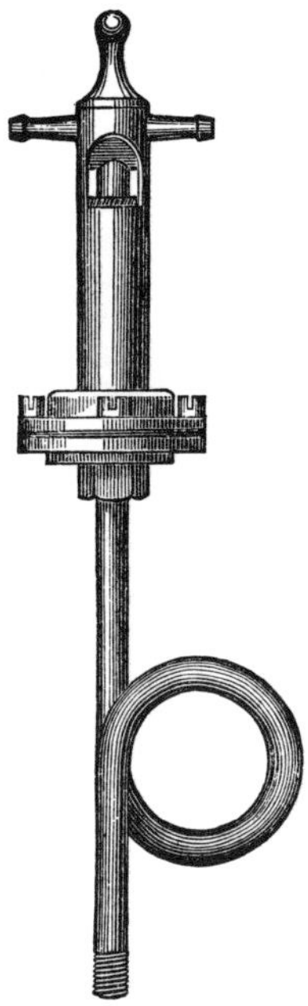

GAS REGULATOR FOR VULCANIZERS.

This Cut represents an invention for regulating the flow of gas to the heating apparatus of a Vulcanizer, in connection with the usual Thermometer.

The Coiled Tube being attached to the Vulcanizer, constitutes a steam-trap, from which the steam presses upon the packing in the joint above, and forces up a leaf-spring and a valve rod to which it is connected, the rod extending upward through the cylinder to a cross-tube at the top through which the gas is conducted to the heater. In this cross-tube a piece of small rubber tubing is inserted, which through a slot in the cross-tube is compressed by the valve rod from below, according to the steam pressure, thus reducing or interrupting the flow of gas and diminishing the heat. The degree or limit of heat desired is fixed by raising or lowering the thumb-screw on the valve rod, and this degree is maintained by the action of the Regulator.

Price $8.00

FLASK CLAMP.

FOR CLOSING FLASKS AFTER PACKING.

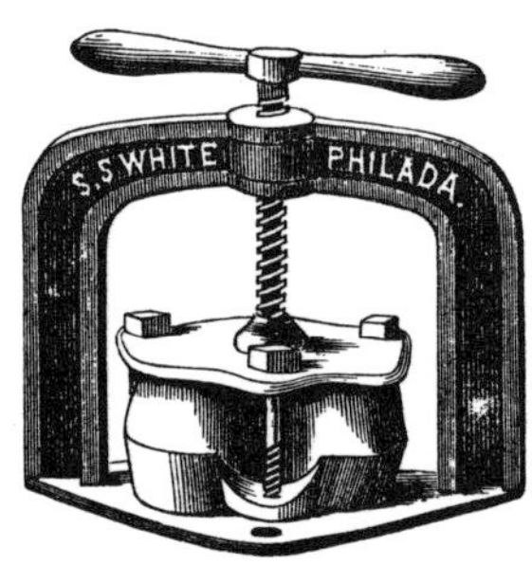

Price $2.00

SOLDER FOR RUBBER WORK.

The advantages are, that it saves time, the discoloring and weakening of the Plate and inconvenience of Vulcanizing. Directions accompany each Ingot.

Per Ingot, 1 oz. $1.00

LIQUID RUBBER SOLDER.

(WELCH'S.)

Put up in 1 oz. bottles . . . . 50 cents.

METALLIC AIR-CHAMBER PATTERNS.

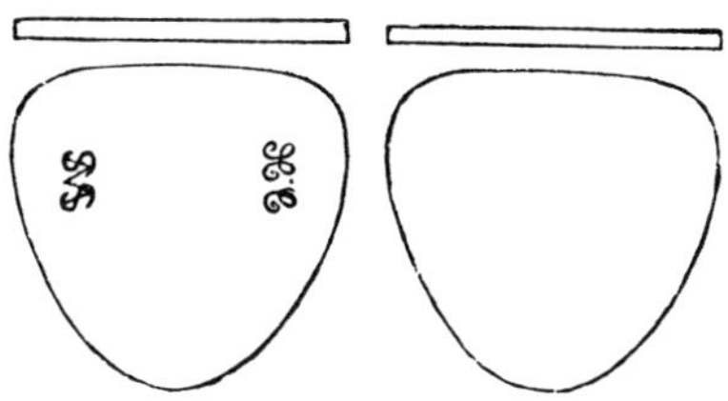

1.

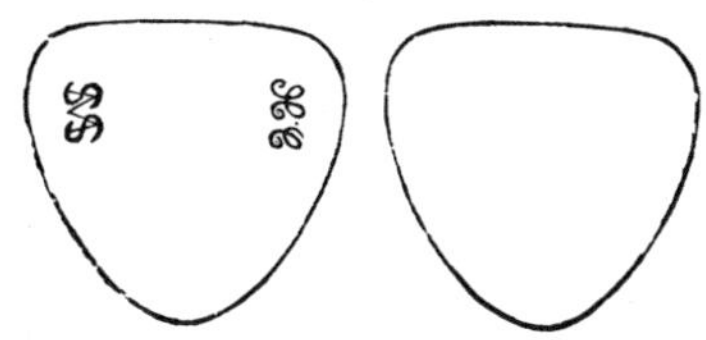

2.

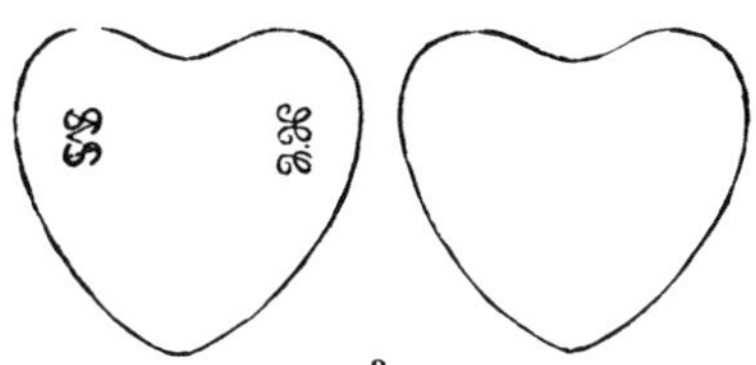

3.

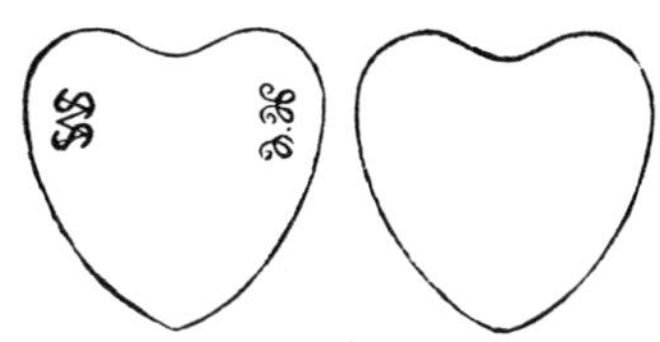

4.

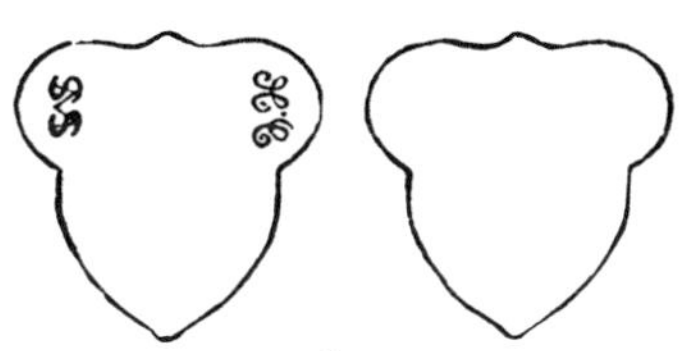

5.

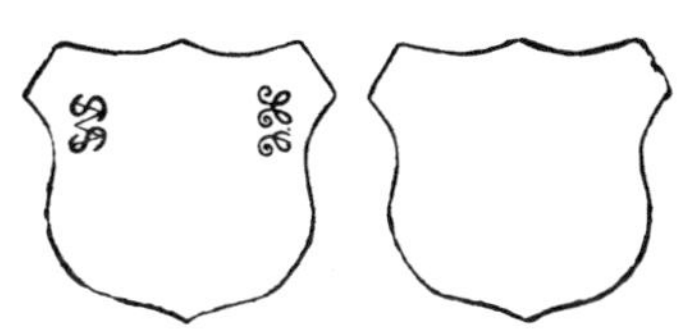

6.

Made from new dies, in which special care has been taken to avoid sharp edges and angles.

The fact, however, which gives them value over those heretofore in the market is, that they are made of METAL THAT WILL NOT BLACKEN THE RUBBER.

This has been a grave objection against their use, but it has been entirely overcome in these.

Of each style there are two thicknesses, represented by the lines over Fig. 1.

They are made so well, and offered at such a price, that no one, after once using them, will feel like cutting his own Patterns.

Both sides of each style are shown in the Cuts.

Thin	per doz. 25 cents.
Thick	" 38 "

VULCANITE FILES.

(SEE OPPOSITE PAGE.)

1 2. 3. 4. 5. 6. A B. C.

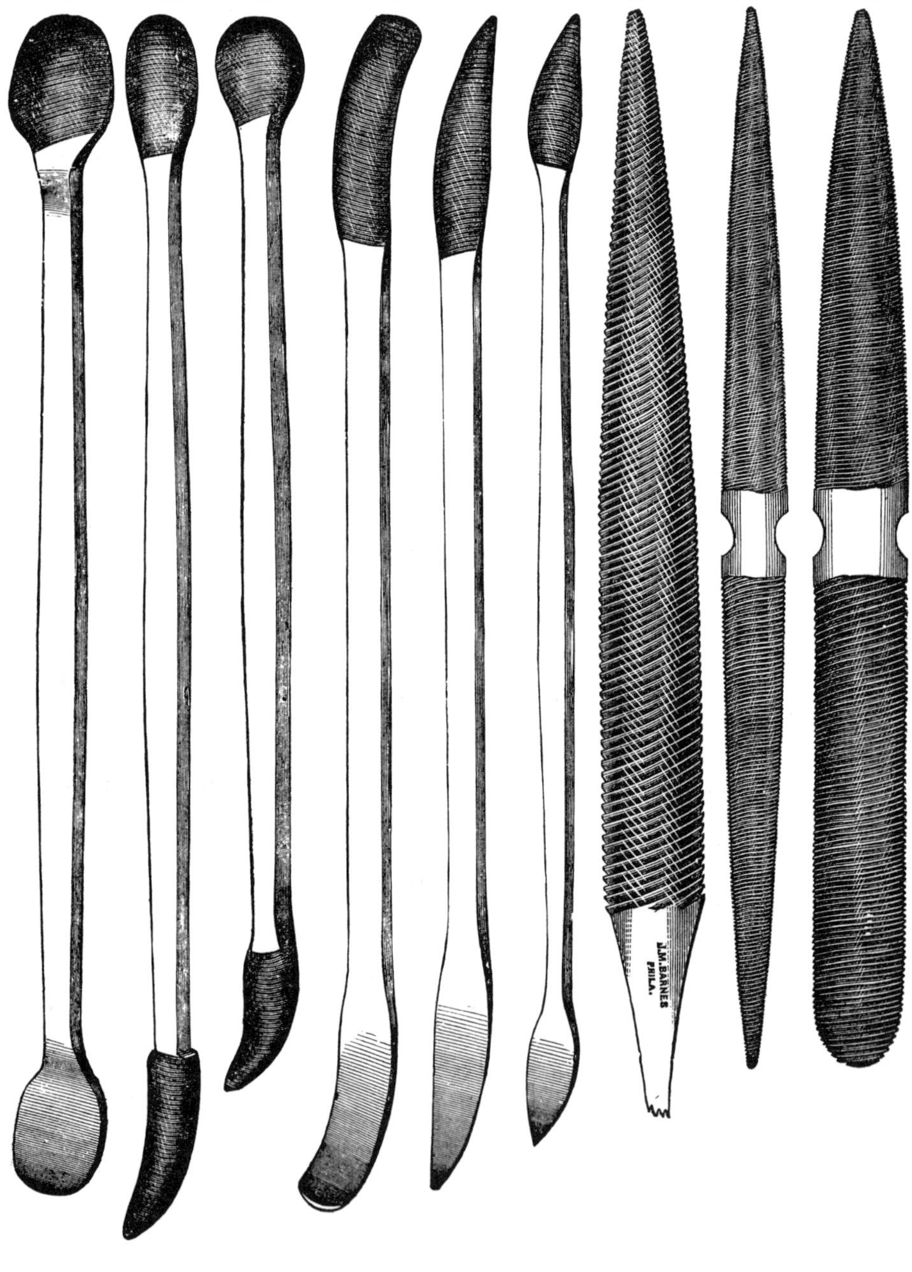

VULCANITE FILES.

(SEE CUTS ON OPPOSITE PAGE.)

Nos. 1, 4, 5, 6, are cut on one side of each end. Nos. 2 and 3 are cut on both sides of each end.

In addition to those delineated, we have the Half-round Coarse-cut Files, $4\frac{1}{2}$, $5\frac{1}{4}$, and 6 inches in length, for the same purpose.

Double-end Rubber Files. Nos. 1 to 6	each	$0.20
Half-round " " $4\frac{1}{2}$ inch. (See Cut A)	"	.17
" " " $5\frac{1}{4}$ " (" A)	"	.20
" " " 6 " (" A)	"	.25
" " " Steel Handle, $4\frac{1}{2}$ inches	"	.20
" " " " $5\frac{1}{4}$ "	"	.25
" " " " 6 "	"	.30
" " Double-end, $7\frac{1}{2}$ inches long, one end coarse and one end fine. (See Cut B)	"	.28
Double-end Fish Belly, one end coarse and blunt, and the other fine cut and pointed. (See Cut C)	"	.42

BOILER FOR HEATING UP FLASKS.

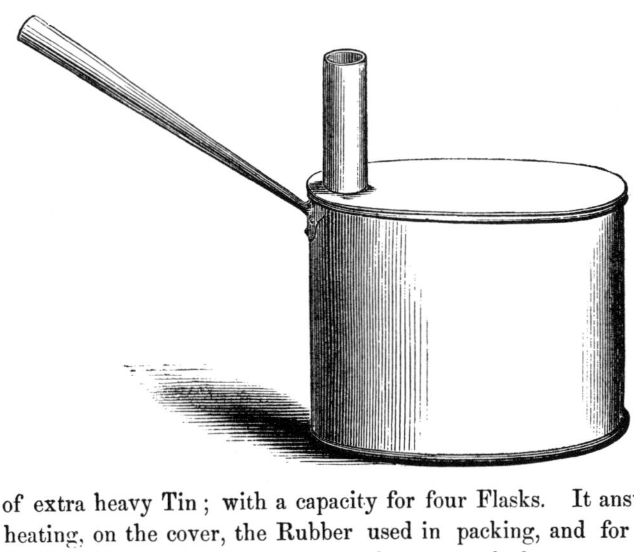

Made of extra heavy Tin; with a capacity for four Flasks. It answers the double purpose of heating, on the cover, the Rubber used in packing, and for heating, in the water, the Flasks to bring them together after they are packed.

Price $1.00

VULCANITE SCRAPERS.

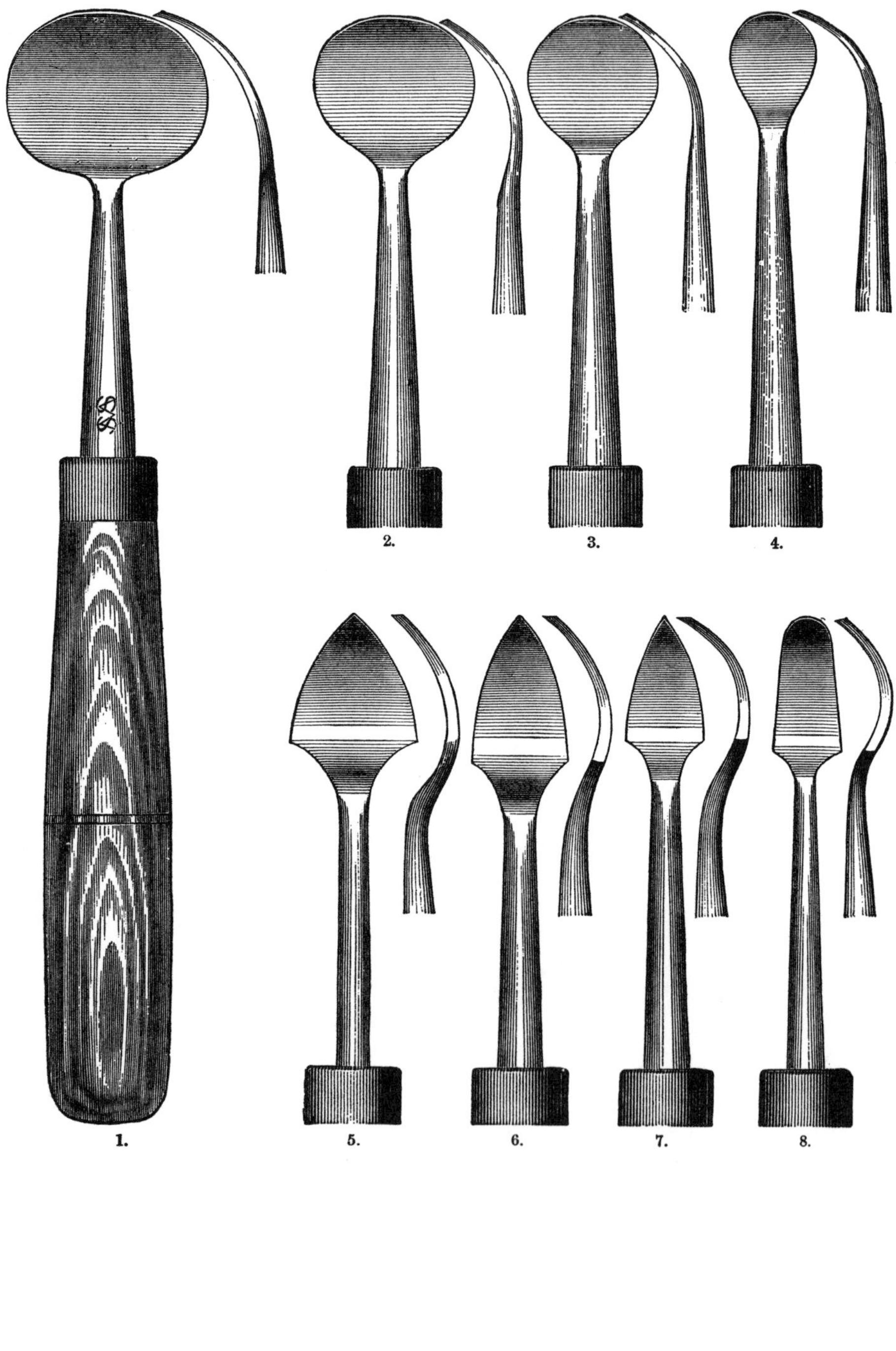

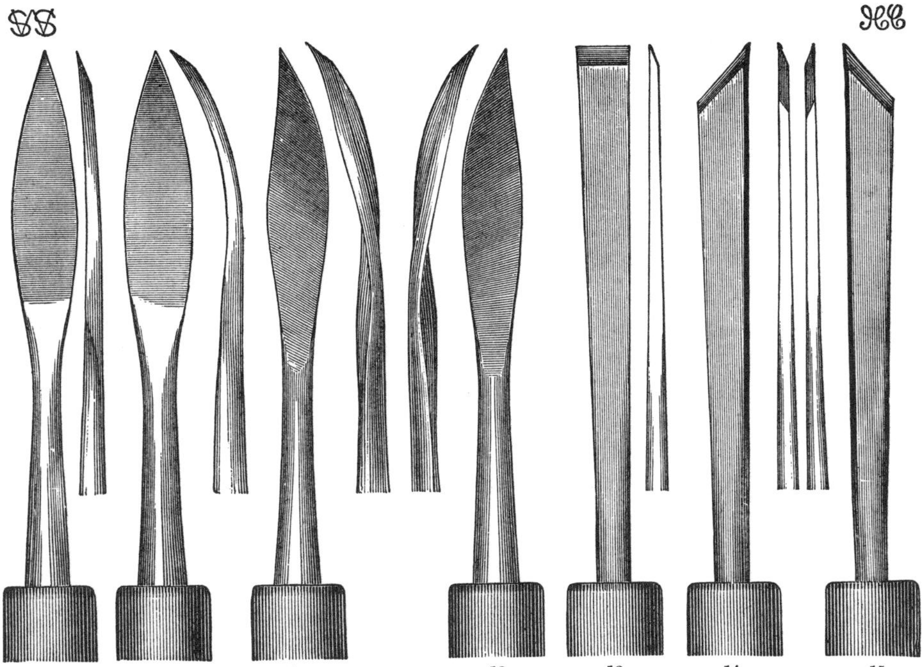

9. 10. 11. 12. 13. 14. 15.

Light Wood Handles, No. 1 . . . . 40 cents.
" " Nos. 2 to 15 . . . . each 25 "

VULCANITE PACKERS.

Set of Five.

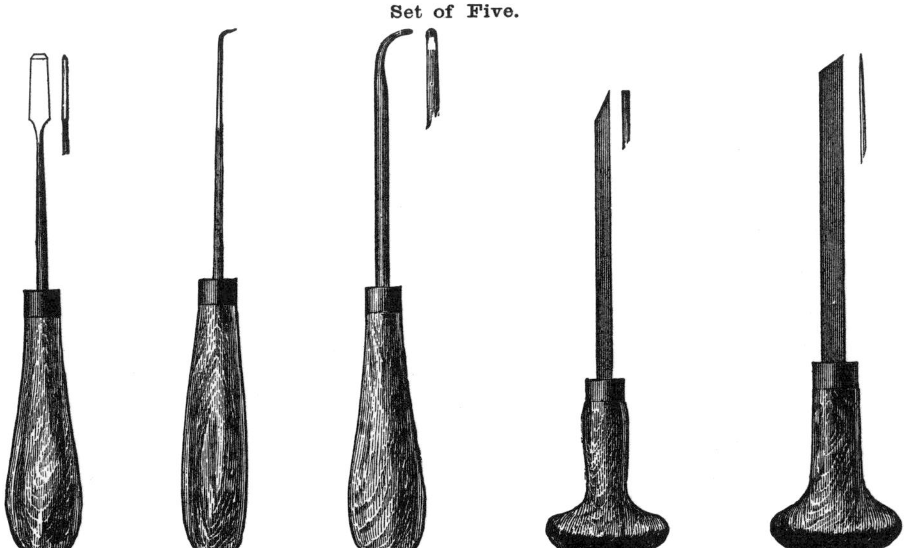

1. 2. 3. 4. 5.

Price . . . . **each 25 cents.**

VULCANITE SCRAPERS.

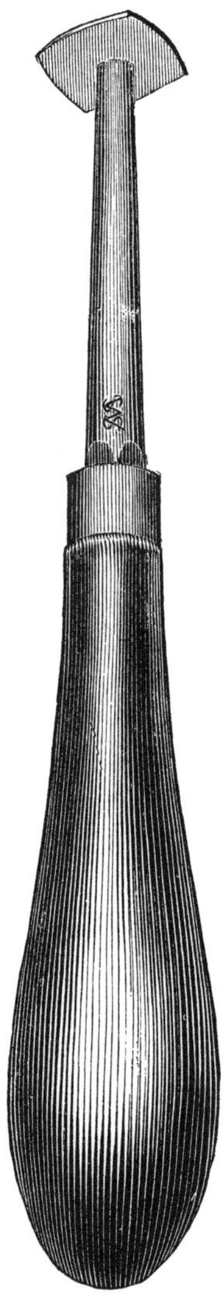

A.

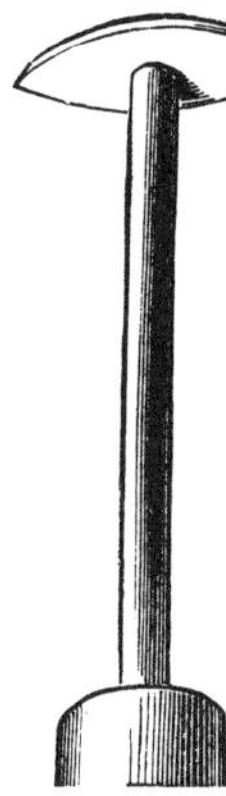

B.

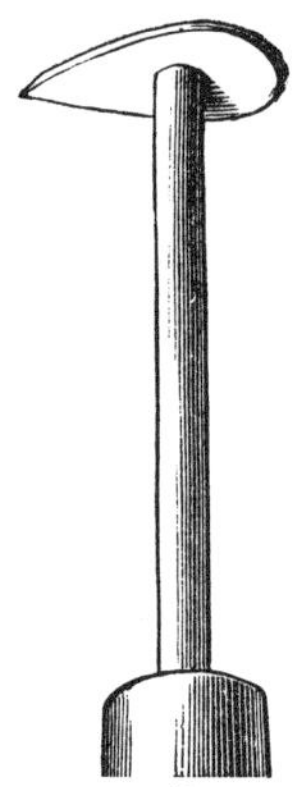

C

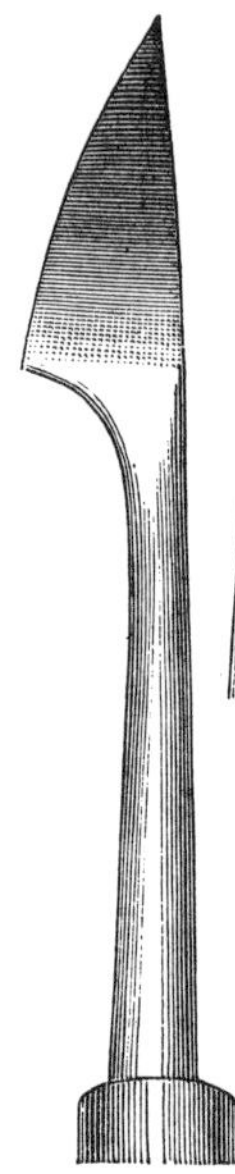

D

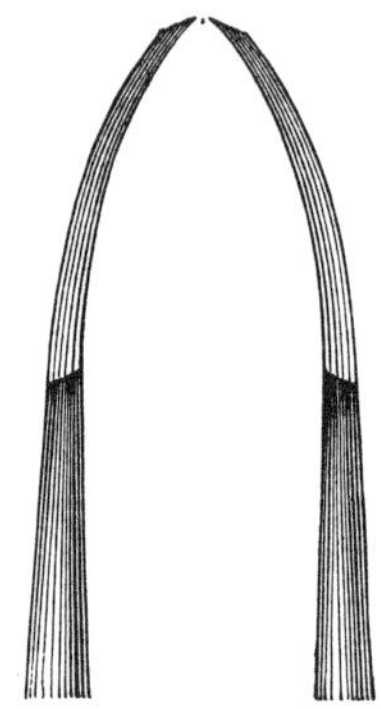

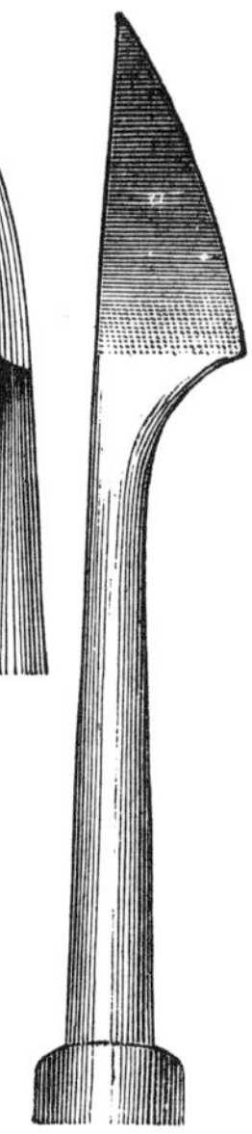

E.

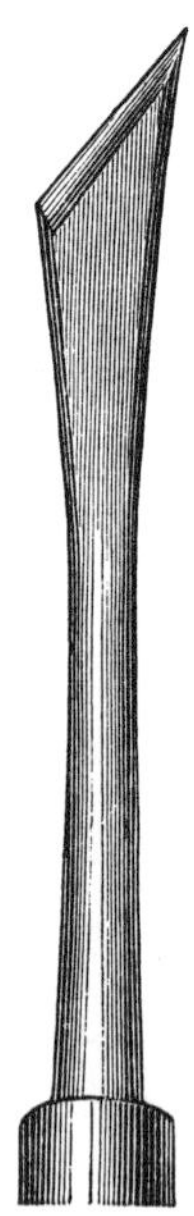

F.

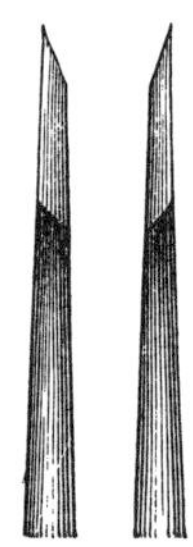

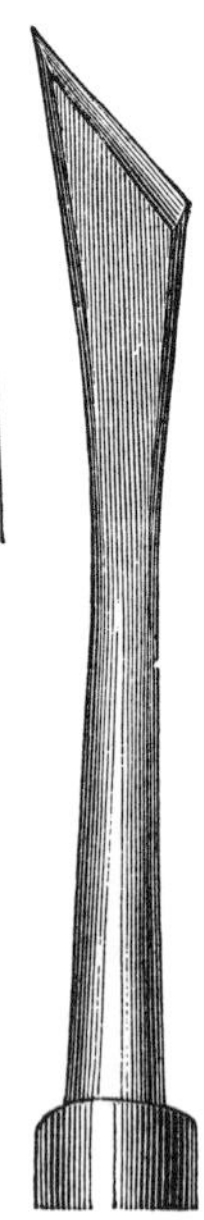

G.

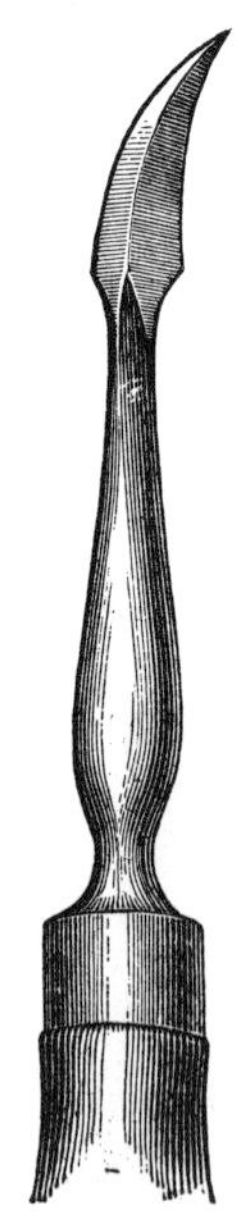

H.

Polished Black Handles, A to H . . . . each 50 cents.

VULCANITE BURS FOR LATHE.

1 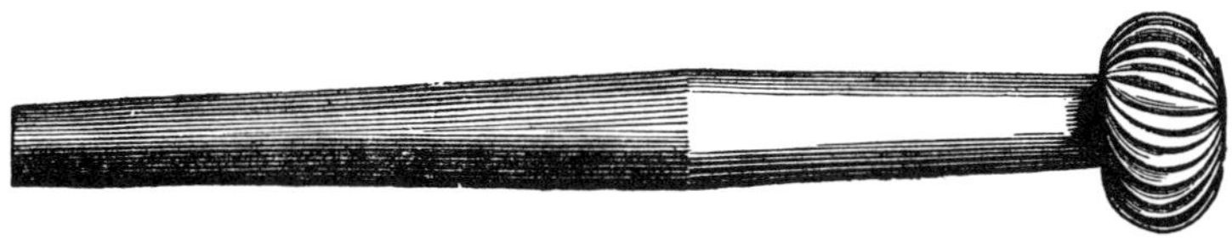

2 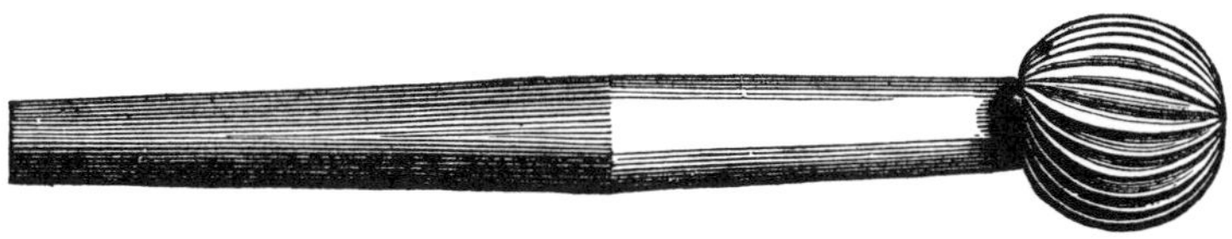

3. 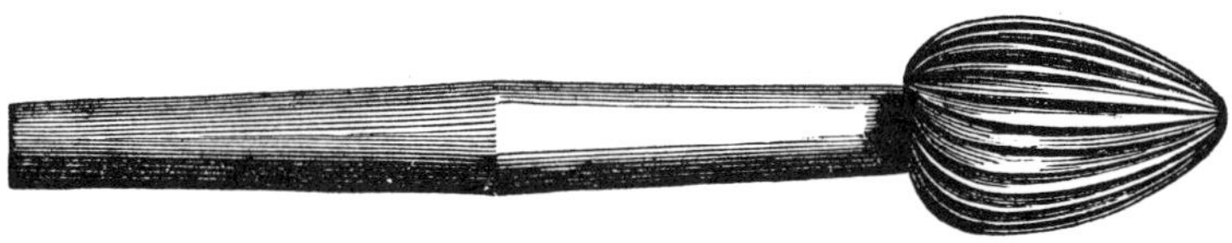

4. 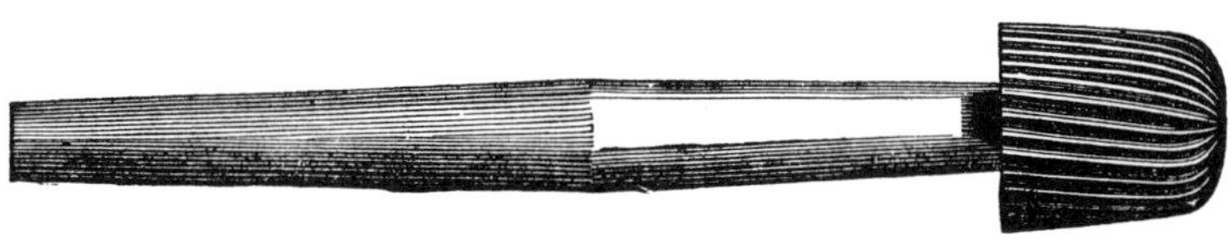

These Burs are cut and finished in the best manner. Four forms are illustrated, each the exact size of the instrument.

Price . . . . each $1.25

CIRCULAR FILES OR FILE-CUT WHEELS.

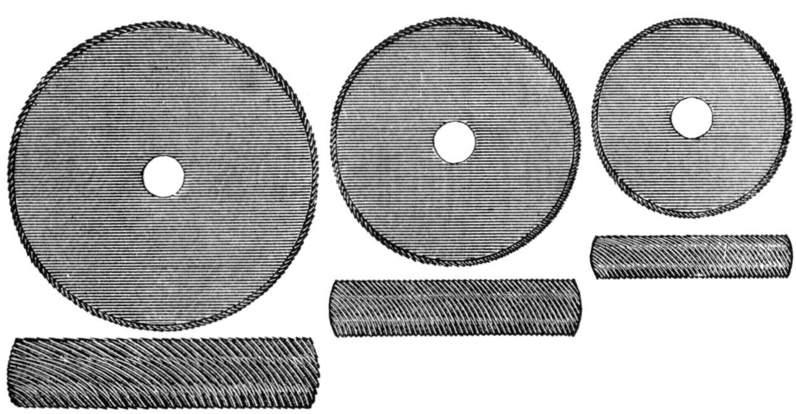

Designed for Vulcanite work. The Cuts illustrate the diameter, width, and cut.

Price . . . . each $1.25

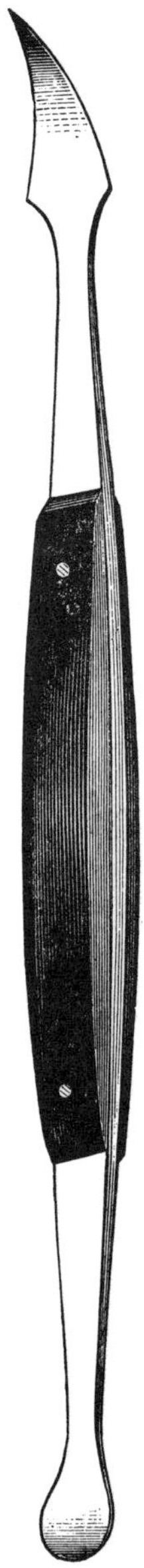

No. 1.

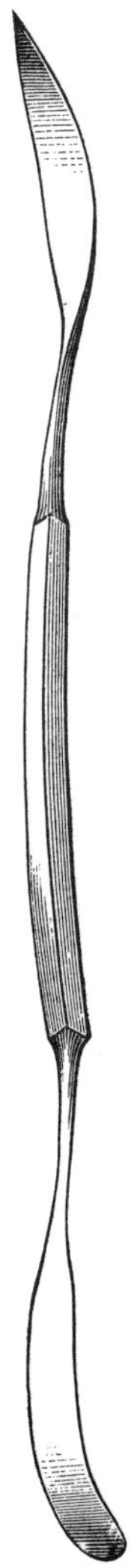

No. 2.

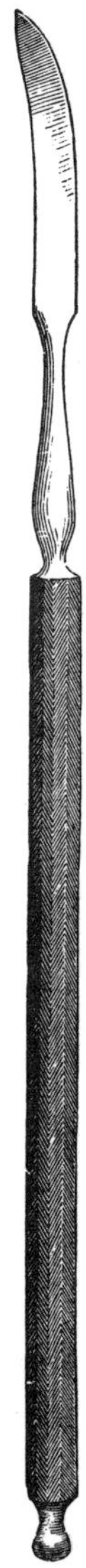

No. 3.

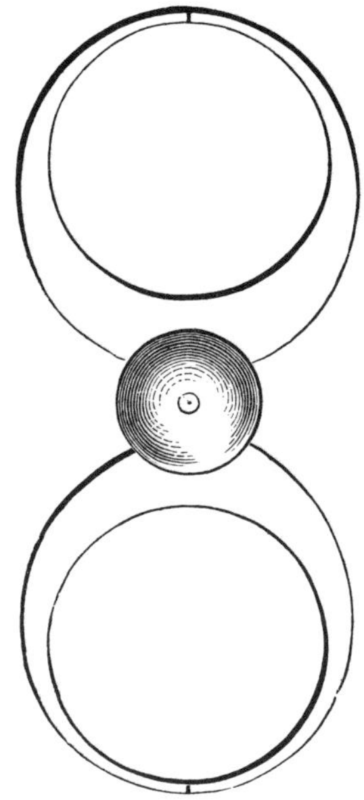

No. 4.

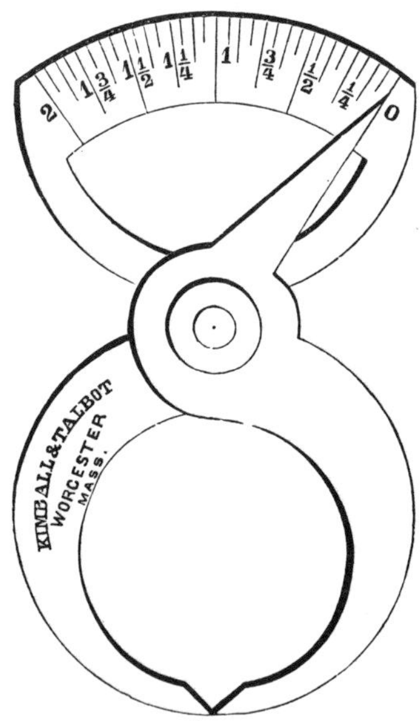

No. 5.

WAX KNIVES OR SPATULAS.

Ebony Mounted, No. 1 . . .	$0.75	File-cut Handle, No. 3 . . .	$0.60
Plain Center, " 2 . . .	.40	Steel Bright	.20
Spoon-shape	.25		

CALLIPERS.

Brass, No. 4	$0.40	Steel, No. 5	$1.00

MISCELLANEOUS.

Anatomical Preparations.

FIRST AND SECOND DENTITION.

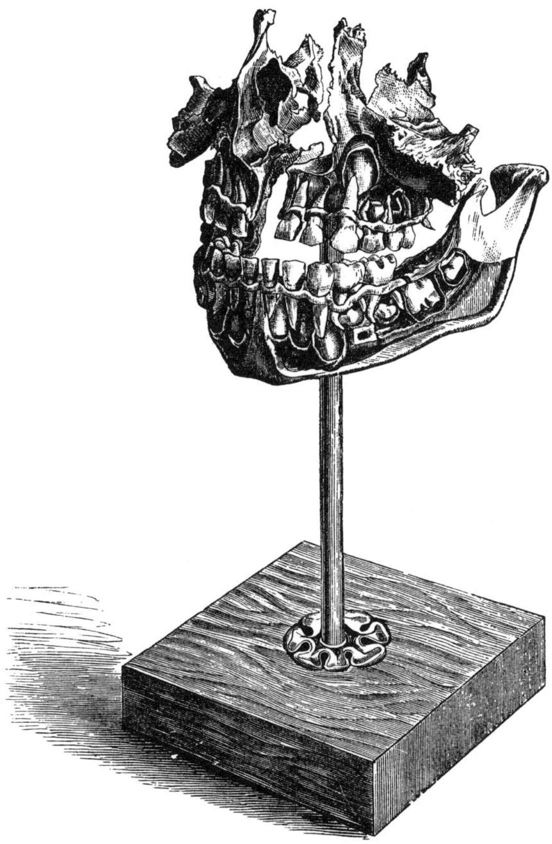

There are two varieties of these preparations; one exhibiting Dentition between the ages of six and seven—the other between the ages of seven and eight years. Mounted on Round Bases and covered with Glass Vases, as illustrated on the following page.

First and Second Dentition, Upper and Lower Maxilla Mounted, with Vase . $15.00
Head, showing First and Second Dentition. Mounted, with Vase . . . 25.00

UPPER AND LOWER MAXILLA.

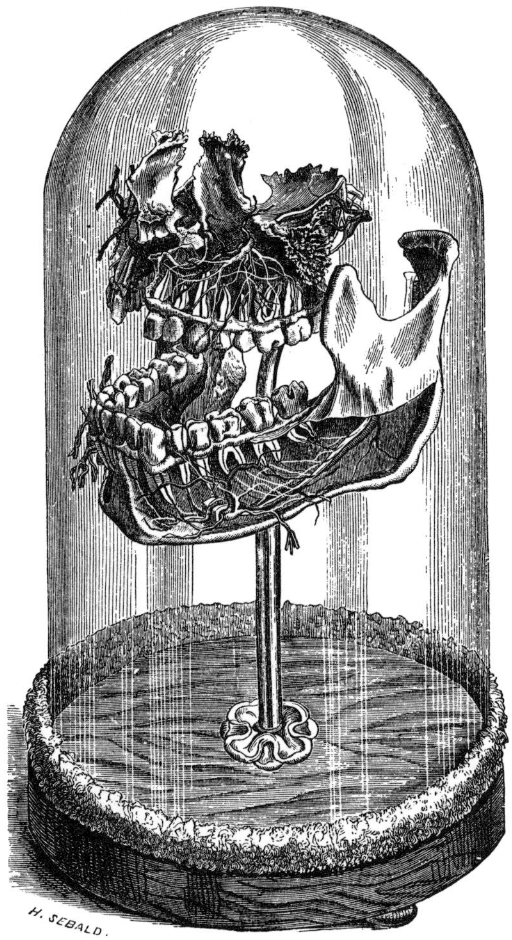

Upper and Lower Maxilla, exhibiting Nerve and Artery on one side, and Artery and Vein on the other, Jaw carved and Teeth split to show the Nerve Cavity. Mounted, with Vase $25.00

Half Upper and Lower Maxilla, showing distribution of Fifth Pair of Nerves. Mounted, with Vase $20.00

SECTION OF HEAD SHOWING FIFTH PAIR OF NERVES.

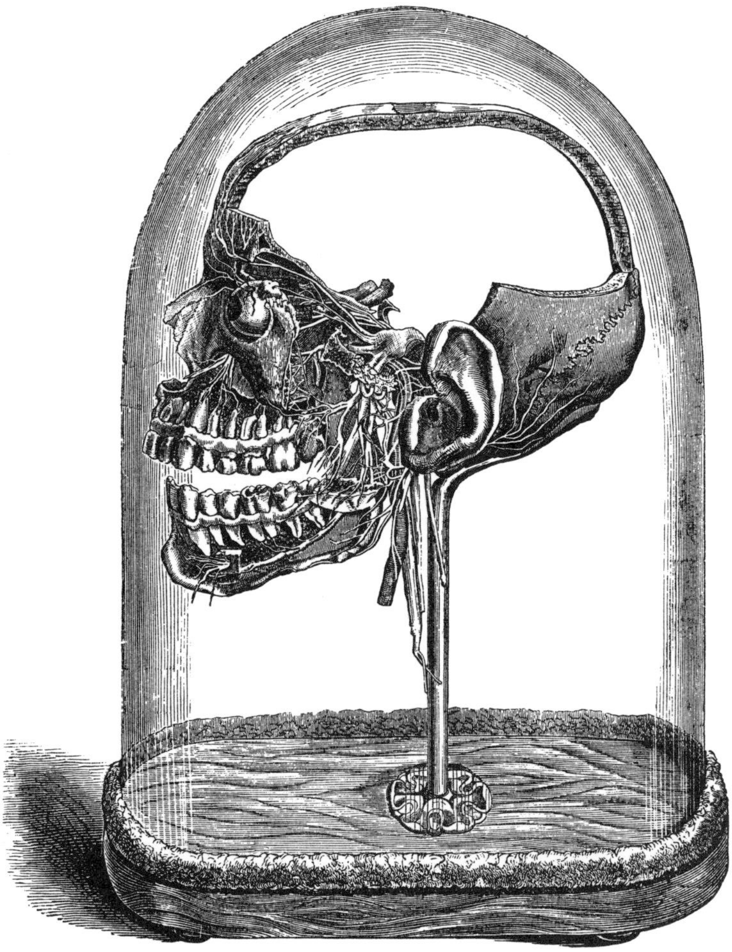

The above Cut gives a general idea of a desirable Preparation, illustrating the distribution of the Fifth Pair of Nerves. They are not always exactly like the one illustrated in the Cut, but are selected with care from the stock of the Artist, with a view to show the principal ramifications of this important Pair of Nerves.

Section of Head, showing distribution of Fifth Pair of Nerves, connected with Teeth and Jaws. Mounted, with Vase $50.00

ANATOMICAL PREPARATIONS.

Fig. 1.

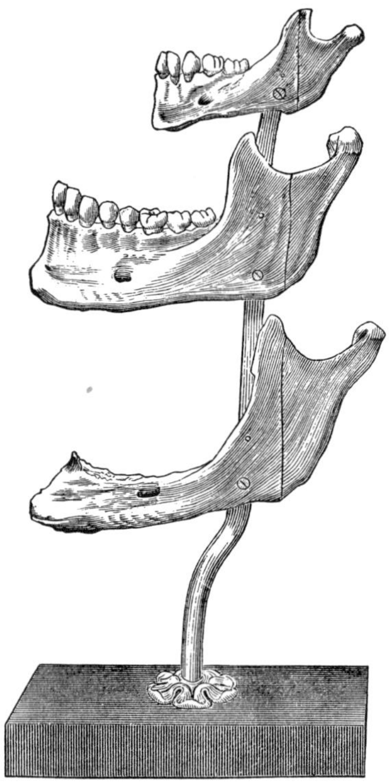

Fig. 2.

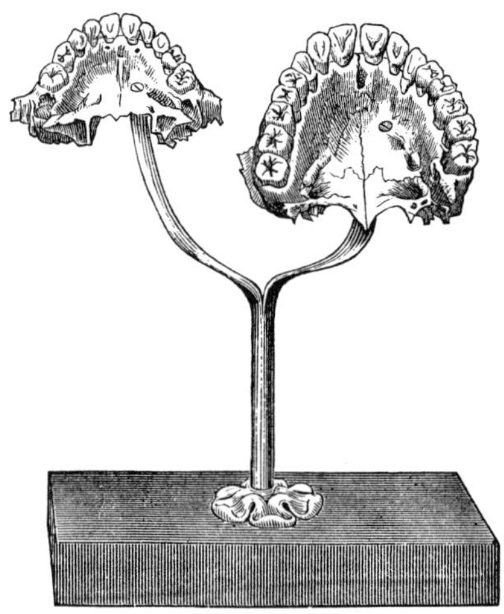

Comparison of the Angle of the Lower Jaw in the Infant, Adult, and Old Age, Fig. 1. Mounted, without Vase	$9.50
Comparison of the Arch of the Upper Jaw in the Infant and the Adult, Fig. 2. Mounted, without Vase	9.50
Skull, No. 1	16.00
" " 2	12.00
" " 3	10.00
" Sawed in seven pieces	30.00
" Disarticulated	125.00
Model of Molar Tooth (Papier-maché)	50.00
Cerebellum (Papier-maché)	26.00
Brain " "	110.00
Eye " "	40.00
Ear " "	52.00
Heart, Fœtal " "	26.00
" Adult " "	26.00

A supply of Adult Jaws and Dentitions always on hand, warranted perfect in every particular, which will be packed to transport safely, with proper handling, to any part of the country.

ANATOMICAL ILLUSTRATION OF THE FIFTH NERVE.

New Edition. Size of plate, 21 by 27 inches.

This Plate gives correct views of the course of the Fifth or Trifacial Nerve, and its connection with the other Cranial Nerves and the Sympathetic; while the arteries and parts accessory to it are clearly displayed. The drawings are the size of life, and faithfully Colored. The same Plate also contains representations of the Microscopical Anatomy of the Teeth. This work is strongly recommended as embracing far more than any Model, however complicated, is made to show, and, as a work of study and reference, will be found invaluable to the Profession.

Accompanying the Plate is a Key in the form of a Pamphlet giving a concise and practical description of the Anatomy of the Fifth Pair of Nerves.

The Plate and description will be put up in pasteboard Boxes, so that they may be transported without injury, and sent free of postage.

Price $1.00
Mounted in Map style 1.75

DIAGRAMS OF THE NERVES OF THE HUMAN BODY.

In two Colors. Exhibiting their origin, divisions, and connections, with their distribution to the various regions of the cutaneous surface and to all their muscles. By William Henry Flower, Fellow of the Royal College of Surgeons; Assistant Surgeon to and Demonstrator of Anatomy at the Middlesex Hospital. Edited, with additions, by William W. Keen, M.D.

The Anatomy of the Nervous System generally meets with less attention than might be usefully bestowed upon it, owing to the difficulties supposed to surround its study. The author's object is to place that knowledge in a form easily accessible, as well to students as to those whose avocations no longer afford time or opportunity for elaborate anatomical investigation.

Sent, free of postage, to any part of the United States, on receipt of the price . $2.00

THE ERUPTION OF THE TEETH.

A Diagram designed by Dr. J. N. Farrar, to illustrate, to popular comprehension, the relation of the sixth-year molar to the permanent set.

The ignorance of parents in regard to their children's teeth, which every practitioner finds so difficult to overcome, makes it desirable to have a ready means of explanation which will impress the facts upon their minds.

The Chart is neatly engraved; size, 13 inches by 10 inches, with good margin.

Heavy Plate Paper, suitable for framing . . . . 20 cents.
Bristol Board, eyeleted for hanging . . . . 25 "
Framed . . . . $1.50, $2.00, and $2.50

Also, the same Diagrams and Letter-press may be had in the form of an Eight-Page Pamphlet, on Heavy Plate Paper, suitable for presentation to patients.

Price . . . . per hundred $3.00

A liberal reduction when ordered in quantities.

Name and address printed, if desired, on last page of cover, at the following rates: for 100, $1.00; for 500, $2.00; for 1000, $3.00.

THE TEETH: NATURAL AND ARTIFICIAL.

BY J. W. WHITE, M.D., D.D.S.

This is a neat little pamphlet of 30 pages, intended to convey popular information in regard to the Teeth; their importance; the necessity of attention to preserve their health and usefulness; the effects of neglect upon them and upon the general health; the eruption of the deciduous and permanent sets as to time and order; hints as to their care; of brushes, powders and washes; a brief description of the materials and processes employed in the manufacture of porcelain teeth; difference between mere mechanical and artistic service in adapting them to individual needs, etc.

It is believed that dentists can not only serve their patients, but advance their own interests, by placing this pamphlet in the hands of their patrons.

Price	per hundred	$3.00
" large margin, fine paper	"	7.00
" large margin, extra fine paper	"	10.00

Name and address printed on cover, at the following rates: for 100, $1.00; for 500, $2.00; for 1000, $3.00.

The cheapest edition has an advertisement of the publisher, giving information of value to the public. The seven- and ten-dollar varieties can be had with or without the advertisement, according to the wish of the purchaser.

Sample copy sent free on application.

DENTAL AND MEDICAL BOOKS.

Aitken's Science and Practice of Medicine. 2 vols. Cloth, $12.00. Sheep	$14.00
Arthur's Treatment and Prevention of Decay of the Teeth. 16mo. Cloth	1.50
Beale's How to Work the Microscope. 400 Plates. Cloth	7.50
Biddle's Materia Medica for Students. Cloth	4.00
Carpenter's Physiology. Cloth, $5.50. Sheep	6.50
Cleveland's Lexicon. " 1.25. Tucks	1.50
Coles's Deformities of the Mouth. Colored Plates. Cloth	2.50
" Dental Mechanics. Cloth	2.50
Dalton's Physiology. Cloth, $5.50. Sheep	6.50
Dental Anomalies. Paper	.25
Dental Cosmos. Bound vols. Half Turkey	3.50
Dentist's Pocket Diary and Appointment-Book, $1.00. Tucks	1.25
Draper's Human Physiology. 1 vol. Cloth, $5.00. Sheep	5.50
Dunglison's Dictionary. Cloth, $6.50. Sheep	7.50
" Physiology. 2 vols. Cloth	7.00
Erichsen's Surgery. 2 vols. Cloth, $9.00. Sheep	11.00
Flower's Nerves of the Human Body. Quarto. Cloth	2.00
Fownes's Chemistry. Cloth, $2.75. Sheep	3.25
Fox and Harris on the Teeth. Sheep	4.00
Garretson's System of Oral Surgery. 1 vol. Cloth, $10.00 Sheep	11.00

Gray's Anatomy. Cloth, $6.00. Sheep	$7.00
Gross's System of Surgery. 2 vols. Sheep	15.00
Handy's Text-Book of Anatomy. Sheep	4.00
Harris's Dictionary of Dental Surgery. Cloth, $6.50. Sheep . . .	7.50
" Principles and Practice of Dentistry. 1 vol. Cloth, $6.50. Sheep.	7 50
Hartshorne's Essentials of the Principles and Practice of Medicine. Cloth .	2.63
" Conspectus of the Medical Sciences. Cloth, $4.25. Sheep .	5.00
Heath's Injuries and Diseases of the Jaws. 1 vol. Cloth	5.00
Huxley's Lessons in Elementary Physiology. 12mo. Cloth . . .	1.50
Kirke's Hand-Book of Physiology. Cloth	5.00
Leber & Rottenstein's Dental Caries. Cloth	1.50
Leidy's Anatomy. Sheep	5.00
Meredith's The Teeth and How to Save Them. Cloth	1.25
Mitchell's Therapeutics. Sheep	4.00
Morton and Leeds's Chemistry. Cloth	2.00
Morton's Anatomy. Cloth	4.00
Neill & Smith's Compend. Cloth, $4.00. Sheep	4.75
Paget's Surgical Pathology. " 7.50. "	8.50
Physician's Med. Compend and Pharmaceutical Formulæ. Tucks, $1.00. Clo.	1.50
Richardson's Mechanical Dentistry. Sheep	4.50
Robertson on Extracting. Cloth	1.50
Salter's Dental Pathology and Surgery. Cloth	4.50
Sansom on Chloroform. Cloth	2.00
Sewill's Student's Guide to Dental Anatomy and Surgery. Cloth . . .	1.75
Sharpey and Quain's Anatomy. 2 vols. Cloth	6.00
Silliman's Chemistry. Cloth	2.00
Stillé's Therapeutics. 2 vols. Cloth, $10.00. Sheep	12.00
Taft's Practical Treatise on Operative Dentistry. Sheep	4.50
Tanner's Practice of Medicine. 1 vol. Cloth, $6.00. Sheep . . .	7.00
Thomas's Medical Dictionary. Cloth, $3.25. Sheep	3.75
Thomas on Nitrous Oxide	1.25
Tomes's Dental Surgery. Cloth	5.00
Tyson's Cell Doctrine. Colored Plate. 1 vol. Cloth	2.00
United States Dispensatory. Sheep	10.00
" " Pharmacopœia. Cloth, $1.75. Sheep	2.25
Waring's Practical Therapeutics. Cloth, $5.00. Sheep	6.00
Watson's Practice of Physic. 2 vols. Cloth, $9.00. Sheep	11.00
Watt's Chemical Essays. Cloth	1.25
Wedl's Pathology of the Teeth. Cloth, $4.50. Sheep	5.50
White's Taking Impressions of the Mouth. Cloth	1.25
Williams's Principles of Medicine. Cloth	3.50
Wilson's Anatomy. Cloth, $4.00. Sheep	5.00
Wood's Practice of Medicine. 2 vols. Sheep	10.00
" Therapeutics and Pharmacology. 2 vols. Sheep	10.00

ALLPORT'S REGISTERING DENTAL LEDGER.

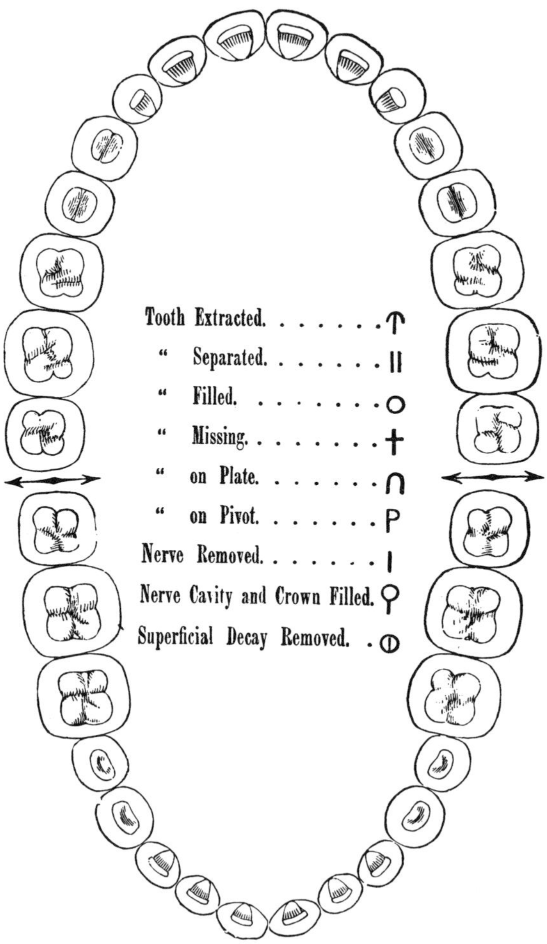

A Ledger for Dentists' use, designed by Dr. Allport, of Chicago, and intended to facilitate the registering of accounts.

The annexed Cut represents a diagram, of which there are two on each page, with space alongside of each, appropriately ruled, for name of patient, reference, date of operations, charge for the same, and credit for amounts paid.

The symbols denote the character and locality of the various operations performed, thus showing at a glance the history and condition of the mouth of each patient.

These Books are got up in neat style, printed on good paper, and substantially bound.

This Ledger has had extensive sale and is still in large demand.

340 pages, half Turkey and Cloth sides (paper extra quality)	$5.00
340 " " Roan	4.00
172 " " "	3.00

Specimen pages sent on application.

CHILD'S DENTAL RECORD.

Containing forms similar to Bill Head No. 2, as described on page 365 of Catalogue. Four forms, 6½ inches long by 2½ inches wide on each page. Printed on good paper and substantially bound. 216 pages.

Price $3.00

DENTISTS' ACCOUNT BOOKS.

Designed to accompany Bill Head No. 1, as described on page 364 of Catalogue. It has a similar Cut over each page, 5 inches in length. Printed on fine paper, paged, and substantially bound in four sizes.

96 pages	$1.25
192 "	2.25
288 "	3.25
384 "	3.75

MEREDITH'S POCKET REGISTER, POCKET JOURNAL, AND POCKET LEDGER.

Price of either: in Leather, with Tuck	$1.50
" " " English Cloth	1.25

For Cut and description, see advertising pages of DENTAL COSMOS for January and February, 1874. Sent postpaid on receipt of price.

DICKINSON'S DENTAL PLATE REGISTER AND LEDGER.

Price $2.00

187

Mr. ....

To Dr.

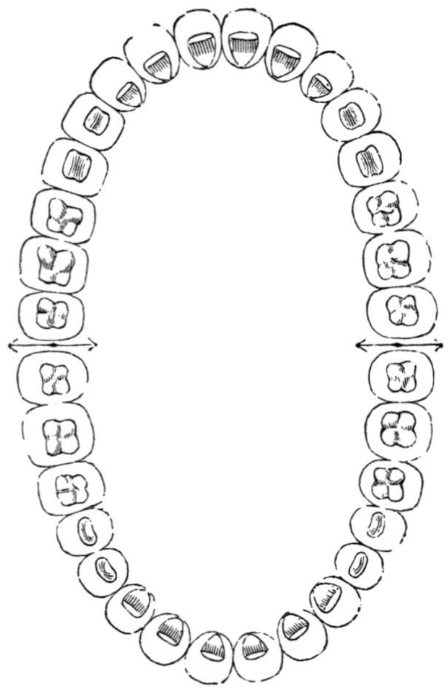

BILL HEAD, No. 1.

This is a form of Bill Head for Dentists, and is so arranged that both Operator and Patient are freed from all danger of imposition.

For example: for any tooth operated upon, a mark within the circle of the corresponding tooth in the diagram will designate the operation, so that the patient will know by a glance if the charge be correct. It is assumed that the operator will use in connection with this form a book containing forms similar to the diagram. Size of Bill Head, 8½ inches wide by 7 inches long.

Printed on Fine Paper . per hundred 75 cents.

ELECTROTYPES of the Diagram of Teeth for those who wish to print their own Bill Heads will be furnished at $1.00 each.

BILL HEAD, No. 2.

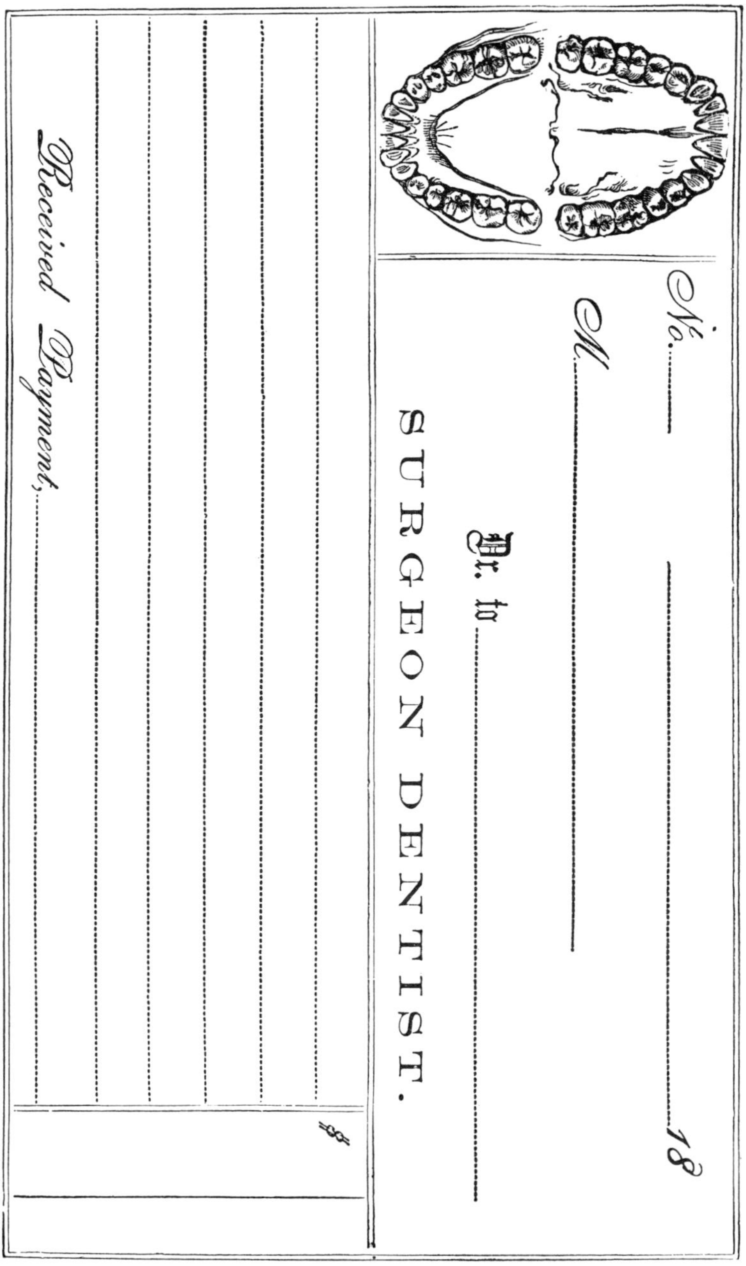
No. ____ 18
M ____
Dr. to ____
SURGEON DENTIST.
$
Received Payment, ____

The above is a fac-simile of Bill Head . . . . . . per hundred 50 cents.

187

M.

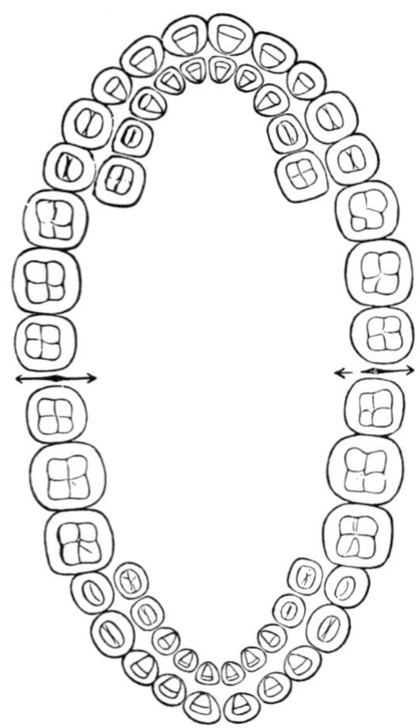

BILL HEAD, No. 3.

NEW STYLE.

SUGGESTED BY DR. ROBERT H. MOFFITT.

The Diagram, of which a miniature copy is here given, is of the same size as is used in Allport's Ledger (page 362), and contains the signs used therein. The addition of the deciduous teeth, upper and lower, makes it convenient for recording operations upon children's teeth.

Size of Bill Head, 8½ by 7 inches. Price per hundred, 75 cents.

DENTISTS' POCKET DIARY AND APPOINTMENT-BOOK.

For Registering Appointments for Dental Operations.

MONDAY,			187
8		1	
9		2	
10		3	
11		4	
12		5	

TUESDAY,			
8		1	
9		2	
10		3	
11		4	
12		5	

The above Diagram shows the exact size and style of two-thirds of a page of the Pocket Diary, presenting, when open, engagements for one week. The figures denote the hour of the engagement. It contains blanks for 54 weeks, and, being without date, is good for any time. It has also a neat memorandum attached.

Flexible Cover, Gilt Edge $1.00
" " " " with Pocket and Tuck 1.25

DENTAL CUTS.

No. 2.

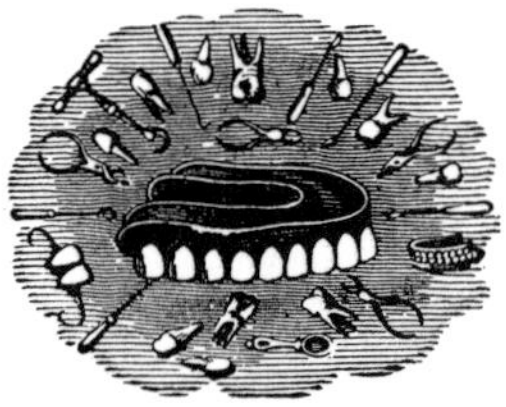

No 5.

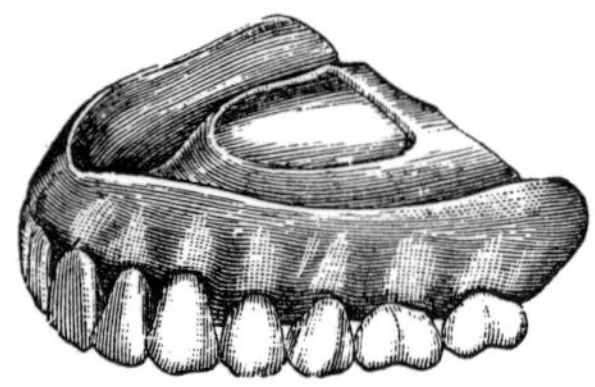

No. 6.

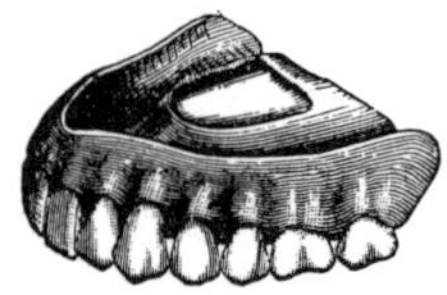

No. 4.

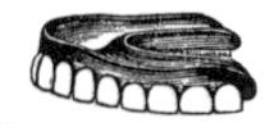

No. 7.

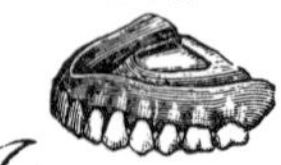

No. 3.

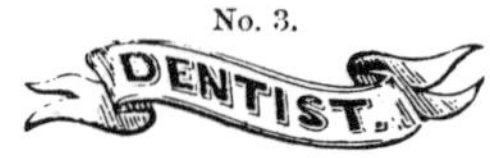

No. 9.

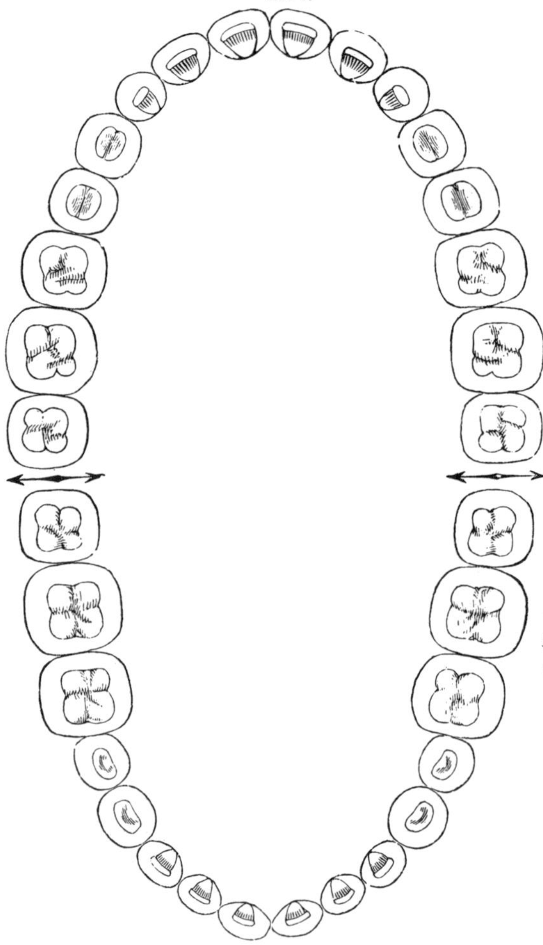

No. 8.

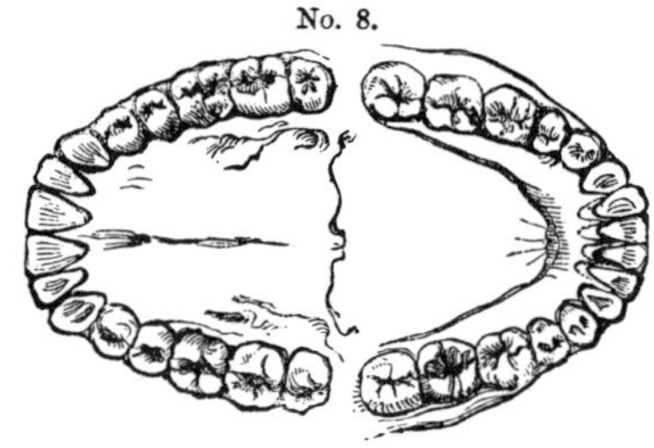

No. 1.

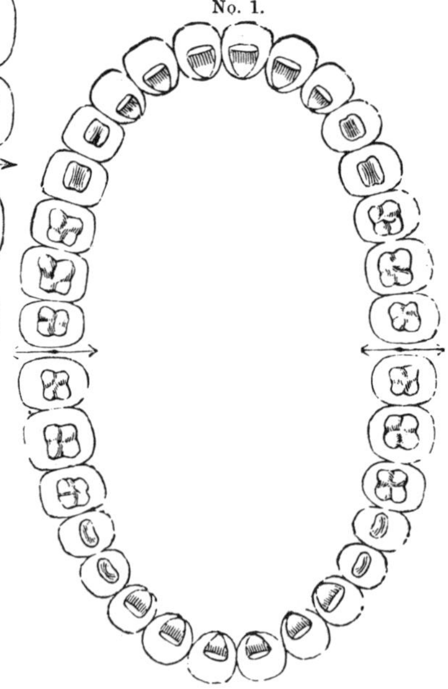

The above Cuts represent such as are used for Advertisements and Business Cards; they are the exact height of type, and can be furnished at the following prices:

No. 1.	Electrotype	$1.00	No. 5.	Electrotype	$0.75	No. 7.	Stereotype	$0.37
" 2.	"	.75	" 6.	"	.60	" 8.	Electrotype	.75
" 3.	Stereotype	.40	" 6.	Stereotype	.45	" 9.	"	1.50
" 4.	"	.37	" 7.	Electrotype	.45			

GLASS BOXES AND JARS FOR TOOTH POWDERS AND PASTES.

White Enamel or Pearl Color Boxes, with Britannia Covers, $2\frac{3}{4}$ inches in diameter by $1\frac{1}{8}$ in. high . . . . per doz. $1.25

White Enamel or Pearl Color Boxes, all Glass, $2\frac{1}{4}$ in. diameter, 1 in. high " 1.00

" " " " $2\frac{1}{2}$ " " $1\frac{1}{4}$ " " 1.25

" " " " 3 " " $1\frac{1}{4}$ " " 1.50

" " " " 3 " square, 1 " " 1.75

Alabaster Boxes, Oval, $3\frac{1}{2}$ in. long by $2\frac{1}{2}$ in. wide and $1\frac{1}{4}$ in. high . " 1.00

White Enamel or Pearl Color Boxes, with Gilt Rim, on feet, 3 in. diameter " 5.00

Flint Glass Boxes, on feet, 3 in. diameter . . . . . . " 3.50

White Enamel Boxes, Gilt Rim, $3\frac{1}{4}$ in. diameter, $1\frac{3}{4}$ in. high . . " 4.00

White Enamel or Pearl Color Boxes, Octagon, $3\frac{1}{2}$ in. long by $2\frac{1}{2}$ in. wide and $1\frac{1}{2}$ in. deep . . . . per doz. 2.50

Flint Glass Boxes, Octagon, $3\frac{1}{2}$ in. long by $2\frac{1}{2}$ in. wide and $1\frac{1}{2}$ in. deep " 2.50

White Enamel or Pearl Color Boxes, Octagon, dimensions as above, with one Gilt Line on Lid . . . . per doz. 4.50

White Enamel or Pearl Color Boxes, Octagon, dimensions as above, with three Gilt Lines on Lid . . . . per doz. 5.00

Semi-Transparent 6 oz. Jars, 3 in. diameter by 3 in. high . . . " 2.25

Flint Glass 1 oz. Jars . . . . " 1.25

WOOD TOOTH-POWDER BOXES.

Boxwood, Varnished, labeled Tooth-Powder, without name, $2\frac{1}{4}$ in. diameter, $1\frac{1}{8}$ in. deep, designated as No. 2 . . . . per doz. $0.50

Boxwood, Varnished, labeled Tooth-Powder, without name, $2\frac{1}{2}$ in. diameter, $1\frac{1}{4}$ in. deep, designated as No. 3 . . . . . . per doz. .60

Boxwood, Varnished, labeled Tooth-Powder, without name, $2\frac{3}{4}$ in. diameter, $1\frac{1}{4}$ in. deep, designated as No. 4 . . . . . . per doz. .70

FINE CARD BOARD AND PAPER TOOTH-POWDER BOXES.

No. 1. Paper, Round, covered with Gilt and Star Paper, lined with Silver Paper, $2\frac{1}{2}$ in. diameter, $\frac{7}{8}$ in. high . . . . per doz. $0.40

No. 2. Fine Card Board, Round, covered with Enameled Paper, edged with Gold Paper, $2\frac{1}{2}$ in. diameter, $\frac{7}{8}$ in. high . . . . . per doz. .50

No. 3. Fine Card Board, Oval, covered with Gelatin Paper, edged with Gold Paper, $2\frac{7}{8}$ in. long, 2 in. wide, $\frac{7}{8}$ in. high . . . . per doz. .60

No. 4. Fine Card Board, Round, covered with Gelatin Paper, edged with Gold Paper, $2\frac{1}{2}$ in. diameter, $\frac{7}{8}$ in. high . . . . . per doz. .60

No. 5. Paper, Half Oval, covered with Gelatin Paper, edged with Gilt Paper, $2\frac{3}{8}$ in. long, $2\frac{1}{4}$ in. wide, $1\frac{1}{8}$ in. high . . . . . per doz. .65

No. 6. Paper, Half Oval, covered with Gelatin Paper, edged with Gilt Paper, $2\frac{3}{8}$ in. long, $2\frac{1}{4}$ in. wide, $\frac{15}{16}$ in. high . . . . . per doz. .65

All the above are without Labels.

No. 7. Paper Top and Bottom, Card Board Side, Round, covered with Enameled Paper, edged with Gilt Paper, $2\frac{1}{2}$ in. diameter, $\frac{7}{8}$ in. high . per doz. $0.50

No. 8. Paper, Round, covered with Enameled Paper, lined with Silver Paper, edged with Gilt Paper, $2\frac{1}{2}$ in. diameter, $\frac{7}{8}$ in. high . . per doz. .60

No. 9. Fine Card Board, Round, covered with Enameled Paper, edged with Gold Paper, $2\frac{1}{2}$ in. diameter, $\frac{7}{8}$ in. high . . . . . . per doz. .60

No. 10. Fine Card Board, Oval, covered with Enameled Paper, edged with Gold Paper, $2\frac{7}{8}$ in. long, 2 in. wide, $\frac{7}{8}$ in. high . . . . . per doz. .60

No. 11. Paper, Half Oval, covered with Enameled Paper, edged with Gilt Paper, $2\frac{3}{8}$ in. long, $2\frac{1}{4}$ in. wide, $1\frac{1}{8}$ in. high . . . . . . per doz. .70

No. 12. Paper, Half Oval, covered with Enameled Paper, edged with Gilt Paper, $2\frac{3}{8}$ in. long, $2\frac{1}{4}$ in. wide, $1\frac{5}{16}$ in. high . . . . . . per doz. .70

The above (from Nos. 7 to 12) are labeled "Tooth-Powder," in fancy gilt letters.

We will fill any of our Round Boxes with our best Tooth-Powder (No. 1) at $1.00 per doz. additional, and the Half Oval at $1.30 per doz. additional.

STAND FOR OFFICE PREPARATIONS.

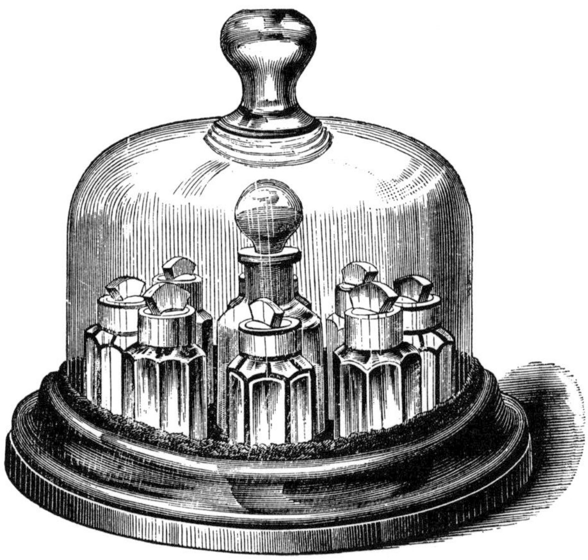

This is intended for the clean and convenient keeping of Dental Polychrests, such as Carbolic Acid, Iodine, etc. The Base is of wood, highly polished, $7\frac{1}{2}$ inches in diameter, $1\frac{1}{2}$ inches high. Vase of fine glass, 6 inches in diameter, $6\frac{3}{4}$ inches high. Containing 8 Cut-glass Bottles with ground stoppers, and a Drop Bottle in the center. Chenille around the Vase.

Price $6.00

CHAMOIS SKINS.

Prices from 50 cents to $1.50 each.

TOOTH-POWDER BOTTLE.

Patented Nov. 19, 1867, by Dr. J. B. Da Camara.

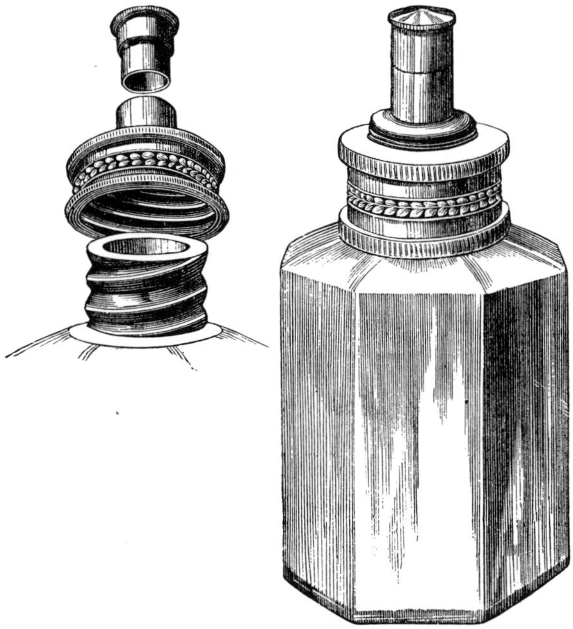

The Bottle has a Nickel-Plated Metallic Cap, which is retained by a thread on the neck, and is easily removed to fill the bottle.

The tube in the center allows the nice distribution of the powder on the brush, and is closed by a neatly-fitted sliding cap.

This convenient manner of keeping Tooth-Powder meets with general favor. It avoids waste, can be readily carried when traveling, retains the fragrance of the powder, and several may use from the same bottle with propriety.

PRICES.

Glass Bottle and Cap (as per Cut), without boxes . . . . . per doz. $2.00
" " " " " with elegantly finished Round Boxes, Gilt Rim size of bottle . . . . per doz. 2.60
Glass Bottle and Cap (as per Cut), without boxes, filled with S. S. White's Tooth Powder No. 1 . . . . per doz. 3 25
Glass Bottle and Cap (as per Cut), with elegantly finished Round Boxes, Gilt Rim, size of Bottle, filled with S. S. White's Tooth-Powder No. 1 . per doz. 3.75

Dentists can affix their own Labels.

SMALL CUT-GLASS BOTTLES, WITH GROUND-GLASS STOPPERS.

Direct importation of these convenient small Bottles for Office Preparations, etc., of various patterns, colors, and sizes.

Prices ranging from 15 cents to 30 cents each.

GOLD FOIL STAND.

This is a neat and useful little piece of Office Furniture. It is intended for preserving gold prepared for fillings from dust and moisture. The Stand for Office Preparations, illustrated on page 370, will give a general idea of the article. The Base is of polished wood, covered on the upper surface with soft spunk, and protected by a Glass Vase fitted into the Base, the joint protected by a ring of Chenille. There are four sizes, the Vases respectively measuring 3, 4, 4½, and 5 inches in diameter; the height, inclusive of base, from 3 to 4 inches.

Price of the 3 and 4 inch	**each** $1.50
" " 4½ " 5 "	" 2.00

SCALES.

A fine assortment of Scales suitable for Physicians and Dentists, so arranged that the Apparatus can be mounted on the box or inclosed within it.

Oval Tin Box, to hold in hand		$1.20
Oak Box, 5 inch, to hold in hand		1.25
" 6 " " "		1.50
Walnut Box, Pocket, 6 inches by 2 inches	No. 1552	3.90

This is a very compact arrangement. The Beam swings on the Lid, and but a single movement is required to adjust the Scales ready for use.

Mahogany Box, 8¼ inches by 4¼ inches	No. 1510–9	$4.00
" " 8½ " 4¼ "	" 1511–22	6.00
" " 9¾ " 5¾ "	" 1511–24	6.00
Marble-top " 8½ " 4 "	" 1513–22	6.25
Mahogany " 10½ " 5¼ "	" 1512–27	6.75

MICROSCOPICAL OBJECTS.

A large assortment of Mounted Preparations for the Microscope.

Price . . . . each 45 cents.

BECK'S ECONOMIC MICROSCOPES.

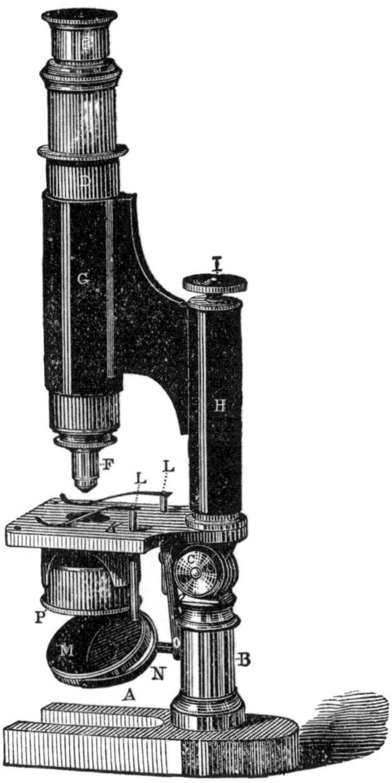

No. 1.

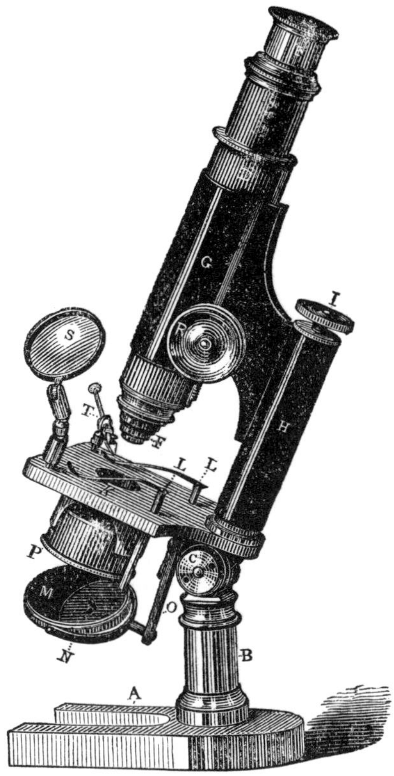

No. 2.

These Instruments have been especially constructed to meet the requirements of Physicians, Students, and others who desire a Stand of perfect workmanship, combined with Objectives of first-rate quality. The body is supplied with a lengthening tube, and the sub-stage is fitted for carrying Polariscope and other illuminating apparatus.

With the exception of the substitution of a Rackwork Coarse Adjustment for the sliding movement by hand, the Stand of No. 2 in no way differs from that of No. 1. The Coarse Adjustment, R, is produced by a rack and pinion, which moves the Body-Tube, D, carrying the Object-Glass, F, and Eye-Piece, E, up and down with greater precision.

No. 1, with one Eye-Piece and two Object-Glasses (the 1 inch and the ¼ inch), magnifying from 45 to 240 Diameters, packed in neat Mahogany Case, with lock and key $45.00

No. 2, with two Eye-Pieces and two Object-Glasses (as above), magnifying from 45 to 330 Diameters, a Side Condensing Lens for the illumination of opaque objects, a pair of Stage Forceps, a pair of Brass Pliers, and a Glass Plate with a ledge for the examination of fluids, packed in a Mahogany Case, with lock and key 55.00

QUEEN'S "HOLMES'S" CLASS MICROSCOPE.

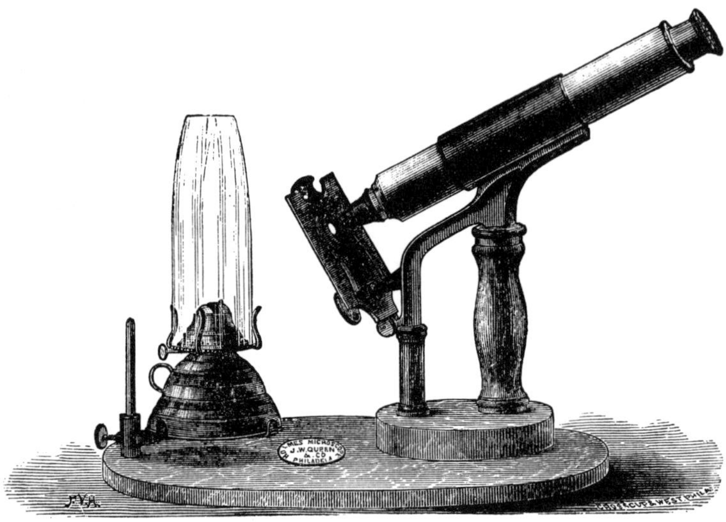

This Microscope was originally designed by Dr. O. W. Holmes, of Boston, for use in his own Class. By slight modifications of his original plan, and the substitution of metal for wood in some of the parts (without, however, increasing the weight), the Instrument is produced in an improved form. It fills a long-felt want, combining as it does a perfect Class Microscope, with a very excellent and practical Stand for all ordinary table use. Supported on a base of polished walnut by two columns of the same wood (one of which forms the handle for Class use) is a light frame of bronzed iron, bearing upon its upper surface, at an angle most convenient for observation, a short split tube through which the compound body slides with perfect smoothness, forming the Coarse Adjustment for focus. The Fine Adjustment is effected by a micrometer screw and lever beneath the stage. The latter is furnished with light spring clips, for holding the object, and a revolving diaphragm with different-sized openings. The compound body is furnished with a first-class Eye-Piece, and the "Society Screw," whereby any objective of standard English or American make can be used on it. A Coal-Oil Lamp on adjustable stand, firmly secured to the base of the Instrument, furnishes the illumination. For transparent objects, the light from the edge or width of the flame is allowed to fall directly upon the object, through the central aperture of the stage. For opaque objects, the Lamp is raised to the top of its stand, and its rays are allowed to fall upon a small concave mirror attached to the iron frame by a universal joint, whence they are reflected upon the object. If it is desired to use the Instrument upon the table by daylight, a mirror properly hung on universal joints can be substituted for the Lamp. The entire height of the Instrument is about twelve inches; size of base, twelve by four inches; weight, three and a quarter pounds.

Price, without Mirror	$20.00
" with "	25.00
Black Walnut Case, with fittings for Microscope and all accessories . . .	7.50

APPENDIX.

In this Department will be found various New Articles which have been added to our Stock during the compilation of the Catalogue, together with others which were inadvertently omitted from the departments to which they properly belong.

CHAPPELL'S GOLD BUILDERS.

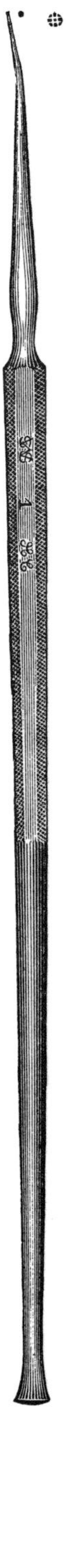

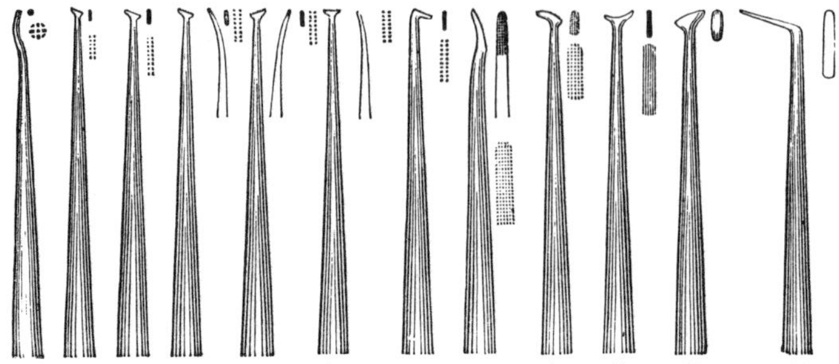

2. 3. 4. 5 6. 7. 8. 9. 10. 11. 12. 13.

Our Cuts give only the shapes and sizes of these new Instruments for filling Teeth with Gold. The enlarged side Cuts (to exhibit serrations by count) will indicate how fine and delicate the workmanship must be which puts in the small space of these plugging faces so many serrates accurately divided.

These points and faces have many variations and differences which will clearly distinguish them from those in other sets to which they bear resemblance. Nearly every one of them is in some special way unique. They are designed to be used with adhesive Gold; Dr. Chappell prefers "No. 30 Rolled Cohesive Gold, cut in strips $\frac{1}{16}$, $\frac{1}{8}$, $\frac{3}{16}$ in. wide, and 1 in. long, re-annealing as used."

They are Malleting Shaft Pluggers. We request attention to the forms of points as regards face-angles, and the double-foot or foot-and-heel form, and how the insteps are cut away. These enable the Operator to enter the cavity freely, and work the Gold to the contour surface, into the retaining canals, and against the walls, from the beginning of the gold building. The serrations are *peculiar* in the angle of the valley cut. Dr. Chappell says of this peculiarity, that "the interdigitations made by the serrations will range as seats in an amphitheatre, and the shape of these steps firmly secures the metal in place, until the welding force is applied to the instrument, when the metal becomes a solid mass, by cohesive force, free from 'seams' or 'balling up.'"

Nos. 11 and 12 of this set are designed for convex and concave contour building and surface finishing for No. 13, which is a smooth Planisher.

PRICES.

Set of 13, Varney Handle, as shown in Cut	per set	$20.00
Nos. 1 and 13	each	1.00
No. 2	"	1.10
" 12	"	1.25
Nos. 3, 4, and 7	"	1.50
" 5 and 6	"	1.60
" 8 and 11	"	1.75
No. 9	"	2.00
" 10	"	2.50
Set of 13, Octagon, Taper End, $6\frac{3}{4}$ inches long	per set	17.40

HARD PLATINUM INSTRUMENTS.

FOR CHLORIDE OF ZINC.

SUGGESTED BY DR. C. E. FRANCIS.

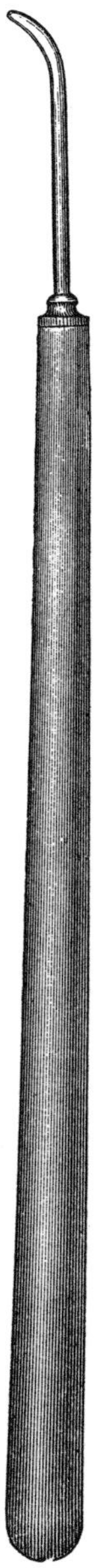

1.

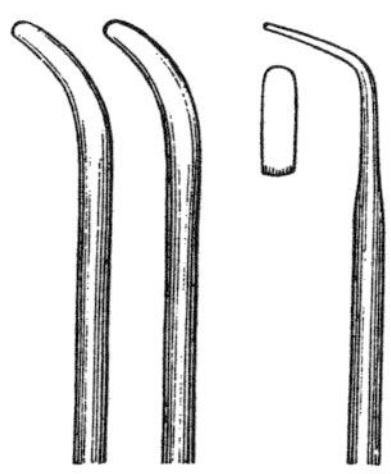

2. 3. 4.

These Instruments are intended to be used to mix, convey, and manipulate Oxychloride, Os-Artificiel, Cement-Plombe, and other Plastic Zinc Stoppings. The hard alloy of Platinum with Iridium is firm enough for these uses, and withstands the corrosive action of the Zinc-Chloride.

Our set consists of four convenient points with fine Ivory Handles, size of Cut, set firmly against a solid Silver Collar.

Nos. 1, 2, and 3 differ only in size.

Price . . . . per set $9.00

PLASTIC FILLING INSTRUMENTS.

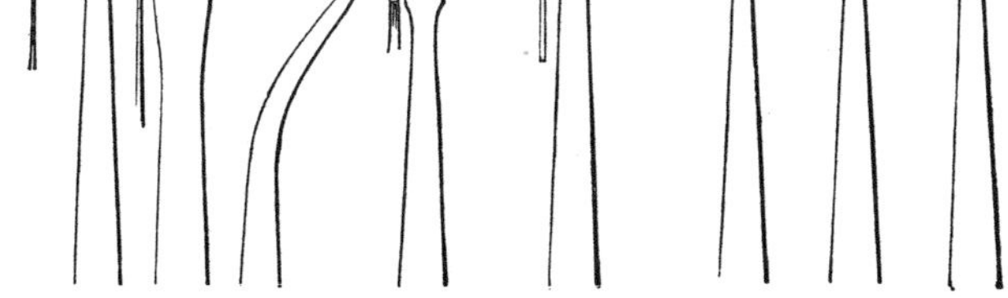

2. 3. 4. 5. 6. 7. 8. 9.

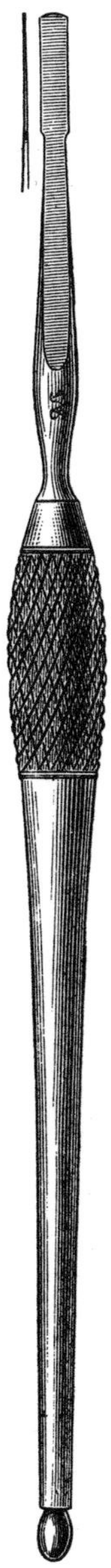

1.

Our Cuts represent a set of nine Steel Instruments intended for use with Oxychloride and Gutta-Percha stoppings. They are suitable for mixing, carrying, packing, and burnishing these materials in crown, labial, and proximal cavities.

We have used great care in the selection of these points, and believe that the Set is complete for the varied cases, materials and locality, without any useless ones. Mounted as shown in Cut No. 1.

Long Tapered Ebony Handles, Checkered Finger Hold,	per set	$9.00
" " " " "	each	1.00
Octagon Handles, High-Blue	per set	4.50
" "	each	.50

AMALGAM CARRIER AND BURNISHER COMBINED.

PATTERN FURNISHED BY DR. JAMES B. WILLMOTT.

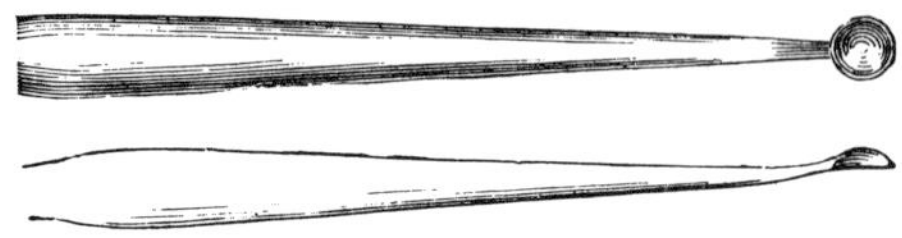

Used for carrying Amalgam to the cavity, and also as a Burnisher in finishing.

Octagon Steel, Plain Handle, Bronzed	50 cents.
¼-inch File-Cut Handle, Bronzed	60 "

BARBED SCALERS.

INVENTION OF DR. L. T. SHEFFIELD.

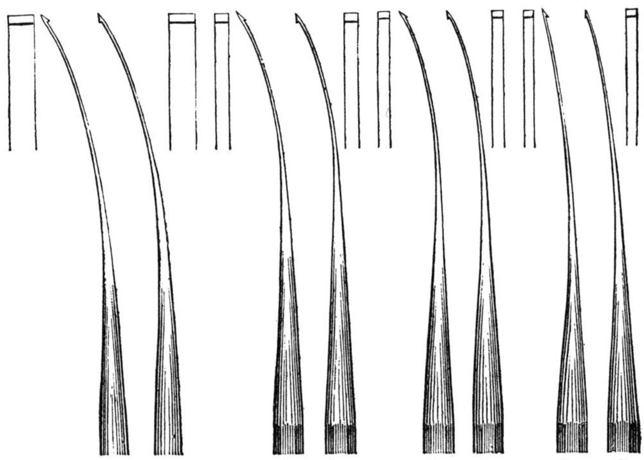

1. 2. 3. 4. 5. 6. 7. 8.

These Instruments are designed to pass between and around the necks of teeth which are loosened by old deposits of tartar. Being in pairs, with the barbed edges on opposite faces, they admit of application right and left, and on proximal surfaces. While holding the tooth with the finger upon it firmly in the socket, they can be used either by pushing to scale with the Chisel edge, or by making the draw-cut with the Barbed edge.

They are so thin and flexible that they work easily under loosened gums and around exposed fangs. The Large Pair are designed for use on the broad surfaces of back molars.

Elegantly made with Stoned Edges and Spring Tempered blades. Plain Octagon Handles of graded sizes. Polished, Blued, and Lacquered.

Price	per set $5.00
Large Pair, Nos. 1 and 2	each .75
3 Smaller Pairs, Nos. 3, 4, 5, 6, 7, 8	" .60

ENGINE HAND-PIECE SHIELD.

INVENTED AND PATENT APPLIED FOR BY DR. J. E. SWALLOW.

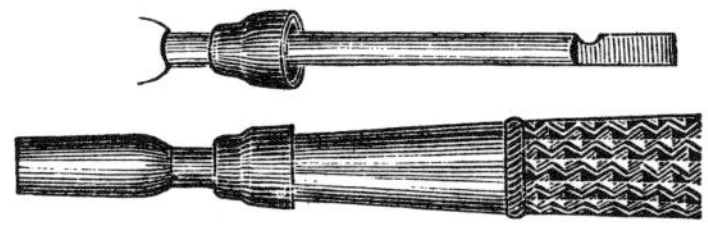

This device is made of soft rubber. It is slipped over the Mandrel far enough to allow the cup end to cover the nose of the Hand-Piece, and revolves with the instrument, preventing moisture or dust from getting into and wearing away the nose of Hand-Piece.

Price . . . . per doz. 75 cents.

VULCANITE BURS.

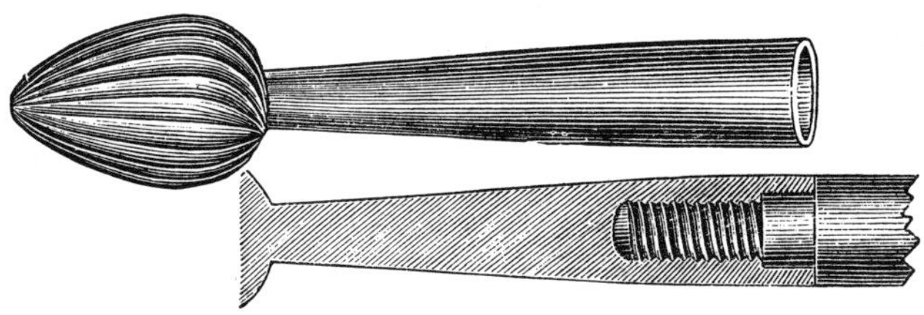

These Burs are made with a plain collar on the inner end of shaft, and a screw at the lower end, so as to adapt them to our Laboratory Lathes Nos. 3 and 4.

The upper Cut shows full size of Bur, and the sectional Cut represents it as screwed on the Lathe Mandrel.

They are made in four shapes, as shown on page 351.

Price . . . . each $1.25

PACK'S GOLD.

Eureka Gold Filling . . . .
Soft Gold Foil . . . .
Cohesive Foil . . . .
Pellets . . . .

BRASS CHUCK, No. 5.

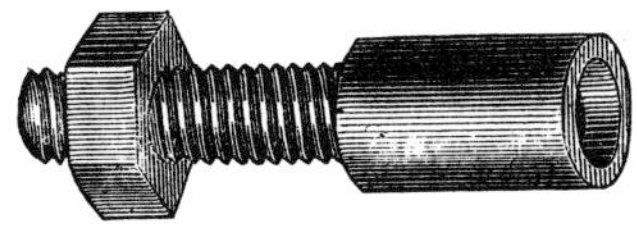

This Chuck is also adapted to our Laboratory Lathes Nos. 3 and 4, and is intended to carry Brush Wheels, Cotton Wheels, etc.

It is represented full size, and is secured to the Lathe Mandrel in the same manner as the Vulcanite Bur.

Price . . . . each 50 cents.

SCRATCH BRUSHES.

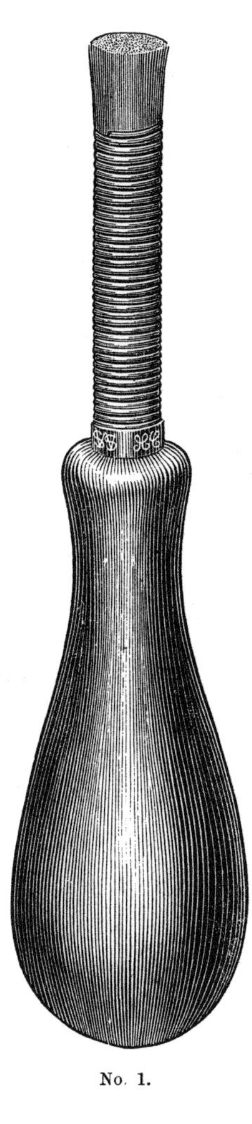

No. 1.

No. 1, Brass Brush Wire, for cleaning burs, files, and the serrations of pluggers.

No. 2, Steel Brush Wire, with cone-shaped end for scrubbing celluloid plates before polishing; suggested by Dr. Rehwinkel. We have succeeded in obtaining a smaller size of No. 2, very desirable for plate scrubbing. They are stamped "No. 2 S."

No. 3, Steel Brush Wire, similar to No. 2, but made of extra fine Wire. Many Operators prefer the coarser sort.

All have the wrapper wire tinned, so that they can be safely cut down to expose more Brush. Fine Polished, Ebonized Handles.

For laboratory use, with Handles of Natural Wood, Nos. 2 and 3 are 10 cents less in price.

To dress the points of Wire Brushes, pull off the wrapper wire to the length desired, then take a flat bastard file, holding the handle in the left hand with the point resting on the bench or table, and draw the Brush upon the flat side of the file until the point is shaped to suit.

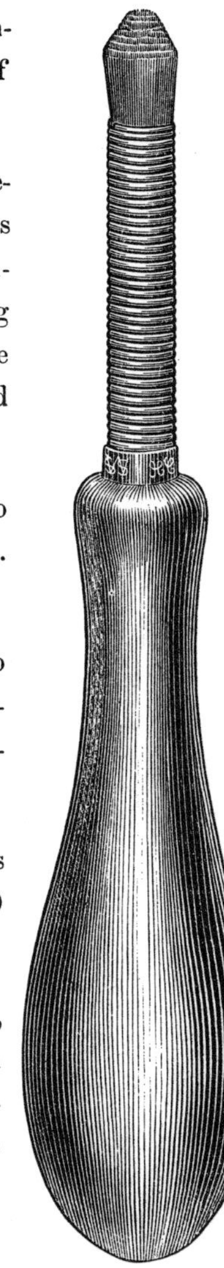

Nos. 2 and 3.

PRICES.

No. 1	each 50 cents.
" 2 and No. 2 S	" 65 "
" 3	" 75 "

CORUNDUM HONES.

FOR SHARPENING CARVING KNIVES, ETC.

These Hones are of the best Corundum, with an iron rod passing through the center, insuring strength and durability. The blade, or Corundum portion, is 9¼ inches long; round, tapering from ¾ inch at the base to $\frac{9}{16}$ inch at the point; handle is wood, 5 inches long, full length 14 inches. Highly recommended for the purposes for which they are designed.

Grooved Wood Handles	each	$0.75
Ebony Handles, Nickel-Plated Nut	"	1.00

DENTAL BIBS.

Horton's White Rubber, with Wire Frame	each	$2.00
Winn's " " " Cord	"	.80

RELYEA'S COMPOUND DENTAL PLATE RETAINER.

Put up in Boxes, containing a half-dozen . . . . per box $3.50

DENTAL FLOSS SILK HOLDERS.

CODMAN & SHURTLEFF'S.

No. 1	each	$0.50
" 2	"	1.00

MISCELLANEOUS.

Gauges for Pivot Wood, Polished Steel	each	$0.50
" " " Ivory	each .50 to	1.00
Camel's-Hair Pencils	each .05; per doz.	.50
Scrubbers for Cleaning Rubber Plates	each	.30
Screw Plates, 5 space	"	1.00
" " 6 "	"	1.38
" " 7 "	"	1.70
" " 8 "	"	2.10
" " 9 "	"	2.40
" " 10 "	"	2.75
Lukens's Body, "A"	per lb.	2.50
Williams's Gold, all varieties		

INSTRUCTIONS IN THE MANIPULATION OF HARD RUBBER OR VULCANITE FOR DENTAL PURPOSES.

By E. Wildman, M.D., D D.S., late Professor of Mechanical Dentistry in the Pennsylvania College of Dental Surgery. Sixth Edition. Got up in handsome style. Bound in cloth.

Price $1.25

THE WESTON AMALGAMS.

THREE VARIETIES, Nos. 1, 2, and 3.

Directions for Use.—These Amalgams should not be washed.

No. 1. SOFT AMALGAM. A substitute for Tin, Hill's Stopping, Oxychloride of Zinc, etc.

Place in the palm of the left hand a small quantity of re-distilled mercury. To this add the requisite amount of the alloy, and with the forefinger of the right hand work it into a stiff paste. If for a temporary filling in a proximal cavity, it will be sufficient to press out the excess of mercury between the thumbs and forefingers of both hands. If for a permanent filling, the mass should be squeezed with a pair of stout broad-nose pliers through strong, closely-woven linen duck, or similar material. (Towels or napkins are apt to leave their fibers imbedded in the Amalgam.)

After submitting the mass to the requisite pressure, cut it into small blocks. To insert it, use well-worn, foot-shaped instruments, with such others as the special case may require. Fill the undercuts and the entire circumference of the cavity with the smallest and softest blocks,—those cut from the edges of the pellet,—leaving the center depressed, to be filled with the larger and denser ones. This should invariably be done with all slow-setting Amalgams. When the cavity has been thoroughly filled, and a sufficient amount added for finishing, condense, trim, and burnish; but, if convenient, the filling would be better if burnished at a subsequent sitting.

No. 2. MEDIUM AMALGAM. Especially adapted for permanent fillings in proximal cavities of bicuspids and molars, and crown fillings where the walls are intact.

Mix as directed for the No. 1 Amalgam. If for a crown filling, make the mass into two pellets; press the mercury from one with the fingers, and from the other with the pliers. (Eight grains of the mass after the mercury has been expressed by the pliers will contain about two and one-half grains of the latter.) Cut both pellets into blocks; fill the bottom of the cavity and the undercuts with the soft blocks, and finish with the hard. Trim and condense, postponing the burnishing, if possible, until a subsequent sitting. With a little practice sufficient pressure can be made with the thumbs and fingers in preparing this Amalgam, thus dispensing with the aid of pliers.

No. 3. HARD, QUICK-SETTING AMALGAM. To 2½ grains of mercury, held in the palm of the hand, add 6 grains of the alloy.* Work the two together with the forefinger of the other hand until thoroughly combined, forming a stiff, crumbling mass. Compress with the thumb and finger into a solid pellet. Without expressing the mercury, divide into small portions, and proceed as before directed.

After the expiration of twenty minutes, if these instructions have been closely followed and the walls of the cavity be intact, the parts having been thoroughly dried, the filling may be finished and burnished. If the case be one which has required quite extensive building up, the finishing may preferably be postponed until the following day.

No. 1	per oz.	$3.00
" 2	"	4.00
" 3	"	5.00

*A little experience will enable the Operator to dispense with the scales.

GENERAL NOTICE.

We quote the prices of a great many Instruments with BRONZED HANDLES, because that style of finish has been the most acceptable to Dentists for many years. The varnish used in fixing the Bronze protects the handle from rust and the Dentist from stained fingers, even after the brightness has worn off. But we supply all the standard instruments which have plain Octagon Handles finished "Black" or "Blued" at the same price as "Bronzed," on large or small orders.

For File-Cut and Checkered Handles, Blueing rusts so quickly in the valleys as to be undesirable. Finer kinds of work which require high polish—such as Fire-Gray Lacquered on Varney Pluggers, and the High-Blue on our Taper Handled Excavators—would cost extra.

CORRECTIONS.

Page 88, Screw Mandrel without Shoulder, priced at 13 cents should be 7 cents.
Page 223, Hand Mirror, 5½ inches, priced at $1.50 should be $1.00.
Page 330, Small Corundum Cup, priced at 25 cents should be 20 cents.

NOTICE.

NEW INVENTIONS OR MANUFACTURES

APPLICABLE TO THE

PRACTICE OF DENTISTRY

WILL BE NOTICED AS THEY APPEAR,

IN THE

ADVERTISING PAGES

OF THE

DENTAL COSMOS.

(See page 8.)

PRESS OF
J. B. LIPPINCOTT & CO.
PHILADELPHIA.

INDEX.

A.

B.

C.

D.

F.

G.

H.

I.

J.

K.

L.

M.

N.

O.

P.

Q.

R.

S.

T.

U.

V.

Z.

COLOPHON

Collaborators on

S. S. White Catalogue of Dental Instruments and Equipment:

Heather Austin, Editorial Assistant
Data Reproductions Corporation, Printer and Binder
Steve Renick/Anselm Design, Designer
Martha Nicholson Steele, Editor, Project Manager, and Electronic Typesetting
Tiki Bob Publishing & Design, Spine Design and Electronic Typesetting

The text type is Adobe Garamond
from Adobe Systems.

This edition is limited to 300 copies.